Breast Imaging

SERIES EDITOR **James H. Thrall, MD**
Radiologist-in-Chief
Massachusetts General Hospital
Juan M. Taveras Professor of Radiology
Harvard Medical School
Boston, Massachusetts

OTHER VOLUMES IN
THE REQUISITES IN RADIOLOGY SERIES

Breast Imaging

Second Edition

Debra M. Ikeda, MD

Professor
Department of Radiology
Stanford University School of Medicine
Stanford, California

ELSEVIER
MOSBY

3251 Riverport Lane
St. Louis, Missouri 63043

BREAST IMAGING: THE REQUISITES
Copyright © 2011, 2004 by Mosby, Inc., an affiliate of Elsevier Inc.

ISBN: 978-0-323-05198-9

Library of Congress Cataloging-in-Publication Data

Ikeda, Debra M.
    Breast imaging / Debra M. Ikeda. – 2nd ed.
        p. ; cm. – (Requisites)
    Includes bibliographical references and index.
    ISBN 978-0-323-05198-9 (hardcover : alk. paper)
    1. Breast—Radiography. 2. Breast—Imaging. 3. Breast—Diseases—Diagnosis.
I. Title. II. Series: Requisites series.
    [DNLM: 1. Mammography. 2. Breast Diseases—diagnosis. 3. Magnetic Resonance Imaging—methods. 4. Ultrasonography, Mammary. WP 815]
    RG493.5.R33I346 2011
    618.1'907572—dc22

                                                                    2010028629

Acquisitions Editor: Rebecca Schmidt Gaertner
Publishing Services Manager: Pat Joiner-Myers
Senior Project Manager: Joy Moore
Designer: Steven Stave

Printed in the United States of America

Last digit is the print number: 9 8 7 6 5 4 3 2 1

For my mom, Dorothy Yoshie Kishi Ikeda;
for women with breast cancer, their families, their loved ones and supporters; and
for physicians, health care givers, scientists, engineers, and physicists who
support them and battle breast cancer on their behalf.

Contributors

Bruce L. Daniel, MD
Associate Professor
Department of Radiology
Stanford University School of Medicine
Stanford, California

Frederick M. Dirbas, MD
Associate Professor of Surgery
Stanford University School of Medicine
Leader, Breast Disease Management Group
Stanford Cancer Center
Stanford, California

R. Edward Hendrick, PhD, FACR
Clinical Professor of Radiology
University of Colorado-Denver School of Medicine
Aurora, Colorado

Kathleen C. Horst, MD
Assistant Professor
Department of Radiation Oncology
Stanford University School of Medicine
Stanford, California

Debra M. Ikeda, MD
Professor
Department of Radiology
Stanford University School of Medicine
Stanford, California

Andrew Quon, MD
Chief, Clinical PET-CT
Assistant Professor of Radiology
Stanford University School of Medicine
Stanford, California

Foreword

The first edition of *Breast Imaging: The Requisites* was an outstanding addition to the Requisites in Radiology series. In its second edition, Dr. Debra Ikeda and her contributors have again done a truly outstanding job in presenting a very challenging topic in a manner that is straightforward and readily accessible to the reader. Part of the challenge in writing a book on breast imaging is that the topic encompasses screening, diagnostic and interventional procedures, and a multiplicity of imaging methods. Dr. Ikeda's approach is logical, and readers will have no trouble finding and going immediately to the chapter or material of interest.

The material covered in the second edition of *Breast Imaging: The Requisites* reflects the rapid development of technology for breast imaging. Along with continued technologic breakthroughs in ultrasound and magnetic resonance imaging, positron emission tomography and PET/CT have shown potential in the diagnosis and management of breast disease.

While technologic advances have changed the practice of breast imaging over the last decade, the special responsibility of radiologists has not changed. Radiologists remain the critical stewards of a patient's care in going from a screening study to a diagnostic study and then to an interventional procedure. The intimate relationship between patients with breast disease and the radiologist is unique in radiology practice. *Breast Imaging: The Requisites* captures the importance of this relationship.

Dr. Ikeda and her colleagues have done a meticulous job in illustrating and cross referencing *Breast Imaging: The Requisites*. The quality of the illustrations is superb and increased in value by equally excellent line drawings and diagrams designed to simplify and bring out basic concepts. The utility of the work is further increased by the use of tables and boxes that summarize key points covered in the text.

In their second edition, Dr. Ikeda and colleagues have again succeeded in producing a book that exemplifies the philosophy and goals of the Requisites in Radiology series. The authors have captured the important conceptual, factual, and practical aspects of breast imaging including new advances in technology in a way that is both concise and authoritative. Dr. Ikeda and her invited co-authors are to be congratulated on doing such an outstanding job for the benefit of their readers and for the benefit of both physicians and patients engaged in providing and receiving breast imaging services.

The Requisites in Radiology series is now an old friend for a generation of radiologists. The intent of the series is to provide the resident, fellow, or practicing physician with an authoritative textbook that can be reasonably read within several days, and for trainees, perhaps reread several times during clinical rotations or during board preparation. The Requisites in Radiology series is not intended to be exhaustive but to provide the material required for clinical practice.

Dr. Ikeda and colleagues have done an outstanding job in sustaining the philosophy of the Requisites series. *Breast Imaging: The Requisites* is again a truly outstanding and contemporary text for breast imaging.

James H. Thrall, MD

Preface

An explosion of scientific data regarding breast cancer gene signatures and tissue microarrays, stromal-epithelial signaling, breast cancer stem cell research, reporter genes and probe development, and therapeutic diagnostics changed the way we view breast cancer. We once looked at breast cancer by its morphology alone, using mammography and ultrasound. Now we look at breast cancer morphology and contrast enhancement characteristics on magnetic resonance imaging scans routinely. We look at patient risk factors and genetic predisposition to cancer. We look at breast cancer estrogen, progesterone, and HER2/neu receptors. We look at the genetic profile of the cancer itself. The world has changed.

However, what has *not* changed are the basic premises of breast cancer management:

Detect breast cancer
Differentiate cancer from benign findings
Get tissue
Stage the patient (find all the cancer, everywhere)
Help plan patient management and treatment
See if treatment is working (drug response)
Help the surgeon plan to excise all cancer after neoadjuvant chemotherapy
Make sure all the cancer is gone after treatment (surgery, chemotherapy)
Find cancer if it comes back (anywhere)

The second edition of *Breast Imaging: The Requisites* is a simple book, written so that residents can finish it within a month during their breast imaging rotation. With this book, residents should be able to tackle easy cases, and work up to harder diagnostic problems. Readers will learn tools to help with the hard cases, and tricks to find cancers that hide or mimic benign disease. But not all cases are easy. There is adversity in cancer detection, diagnosis, and management. Adversity should be expected. There is adversity in life. There is adversity in everything. Get over it. Welcome adversity. View adversity as a challenge to overcome, as an opportunity to try new things and to learn. It's the only way to get better as a breast imager.

ACKNOWLEDGMENTS

No book is finished without tremendous help; I would like to thank several people who did heroic work to make the book what it is. First, I acknowledge the superb administrative support, sharp editorial advice, and cheery demeanor from Heidi Fisher and Joe Hubbard, whose organizational skills and meticulous attention to detail kept me and the book on track and moving forward. Bravo, Heidi and Joe!

I thank my co-authors, Dr. R. Edward Hendrick, Dr. Frederick Dirbas, Dr. Kathleen Horst, Dr. Bruce Daniel, and Dr. Andrew Quon for their invaluable scientific and educational contributions to their chapters. Rebecca Jacoubowsky, Mark Reisenberger, and Dr. Sunita Pal all helped tremendously with the illustrations and technical support. I thank my partners Drs. Sunita Pal, Roger Jackman, Jennifer Kao, and Lisa Schmelzel for showing me cases and sharing ideas of what might be good tools or illustrations for teaching residents. I especially thank my chairman, Gary Glazer, for his vision for breast imaging at Stanford and his determination to make it happen.

I thank my friends Lisa Schmelzel and Mark Elpers, Kathy Fong and Eric Bain, Linda and Steve Folkman, Bev Abbott and J.R. Elpers, Donna Ito and Joost Ruck, Naomi Kane, Judy and Machiel van der Loos, Jennifer and John Hausler, Valerie Ito and Bob Schubert, Kathy and Ron Emery, Marlene and Hank Stern, Nancy Stern, Tracy Hughes, Lucy Harris, Angelena Ho, Jessica Leung, Lynne Steinbach and Eric Tepper, Kevin and Jennifer Griffin, Warren Garner and Vicki Marx, Kathy and Andy Switky, Laurie Torres, Betty-Anne Stenmark, and Rick Sturza and Mary Aiken for their unflagging support and belief in me through the tough years between 2005 and 2010. Thank you!

I thank Glenn Carpenter for his much appreciated and beloved support as SSO and second mouse.

I thank, respect, and am grateful to the women who are treated at Stanford University Medical Center. I am thankful for their families and supporters. Each woman faces her own breast cancer in her own way. Some can barely struggle through. Others just do what they have to do and soldier through treatment. Still others find the strength to volunteer for our Stanford imaging research studies, designed to study cancer and help women with breast cancer 10 years from now.

I remember a woman with breast cancer who agreed to participate in an imaging study. She said, "I am going to do this study because the secret to breast cancer is inside me." I felt chills because she was right: The secret to curing breast cancer is partly answered in each woman. Thus, I am grateful to the scientists, physicists, chemists, and engineers who design and conduct breast cancer studies aiming to save women and the women who participate in the studies to save other women.

I hope that you will learn the essentials of breast imaging and use your knowledge to find breast cancer and save women's lives, to their benefit and to the benefit of their families and loved ones. Then I hope you will take what you have learned and use it to develop new ideas and techniques to help others and advance this field. Remember, never, ever give up!

Good luck and bon voyage!

—*Deb*

Contents

CHAPTER 1

Mammography Acquisition
Screen-Film and Digital Mammography, the Mammography Quality Standards Act, and Computer-Aided Detection

R. Edward Hendrick and Debra M. Ikeda

Mammography is one of the most technically challenging areas of radiography, requiring high spatial resolution, excellent soft-tissue contrast, and low radiation dose. In thicker and denser breasts, wide image latitude is also needed. Specialized x-ray imaging equipment, screen-film image receptors, processors, digital image receptors, review workstations, and computer-aided detection (CAD) systems specific to mammography have been developed to meet these challenges.

Randomized, controlled trials (RCTs) of women invited to mammography screening conducted between 1963 and 1990 showed that early detection and treatment of breast cancer led to a 25% to 30% decrease in breast cancer mortality. More recent studies of service screening in Sweden and Canada have shown that screening mammography can reduce breast cancer mortality by 40% to 50% compared to unscreened women (Tabar et al., Duffy et al., Coleman et al.). As a result, the American Cancer Society recommends that asymptomatic women age 40 years and older have an annual mammogram and receive a clinical breast examination as part of a periodic health examination, preferably annually (Saslow et al.) (Box 1-1).

In all of these studies, image quality was demonstrated to be a critical component of early detection of breast cancer. To standardize and improve the quality of mammography, in 1987 the American College of Radiology (ACR) started a voluntary ACR Mammography Accreditation Program (MAP). In 1992, the U.S. Congress passed the Mammography Quality Standards Act (MQSA; P.L. 102-539), which went into effect in 1994 and remains in effect today through reauthorizations in 1998, 2004, and 2007. MQSA mandates requirements for facilities performing mammography, including equipment and quality assurance requirements, as well as personnel qualifications for physicians, radiologic technologists, and medical physicists involved in the performance of mammography in the United States, whether screening or diagnostic, screen-film or digital (Box 1-2).

This chapter outlines the basics of image acquisition using screen-film and digital mammography, describes the essentials of CAD in mammography, and reviews the quality assurance requirements for mammography stipulated by the MQSA.

TECHNICAL ASPECTS OF MAMMOGRAPHY IMAGE ACQUISITION

Mammograms are obtained on specially designed, dedicated x-ray machines using either x-ray film and paired fluorescent screens or digital detectors to capture the image. All mammography units are comprised of a rotating anode x-ray tube with matched filtration for soft-tissue imaging, a breast compression plate, a moving grid, an x-ray image receptor, and an automatic exposure control (AEC) device that can be placed under or detect the densest portion of the breast, all mounted on a rotating C-arm (Fig. 1-1). A technologist compresses the patient's breast between the image receptor and compression plate for a few seconds during each exposure. Breast compression is important because it spreads normal fibroglandular tissues so that cancers, which have similar attenuation properties to fibroglandular tissues, can be better seen. Breast compression also decreases breast thickness, thereby decreasing exposure time, radiation dose to the breast, and the potential for image blurring as a result of patient motion and unsharpness.

Women worry about breast pain from breast compression and about the radiation dose from mammography. Breast pain during compression varies among individuals and can be decreased by obtaining the mammogram 7 to 10 days after the onset of menses, when the breasts are least painful. Breast pain can also be minimized by taking oral analgesics such as acetaminophen before the mammogram or by using appropriately designed foam pads that cushion the breast without adversely affecting image quality or increasing breast dose.

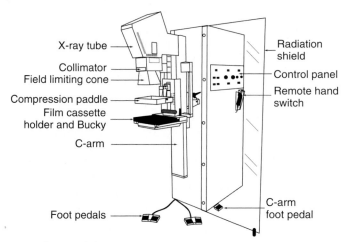

FIGURE 1-1. Components of an x-ray mammography unit.

Current mammography delivers a low dose of radiation to the breast. The most radiosensitive tissues in the breast are the fibroglandular tissues. The best measure of breast dose is mean glandular dose, or the average absorbed dose of ionizing radiation to the radiosensitive fibroglandular tissues. The mean glandular dose received by the average woman is approximately 2 mGy (0.2 rad) per exposure, or 4 mGy (0.4 rad) for a typical two-view examination. Radiation doses to thinner compressed breasts are substantially lower than doses to thicker breasts.

The main radiation risk from mammography is the possible induction of breast cancer 5 to 30 years after exposure. The estimated risk of inducing breast cancer is linearly proportional to the radiation dose and inversely related to age at exposure. The lifetime risk of inducing a fatal breast cancer as a result of two-view mammography

in women age 45 at exposure is estimated to be about 1 in 100,000. For a woman age 65 at exposure, the *risk* is less than 0.3 in 100,000. The *benefit* of screening mammography is the detection of breast cancer before it is clinically apparent. The likelihood of an invasive or in-situ cancer being present in a woman at age 45 is about 1 in 500. The likelihood that the cancer would be fatal in the absence of mammography screening is about 1 in 4, and the likelihood that screening mammography will convey a mortality benefit is 15% (RCT estimates) to 40% (service screening estimates). Hence, the likelihood of screening mammography saving a woman's life at this age is about 1 in 5000 to 1 in 13,000, yielding a benefit-to-risk ratio of 8:1 to 20:1. For a woman age 65 at screening, the likelihood of a mortality benefit from mammography is about 1 in 2000 to 1 in 4000 (assuming a 25% to 50% mortality benefit), yielding a benefit-to-risk ratio of approximately 90:1 to 180:1. Screening mammography is only effective when regular periodic examination is performed.

The generator for a mammography system provides power to the x-ray tube. The peak kilovoltage (kVp) of mammography systems is lower than that of conventional x-ray systems, because it is desirable to use softer x-ray beams to increase both soft-tissue contrast and the absorption of x-rays in the cassette phosphor (absorption efficiency), especially for screen-film mammography (SFM). Typical kVp values for mammography are 24 to 32 kVp for molybdenum targets, 26 to 35 kVp for rhodium or tungsten targets. A key feature of mammography generators is the electron beam current (milliampere [mA]) rating of the system. The higher the mA rating, the shorter the exposure time for total tube output (milliampere second [mAs]). A compressed breast of average thickness (5 cm) requires about 150 mAs at 26 kVp to achieve proper film densities in SFM. If the tube rating is 100 mA (typical of the larger focal spots used for nonmagnification mammography), the exposure time would be 1.5 seconds. A higher-output system with 150-mA output would cut the exposure time to 1 second for the same compressed breast thickness and kVp setting. Because of the wide range of breast thicknesses, exposures require mAs values ranging from 10 to several hundred mAs. Specifications for generators are listed in Box 1-3.

The most commonly used anode/filter combination is Mo/Mo: a molybdenum (Mo) anode (or target) and a Mo filter (25–30 microns thick), especially for thinner compressed breasts (<5 cm thick). Most current manufacturers also offer a rhodium (Rh) filter, to be used with the Mo target (Rh/Mo), to produce a slightly more penetrating (harder) x-ray beam for use with thicker breasts. Some manufacturers offer other target materials, such as Rh/Rh: a rhodium target paired with a rhodium filter, or tungsten (W), which is paired with a rhodium filter (W/Rh) or aluminum (Al) filter (W/Al). These anode/filter combinations are designed for thicker (>5 cm) and denser breasts. Typically, higher kVp settings are also used with these alternative target/filter combinations to result in a harder x-ray beam for thicker breasts, because fewer x-rays are attenuated with a harder x-ray beam (Box 1-4). One of the best parameters to measure the hardness or penetrating capability of an x-ray beam is the half-value layer (HVL), which represents the thickness of aluminum that reduces the exposure by one half. The harder the x-ray beam, the higher the HVL. The typical HVL for mammography is 0.3 to 0.5 mm of Al. The Food and Drug Administration (FDA) requires that the HVL for mammography cannot be less than kVp/100 ± 0.03 (in mm of Al), so that the x-ray beam is not too soft. For example, at 28 kVp, the HVL cannot be less than 0.31 mm of Al. There is also an upper limit on the half-value layer that depends on the target-filter combination. For the upper limit of Mo/Mo, the HVL must be less than kVp/100 + 0.12 (in mm of Al); so for 28 kVp, the HVL must be less than 0.4 mm of Al.

The size of the larger mammography focal spot used for standard, contact (i.e., nonmagnification) mammography is typically 0.3 mm. Magnification mammography requires a smaller focal spot, about 0.1 mm, to reduce penumbra (geometric blurring of structures in the breast produced due to the breast being closer to the x-ray source and farther from the image receptor to produce greater "geometric" magnification). The effect of focal spot size on resolution in the breast is tested by placing a line pair pattern in the location of the breast, at a specific distance (4.5 cm) from the breast support surface. For SFM, the larger mammography focal spot used for standard, contact mammography should produce an image that resolves at least 11 line pairs/millimeter (11 lp/mm) when the lines of the test pattern run in the direction perpendicular to the length of the focal spot (this measures the blurring effect of the length of the focal spot) and at least 13 lp/mm when the lines run parallel to the focal spot (measuring the blurring effect of the width of the focal spot). Thus, although the SFM image receptor can resolve 18 to 21 lp/mm, the geometry of the breast in contact mammography and the finite-sized larger focal spot reduce the limiting spatial resolution of the system to 11 to 15 lp/mm *in the breast*. The

limiting spatial resolution of digital mammography systems is less (5–10 lp/mm), due to pixelization of the image by the digital image receptor. In digital, a "line" is 1 pixel width, and a line pair is 2 pixels. For example, for a digital detector with 100 micron (0.1 mm) pixel size or pitch (the center-to-center distance between adjacent pixels), a line pair consists of 2 pixels or 200 microns (0.2 mm). Therefore, one can fit 5 line pairs (at 0.2 mm each) into a 1 mm length, or the detector has a limiting spatial resolution of 5 lp/mm. By similar reasoning, a digital detector with 50 micron pixels has a limiting spatial resolution of 10 lp/mm.

The x-ray tube and image receptor are mounted on opposite ends of a rotating C-arm to obtain mammograms in almost any projection. The source-to-image receptor distance (SID) for mammography units must be *at least* 55 cm for contact mammography. Most systems have SIDs of 65 to 70 cm.

Geometric magnification is achieved by moving the breast farther from the image receptor (closer to the x-ray tube) and switching to a small focal spot (Fig. 1-2). Placing the breast halfway between the focal spot and the image receptor (as in Fig. 1-2B) would magnify the breast by a factor of 2.0 from its actual size to the image size because of the divergence of the x-ray beam. The MQSA requires that mammography units with magnification capabilities must provide at least one fixed magnification factor of between 1.4 and 2.0 (Table 1-1). Geometric magnification makes small, high-contrast structures such as microcalcifications more visible by making them larger relative to the noise pattern in the image (increasing their signal-to-noise ratio [SNR]). Optically or electronically magnifying a contact image, as would be done with a magnifier on SFM or using a zoom factor greater than 1 on a digital mammogram, does not increase the SNR of the object relative to the background, because both are increased in size equally. To avoid excess blurring of the image with geometric magnification, it is important to use a sufficiently small focal spot (usually 0.1 mm nominal size) and not too large a magnification factor (2.0 or less). When the small focal spot is selected for geometric magnification, the x-ray tube output is decreased by a factor of 3 to 4 (to 25–40 mA) compared to that from a large focal spot (80–150 mA). This can extend imaging times for magnification mammography, even though the grid is removed in magnification mammography. The air gap between the breast and image receptor provides adequate scatter rejection in magnification mammography without the use of an antiscatter grid.

Collimators control the size and shape of the x-ray beam to decrease patient exposure to tissues beyond the compressed breast and image receptor. In mammography, the x-ray beam is collimated to a rectangular field to match the image receptor rather than the breast contour, because x-rays striking the image receptor outside the breast do not contribute to breast dose. By federal regulation, the x-ray field cannot extend beyond the chest wall of the image receptor by more than 2% of the SID. So, for a 60-cm SID unit, the x-ray beam can extend beyond the chest wall edge of the image receptor by no more than 1.2 cm.

The compression plate and image receptor assembly hold the breast motionless during the exposure, decreasing the breast thickness and providing tight compression, better separating fibroglandular elements in the breast

---

BOX 1-4. Anode-Filter Combinations for Mammography

Mo/Mo
Mo/Rh
Rh/Rh
W/Rh, W/Ag, or W/Al

Ag, silver; Al, aluminum; Mo, molybdenum; Rh, rhodium; W, tungsten.

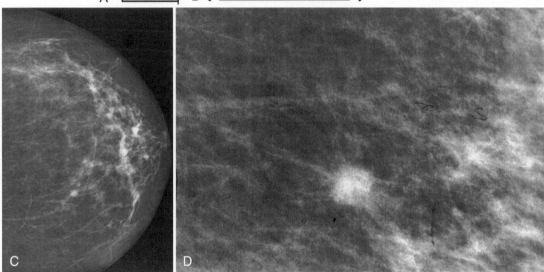

FIGURE 1-2. Magnification mammography improves resolution. Nonmagnified, or contact, mammography (**A**) and geometrically magnified mammography (**B**). Using a small or microfocal (0.1 mm) focal spot with the configuration shown in part **B**, higher spatial resolution can be obtained in the breast compared to part **A**, where a larger (0.3 mm) focal spot is used. **C,** Craniocaudal mammogram shows a possible benign mass in the inner breast. **D,** Microfocal magnification shows irregular borders not seen on the standard view.

(Fig. 1-3). The compression plate has a posterior lip that is more than 3 cm high and usually is oriented at 90 degrees to the plane of the compression plate at the chest wall. This lip keeps chest wall structures from superimposing and obscuring posterior breast tissue in the image. The compression plate must be able to compress the breast for up to 1 minute with a compression force of 25 to 45 pounds. The compression plate can be advanced by a foot-controlled motorized device and adjusted more finely with hand controls.

TABLE 1-1. Mammography Focal Spot Sizes and Source-to-Image Distances

Mammography Type	Nominal Focal Spot Size (mm)	Source-to-Image Distance (cm)
Contact film-screen	0.3	≥55
Magnification	0.1	≥55

The Mammography Quality Standards Act requires magnification factors between 1.4 and 2.0 for systems designed to perform magnification mammography.

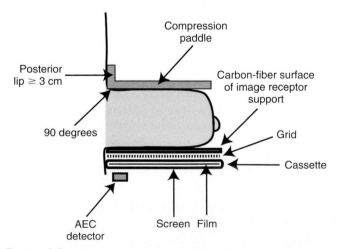

FIGURE 1-3. Schematic of a compression paddle and image receptor showing the components of the cassette holder, the compression plate, and the breast. The film emulsion faces the screen. AEC, automatic exposure control. (Adapted from Farria DM, Kimme-Smith C, Bassett LW: Equipment, processing, and image receptor. In Bassett LW, editor: *Diagnosis of diseases of the breast*, Philadelphia, WB Saunders, 1997, pp 32 and 34.)

Screen-Film Mammography Image Acquisition

In SFM, the image receptor assembly holds a screen-film cassette in a carbon-fiber support with a moving antiscatter grid in front of the cassette and an AEC detector behind it. Screen-film image receptors are required to be 18 × 24 cm and 24 × 30 cm in size to accommodate various sized breasts (Box 1-5). Each size image receptor must have a moving antiscatter grid composed of lead strips with a grid ratio (defined as the ratio of the lead strip height to the distance between strips) between 3.5:1 and 5:1. The reciprocating grid moves back and forth in the direction perpendicular to the grid lines during the radiographic exposure to eliminate grid lines in the image by blurring them out. One manufacturer uses a hexagonal-shaped grid pattern to improve scatter rejection; this grid is also blurred by reciprocation during exposure. Use of a grid improves image contrast by decreasing the fraction of scattered radiation reaching the image receptor. Grids increase the required exposure to the breast by approximately a factor of 2 (the Bucky factor), due to attenuation of primary as well as scattered radiation. Grids are not used with magnification mammography. Instead, in magnification mammography, scatter is reduced by collimation and by rejection of scattered x-rays due to a significant air gap between the breast and the image receptor.

The AEC system, also known as the *phototimer*, is calibrated to produce a consistent film optical density (OD) by sampling the x-ray beam after it has passed through the breast support, grid, and cassette. The AEC detector is usually a D-shaped sensor that lies along the midline of the breast support and can be positioned by the technologist closer to or farther from the chest wall. If the breast is extremely thick or inappropriate technique factors are selected, the AEC will terminate exposure at a specific backup time (usually 4–6 seconds) or mAs (300–750 mAs) to prevent tube overload or melting of the x-ray track on the anode.

Screen-film cassettes used in mammography have an inherent spatial resolution of 18 to 21 lp/mm. Such resolution is achieved typically by using a single-emulsion film placed emulsion side down against a single intensifying screen that faces upward toward the breast in the film cassette. The single-emulsion film with a single intensifying screen is used to prevent the parallax unsharpness and cross-over exposure that occur with double-emulsion films and double-screen systems. One manufacturer has introduced a double-emulsion film with double-sided screens (EV System, Carestream Health, Toronto; formerly Eastman Kodak Healthgroup) with a thinner film emulsion and screen on top to minimize parallax unsharpness. Most screen-film processing combinations have relative speeds of 150 to 200, with speed defined as the reciprocal of the x-ray exposure required to produce an OD of 1.0 above base plus fog (which is 1.15–1.2, because base plus fog OD is 0.15–0.2).

Film processing involves development of the latent image on the exposed film emulsion. The film is placed in an automatic processor that takes the exposed film and rolls it through liquid developer to amplify the latent image on the film, reducing the silver ions in the x-ray film emulsion to metallic silver, thereby resulting in film darkening in exposed areas. The developer temperature ranges from 92°F to 96°F. The film is then run through a fixer solution containing thiosulfate (or *hypo*) to remove any unused silver and preserve the film. The film is then washed with water to remove residual fixer, which if not removed can cause the film to turn brown over time. The film is then dried with heated air.

Film processing is affected by many variables, the most important of which are developer chemistry (weak or oxidized chemistry makes films lighter and lower contrast), developer temperature (too hot may make films darker, too cool lighter), developer replenishment (too little results in lighter, lower-contrast films), inadequate agitation of developer, and uneven application of developer to films (causes mottling) (Table 1-2).

For positioning, the technologist tailors the mammogram to the individual woman's body habitus to get the best image. The breast is relatively fixed in its medial borders near the sternum and the upper breast, whereas the lower and outer portions of the breast are more mobile. The technologist takes advantage of the mobile lower outer breast to obtain as much breast tissue on the mammogram as possible. The two views obtained for screening mammography are the craniocaudal (CC) and mediolateral oblique (MLO) projections. The names for the mammographic views and abbreviations are based on the ACR Breast Imaging Reporting and Data System (ACR

BOX 1-5. Compression Plate and Imaging Receptor

Both 18 × 24-cm and 24 × 30-cm sizes are required
A moving grid is required for each image receptor size
The compression plate has a posterior lip >3 cm and is oriented 90 degrees to the plane of the plate
Compression force of 25–45 pounds
Paddle advanced by a foot motor with hand compression adjustments
Collimation to the image receptor, not the breast contour

TABLE 1-2. Variables Affecting Image Quality of Screen-Film Mammograms

Film too dark	Developer temperature too high Wrong mammographic technique (excessive kVp or mA) Excessive plus-density control
Film too light	Inadequate chemistry or replenishment Developer temperature too low Wrong mammographic technique
Lost contrast	Inadequate chemistry or replenishment Water to processor turned off Changed film
Film turns brown	Inadequate rinsing of fixer
Motion artifact	Movement by patient Inadequate compression applied Inappropriate mammographic technique (long exposures)

BI-RADS®), a lexicon system developed by experts for standard mammographic terminology. The first word in the mammographic view indicates the location of the x-ray tube, and the second word indicates the location of the image receptor. Thus, a CC view would be taken with the x-ray tube pointing at the breast from the head (cranial) down through the breast to the image receptor in a more caudal position.

To pass ACR accreditation clinical image review, the MLO mammogram must show most of the breast tissue in one projection, with portions of the upper inner and lower inner quadrants partially excluded (Fig. 1-4). Clinical evaluation of the MLO view should show fat posterior to the fibroglandular tissue and a large portion of the pectoralis muscle, which should be concave and extend inferior to the posterior nipple line (PNL). The PNL describes an imaginary line drawn from the nipple to the pectoralis muscle or film edge and perpendicular to the pectoralis muscle. The PNL should intersect the pectoralis muscle in the MLO view in more than 80% of women. Although the technologist tries to avoid producing skin folds on the film when possible, they are seen occasionally but do not usually cause problems for the radiologist reading the film. The MLO view should show adequate compression, exposure, contrast, and an open inframammary fold, in which both the lower portion of the breast and a portion of the upper abdominal wall should be seen.

To pass ACR accreditation clinical image review, the CC view should include the medial posterior portions of the breast without sacrificing the outer portions (Figs. 1-5 and 1-6). With proper positioning technique, the technologist should be able to include the medial portion of the breast without rotating the patient medially by lifting the lower medial breast tissue onto the image receptor. The pectoralis muscle should be seen when possible on the CC view. On the CC view, the PNL extends from the nipple to the pectoralis muscle or the edge of the film, whichever comes first, perpendicular to the pectoralis muscle or film edge. For a given breast, the length of the PNL on the CC view should be within 1 cm of its length on the MLO view.

Clinical images are evaluated on positioning, compression, contrast, proper exposure, random noise (radiographic mottle or quantum mottle produced by varying numbers of x-rays contributing to the image in different locations, even with a uniform object), sharpness, and artifacts (or structured noise). Imaging on a phantom is helpful in evaluating most of these factors, except for positioning and compression (Fig. 1-7). Adequate exposure (to achieve adequate film OD) and adequate contrast (OD difference) are important to ensure detection of subtle abnormalities (Fig. 1-8). Artifacts seen on clinical images include processing artifacts (roller marks, wet pressure marks, guide shoe marks), white specklike artifacts from dust or lint between the fluorescent screen and film emulsion, grid

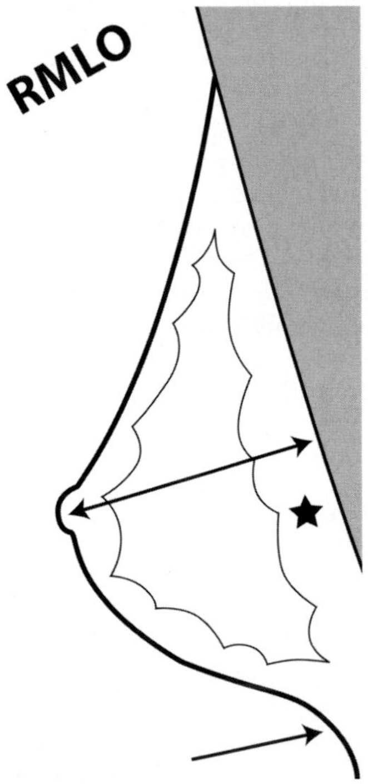

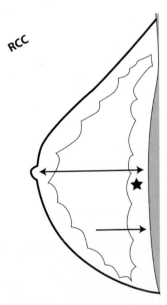

FIGURE 1-4. Positioning for a normal mediolateral oblique (MLO) mammogram. By convention, the view type and side (R, L) labels are placed near the axilla. On a properly positioned MLO view, the inferior aspect of the pectoralis muscle should extend down to the posterior nipple line, an imaginary line drawn from the nipple back to and perpendicular to the pectoral muscle (*double arrow*). The anterior margin of the pectoralis muscle should be convex in a properly positioned MLO view. Ideally, the image shows fat posterior to the glandular tissue (*star*). The open inframammary fold (*arrow*) and abdomen are displayed with the breast pulled up and away from the chest.

FIGURE 1-5. Normal craniocaudal (CC) mammogram. The posterior nipple line (PNL) on the CC view is the distance between the nipple and the posterior aspect of the image. The PNL on the CC view (*double arrow*) should be within 1 cm of the PNL on the mediolateral oblique (MLO) view. The goal is to include posterior medial tissue (excluded on the MLO view) (*arrow*) and as much retroglandular fat (*star*) as possible.

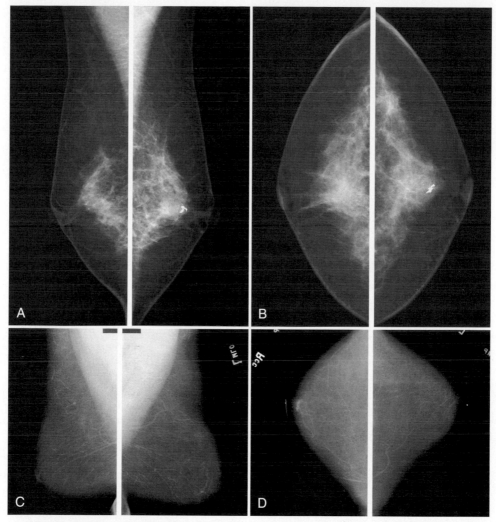

FIGURE 1-6. Improper positioning. **A,** Inadequate pectoralis muscle and sagging breast tissue on this full-field digital mediolateral oblique view show that the posterior nipple line (PNL) requirements are not met, and the craniocaudal (CC) view is rotated laterally (**B**). Note the calcifying fibroadenoma on the left. **C,** In a second patient with a fatty breast, the pectoralis muscle is concave but just barely meets PNL requirements. **D,** The CC views are adequate.

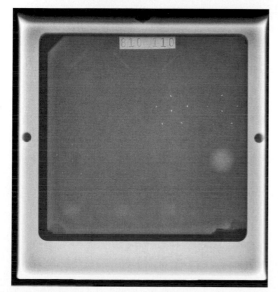

FIGURE 1-7. Phantom image. Fibers, speck groups, and masses in graduated sizes embedded in a 4.5-cm thick phantom are used to evaluate the mammography system; phantom images are obtained at least weekly and after calibration or servicing of equipment. Minimum score: four fibers, three speck groups, and three masses.

lines from incomplete grid motion, motion artifacts from patient movement (made more likely by longer exposure times), skin folds from positioning, tree static caused by static electricity from low humidity in the dark room, or film handling artifacts (fingerprints, crimp marks, or pressure marks) (Figs. 1-9 to 1-12).

Film labeling is important (Box 1-6) because proper labeling ensures accurate facility, patient, laterality, and projection identification. Guidelines from the ACR Mammography Accreditation Program for mammogram labeling state that an identification label on the mammogram should specify the patient's first and last name, unique identification number, facility name and address, date, view and laterality, an Arabic number indicating the cassette used, and the technologist's initials. The laterality and projection marker should be placed near the axilla on all screen-film views.

Digital Mammography Image Acquisition

In digital mammography, the image is obtained in the same manner as in screen-film mammography, using a compression plate and an x-ray tube, with the screen-film

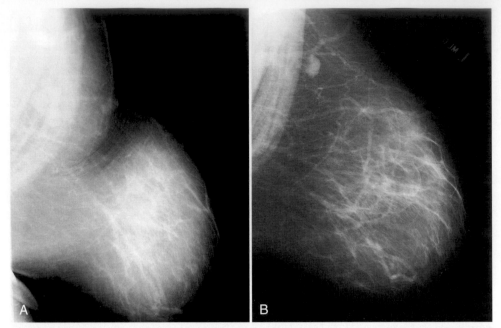

FIGURE 1-8. **A,** Underpenetration and an inadequately exposed and compressed breast produce a light film and poor separation of breast tissue; even though the pectoralis muscle is adequately included, skin folds are apparent in the lower portion of the image. **B,** A mammogram of a properly exposed and compressed breast shows normal glandular tissue.

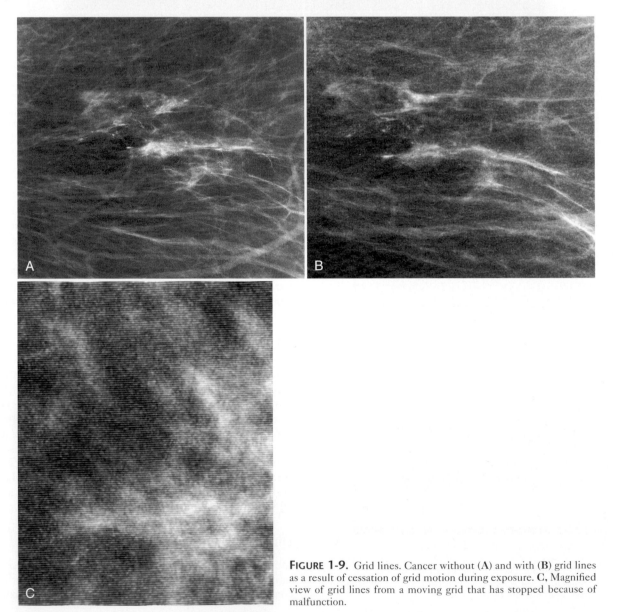

FIGURE 1-9. Grid lines. Cancer without (**A**) and with (**B**) grid lines as a result of cessation of grid motion during exposure. **C,** Magnified view of grid lines from a moving grid that has stopped because of malfunction.

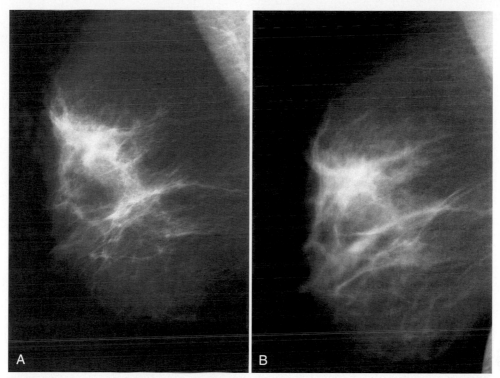

FIGURE 1-10. Dust. **A,** Blurring is caused by a large dust particle shown as a white dot in the upper part of the breast and is due to poor film-screen contact as the dust lifts the film off the screen. **B,** After the large dust particle is removed, the dust artifact and blur are gone.

cassette replaced by a digital detector (Figs. 1-13 and 1-14). Digital image acquisition has several potential advantages in terms of image availability, image processing, and CAD (Fig. 1-15). One advantage is elimination of the film processor, which eliminates artifacts and image noise added by processing films.

Digital mammography uses indirect or direct digital detectors. Indirect digital detectors use a fluorescent screen made of materials such as cesium iodide (CsI) to convert each absorbed x-ray to hundreds of visible light photons. Behind the fluorescent material, light-sensitive detector arrays made of materials such as amorphous silicon diodes or charge-coupled devices (CCDs) measure the produced light pixel by pixel. The weak electronic signal measured in each pixel is amplified and sent through an analog-to-digital converter, enabling computer storage of each pixel's measured detector signal.

Direct digital detectors use detector elements that capture and count x-rays directly, although amplification and analog-to-digital conversion are still applied. Another method to produce digital mammograms involves amorphous selenium. An amorphous selenium plate is an excellent absorber of x-rays and an excellent capacitor, storing the charge created by ionization when x-rays are absorbed. After exposure, an electronic device is used to read out the charge distribution on the selenium plate, which is in proportion to local exposure. This can be done by scanning the selenium plate with a laser beam or by placing a silicon diode array in contact with one side of the plate, with bias voltage applied, to read out the stored charge. Each of these methods allows production of high-resolution digital images.

Another approach to full-field digital mammography (FFDM) is computed radiography (CR), which uses a photostimulable phosphor composed of barium fluorobromide doped with europium (BaFBr:Eu). CR uses the same dedicated mammography units as screen-film, replacing the screen-film cassettes and film processor with CR cassettes (in sizes of 18×24 cm and 24×30 cm) and a CR processor. The phosphor plate within the CR cassette is used to absorb x-rays just as the screen in a screen-film cassette does. Rather than emitting light immediately after exposure (through fluorescence), x-ray absorption in the phosphor causes electrons within the phosphor crystals to be promoted to higher energy levels (through photostimulation). The plate is removed from the cassette in the CR processor and a red laser light scans the phosphor plate point by point, releasing electrons and stimulating emission of a higher energy (blue) light in proportion to x-ray exposure. In conventional x-ray systems, CR phosphor plates have an opaque backing and are read from only one side. In the one FDA-approved CR system for mammography (Fuji 5000D CR, Fujifilm Medical Systems USA), the CR cassette base is transparent and light emitted from the plate during laser scanning is read from both sides to increase reading efficiency.

No matter which digital detector is used, its job is to measure the quantity of x-rays passing through the breast, compression plate, grid (in most cases), and breast holder. The signal measured in each pixel is determined by the total attenuation in the breast along a given ray.

The choice of an analog-to-digital converter determines how many bits of memory will be used to store the signal for each pixel; the more bits per pixel, the more dynamic

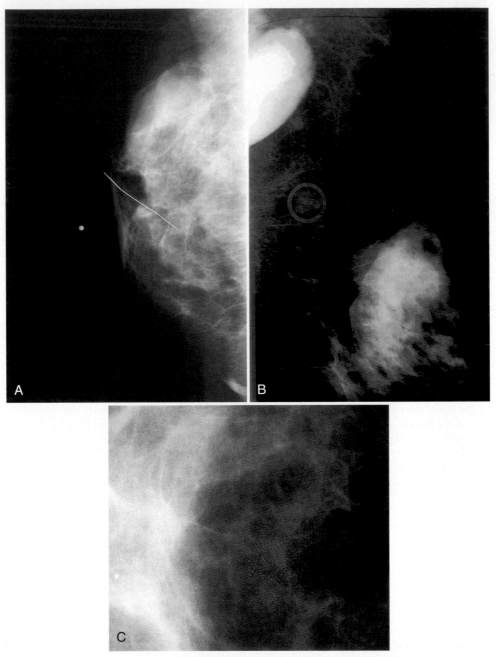

Figure 1-11. Artifacts. **A,** A mediolateral oblique view after biopsy and radiation therapy shows tiny bright white specks over the biopsy scar compatible with dust on the film. Dust can interfere with a search for microcalcifications. Note the nipple marker and linear scar marker showing the previous biopsy site. **B,** Patient's fingertip is visible in the film. **C,** Magnified view of a minus-density (white) fingerprint artifact, usually caused by contact with the film before exposure.

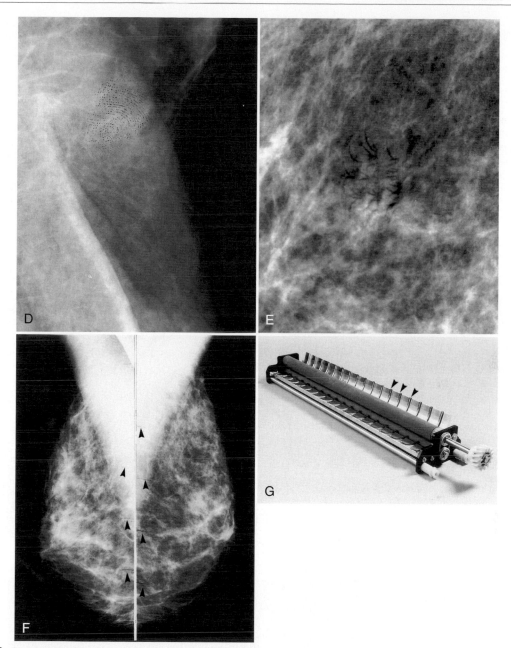

FIGURE 1-11, cont'd. D, Magnified view of a plus-density (dark) fingerprint artifact, usually caused by contact with the film after exposure but before processing. **E,** Subtle plus-density tree static artifacts caused by static discharge in a limited region of the film. The light emitted from the static discharge causes localized film exposure before processing. **F,** Guide shoe marks. Dark lines (*arrowheads*) at the edge of the film in the direction of film travel that are evenly spaced are caused by excessive pressure on the film emulsion from guide shoes as the film travels through the processor. Guide shoe marks can sometimes result in minus-density linear artifacts in the direction of film travel as well. **G,** A film guide that turns the film as it passes through the processor. Such guides (*arrowheads*) are located at the top and bottom of each tank. Improperly adjusted film guides can lead to excessive pressure on the film emulsion and result in guide shoe artifacts.

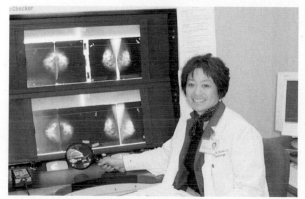

FIGURE 1-12. Film viewing conditions. Because mammography viewboxes have high luminance levels (>3000 candela/m^2 [3000 nit]), mammograms should be masked so that no light strikes the radiologist's eye without passing through the exposed film. That is also why film collimation should be rectangular and extend slightly beyond the edge of the image receptor, so that film is darkened to its edges. Viewbox luminance should be reasonably uniform across all viewbox panels. In addition, the ambient room illumination should be low (<50 lux, and preferably less) to minimize "dazzle glare" from film surfaces. Both viewbox luminance and room illumination should be checked annually by the medical physicist as part of the site quality control program (see the *ACR Mammography Quality Control Manual,* 1999 edition).

range for the image, but at higher storage cost. Specifically, if 12 bits per pixel are used, 2^{12} or 4096 signal values can be stored. If 14 bits per pixel are used, 2^{14} or 16,384 signal values can be stored. Usually 12- to 14-bits storage per pixel is used. In either case, 2 bytes per pixel are required (8 bits = 1 byte) to store the image. For example, the GE Senographe 2000D and DS digital detectors have 1920 × 2304 pixel arrays, or 4.4 million pixels, requiring 8.8 million bytes (8.8 megabytes, MB) of storage per image. Other FFDM systems require up to 52 MB of storage per image.

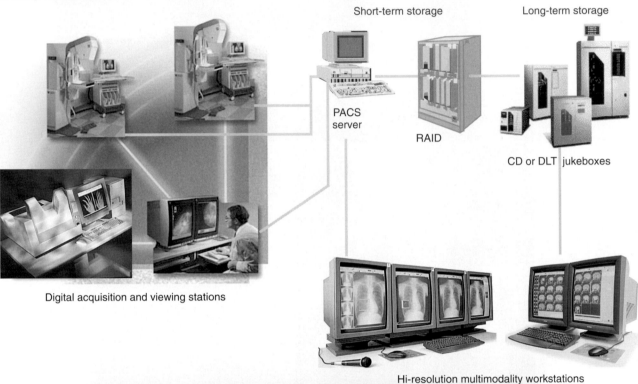

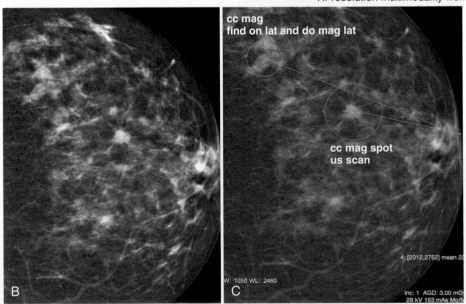

FIGURE 1-13. **A,** Schematic of a full-field digital mammography unit, workstation, picture archiving and communication system (PACS) or long-term storage, and workstation displays. Using digital mammography and PACS for screening recall, two spiculated masses representing infiltrating ductal carcinoma on the craniocaudal view (**B**) were marked by computer-aided detection and were recalled. The radiologist annotates the images and sends them to PACS for the technologist to retrieve when the patient returns for workup (**C**). CD, compact disk; DLT, digital linear tape; RAID, redundant array of independent disks. (**A** adapted from figures provided by GE Medical Services, Waukasha, WI.)

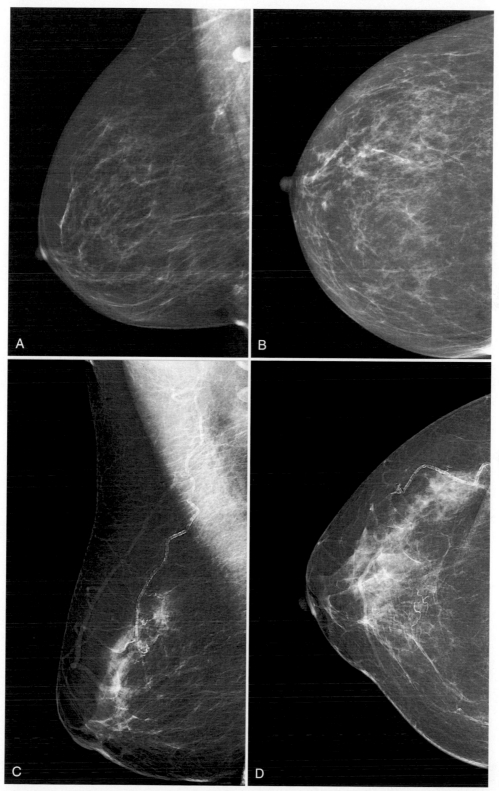

FIGURE 1-14. Full-field digital mammography showing fatty breast tissue (**A** and **B**) and scattered fibroglandular densities on mediolateral oblique and craniocaudal views (**C** and **D**).

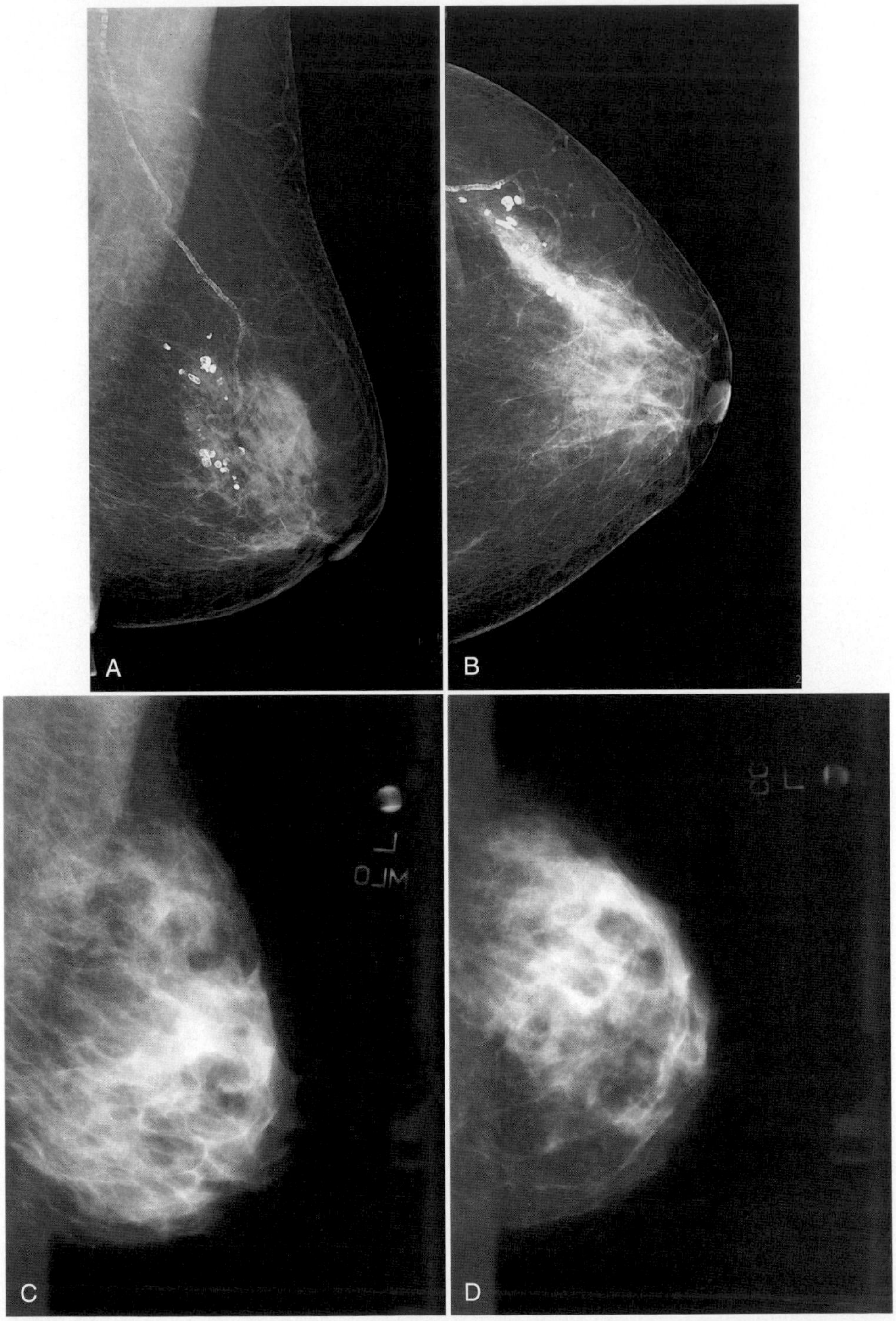

FIGURE 1-15. Calcifications seen on mediolateral oblique and craniocaudal full-field digital mammograms represent fat necrosis from previous trauma that was noted on a screening mammogram. Heterogeneous (**A** and **B**) and dense (**C** and **D**).

Screen-film image receptors used for mammography have a line-pair resolution of 18 to 21 lp/mm. To equal this spatial resolution, a digital detector would require 25-micron pixels, which would yield noisier images and pose a storage issue due to the large data sets required to store those images. FFDM systems have spatial resolutions ranging from 5 lp/mm (for 100-micron pixels) to 10 lp/mm (for 50-micron pixels). In digital mammography systems, it is the size of the pixels, or more correctly their center-to-center distance (pitch), that determines (and limits) the spatial resolution of the imaging chain.

The lower limiting spatial resolution of FFDM systems compared to film is offset by the increased contrast resolution of FFDM systems. Unlike SFM, in which the image cannot be manipulated after exposure and processing, FFDM images can be optimized after image capture by image postprocessing and adjustment of image display. For fixed digital detectors, such as CsI and silicon diode arrays (used by GE) and selenium and amorphous silicon diode arrays (used by Hologic and Siemens), one image processing step that can minimize image noise and structured artifacts is flat-field correction, or "gain correction" of each acquired digital image. This is done by making and storing a sensitivity map of the digital detector and using that map to correct all exposures. Typically, slot-scanning devices (such as the older SenoScan digital system, Fischer Medical Systems) and CR systems do not have the ability to perform flat-field correction of digital images. Beyond this, all digital systems have the ability to process the acquired digital image to minimize or eliminate the signal difference that results from the roll-off in thickness of the breast toward the skin line (thickness equalization); some add processing to help enhance the appearance of microcalcifications (e.g., GE Premium View and FineView). The window width and window level for all digital images viewed with soft copy display on review workstations can be adjusted, changing the contrast and brightness of the images, respectively, as well as digitally magnifying images.

Another important difference between SFM and FFDM is that screen-film images have a linear relationship between the logarithm of x-ray exposure and film OD only in the central portion of the characteristic curve. In FFDM, there is a linear relationship between x-ray exposure and signal over the entire dynamic range of the detector. Thus, digital images do not suffer contrast loss in underexposed or overexposed areas of the mammogram (as long as detector saturation does not occur), and instead show similar contrast over the full dynamic range of signals. FFDM also eliminates the variability and noise added by film processing.

In terms of breast dose, FFDM has a mean glandular dose lower than, or comparable to, the radiation dose of SFM. Recent results from the American College of Radiology Imaging Network (ACRIN) Digital Mammographic Imaging Screening Trial (DMIST) found the average single-view mean glandular dose for FFDM to be 1.86 mGy, 22% lower than the average SFM mean glandular dose of 2.37 mGy (Hendrick et al., 2010). Specific manufacturers, especially those using slot-scanning techniques, produce lower doses than SFM. Slot-scanning systems, such as the Fischer SenoScan, have a narrow slot of detector elements that are scanned under the breast in synchronization with a narrow fan beam of x-rays swept across the breast. This design, although more technically difficult to implement, has the advantage of eliminating the need for a grid to reduce scattered radiation. Scatter is partially eliminated by the narrow slot itself. The absence of a grid reduces the amount of radiation to the breast needed to get the same SNR in the detector. Some full area detectors with AEC systems have also demonstrated lower breast doses compared to SFM, especially for thicker breasts.

Once captured and processed, the image data are transferred to a reading station for interpretion on high-resolution (2048 × 2560, or 5 Mpixel) monitors or printed on films by laser imagers (with approximately 40-micron spot sizes) for interpretation of hardcopy images on film viewboxes or alternators. Digital data can be stored on optical disks, magnetic tapes, Picture Archiving and Communication Systems (PACS), or on CD-ROMs for later retrieval.

The MQSA states that FFDM images must be made available to patients as hardcopy films, as needed, which means the facility must have access to an FDA-approved laser printer for mammography that can reproduce the gray scale and spatial resolution of FFDM films. The images may also be given to the patient on a CD, if acceptable to the patient.

A number of studies have evaluated the performance of FFDM compared to SFM for screening asymptomatic women for breast cancer. Early studies showed comparable or slightly worse results (but not statistically significant differences) for receiver operating characteristic (ROC) curve area and sensitivity (Lewin et al.) or cancer detection rate (Skaane and Skjennald) of FFDM compared to SFM. Larger studies, however, showed some benefits of FFDM compared to SFM. The ACR Imaging Network Digital Mammographic Imaging Screening Trial (ACRIN DMIST) paired study (Pisano and colleagues), showed no difference overall, but found that FFDM had statistically significantly higher ROC curve areas than SFM for women under age 50, for premenopausal and perimenopausal women, and for women with denser breasts (BI-RADS® density categories 3 and 4). The Oslo II trial (Skaane et al.) showed that digital mammography had a significantly higher cancer detection rate (5.9 cancers per 1000 women screened) than SFM (3.8 cancers per 1000 women screened).

As of May 2010, about two thirds (65.4%) of the mammography units in the United States were digital mammography systems. The FDA-approved manufacturers for digital mammography and their unit properties are listed in Table 1-3.

QUALITY ASSURANCE IN MAMMOGRAPHY AND THE MAMMOGRAPHY QUALITY STANDARDS ACT

MQSA, a federal law regarding mammography that is enforced by the FDA, stipulates that all institutions performing mammography must be certified by the FDA. A prerequisite to FDA certification is accreditation to perform mammography by an FDA-approved accrediting body, such as the ACR or an FDA-approved state accrediting body. Arkansas, Iowa, and Texas are approved to accredit mammography facilities in their own states. MQSA regulations are listed in the *Federal Register*. To update facilities

TABLE 1-3. Food and Drug Administration–Approved Manufacturers for Digital Mammography and Unit Properties

Manufacturer	Unit Names	Image Receptor Sizes (cm)	Pixel Size (microns)	Target-Filter Combinations*
GE Healthcare	Senographe 2000D	19 × 23	100	Mo-Mo, Mo-Rh, Rh-Rh
	Senographe DS	19 × 23	100	Mo-Mo, Mo-Rh, Rh-Rh
	Senographe Essential	24 × 30.7	100	Mo-Mo, Mo-Rh, Rh-Rh
Fischer Medical	SenoScan (no longer sold)	24 × 29	50	(W-Re)-Al*
Hologic	Selenia	24 × 30	70	Mo-Mo, Mo-Rh
	Dimension	24 × 30	70	W-Rh, W-Ag
Siemens	Mammomat Novation DR	24 × 30	70	Mo-Mo, Mo-Rh, W-Rh, W-Al
Fujifilm	5000D (CR)	18 × 24	50	Depends on screen-film mammography
		24 × 30	50	unit used with CR cassettes

*Fischer target material is a combination of tungsten and rhenium.
Al, aluminum; Ag, silver; CR, computed radiography; Mo, molybdenum; Re, rhenium; Rh, rhodium; W, tungsten.

on the latest regulation changes and updates, the FDA maintains a Web site on MQSA (www.fda.gov/cdrh/mammography/) that includes a section to guide users who have questions on MQSA compliance (www.fda.gov/cdrh/mammography/guidance-rev.html).

MQSA certification involves an initial application to the FDA and FDA approval to perform mammography, continuous documentation of compliance, and yearly facility inspection by an MQSA or state inspector. Noncompliance with regulations may result in FDA citations, with time limits on deficiency corrections. Serious noncompliance issues may result in facility closure. Falsification of data submitted to the FDA can result in monetary fines and jail terms.

MQSA equipment requirements for mammography are summarized in Box 1-7. MQSA qualification requirements for radiologists, technologists, and medical physicists are outlined in Boxes 1-8 to 1-10.

One radiologist at each facility must be designated the *supervising interpreting physician* to oversee the facility's quality assurance (QA) program (Boxes 1-11 and

1-12). The supervising physician oversees assessment of mammography outcomes to evaluate the accuracy of interpretation. The facility must have a method for recording outcomes on interpretation of all abnormal mammographic findings and tallying these interpretations for each

---

BOX 1-7. Mammography Quality Standards Act Equipment Requirements for Mammography

Be specifically designed for mammography

Have a breast compression device and have additional hand-operated compression to augment motor-driven compression

Have provision for operation with a removable grid for either 18 × 24-cm or 24 × 30-cm image receptors (screen-film only)

The mean glandular dose to a 4.5-cm thick breast is less than 3 mGy (0.3 rad) when the site's clinical technique is used

Can angulate 180 degrees from craniocaudal orientation in at least one direction

Other minimum standards for beam limitation and light field, magnification capability, display of focal spot selection, technique factor selection and display, automatic exposure control, x-ray film, intensifying screens, film processing solutions, lighting and hot lights, film masking devices

Modified from *The federal register*. Available at www.fda.gov/cdrh/mammography/.

BOX 1-8. Mammography Quality Standards Act Qualifications for Interpreting Physicians

Be licensed to practice medicine in the state

Be certified by a body approved by the FDA to certify interpreting physicians or have 3 months' full-time training in mammography interpretation, radiation physics, radiation effects, and radiation protection *and*

Have earned 60 hours of documented mammography continuing medical education (CME) (time in residency will be accepted if documented in writing) and 8 hours of training in each modality (such as screen-film or digital mammography) *and*

Have read at least 240 examinations in the preceding 6 months under supervision or have read mammograms under the supervision of a fully qualified interpreting physician (see *The Federal Register* for exact requirements) *and*

Have read 960 mammograms over a period of 24 months

Have earned at least 15 Category 1 CME credits in mammography over a 36-month period, with 6 credits in each modality used

To re-establish qualifications, either interpret or double-read 240 mammograms under direct supervision or bring the total to 960 over a period of 24 months and accomplish these tasks within the 6 months immediately before resuming independent interpretation. Regarding CME, if the requirement of 15 hours per 36 months is not met, the total number of CME hours must be brought up to 15 per 36 months before resuming independent interpretation.

Note: To perform a new imaging modality (e.g., digital mammography), the interpreting physician must have 8 CME credits specific to that modality before starting the modality.

Modified from *The federal register*. Available at www.fda.gov/cdrh/mammography/.

BOX 1-9. Mammography Quality Standards Act Qualifications for Radiologic Technologists

Have a license to perform radiographic procedures in their state *or*

Be certified by one of the bodies (such as the American Registry of Radiologic Technologists) approved by the FDA

Have undergone 40 hours of documented mammography training, with 8 hours of instruction in each modality used, and have completed at least 25 examinations *or*

Be exempted by having qualified under interim regulations

Complete 200 examinations in the previous 24 months and teach or complete at least 15 continuing education units (CEUs) in the past 36 months, including 6 in each modality used

To re-establish qualifications, must complete 25 examinations under direct supervision and complete 15 CEUs per 36 months.

Modified from *The federal register*. Available at www.fda.gov/cdrh/mammography/.

BOX 1-10. Mammography Quality Standards Act Qualifications for Medical Physicists

Have a license or approval by a state to conduct evaluations of mammography equipment under the Public Health Services Act or have certification in an accepted area by one of the accrediting bodies approved by the FDA

Have a master's or higher degree in physics, radiologic physics, applied physics, biophysics, health physics, medical physics, engineering, radiation science, or public health with a bachelor's degree in the physical sciences *and*

Have 1 year in training in medical physics specific to diagnostic radiologic physics *and*

Have 2 years' experience in conducting performance evaluation of mammography equipment *and*

Teach or complete 15 hours of continuing medical education in mammography physics every 36 months

Modified from *The federal register*. Available at www.fda.gov/cdrh/mammography/.

BOX 1-11. Quality Assurance Program for Equipment

All programs must establish and maintain a quality assurance (QA) program with periodic monitoring of the dose delivered by the examinations

For screen-film systems, the QA program is the same as described in Hendrick et al: *Mammography Quality Control Manual: Radiologist's Manual* (1999), *Radiological Technologist's Manual*, and *Medical Physicist's Manual* prepared by the American College of Radiology Committee on Quality Assurance in Mammography

Maintenance of log books documenting compliance and corrective actions for each unit

Establish and maintain radiographic images of phantoms to assess performance of the mammography system for each unit

Major changes from the interim regulations include weekly phantom image quality testing and mammography unit performance tests after each relocation of the mobile unit

Modified from *The federal register*. Available at www.fda.gov/cdrh/mammography/.

BOX 1-12. Quality Assurance for Clinical Images

Monitoring of repeat rate for repeated clinical images and their causes

Record keeping, analysis of results, and remedial actions taken on the basis of this monitoring

Modified from *The federal register*. Available at www.fda.gov/cdrh/mammography/.

BOX 1-13. Quality Assurance for Interpretation of Clinical Images

Establishment of systems for reviewing outcome data from mammograms, including

Disposition of all positive mammograms

Correlation of surgical biopsy results with mammogram reports

Designation of a specific physician to ensure data collection and analysis and show that the analysis is shared with the facility and individual physicians

Modified from *The federal register*. Available at www.fda.gov/cdrh/mammography/.

---

individual physician and for the group as a whole, providing feedback to each radiologist on a yearly basis (Box 1-13). A portion of the medical audit includes review of the pathology in cases recommended for biopsy.

One radiologic technologist designated the *QC technologist* oversees the quality control (QC) tasks outlined in Table 1-4, which specifies the minimum frequency of each QC test and action limits for test performance. One important test performed by the QC technologist and reviewed by the interpreting physician is evaluation of the mammography phantom image; this test is performed at least weekly and evaluates the entire imaging system. The phantom consists of fibers, speck clusters, and masses of various sizes imbedded in a uniform phantom material. The technologist takes a phantom radiograph using the

site's clinical technique for a 4.5-cm thick compressed breast, the radiograph is processed on the site's film processor, and the image is evaluated for the number of objects seen in each category. To pass accreditation and meet MQSA requirements, the phantom should show a minimum of four fibers, three speck groups, and three masses (Box 1-14). The phantom image should also be free of significant artifacts. These and other tests are used to evaluate the entire imaging system.

The medical physicist surveys the equipment just after installation, after important major equipment repairs or upgrades, and annually, performing the QC tests outlined in Box 1-15. The medical physicist's survey report is an

TABLE 1-4. Technologist Quality Control Tests for Screen-Film Mammography

Periodicity	Quality Control Test	Desired Result
Daily	Darkroom cleanliness	No dust artifacts
Daily	Processor quality control	Density difference and mid-density changes not to exceed control limits of ±0.15
Weekly	Screen cleanliness	No dust artifacts on films
Weekly	View box cleanliness	No marks on panels, uniform lighting
Weekly	Phantom image evaluation	Film density >1.4 with control limits of ±0.20 Densities do not vary over time or between units Minimum test objects seen: 4 largest fibers, 3 largest speck groups, 3 largest masses
Monthly	Visual checklist	Each item on checklist present and functioning properly
Quarterly	Repeat analysis	Overall repeat rate of <5% Percent repeats similar for each category
Quarterly	Analysis of fixer retention	Residual sodium thiosulfate (hypo) ≤0.05 $\mu g/cm^3$
Semiannually	Darkroom fog	Fog ≤0.05 optical density difference for 2-min exposure in darkroom
Semiannually	Screen-film contact	Large areas (>1 cm) of poor contact unacceptable
Semiannually	Compression	Power mode: 25–45 pounds Manual mode: >25 pounds

From Hendrick et al: *Mammography quality control manual.* Reston, VA, 1999, American College of Radiology, p. 119.

BOX 1-14. Phantom Image

Evaluates the entire mammographic imaging chain (other than technologist positioning)
Performed at least weekly
Must see 4 fibers, 3 speck groups, 3 masses
Must be free of significant artifacts

From Hendrick et al: *Mammography quality control manual,* Reston, VA, 1999, American College of Radiology, p 119.

---

important component of the QA program and is reviewed by the supervising physician to ensure high-quality mammography. The facility is responsible for correcting deficiencies pointed out by the site medical physicist.

Each year, the mammography facility is inspected by state or federal inspectors who evaluate compliance with

---

BOX 1-15. Medical Physicist's Screen-Film Mammography Quality Control Tests (Annually and after Major Equipment Changes)

1. Unit assembly evaluation
2. Assessment of collimation
3. Evaluation of system resolution
4. Automatic exposure control (AEC) assessment of performance
5. Uniformity of screen speed
6. Artifact evaluation
7. Evaluation of image quality
8. kVp accuracy and reproducibility
9. Assessment of beam quality (half-value layer measurement)
10. Breast entrance exposure, AEC reproducibility, average glandular dose, and radiation output rate
11. View box luminance and room luminance

BOX 1-16. Educational Requirements for New Personnel Using Digital Mammography

8 hours of training specific to digital mammography before its use
6 hours of Category 1 continuing medical education or continuing education unit credits in this new modality every 3 years (FDA has delayed enforcement of this requirement indefinitely)
The 6 hours can be part of the required 15 hours of continuing education in mammography required by the Mammography Quality Standards Act

---

MQSA regulations. Site QA records and site personnel qualifications are routinely checked by the MQSA inspector. Correction of deficiencies specified in the medical physicist's report is an important item checked by MQSA inspectors. Noncompliance with MQSA requirements may result in warnings requiring corrective actions or, in extreme cases, facility closure.

Screen-Film Mammography Quality Control

For SFM, MQSA specifies the QA/QC tests to be carried out by the QC technologist and the site medical physicist, as well as how frequent these tests must be performed. Technologist test frequencies range from daily to semiannually, as specified in Table 1-4. Medical physicist tests are required annually, on acceptance of new equipment, or after major equipment changes and before its use on patients or volunteers (see Box 1-15). The technologist and medical physicist tests for SFM are described in detail in the 1999 edition of the ACR *Mammography Quality Control Manual* (Hendrick et al. 1999).

Full-Field Digital Mammography Quality Assurance and Quality Control

To comply with MQSA requirements, all personnel must have 8 hours of training specific to digital mammography documented in writing before clinical use of FFDM units in that facility (Box 1-16). Specifically, the radiologist must receive 8 hours of training in interpretation of digital mammography, with the strong recommendation from the FDA that training include instruction from a radiologist experienced in digital mammography interpretation on the specific system used. Technologists and medical physicists must also have documented training by appropriately qualified individuals; for example, the manufacturer's application specialists or other qualified individuals should train technologists, and medical physicists qualified in digital mammography should provide hands-on training for medical physicists. It was originally specified that after initial certification, all personnel involved in digital mammography should receive 6 hours of Category I continuing medical education (CME) or continuing educational units (CEU) every 3 years, which could be part of the required 15 hours of continuing education required for all personnel in mammography. The completion of the required 15 hours of Category I CME in mammography every 3 years must be documented in writing.

MQSA requires that QC testing for FFDM be performed by the facility "according to the image receptor manufacturer's specification." Each digital manufacturer has a detailed QC manual specifying tests, test frequencies, and pass-fail criteria. All manufacturers' QC manuals differ in the specific tests, frequencies, and criteria.

For some tests, such as mean glandular dose to the ACR phantom being less than 3 mGy, the FDA specifies that failures must be corrected immediately before that component of the FFDM system (e.g., the digital mammography unit, review workstation, or laser imager) can be used. Test failures that must be corrected immediately include phantom image quality, contrast-to-noise ratio, radiation dose, and review workstation calibration. For other test failures, such as repeat analysis, collimation assessment, and other physics tests, 30 days are permitted for correction after problem identification. Typical digital mammography QC tests are listed in Box 1-17, although these vary by digital manufacturer.

■ COMPUTER-AIDED DETECTION

Radiologists are trained to detect early, subtle signs of breast cancer, such as pleomorphic calcifications and spiculated masses on mammograms. CAD systems use algorithms to review mammograms for bright clustered specks and converging lines, which represent pleomorphic calcifications and spiculated masses, respectively. These programs were developed to help radiologists search for signs of cancer against the complex background of dense breast tissue and fat.

Some facilities use CAD as a *second reader*. *Double reading* in screening mammography involves two observers reviewing the same mammograms to increase detection of cancer, decrease the false-negative rate or, in some facilities, decrease the false-positive recall rate by using a consensus. Studies have shown that double reading, depending on its implementation, increases the rate of detection of cancer by 5% to 15%. However, the expense and logistic problems of implementing a second interpreting radiologist limit the practice of double reading of mammography in clinical practice in the United States.

Box 1-17. Medical Physicist's Digital Mammography Quality Control Tests (Annually and after Major Equipment Changes)

1. Full-field digital mammography (FFDM) unit assembly evaluation
2. Flat-field uniformity test*
3. Artifact evaluation
4. Automatic exposure control mode and signal-to-noise ratio check*
5. Phantom image quality test*
6. Contrast-to-noise ratio test*
7. Modulation transfer function measurement*
8. Assessment of collimation
9. Evaluation of focal spot size
10. kVp accuracy and reproducibility
11. Assessment of beam quality (half-value layer measurement)
12. Breast entrance exposure, mean glandular dose,* and radiation output rate
13. Image quality of the display monitor

*Indicates immediate correction required before using the FFDM unit.

Mammography data used for CAD algorithms are obtained digitally from FFDM units or are digitized from screen-film mammograms. The digital or digitized mammograms undergo analysis by computer schemes, which mark potential abnormal findings on a low-resolution paper print or monitor image (Fig. 1-16). For FFDM, CAD marks potential abnormalities directly on the image displayed on the workstation monitor. The radiologist interprets and analyzes the marked findings, and each finding is dismissed as insignificant or recalled for further workup (Fig. 1-17).

CAD algorithms detect microcalcifications, masses, and parenchymal distortions on images using computer schemes derived from large numbers of mammograms in which biopsy results are known. The computer scheme's ability to mark true cancers is optimized by reviewing the "true positive" and "false positive" marks on the training set of mammograms. These optimized algorithms are later tested on both known subtle and obvious cancers. Using the optimized schemes, commercial CAD systems mark abnormalities that represent cancers ("true positive" marks, a measure of CAD sensitivity), and findings that do *not* represent cancer or where no known cancer has occurred ("false positive" marks, a measure of CAD specificity) (Fig. 1-18). Because detection of masses or calcifications by the CAD scheme is directly affected by image quality, good-quality mammograms are required to obtain good CAD output. Mammograms of suboptimal quality will result in poor CAD output. CAD output also can be affected by the type and reproducibility of the digitizer if the data is from digitized SFM. Thus, it is essential to have high-quality mammograms since CAD cannot overcome poor image quality.

The FDA has approved CAD systems for breast cancer detection in both screening and diagnostic mammography using both screen-film and digital mammography, including the Fuji CR digital system.

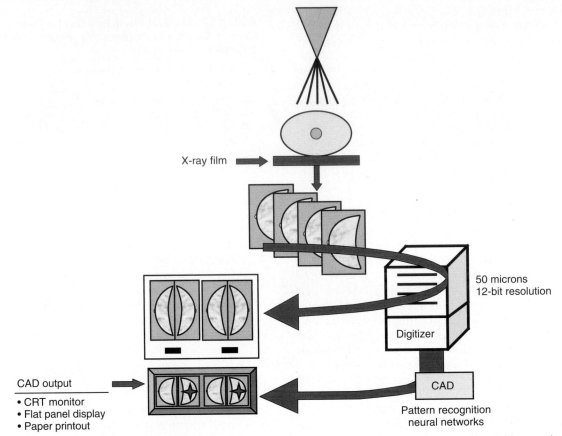

X-ray film

50 microns
12-bit resolution

Digitizer

CAD output
• CRT monitor
• Flat panel display
• Paper printout

CAD

Pattern recognition
neural networks

FIGURE 1-16. Computer-aided detection (CAD) schematic for screen-film and full-field digital mammograms. Film digitizers typically operate at 50-micron pixel (or 10 lp/mm) spatial resolution. Digital spatial resolution is set by the digital detector (see Table 1-3). CRT, cathode ray tube. (Courtesy of R. Castellino, R2 Technology, San Jose, CA.)

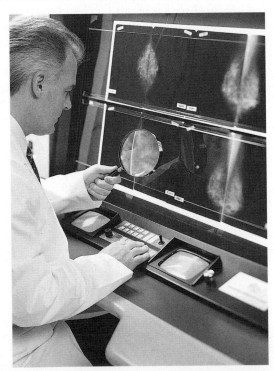

FIGURE 1-17. Mammograms and computer-aided detection output. For screen-film mammography, the technologist digitizes the mammograms and then mounts the images on an alternator for the radiologist to interpret. A computer marks potential findings on the mammogram and displays the findings on low-resolution images on the monitor below the films. (Courtesy of R. Castellino, R2 Technology, San Jose, CA.)

A retrospective study of breast cancers found on mammography by Warren-Burhenne and colleagues determined that a CAD program marked 77% (89/115) of screening-detected breast cancers. Birdwell and colleagues reviewed "negative" mammograms obtained the year before the diagnosis of 115 screen-detected cancers in 110 patients. They reported that a CAD program marked reader-missed findings in 77% (88/115) of false-negative mammograms. Specifically, CAD marked 86% (30/35) of missed calcifications and 73% (58/80) of missed masses.

Freer and Ulissey reported that in a prospective community breast center study of 12,860 women undergoing screening mammography, CAD increased their cancer detection rate by 19.5%. Radiologists detected 41 of 49 cancers and missed 8 cancers found by the CAD system (7 of 8 were calcifications). CAD detected 40 of the 49 cancers, but it did not mark 9 radiologist-detected masses that were proven to be cancers.

It is important to note that CAD systems did not diagnose all cancers, nor should they be used as the only evaluator of screening mammograms. In Freer and Ulissey's study, radiologists initially made a decision about the mammogram and then used CAD and re-reviewed the marked mammogram. The radiologist's decision to recall a potential abnormality could not be changed by failure of the CAD system to mark the potential finding. Findings marked by CAD could be recalled even if the finding was not initially detected by the radiologist but was judged to be abnormal in retrospect. This means that radiologists

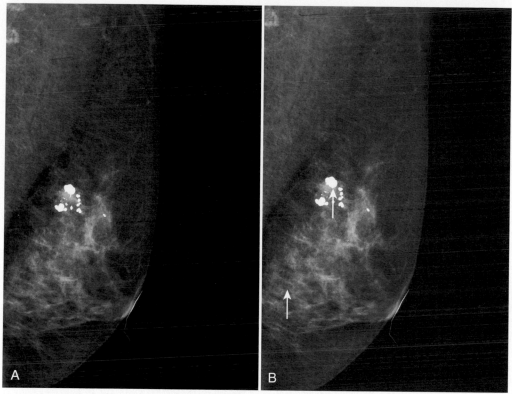

FIGURE 1-18. A, Left digital mediolateral oblique mammogram before computer-aided detection (CAD) shows calcifications. **B,** The CAD scheme puts a triangular mark on the calcification clusters in the upper and lower breast (*arrows*).

should read the mammogram first so they are not influenced by CAD marks initially because not all cancers are marked by CAD.

CAD marks have low specificity inasmuch as approximately 97.6% of the CAD marks were dismissed by the interpreting radiologists in the study by Freer and Ulissey. The radiologist had identified almost all of the 2.4% of CAD-marked findings that were selected for recall, which means that high-sensitivity CAD systems will mark significant potential findings as well as numerous insignificant findings, thus identifying tumors but marking a number of normal findings that must be dismissed. Accordingly, it is expected that many insignificant findings will be marked by the CAD system, most of which can be dismissed readily, and yet the radiologists' attention will still be drawn to overlooked suspicious areas.

Other CAD studies have shown somewhat less positive results. Gur and colleagues assessed changes in screening mammography recall rate and cancer detection rate after the introduction of a CAD system into a single academic radiology practice. Based on 56,432 cases interpreted without CAD and 59,139 cases interpreted with CAD by 24 radiologists, recall rates were identical without and with CAD (11.39% versus 11.40%, respectively; $p = 0.96$), as were breast cancer detection rates without and with CAD (3.49 versus 3.55 per 1000 women screened, respectively; $p = 0.68$). Feig and colleagues used Gur's data to point out that lower-volume readers benefited from CAD by having a 19.7% higher cancer detection rate, but at the price of a 14% increase in recall rate, from 10.5% to 12%.

Fenton and colleagues conducted a retrospective study comparing SFM without and with CAD in early imple-

mentation (2–25 months). They showed that adding CAD led to a nonsignificant increase in sensitivity (from 80.4% without CAD to 84% with CAD; $p = 0.32$), a significant decrease in specificity (from 90.2% without CAD to 87.2% with CAD; $p < 0.001$), and a significant decrease in accuracy (area under the ROC curve decreased from 0.919 without CAD to 0.871 with CAD; $p = 0.005$).

A study by Gromet compared CAD-aided reading of screening mammograms to double-reading without CAD. He found that CAD-aided reading had a nonsignificantly higher sensitivity than double-reading (90.4% versus 88.0%), with a significantly lower recall rate (10.6% versus 11.9%, respectively; $p < 0.0001$).

CAD programs have the potential to increase detection of cancer, particularly for readers with less experience or lower reader volumes, perhaps at the price of somewhat lower specificity and slightly longer interpretation times. In the end, however, it is the radiologist's knowledge and interpretive skills that have an impact on cancer detection, whether CAD is used or not.

CONCLUSION

Mammography acquisition is affected by a number of variables, including factors affecting image quality, such as the x-ray equipment, processing technique, technologist positioning, breast compression, patient differences such as breast density, lesion type, and the skills of the interpreting radiologist. It is important for radiologists to understand equipment requirements and the effect of imaging parameters on image quality; in addition, practitioners should be able to solve imaging problems that occur in everyday clinical practice. MQSA regulations were put into effect to mandate many of the factors that are known to affect image quality and to improve the quality of mammography. Every radiologist who performs breast imaging should understand MQSA requirements and be able to supervise a high-quality mammography practice, working toward improved technical quality and interpretive skills based on follow-up and feedback from sound quality assurance practices.

■ KEY ELEMENTS

American Cancer Society Guidelines for breast cancer screening of asymptomatic women include annual mammography starting at age 40.

The Mammography Quality Standard Act of 1992 is a congressional act enforced by the FDA under which mammography facilities in the United States are regulated.

The usual exposure for a mammogram is 24 to 32 kVp at 25 to 200 mA.

Screen-film and digital systems deliver a mean glandular breast dose of about 2 mGy per exposure (4 mGy per two-view examination) to a woman of average breast thickness and glandularity; mean glandular dose is lower for thin breasts, higher for thick breasts.

Anode/filter combinations for mammography are Mo/Mo, Mo/Rh, Rh/Rh, and W/Rh.

Screen-film image receptors are 18×24 cm and 24×30 cm in size.

Focal spot sizes for contact mammography and magnification mammography are nominally 0.3 and 0.1 mm, respectively.

Magnification mammography should produce $1.4\times$ to $2.0\times$ magnification.

Moving grids with grid ratios between $3.5:1$ and $5:1$ are used for contact mammography; no grid is used for magnification mammography.

The phantom image using the ACR mammography phantom evaluates the entire mammography imaging chain, is performed weekly, and at a minimum should detect four fibers, three speck groups, and three masses.

Film labeling includes the patient's first and last names and unique identification number, the name and address of the facility, the date, the view and laterality positioned near the axilla, numbers indicating the cassette and the mammography unit, and the technologist's initials.

The mediolateral oblique view should show good compression, contrast, exposure, sharpness, little noise, a posterior nipple line that intersects a concave pectoralis muscle, and an open inframammary fold.

The craniocaudal view should show good compression, contrast, exposure, sharpness, little noise, and a PNL that has a distance within 1 cm of the mediolateral oblique PNL length, and it should include medial breast tissue without sacrificing lateral breast tissue.

The MQSA requires specific training, experience, and continuing education for technologists, radiologists, and medical physicists.

To use a new modality, such as digital mammography, technologists, radiologists, and medical physicists are all required to have an initial 8 hours of training on that new modality prior to use.

Digital mammography detectors are composed of cesium iodide plus amorphous silicon diodes, cesium iodide plus arrayed charge-coupled devices, charged selenium plate read by silicon diodes, or CR plates consisting of a barium fluorobromide plate, which is read by a CR laser scanner.

Digital mammograms may be interpreted on printed films or on high-resolution $2K \times 2.5K$ (5 Mpixel) monitors.

CAD programs can detect subtle but suspicious mammographic findings in dense or complex breast tissue.

CAD programs do not detect every breast cancer.

When CAD is used for interpretation of mammograms, the decision to recall a finding on a mammogram rests solely on the radiologist's experience and judgment in interpretation of films.

■ SUGGESTED READINGS

American College of Radiology: *ACR BI-RADS®—Mammography*, ed 4, Reston, VA, 2003, American College of Radiology.

Baker JA, Rosen EL, Lo JY, et al: Computer-aided detection (CAD) in screening mammography: Sensitivity of commercial CAD systems for detecting architectural distortion, *AJR Am J Roentgenol* 181:1083–1088, 2003.

Bassett LW, Feig SA, Hendrick RE, et al: *Breast Disease (Third Series) Test and Syllabus*, Reston, VA, 2000, American College of Radiology.

Berns EA, Hendrick RE, Cutter GR: Performance comparison of full-field digital mammography to screen-film mammography in clinical practice, *Med Phys* 29:830–834, 2002.

Berns EA, Hendrick RE, Solari M, et al: Digital and screen-film mammography: comparison of image acquisition and interpretation times, *AJR Am J Roentgenol* 187:38–41, 2006.

Birdwell RL, Ikeda DM, O'Shaughnessy KF, Sickles EA: Mammographic characteristics of 115 missed cancers later detected with screening mammography and the potential utility of computer-aided detection, *Radiology* 219:192–202, 2001.

Ciatto S, Del Turco MR, Risso G, et al: Comparison of standard reading and computer aided detection (CAD) on a national proficiency test of screening mammography, *Eur J Radiol* 45:135–138, 2003.

Coldman A, Phillips N, Warren L, Kan L: Breast cancer mortality after screening mammography in British Columbia women, *Int J Cancer* 120:1076–1080, 2007.

Curry TS, Dowdy JE, Murray RC: *Christensen's Physics of Diagnostic Radiology*, ed 4, Malvern, PA, 1990, Lea & Febiger.

Duffy SW, Tabar L, Chen THH, et al., for The Swedish Organized Service Screening Evaluation Group: Reduction in breast cancer mortality from organized service screening with mammography: 1. Further confirmation with extended data, *Cancer Epidemiol Biomarkers Prev* 15:45–51, 2006.

Feig SA, Sickles EA, Evans WP, Linver NM: Re: Changes in breast cancer detection and mammography recall rates after the introduction of a computer-aided detection system, *J Natl Cancer Inst* 96:1260–1261, 2004.

Fenton JJ, Taplin SH, Carney PA, et al: Influence of computer-aided detection on performance of screening mammography, *N Engl J Med* 356:1399–1409, 2007.

Freer TW, Ulissey MJ: Screening mammography with computer-aided detection: prospective study of 12,860 patients in a community breast center, *Radiology* 220:781–786, 2001.

Galen B, Staab E, Sullivan DC, Pisano ED: Congressional update: Report from the Biomedical Imaging Program of the National Cancer Institute. American College of Radiology Imaging Network: The digital mammographic imaging screening trial—an update, *Acad Radiol* 9:374–375, 2002.

Gur D, Sumkin JH, Rockette HE: Changes in breast cancer detection and mammography recall rates after the introduction of a computer-aided detection system, *J Natl Cancer Institute* 96:185–190, 2004.

Gromet M: Comparison of computer-aided detection to double reading of screening mammograms: review of 231,221 mammograms, *AJR Am J Roentgenol* 190:854–859, 2008.

Hemminger BM, Dillon AW, Johnston RE, et al: Effect of display luminance on the feature detection rates of masses in mammograms, *Med Phys* 26:2266–2272, 1999.

Hendrick RE, Bassett LW, Botsco MA, et al: *Mammography Quality Control Manual*, Reston, VA, 1999, American College of Radiology.

Hendrick RE, Cole E, Pisano ED, et al: ACRIN DMIST retrospective multi-reader study comparing the accuracy of softcopy digital and screen-film mammography by digital manufacturer, *Radiology* 247:38–48, 2008.

Hendrick RE, Cutter G, Berns EA, et al: Community-based screening mammography practice: services, charges and interpretation methods, *AJR Am J Roentgenol* 84:433–438, 2005.

Hendrick RE, Pisano ED, Averbukh A, et al: Comparison of acquisition parameters and breast dose in digital mammography and screen-film mammography in the American College of Radiology Imaging Network Digital Mammographic Screening Trial, *Am J Roentgenology* 194:362–369, 2010.

Lewin JM, D'Orsi CJ, Hendrick RE, et al: Clinical comparison of full-field digital mammography and screen-film mammography for detection of breast cancer, *AJR Am J Roentgenol* 179:671–677, 2002.

Lewin JM, Hendrick RE, D'Orsi CJ, et al: Comparison of full-field digital mammography with screen-film mammography for cancer detection: Results of 4,945 paired examinations, *Radiology* 218:873–880, 2001.

Linver MN, Osuch JR, Brenner RJ, Smith RA: The mammography audit: A primer for the Mammography Quality Standards Act (MQSA), *AJR Am J Roentgenol* 165:19–25, 1995.

Markey MK, Lo JY, Floyd CE Jr: Differences between computer-aided diagnosis of breast masses and that of calcifications, *Radiology* 223:489–493, 2002.

Monsees BS: The Mammography Quality Standards Act. An overview of the regulations and guidance, *Radiol Clin North Am* 38:759–772, 2000.

MQSA (Mammography Quality Standards Act) final rule released. American College of Radiology, *Radiol Manage* 20:51–55, 1998.

Nass SJ, Henderson IC, Lashof LJ, editors: *Mammography and Beyond: Developing Technologies for the Early Detection of Breast Cancer*, Washington, DC, 2001, National Academy Press.

Pisano ED, Cole EB, Kistner EO, et al: Interpretation of digital mammograms: comparison of speed and accuracy of soft-copy versus printed-film display, *Radiology* 223:483–488, 2002.

Pisano ED, Cole EB, Major S, et al: for the International Digital Mammography Development Group: Radiologists' preferences for digital mammographic display, *Radiology* 216:820–830, 2000.

Pisano ED, Gatsonis CA, Yaffe MJ, et al: American College of Radiology Imaging Network Digital Mammographic Imaging Screening Trial: objectives and methodology, *Radiology* 236:404–412, 2005.

Pisano ED, Gatsonis CA, Hendrick RE, et al: Diagnostic performance of digital versus film mammography for breast-cancer screening: the results of the American College of Radiology Imaging Network (ACRIN) Digital Mammographic Imaging Screening Trial (DMIST), *N Engl J Med* 353:1773–1783, 2005.

Pisano ED, Hendrick RE, Yaffe MJ, et al: Diagnostic accuracy of digital versus film mammography: exploratory analysis of selected population subgroups in DMIST, *Radiology* 246:376–383, 2008.

Pisano ED, Yaffe MJ: Digital mammography, *Radiology* 234:353–361, 2005.

Quek ST, Thng CH, Khoo JB, Koh WL: Radiologists' detection of mammographic abnormalities with and without a computer-aided detection system, *Australas Radiol* 47:257–260, 2003.

Rong XJ, Shaw CC, Johnston DA, et al: Microcalcification detectability for four mammographic detectors: flat-panel, CCD, CR, and screen/film, *Med Phys* 29:2052–2061, 2002.

Rothenberg LN, Feig SA, Hendrick RE, et al: *A Guide to Mammography and Other Breast Imaging Procedures*, NCRP Report #149, Bethesda, MD, 31 December 2004, National Council of Radiation Protection and Measurements.

Saslow D, Boetes C, Burke W, et al, for the American Cancer Society Breast Cancer Advisory Group: American Cancer Society guidelines for breast screening with MRI as an adjunct to mammography, *CA Cancer J Clin* 57:75–89, 2007.

Skaane P, Hofvind S, Skjennald A: Randomized trial of screen-film versus full-field digital mammography with soft-copy reading in population-based screening program: follow-up and final results of Oslo II study, *Radiology* 244:708–717, 2007.

Skaane S, Skjennald A: Screen-film mammography versus full-field digital mammography with soft-copy reading: randomized trial in a population-based screening program—the Oslo II study, *Radiology* 232:197–204, 2004.

Smith RA, Saslow D, Sawyer KA, et al: American Cancer Society guidelines for breast cancer screening: update 2003, *CA Cancer J Clin* 53:141–169, 2003.

Tabar L, Yen MF, Vitak B, et al: Mammography service screening and mortality in breast cancer patients: 20-year follow-up before and after introduction of screening, *Lancet* 361:1405–1410, 2003.

U.S. Department of Health and Human Services. Food and Drug Administration: Compliance Guidance: The Mammography Quality Standards Act Final Regulations Document #1; Availability. Notice, *Fed Reg* 64(53):13590–13591, 1999.

U.S. Department of Health and Human Services. Food and Drug Administration: State certification of mammography facilities. Final rule, *Fed Reg* 67(25):5446–5469, 2002.

Vedantham S, Karellas A, Suryanarayanan S, et al: Breast imaging using an amorphous silicon-based full-field digital mammographic system: stability of a clinical prototype, *J Digit Imaging* 13:191–199, 2000.

Vedantham S, Karellas A, Suryanarayanan S, et al: Full breast digital mammography with an amorphous silicon-based flat panel detector: physical characteristics of a clinical prototype, *Med Phys* 27:558–567, 2000.

Venta LA, Hendrick RE, Adler YT, et al: Rates and causes of disagreement in interpretation of full-field digital mammography and film-screen mammography in a diagnostic setting, *AJR Am J Roentgenol* 176:1241–1248, 2001.

Warren Burhenne LJ, Wood SA, D'Orsi CJ, et al: Potential contribution of computer-aided detection to the sensitivity of screening mammography, *Radiology* 215:554–562, 2000.

Zheng B, Shah R, Wallace L, et al: Computer-aided detection in mammography: an assessment of performance on current and prior images, *Acad Radiol* 9:1245–1250, 2002.

Zhou XQ, Huang HK, Lou SL: Authenticity and integrity of digital mammography images, *IEEE Trans Med Imaging* 20:784–791, 2001.

CHAPTER 2

Mammogram Interpretation

The incidence of breast cancer in women in the United States has continued to rise. The rate of increase has slowed recently, however, with the exception of in situ breast cancer, which has continued to increase. Breast cancer death rates have decreased since the early 1990s, with decreases of 2.5% per year among white women. Decreased breast cancer deaths have been attributed in part to breast cancer screening, adjuvant chemotherapy, and adoption of a healthy standard of living that includes exercise, maintenance of an appropriate body mass index, and decreased alcohol consumption. Randomized, population-controlled breast cancer screening trials using mammography have shown an approximately 30% reduction in breast cancer deaths in the women invited to screening compared to women in the control group. Because of this data, the American Cancer Society recommends annual screening mammography for women age 40 years and older.

This chapter reviews breast cancer risk factors, signs, and symptoms of breast cancer, the normal mammogram, mammographic findings of breast cancer, basic interpretation of screening mammograms, and workup of findings detected at screening with additional mammographic views.

BREAST CANCER RISK FACTORS

Risk factors for breast cancer are important to consider when reading mammograms, because they indicate a pretest probability of breast cancer. Compiling risk information on the breast history sheet provides the interpreting radiologist quick and easy-to-use access to this information (Fig. 2-1). Breast cancer risk factors are listed in Box 2-1. The most important risk factors are older age and female gender; U.S. statistics indicate that breast cancer will develop in one in eight women, if the women have a 90-year life span. Men also develop breast cancer, but only 1% of all breast cancers occur in men.

The risk for breast cancer increases with increasing age and drops off at age 80. Women with a personal history of breast cancer have a higher risk of developing breast cancer in the ipsilateral or contralateral breast than does the general population. In women undergoing breast conservation, the conservatively treated breast has a 1% per year risk of developing cancer.

A family history of breast or ovarian cancer is a particularly important risk factor. The age, number, and cancer type in the affected relative is especially significant. Women with a first-degree relative (mother, daughter, or sister) with breast cancer have about double the risk of the

general population and are at particularly high risk if that cancer was premenopausal or bilateral. If many relatives had breast or ovarian cancer, the woman may be a carrier of *BRCA1* or *BRCA2*, the autosomal dominant breast cancer susceptibility genes. Genetic testing for these genes is possible. However, genetic testing is most appropriate when combined with the counseling, evaluation, and support provided by a genetic screening center because of the untoward social effects of positive (or negative) results. Carriers of the breast cancer susceptibility gene *BRCA1* on chromosome 17 have a breast cancer risk of 85% and an ovarian cancer risk of 63% by age 70. Women with *BRCA2* on chromosome 15 have a high risk of breast cancer and a low risk of ovarian cancer. These genes account for 5% of all breast cancers in the United States and for 25% of breast cancers in women younger than age 30. Women of Ashkenazi (Eastern European) Jewish heritage have a slightly higher risk of breast cancer than does the general population (Box 2-2), but additional work is being done to determine whether this population has a higher rate of breast and ovarian cancer related to *BRCA1* and *BRCA2* mutations. Other genetic syndromes that have a higher risk of breast cancer include the Li-Fraumeni, Cowden, and ataxia-telangiectasia syndromes.

Early menarche (before age 12), late menopause (after age 55), nulliparity, and first live birth after age 30 bestow a slightly higher risk for breast cancer, as a result of having more menstrual cycles and longer exposure to estrogen and progesterone. Data from a 2003 study, part of the Women's Health Initiative, a randomized, controlled trial of the effects of estrogen plus progestin (combination hormone replacement therapy [CHRT]) versus placebo, showed a 24% greater incidence of breast cancer in women receiving CHRT versus the control group. Whereas previous data showed an adjusted relative risk of 1.46 for the development of breast cancer in women receiving CHRT for more than 5 years, the 2003 analysis showed the risk for breast cancer rising within 5 years of starting CHRT; in addition, it showed more difficulty in detecting cancers by mammography in this group.

A breast biopsy showing atypical ductal hyperplasia (ADH) histology increases the risk for breast cancer to four to five times that of the general population. The presence of lobular carcinoma in situ (LCIS) also increases the risk for breast cancer, but at a much higher rate than ADH, about 10 times that of the normal population. LCIS is a misnomer and not a cancer at all. Rather, LCIS is a high-risk marker for developing breast cancer. A woman with LCIS has a 27% to 30% chance of developing invasive ductal or lobular cancer in the ipsilateral or contralateral breast over a 10-year period. Thus, a biopsy showing LCIS

STANFORD HOSPITAL AND CLINICS
DEPARTMENT OF RADIOLOGY
MAMMOGRAM HISTORY

Tech:_____

KVP: _____ Density: _____

DAY TELEPHONE#: (   ) _____
PLEASE CHECK

YES	NO	
		Do you have any current breast complaints or problems?

Indicate below any scars, lumps, moles, and/or areas of concern:

	Right	Left
☐ Scars	____	____
☐ Lump or Mass	____	____
☐ Moles	____	____
☐ Tissue Thickening	____	____
☐ Skin Thickening or Retraction	____	____
☐ Nipple Discharge	____	____
☐ Nipple Inversion or Retraction	____	____
☐ Pain	____	____
☐ Other _____	____	____
☐ Comments _____	____	____

YES	NO	
		Have you had a mammogram before? Location: _____ Date: _____ If your last mammogram was NOT at Stanford, please complete a FILM RELEASE FORM
		Have you had a breast *physical* examination by a health care professional? If yes when?_____ If you have *not* had a breast *physical* exam, *you should have one within a month* of this mammogram by your own health care professional to complete the evaluation of your breasts.
		Do you have children? *Your* age at the birth of your first child_____ **DO YOU HAVE BREAST IMPLANTS?**
		Date of the beginning of your last period, or _____ Date of menopause, or _____ Date of your hysterectomy _____ **YES ____ NO ____**
		Are you taking birth control or fertility drugs? If yes, began in 19 _____
		Are you taking hormones (estrogen/Premarin)? If yes, began in 19 _____ IF YES, WHY? ☐ menopause ☐ heart condition ☐ osteoporosis ☐ prior hysterectomy ☐ other
		Do you have rheumatoid arthritis?
		Have you or anyone in your family ever had breast cancer? ☐ Don't know ☐ MYSELF at age ____ ☐ MOTHER at age ____ ☐ GRANDMOTHER at age ____ ☐ SISTER at age ____ ☐ AUNT at age ____ ☐ DAUGHTER at age ____
		Have you had cancer? If yes, please describe what type: _____ Type of treatment: ☐ Radiation ☐ Chemotherapy ☐ Surgery
		Have you ever had breast surgery? IF YES, SEE BELOW.

If you answered yes to the question above, please indicate date, reason for surgery, and type of surgery below:

	Right	Date and reason, benign or malignant	Left	Date and reason, benign or malignant
Surgical biopsy	Right	_____	Left	_____
Needle biopsy	Right	_____	Left	_____
Cyst aspiration	Right	_____	Left	_____
Lumpectomy	Right	_____	Left	_____
Mastectomy	Right	_____	Left	_____
Breast Implants	Right	_____	Left	_____
Breast Reduction	Right	_____	Left	_____

FIGURE 2-1. Breast history form. Includes a diagrammatic breast template and places to record the patient's history and current problems or complaints.

Box 2-1. Breast Cancer Risk Factors

Female
Older age
Personal history of breast cancer
First-degree relative with breast cancer
Early menarche
Late menopause
Nulliparity
First birth after age 30
Atypical ductal hyperplasia
BRCA1, BRCA2
Radiation exposure
Lobular carcinoma in situ

Box 2-2. Family History Suggesting an Increased Risk of Breast Cancer

>2 relatives with breast or ovarian cancer
Breast cancer in relative age <50 years
Relatives with breast and ovarian cancer
Relatives with 2 independent breast cancers or breast plus ovarian cancer
Male relative with breast cancer
Family history of breast or ovarian cancer and Ashkenazi Jewish heritage
Li-Fraumeni syndrome
Cowden syndrome
Ataxia-telangiectasia

---

results in patient management of either "watchful waiting" with increased surveillance by frequent imaging and physical examination, or bilateral mastectomy.

Women who had an early exposure to radiation also have an increased risk for breast cancer. A medical history of radiation therapy for Hodgkin disease, multiple fluoroscopic examinations for tuberculosis, ablation of the thymus, or treatment of acne with radiation infers possible scattered radiation to the breasts, which may induce breast cancer. In fact, the risk for developing breast cancer is so high in women with Hodgkin disease that in 2008 the American Cancer Society recommended magnetic resonance screening for Hodgkin's disease survivors.

Extensive mammographic breast density, or a large amount of fibroglandular tissue within the breast by volume as measured on the mammogram, is strongly associated with the risk of breast cancer. However, the association and the reasons for this finding, as well as its relative association among different ethnicities, are still being studied.

Other lifestyle choices also affect breast cancer risk. One is drinking alcohol. One drink per day bestows a very small risk, but two to five drinks per day increases the risk to 15 times that of women who do not drink. Being overweight or obese also increases the risk of cancer, especially if the weight gain happens after menopause and the fat is around the abdomen. A woman with an "apple-shaped" body is at higher risk than one with a "pear-shaped" body. Exercise

has been shown to reduce breast cancer risk after menopause, with one study suggesting that cancer risk was reduced at least in part via hormonal pathways. However, more study of these changeable risk factors is needed.

Quantitative statistical models that estimate the short-term or lifetime risk for breast cancer include the Claus model and the Gail statistical model. These models compile individual risk factors and combine them into an estimate of the lifetime risk for breast cancer for individual women.

Despite all these risk factors, it remains true that 70% of all women with breast cancer have none of these risk factors other than older age and female gender.

■ SIGNS AND SYMPTOMS OF BREAST CANCER

Women, or their partners, often find their own breast cancer by discovering a palpable hard breast lump. Breast lumps are a common symptom for which women seek advice (Box 2-3). Of particular concern are new, growing, or hard breast masses. Masses that are stuck to the skin or chest wall are particularly worrisome for an invasive breast cancer.

Nipple discharge is another finding for which women often seek advice. Nipple discharge is usually benign, especially if it is whitish, green, or yellow and is produced from several ducts. Nipple discharge is suspicious for cancer if it is new, expressed from only one duct, bloody or serosanguineous, spontaneous, copious, or serous. An example of a suspicious history is a woman finding new bloody or serous nipple discharge on her nightgown or undergarments.

Nipple inversion is a sign of breast cancer if it is new. Longstanding nipple inversion is not uncommon, however; inverted nipples may be present at birth and are benign. On the other hand, new nipple inversion is of concern because a retroareolar tumor can produce nipple retraction.

Similarly, skin retraction or dimpling is a sign of breast cancer, due to tethering of the skin by cancer. On physical examination, skin retraction or tethering may be seen with the patient's arms at her sides when she inspects her breasts in the mirror. Raising the patient's arms or placing her hands on her hips pulls in the pectoralis muscle and may show skin tethering under the breasts that was previously invisible or may make the tethering more apparent.

Box 2-3. Signs and Symptoms of Breast Cancer

Breast lump
Nipple discharge (new and spontaneous)
  Bloody
  Serosanguineous
  Serous but copious
New nipple inversion
Skin retraction or tethering
Peau d'orange
Nothing (cancer detected on screening mammography)

Peau d'orange is a physical finding indicating breast edema; it is caused by skin edema rising around the bases of tethered hair follicles, resulting in skin pitting, or "orange peel" skin. Breast edema is a nonspecific finding and may indicate inflammatory cancer, mastitis, or axillary lymph node obstruction.

Despite all these signs and symptoms of breast cancer, some women have no physical findings or symptoms at all despite having breast cancer. Their breast cancers are detected on screening mammography.

Breast pain is not generally caused by cancer, but it deserves mention because it is a common cause of morbidity. If cyclic, breast pain is usually endocrine in nature. Although breast pain is usually due to benign etiologies, unfortunately, both breast pain and breast cancer are common. Thus, the physician's goals are to reassure patients with breast pain, search for treatable causes of breast pain such as cysts, and exclude coexistent malignancy.

THE NORMAL MAMMOGRAM

A normal breast is composed of a honeycomb supporting fibrous structure made up of Cooper ligaments that houses fatty tissue, which in turn supports the glandular elements of the breast (Fig. 2-2A). The glandular elements are composed of lactiferous ducts leading from the nipple and branching into excretory ducts, interlobular ducts, and terminal ducts leading to the acini that produce milk. The ducts are lined throughout their course by epithelium composed of an outer myoepithelial layer of cells and an inner secretory cell layer. The ducts and glandular tissue extend posteriorly in a fanlike distribution consisting of 15 to 20 lobes draining each of the lactiferous ducts, with most of the dense tissue found in the upper outer quadrant. Posterior to the glandular tissue is retroglandular fat, described by Dr. Laszlo Tabar as a "no man's land," in which no glandular tissue should be seen. The pectoralis muscle lies behind the fat on top of the chest wall.

On the normal mediolateral oblique (MLO) mammogram, the pectoralis muscle is a concave structure posterior to the retroglandular fat near the chest wall. Normal lymph nodes high in the axilla overlie the pectoralis muscle (see Fig. 2-2B and C). Normal lymph nodes are sharply margin-ated, oval, or lobulated dense masses with a radiolucent fatty hilum. They are commonly found in the upper outer quadrant of the breast along blood vessels. Lymph nodes also occur normally within the breast and are known as normal "intramammary" lymph nodes. If the lymph node has the typical kidney bean shape and a fatty hilum, it should be left alone. If one is uncertain about whether a mass represents an intramammary lymph node, mammographic magnification views may help display the fatty hilum, or ultrasound may show the typical hypoechoic appearance of the lymph node and the echogenic fatty hilum.

Usually fibroglandular tissue occurs symmetrically in the upper outer quadrants of the breasts. The breast tissue is usually distributed fairly symmetrically from left to right. When viewing mammograms, the clinician should place the mammograms back to back so that the chest walls face each other for easy viewing of tissue symmetry (see Fig. 2-5A). Fatty tissue surrounds the glandular tissue.

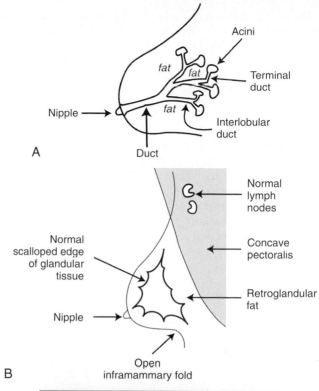

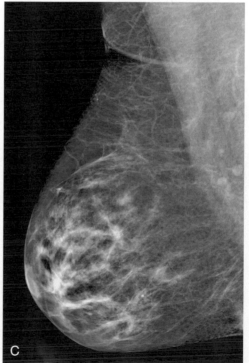

FIGURE 2-2. Normal breast anatomy and correlative mammograms. **A,** Schematic of a normal breast showing the nipple, ducts, and acini containing glands that produce breast milk. **B,** Schematic of a normal mediolateral oblique (MLO) mammogram. Note the normal scalloped edge of glandular tissue, retromammary fat, concave pectoralis muscle, and normal lymph nodes. **C,** Normal MLO mammogram.

On the normal craniocaudal (CC) projection, the pectoralis muscle produces a half-moon–shaped density near the chest wall (Fig. 2-3A and B). Fat lies anterior to the muscle, and the white glandular tissue lies anterior to the fat. In older women, most of the glandular tissue in the medial breast undergoes fatty involution, and therefore most of the residual dense glandular tissue exists in the upper outer breast.

There should be only fatty tissue in the medial breast near the chest wall. The only normal exception is the sternalis muscle, a muscular density near the medial aspect of the chest wall that should not be mistaken for a mass (see Fig. 2-3C and D). If there is a question that the density is a mass instead of the sternalis muscle, a cleavage view (CV) mammogram or ultrasound can prove that the density is a muscle and a normal structure.

Breast "density" is an important feature of the mammogram that describes how much of the breast is filled with glandular tissue, which looks white on the mammogram. Fat is black on the mammogram. Women normally have varying ratios of glandular and fatty tissue in their breasts. A "dense" mammogram has very glandular breast tissue in it and looks mostly white. The opposite of a "dense" mammogram is a "fatty" mammogram, which looks mostly black. Because breast cancer is also white on the mammogram, a white "dense" normal background of glandular tissue can hide a cancer, just like a polar bear can hide in a snowstorm.

The American College of Radiology's (ACR) Breast Imaging Reporting and Data System (BI-RADS®) lexicon separates breast density into quartiles depending on how much glandular tissue the breast contains by volume.

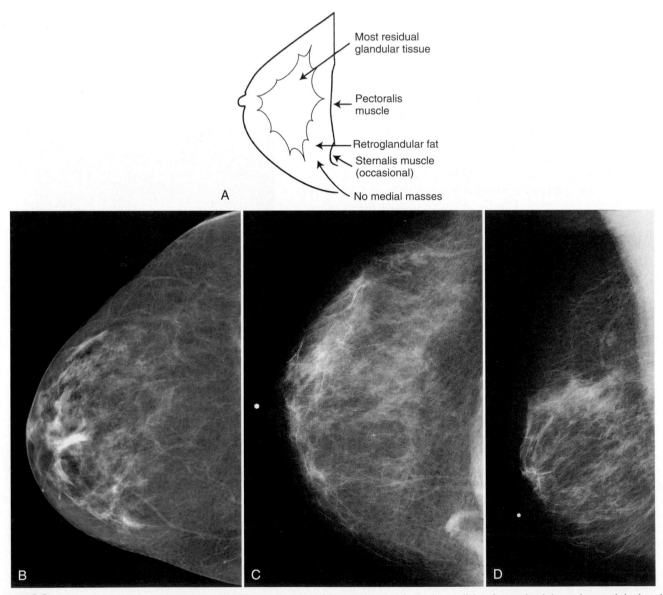

Most residual glandular tissue

Pectoralis muscle

Retroglandular fat

Sternalis muscle (occasional)

No medial masses

FIGURE 2-3. A, Schematic of a normal craniocaudal (CC) mammogram. Note the normal fat in the medial and retroglandular regions and the location of the pectoralis muscles. Most of the residual glandular tissue and the sternalis muscle remains in the upper outer quadrants. **B,** Normal CC mammogram. **C** and **D,** Sternalis muscle. The breast is composed of scattered fibroglandular density. A muscle-like density seen in the right breast medial to the half-moon shape of the pectoralis muscle near the chest wall on the CC view (**C**) but not seen on the mediolateral oblique view (**D**) represents the sternalis muscle.

"Dense" contains the most white (>75% dense), "heterogeneously dense" is less white (50–75% dense), "scattered fibroglandular" is even less white (25–50%), and "fatty" is the least white (<25% dense) (Box 2-4). A "dense" breast does not mean the breast is hard to the touch. Breast density has little correlation to how hard or soft the breast feels on physical examination; that is, you cannot predict how soft a breast will feel by looking at the mammogram. Radiologists describe breast density in the mammogram report so that referring doctors will know how white the breast looks and how confident the radiologist is in excluding cancer.

Young women have mostly glandular breasts, and their mammograms are described as "dense." As women age, the fibroglandular tissue involutes into fat, which is black. The natural progression of the mammogram is mostly white (dense) at a young age when the breasts are filled with glandular tissue, becoming progressively darker as the woman ages and her glandular tissue turns into fat. The amount of remaining glandular tissue varies from woman to woman. Some older women have surprisingly large amounts of dense white tissue on the mammogram; the amount remaining depends on genetics, parity, and exogenous hormone replacement therapy. But generally as women age, the glandular tissue involutes so that there are relatively greater amounts of dense glandular tissue remaining in the upper outer quadrant of the breast and darker fatty areas in the medial and lower part of the breast. In some women, only fatty tissue is left after the menopause (Fig. 2-4).

It is important to know about the relative decrease in breast tissue and breast density over time. Increases in breast density in normal women occur only in pregnant and lactating women, or in women starting exogenous hormone replacement therapy. Unexplained generalized increases in breast density may indicate breast edema or inflammatory cancer. New focal density should prompt investigation because a developing density may represent a cancer.

Breast tissue is usually symmetric, or "mirror image," when comparing left to right mammograms, although 3% of women have normal asymmetric glandular tissue. Normal asymmetric glandular tissue is a larger volume of normal fibroglandular tissue in one breast than in the other, but with one breast not necessarily being larger than the other. One method of evaluating for symmetry is to view the left and right MLO mammograms back to back and the CC mammograms back to back. The glandular tissue pattern is usually fairly symmetric from side to side, and asymmetries are easily identified using this technique (Fig. 2-5A to C).

A normal mammogram does not usually change from year to year after taking into account the normal involution of glandular tissue over time. Because the mammogram stays the same from year to year, comparing old studies with current studies makes it easier to see new or developing changes. For this reason, older films of good quality are placed next to the new films to look for subtle change (see Fig 2-5D to H). Because subtle changes may take longer than a year to become evident, one should compare both last year's films and films more than 2 years old (or the oldest films of comparable quality) to the new ones. If the mammograms are screen-film studies, the images are viewed on a high-intensity view box with the light parts of the films masked to block extraneous light. For full-field digital mammograms (FFDMs) viewed on soft copy, the images are displayed on high-resolution bright monitors in a dark room with little to no ambient light, comparing old mammograms to new ones in the display protocol.

■ MAMMOGRAPHIC FINDINGS OF BREAST CANCER

Mammographic detection of breast cancer depends on the sensitivity of the test, the experience of the radiologist, the morphologic appearance of the tumor, and the background on which it is displayed. Cause for a "missed" breast cancer can usually be traced to one of these factors (Table 2-1).

Radiologists see breast cancers on screening mammography because they see pleomorphic calcifications or spiculations produced by the tumor. Radiologists also may see architectural distortion, asymmetric density, a developing density, a round mass, breast edema, lymphadenopathy, or a single dilated duct, which are the other mammographic signs of breast cancer. The radiologist has to not only see the finding, but to also recognize that the finding is abnormal and correctly interpret the study as needing further action (i.e., is "actionable") (Box 2-5).

TABLE 2-1. Reasons for Missed Cancers

Errors in technique	Poor technique Poor positioning Cancer in location not included in standard field of view
Errors in detection	"Overlooked, missed": characteristic cancer findings, present in retrospect "Unrecognized sign": atypical finding perceived but not acted on, such as round mass or developing focal asymmetry "Nonspecific findings" that look normal (not actionable, not an error)
Errors in interpretation	Radiologist sees and perceives finding, incorrectly interprets finding as nonactionable
Tumor morphology	Tumor shape similar to background fibroglandular tissue displayed on the mammogram
True negative study	Tumor cannot be seen even in retrospect

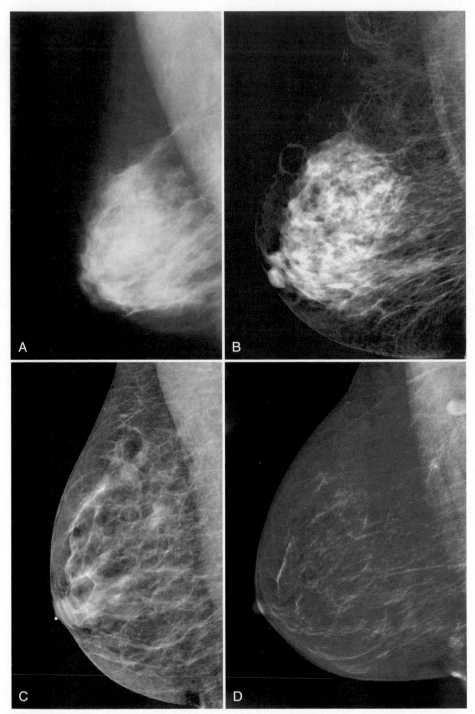

FIGURE 2-4. Mammograms of normal breast density. **A,** Dense glandular tissue of greater than 75% breast tissue by volume in a young woman categorized in BI-RADS® terms as "dense." **B,** A woman with "heterogeneously dense" breast tissue with 50% to 75% glandular tissue. **C,** A woman with "scattered fibroglandular densities" with 25% to 50% glandular tissue. **D,** An older woman with a "fatty" breast composed of less than 25% glandular tissue.

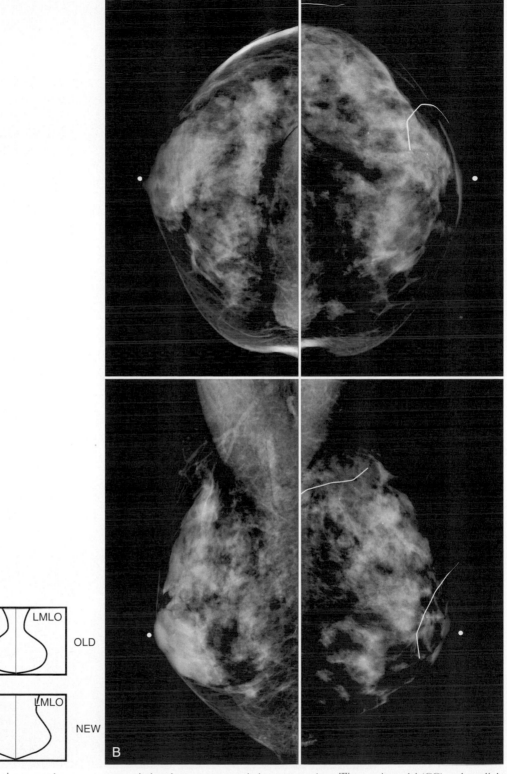

FIGURE 2-5. **A,** Schematic of viewing normal mammograms to judge the symmetry and change over time. The craniocaudal (CC) and mediolateral oblique (MLO) mammograms are viewed with the right and left sides placed back to back. Older mammograms are placed above to check for change from year to year. **B,** Example of normal stable mammograms in viewing scheme. Normal old MLO and CC views are placed back to back above the new views.

Continued

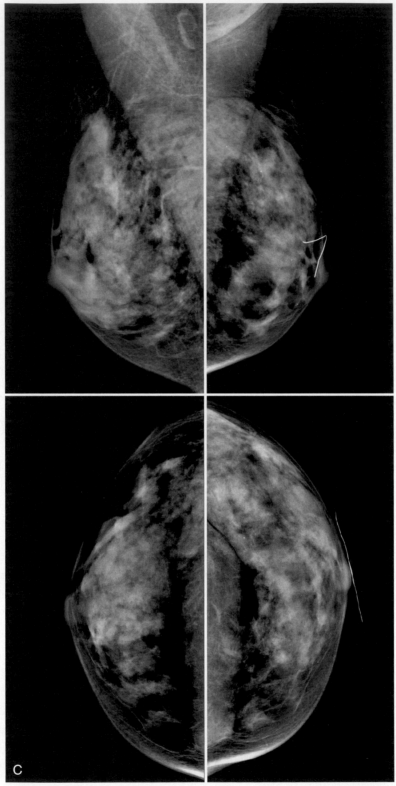

FIGURE 2-5, cont'd. C, Normal new MLO and CC views, also placed back to back. Comparing the new and old studies shows no change in dense tissue and a stable benign nodule in the medial left CC view over a 4-year period.

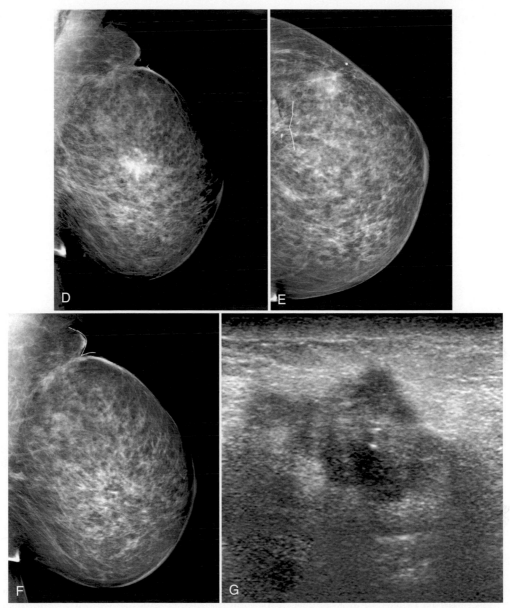

FIGURE 2-5, cont'd. D to H, Example of new developing density (cancer) discovered because of comparing old and new mammograms. A new left MLO (**D**) and CC view (**E**) show a vague new but palpable density in the upper outer left breast, marked with a BB skin marker when compared to the old MLO (**F**). The woman had had an excisional biopsy for cancer near the chest wall 17 years ago, marked by a metallic linear scar marker, and had dense fat necrosis calcification in the biopsy site. New skin thickening was also noted. Ultrasound (**G**) shows an irregular suspicious mass with calcifications. Invasive ductal cancer (new in-breast tumor recurrence) was diagnosed and a mastectomy was done. Incidentally, note the linear metallic scar marker over skin scars in parts **B, C, E,** and **F.**

BOX 2-5. Steps in Radiologists Recognizing Cancer on Mammograms

Radiologist sees the finding

Radiologist recognizes the finding is different from normal tissue

Radiologist correctly interprets the finding as abnormal/possibly abnormal

Radiologist acts on the finding (recall/biopsy)

The mammographic signs of breast cancer listed in Table 2-2 are discussed in further detail in Chapter 3 on breast calcifications, Chapter 4 on breast masses, and Chapter 10 on clinical problems. The trick is to see the cancer, perceive it and have it register in one's mind, then interpret the findings correctly and act on the finding.

Between 10% and 15% of breast cancers are mammographically occult, which means that breast cancer is present but the mammogram is normal. Accordingly, if there are suspicious clinical symptoms or physical findings

TABLE 2-2. Mammographic Findings of Breast Cancer

Finding	Differential Diagnosis
Pleomorphic calcifications	Cancer (most common), benign disease, fat necrosis
Spiculated mass	Cancer, postsurgical scar, radial scar, fat necrosis
Round mass	Cyst, fibroadenoma, cancer, papilloma, metastasis
Architectural distortion	Postsurgical scarring, cancer
Developing density	Cancer, hormone effect, focal fibrosis
Asymmetry: focal or global	Normal asymmetric tissue (3%), cancer (suspicious: new, palpable, a mass containing suspicious calcifications or spiculation)
Breast edema	Unilateral: mastitis, postradiation therapy, inflammatory cancer Bilateral: systemic disease (liver disease, renal failure, congestive heart failure)
Lymphadenopathy	Unilateral: mastitis, cancer Bilateral: systemic disease (collagen vascular disease, lymphoma, leukemia, infection, adenocarcinoma of unknown primary)
Single dilated duct	Normal variant, papilloma, cancer
Mass with calcifications	Cancer, fibroadenoma, papilloma; exclude calcifying oil cyst
Nothing	10% of all cancers are false-negative on mammography

TABLE 2-3. Tools Used for Interpretation of Mammograms

Tool	Use
Breast history, risk factors	Evaluate patient's complaint and risks
Technologist's marks	Show skin lesions, scars, problem areas
Putting images back to back	Detection of asymmetry Look for whitest part of study
Bright light (SFM)	View skin, dark parts of film
Window/level (FFDM)	Contrast for masses, calcifications
Magnifying lens or magnifier	Visualize mass borders, calcifications
Old films	Compare for changes
CAD (if available)	Look for CAD marks *after* initial interpretation

CAD, computer-aided detection; FFDM, full-field digital mammogram; SFM, screen-film mammogram.

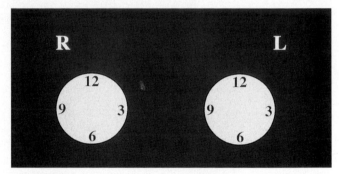

FIGURE 2-6. Clock face. Clock face description of breast lesion locations. The clock face location of breast findings is described by imaging a clock on both the left and the right breast as the woman faces the examiner. Note that the outer portion of the breast on the right is at the 9-o'clock position and the outer portion on the left is at the 3-o'clock position.

and the mammogram is negative, the decision for biopsy should be based on clinical grounds alone.

The ability of mammography to depict breast cancer is optimized by good mammographic technique and positioning, which produces the best chance to display suspicious findings against the normal breast background. Mammographic signs of breast cancer are not seen as well against a dense or fibroglandular background, which hides masses and tiny pleomorphic calcifications. Suspicious masses also may be lost in a "busy" background of round benign cysts or extensive benign calcifications that draw the radiologist's attention away from the cancer. Therefore, the radiologist needs a systematic approach to the mammogram to ensure a consistent, reproducible search pattern. Later, a re-review of "danger zones" where cancers are commonly missed will help the radiologist avoid mistakes.

■ AN APPROACH TO THE MAMMOGRAM

Many tools are available to help the radiologist correctly interpret mammograms (Table 2-3). The first is the breast history and physical findings. The breast history sheet alerts the radiologist to the patient's risk factors for cancer and the patient's pretest probability of cancer (see Fig. 2-1). The history sheet includes the patient's clinical history of breast biopsies and a schematic diagram of their location so that old scars are not misinterpreted as cancer.

A technologist or aide usually interviews the patient, marking the location of any palpable finding on a diagram on the history sheet. Positions of findings in the breast are described in breast quadrants, with the upper outer quadrant representing the breast quadrant nearest the axilla. Another way to describe a breast location is by using the "clock face" method, in which the location of breast findings is described as though a clock were superimposed on each breast as the woman faces the examiner (Fig. 2-6). This means that the upper outer quadrant in the right breast is between the 9- and 12-o'clock positions, but the upper outer quadrant in the left breast is between the 12- and 3-o'clock positions.

The radiologist then reviews the breast history sheet and the technologist's marks (indicating masses, skin moles, biopsies, scars, or implants). The technologist may place special skin markers on moles or palpable masses before taking the mammogram to draw the radiologist's attention for a specific purpose. The technologist should write down why the skin markers were placed to clarify their placement for the radiologist.

The radiologist then starts a targeted systematic review of each film (Table 2-4). The radiologist first evaluates the images for good positioning, contrast, and compression.

TABLE 2-4. Systematic Approach to Interpretation of Mammograms

Search Pattern	Normal Findings
Overall Search	
Evaluation of technique	Good technique
Fibroglandular symmetry	Breast tissue usually symmetric Asymmetric tissue in 3%; be alert for new, palpable, three-dimensional masses or suspicious calcifications
White areas in glandular tissue	No mass or distortion; white areas look like normal tissue on the orthogonal views
Targeted Search	
Edge of glandular tissue	No "pulling in" or tent sign, no concave masses
Nipple/areolar complex	Nipple everted, no skin thickening
Retroareolar region	Normal ducts, vessels, nipple in profile on at least one view
Skin	2–3 mm in thickness, no edema
Axilla	Normal lymph nodes, normal variant axillary breast tissue
Retroglandular fat	All fat, no masses between glandular tissue and chest wall
Medial breast	Mostly fat, normal variant medial sternalis muscle
Film edge	No mass or spiculation from findings lying outside the field of view
Use magnifying lens or magnifier	No pleomorphic calcifications, subtle distortion, or masses
Use bright light (SFM) or adjust window/ level (FFDM)	Evaluate dark areas as needed
Compare with old films	No change; be alert for a developing density, new or changing calcifications or masses
CAD	Do a second look of the marked areas; CAD comes last because it does not pick up all cancers

CAD, computer-aided detection; FFDM, full-field digital mammogram; SFM, screen-film mammogram.

Next, the radiologist looks at the dense breast tissue for symmetry between the left and right breasts, which should be symmetric. The radiologist then looks at the whitest, or densest, part of the mammogram to see whether there is a mass or distortion there.

The radiologist inspects all edges of the glandular tissue where it interfaces with fat. Abnormal findings along the glandular tissue edge include a "pulling in" or tethering of tissue (the *tent sign*) or masses that pop out along the glandular tissue edge. The radiologist looks at the skin/nipple/areolar complex for thickening or retraction. Next, the radiologist makes sure that the retroareolar region, the axilla, retroglandular fat, breast tissue at the film edge, and the skin are normal. The radiologist then searches for calcifications by using a magnifying lens (on screen film mammograms) or an electronic magnifier (digital mammograms). The radiologist then compares the new films with older films of the same quality to evaluate for changes. If computer-aided detection (CAD) devices are used, that

is done so only after the initial review of the mammogram. Computer-provided marks should function as a "second look," because CAD misses some breast cancers that are only detected by the radiologist. In a prospective study of CAD on more than 9000 mammograms in an academic center, CAD and the radiologist found 13 of 19 cancers, CAD found 2 cancers undetected by the radiologist, but the radiologist found 4 cancers not marked by CAD. Because CAD does not find all the cancers, it should not be used alone to read mammograms. The radiologist should read the mammogram and then use CAD as a "second look"; in addition, if the radiologist sees a suspicious finding, he or she should work up that finding no matter what CAD says because CAD misses some cancers that the radiologist sees.

The following section details the individual components of the systematic approach to the mammogram (see Table 2-4). The first step is to look at the mammographic technique for good quality and then to look for symmetry between the breasts, which are usually symmetric. Sometimes breast tissue is asymmetric, meaning that there is more normal glandular tissue in one breast than the other; this is a normal variant, like having one foot bigger than the other. Normal asymmetry consists of a normal asymmetric volume of breast tissue, more in one side than the other. On the CC and MLO views, the glandular asymmetry should "spread out" and not look like a mass (Fig. 2-7). Normal asymmetry can also be caused by removal of fibroglandular tissue from one breast by biopsy, making the other breast look like it has more tissue. Normal asymmetries should have no suspicious calcifications, spiculations, or palpable masses. Normal asymmetries are stable when compared with older studies. They are composed of fibroglandular tissue. If the asymmetry is palpable, has suspicious calcifications or spiculations, is new, or is a mass, the asymmetry may represent cancer and should prompt a workup or biopsy.

The next step is to look at the white parts of the mammograms for masses. Radiologists see masses because they are whiter than the surrounding tissue. Alternatively, a round or spiculated mass edge is seen against fat. If a possible mass is present on one projection, the radiologist looks for the mass on the orthogonal view. To do this the radiologist measures the distance from the nipple to the mass and searches the orthogonal view for the mass at this distance (Fig. 2-8A). If the finding is seen on two views, it is considered a *mass*. If it is seen on only one view, it is called a *density* and represents either a summation shadow (see Fig. 2-8B and C) or a mass (see Fig. 2-8D to H) that is obscured on the second view. The decision to recall this type of finding and prompt a workup is based on the radiologist's experience and the degree of suspicion of the one-view finding.

The radiologist next looks at all the normal glandular tissue edges where they interface with fat. A layer of fat typically surrounds the cone of normal fibroglandular tissue and should contain no masses. As part of the systematic review, the radiologist checks the fat all around the glandular tissue to make sure that no masses are present. These edges should be gently curving, scalloped, and without tethering. Masses at the glandular edge or in breast tissue can "pull in" the fat, producing a tent sign caused by productive fibrosis from cancer retracting the Cooper ligaments and breast ducts. In other cases, tumor

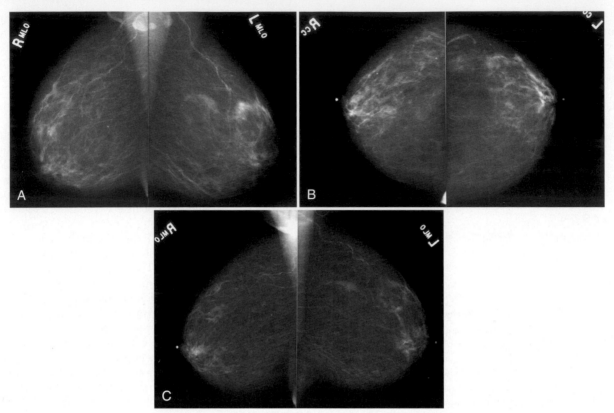

FIGURE 2-7. Normal asymmetry. Mediolateral (MLO) (**A**) and craniocaudal (CC) (**B**) views show an asymmetry in the upper left breast, not as apparent on the CC view, representing normal overlapping tissue. An older MLO mammogram (**C**) shows that the asymmetry is stable.

spiculation produces straight lines extending into the glandular tissue that draw attention to a mass at the center of the radius of spicules (see Fig. 2-8F). Subtle equal-density cancers can be difficult to detect, but looking for secondary signs of straightened lines in glandular tissue or tethering of the glandular tissue edge guides the radiologist to the cancer.

The radiologist then sees if the nipple is everted and reviews the complex structures of ducts and vessels in the retroareolar region. The nipple should be seen in profile on at least one mammographic view. If the nipple is not in profile on at least one view, the nipple may overlie the retroareolar region and obscure a mass, or it might be retracted by cancer. If the nipple is not seen in profile on any view, the mammogram should be repeated with the nipple in profile. If the nipple is truly inverted on the mammogram, the radiologist should check the breast history form to see if it was inverted at birth (normal variant) or if the nipple inversion is new. New nipple inversion is of concern for a retroareolar cancer and prompts a workup.

Normal breast skin is approximately 2 to 3 mm thick on the mammogram, and normal subcutaneous fat is dark. The skin should be smooth all around the breast and not pulled in (Fig. 2-9). Skin thickening greater than 2 to 3 mm that is asymmetric to the contralateral side is abnormal and is especially worrisome if the subcutaneous tissue has become gray and the thin tethering lymphatics and ligaments become thick and trabeculated. This is worrisome for breast edema. In general, skin thickening from cancer should be investigated.

The axilla normally contains lymph nodes, which are smooth oval or kidney bean-shaped masses containing fatty hila on the mammogram (Fig. 2-10A). Lymph nodes that grow larger become dense, round, and lose their fatty hila; they represent lymphadenopathy and are abnormal (see Fig. 2-10B).

Axillary breast tissue is a normal variant and consists of breast tissue in the axilla. Axillary breast tissue develops

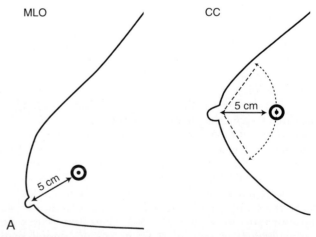

FIGURE 2-8. **A,** Schematic for locating a lesion on two different mammographic projections. The radiologist measures the distance from the finding to the nipple (*left image*) and then inspects the second view at the same distance from the nipple (*right image*) for the finding.

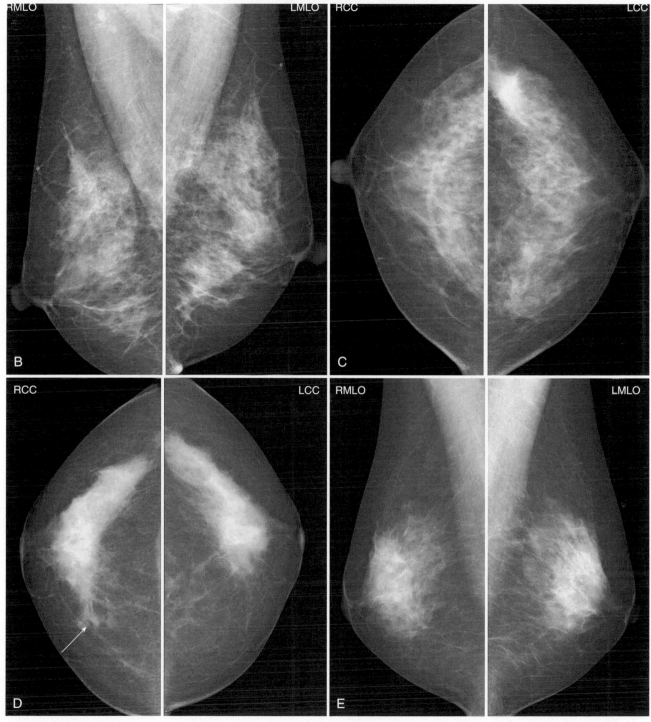

FIGURE 2-8, cont'd. **B** and **C,** Abnormal screening mammograms with a summation shadow on one view. Mediolateral oblique (MLO) (**B**) and craniocaudal (CC) (**C**) screening mammograms of the same patient; an asymmetric density is seen in the outer left CC view. Review of the MLO view shows no mass of the same shape or density at the same distance from the nipple, thus suggesting a confluence of shadows. In addition, the asymmetry has no spiculations or calcifications, was not associated with a palpable finding, and did not appear to be a mass. Workup showed that the density represented a summation shadow. **D** and **E,** Abnormal screening mammograms with cancer seen as an asymmetric density on only one view. CC (**D**) and MLO (**E**) views; more breast tissue is seen in the medial aspect of the right breast on the CC view (*arrow*) than in the medial aspect of the left breast. Closer examination shows the density to have a slightly round shape and possible spiculations, unlike the asymmetric density seen in parts **A** and **B.** It is not seen on the MLO view. Follow-up examination confirmed the density to be a true mass and invasive ductal cancer (IDC).

Continued

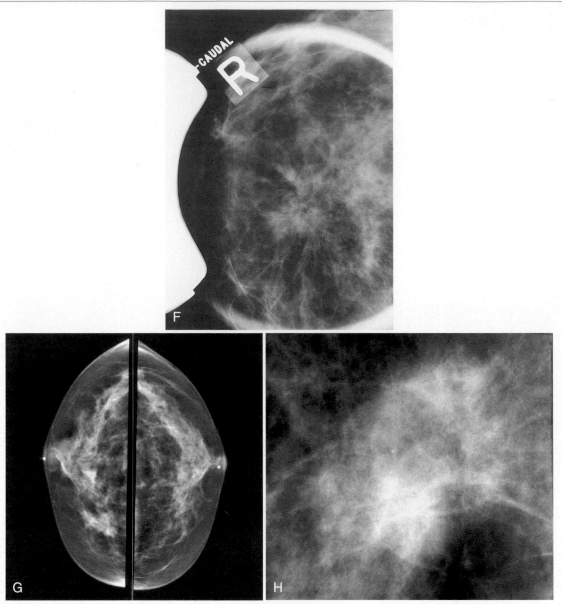

FIGURE 2-8, cont'd. **F**, Use of the surrounding architecture to detect masses. A CC spot magnification view shows an equal-density spiculated mass (radial scar at biopsy) producing subtle distortion of the tissue with straightening of Cooper ligaments. **G** and **H**, Spot magnification workup shows that another mass in the medial breast on the CC view (**G**) persists on the spot magnification view (**H**) and is a spiculated mass (IDC) on biopsy.

along the normal nipple line that extends (in animals) from the axilla along the chest to the abdomen. Axillary breast tissue can be, but is rarely, attached to an extra nipple. Noncompressed axillary breast tissue can simulate a mass, but it can be separated into its normal fibroglandular components by spot compression (see Fig. 2-10C and D). Spiculated masses in the axilla can mimic normal lymph nodes or axillary breast tissue. Any masses in the axilla should be scrutinized carefully to make sure they are normal lymph nodes or axillary tissue and not cancer (see Fig. 2-10E to G).

A few locations in the breast usually contain fat and deserve both special mention and a second look. The first is the medial portion of the breast, which usually becomes fattier over time. Masses or densities in the medial part of the breast are in a "danger zone" and should be scrutinized carefully because usually only fat is present here. The only exception is the normal sternalis muscle seen on the CC

view near the chest wall. A second "danger zone" is the retroglandular fat, or fat between the cone of normal fibroglandular tissue and the chest wall. The area between the glandular tissue and pectoralis muscle should include only fat, with the only exception again being the sternalis muscle. This retroglandular fat is what Dr. Laszlo Tabar called "no man's land." Any masses here are abnormal and should be worked up. The third "danger zone" is the film edge at the chest wall. Here, the hint of a mass edge or spiculations may barely stick out into the field of view and suggest that a tumor is not fully imaged on the mammogram. In these cases, only special mammographic views will display the mass.

The radiologist last looks for pleomorphic calcifications with a magnifying lens (for screen-film studies) or an electronic magnifier (for FFDMs). Radiologists should look at screen-film mammograms with the magnifying lens until they see dust, which ensures that they have looked hard

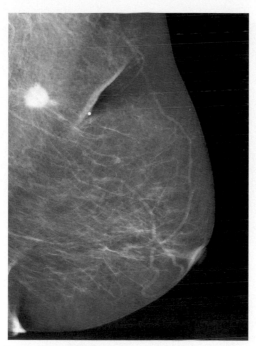

FIGURE 2-9. True axillary mass with a secondary sign of indrawing of the skin, marked by a metallic skin marker. Note the skin fold with the adjacent dark air. This patient had invasive ductal cancer.

enough to find the calcifications that form in breast cancer. For screen-film mammography, the radiologist uses a hot light to illuminate dark portions of the mammogram as needed. For FFDMs, the images are viewed at optimal windowing and leveling to see calcifications, and the radiologist views all portions of the images under electronic magnification that shows skin pores to make sure the films are displayed at a high enough magnification to display tiny calcifications in cancer.

The radiologist then compares the current mammogram with older films of the same quality to check for developing densities and to look for new or progressive changes.

The radiologist last uses CAD (if available) and does a "second look" of findings marked on the mammograms by the CAD system.

By law (Mammography Quality Standards Act [MQSA]; P.L. 102-539), all mammograms must have a summary BI-RADS® code that indicates the radiologist's final impression of the study. Both the BI-RADS® number and the words must be spelled out in the report (Box 2-6). Yearly, federal inspectors read mammographic reports at all U.S. facilities and check them for BI-RADS® summary codes and words. It is against U.S. federal law to exclude the BI-RADS® codes and words on mammogram repeats. Both monetary fines and jail sentences can be imposed on facilities that do not comply with MQSA.

The first BI-RADS® category, category 0, is used for screening recalls or when more studies are needed at the end of a case to make a final assessment. Categories 1 and 2 are used for normal mammograms or for findings requiring no action. Category 3 is used for findings thought to have less than 2% chance of malignancy and for which a short-term, 6-month follow-up mammogram may be implemented, with the expectation that the finding will be stable. Specifically, this category is often used for smooth noncalcified benign-appearing masses, benign-appearing clustered punctate calcifications, or benign-appearing focal densities in appropriate clinical settings. Category 4 encompasses a wide variety of findings for which biopsy is recommended. Category 4 can be further subcategorized into 4A, 4B, and 4C for lesions that require biopsy but with a low, intermediate, or moderate suspicion for cancer, respectively. Category 5 is reserved for mammographic findings highly suggestive of cancer, with a greater than 95% likelihood of cancer. Category 6 is intended for cancers for which a known diagnosis has been established before definite therapy such as surgery or chemotherapy. For example, women with large breast cancers diagnosed by percutaneous core biopsy who will be undergoing subsequent neoadjuvant chemotherapy would be designated category 6.

◼ DIAGNOSTIC VERSUS SCREENING MAMMOGRAPHY

There is a crucial difference between screening and diagnostic mammography. Diagnostic mammography is used for symptomatic women or for women with findings detected on screening mammography (Table 2-5). A radiologist is on-site for diagnostic mammograms to personally guide the workup by using special mammographic views or ultrasound.

Screening mammography is performed without a radiologist on-site. Screening mammography is meant for asymptomatic women. The usual scenario for a screening mammogram is that an asymptomatic woman has her mammogram and goes home. A radiologist reads the mammogram later. In the United States, screening includes two views of each breast—CC and MLO projections of the left and right breasts.

Women with lumps or symptoms need diagnostic mammograms, not screening mammograms. From 10% to 15% of all cancers are not seen at screening mammography; this usually happens in women with palpable breast lumps that

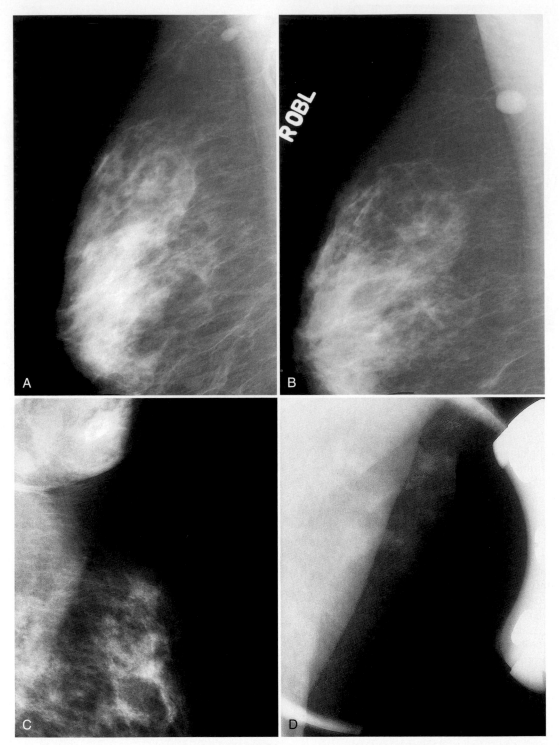

FIGURE 2-10. **A** and **B**, Importance of the axilla on screening. A mediolateral oblique (MLO) view (**A**) shows heterogeneously dense tissue and normal axillary lymph nodes, seen as two oval equal-density masses projected on the pectoralis muscle high in the axilla. The following year one of the lymph nodes was rounder and more dense and did not have any fatty hilum (**B**), findings characteristic of lymphadenopathy in lymphoma. If the axilla had not been reviewed, this finding would have been missed. **C** and **D**, Normal axillary breast tissue. A left screening MLO view (**C**) shows a density high in the axilla over the pectoralis muscle, possibly representing a mass versus normal axillary breast tissue. A spot compression film (**D**) shows that the density represents normal axillary breast tissue because the density does not persist in the same shape and pattern seen on the original screening study.

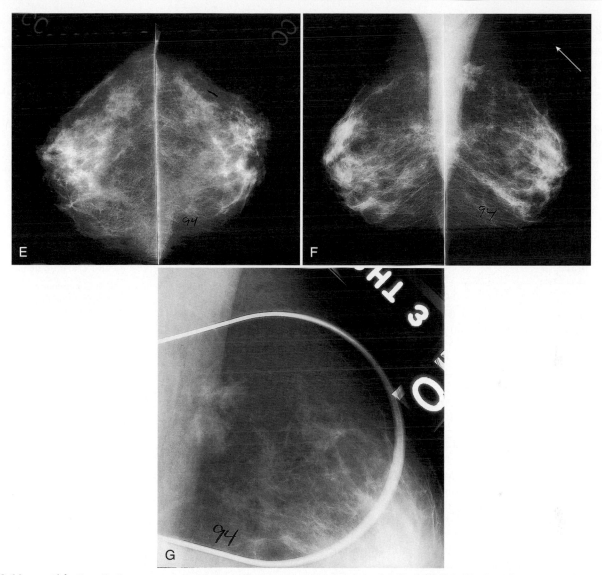

FIGURE 2-10, cont'd. **E to G,** Breast cancer simulating axillary breast tissue. Craniocaudal (**E**) and MLO (**F**) views from a screening study show dense tissue in the axilla (*arrow*). A spot view (**G**) shows that the density retains its shape, does not separate into fibroglandular components, and thus represents a mass—specifically, invasive ductal cancer.

TABLE 2-5. Screening versus Diagnostic Studies

Screening	Asymptomatic women CC and MLO mammograms Films taken and patient released
Diagnostic	Symptomatic women or mammographic finding CC and MLO mammograms Additional mammograms tailored to the problem With or without breast ultrasound Radiologist on-site to guide workup

CC, craniocaudal; MLO, mediolateral oblique.

are the cancer. Screening studies can result in false-negative findings even when the woman has felt her own lump. The false-negative screening mammogram may delay diagnosis. Some cancers that are felt as a lump may need tangential views, spot views, or ultrasound to reveal their presence. The extra studies are only done with a *diagnostic* mammogram, in which the radiologist recognizes the

danger of the palpable mass and gets the other views on ultrasound. Therefore, women with lumps or symptoms need to undergo a *diagnostic* rather than a screening mammogram because the on-site radiologist can recognize the woman's problem and target a dedicated workup to that problem to find the cancer.

ADDITIONAL VIEWS TO CONFIRM OR EXCLUDE THE PRESENCE OF A TRUE LESION

Radiologists use additional mammographic views in three common scenarios: to confirm or exclude a real lesion, to localize or triangulate a true lesion, and to characterize a true lesion (Box 2-7). A common reason to use additional views is in the setting of a "one-view-only" finding. Specifically, the radiologist sees a finding on one view that is not reinforced on the orthogonal view. Additional special views determine whether the finding is real. The first step is to estimate the finding's location on the orthogonal view

---

BOX 2-7. Use of Additional Mammographic Views

To confirm or exclude the presence of a real lesion
To characterize a true lesion
To triangulate or localize a true lesion

BOX 2-8. Views Used to Confirm or Exclude a Lesion (Commonly a One-View-Only Finding)

Lateral view
Spot compression
Spot compression magnification
Rolled views (with or without spot compression or magnification)
Repeat the same view
Step oblique views
Ultrasound

TABLE 2-6. Mammographic Views Used to Visualize and Characterize Findings

Mammographic Problem	Mammographic View
True finding versus summation	Rolled views, spot view, step oblique views; repeat the same view
Triangulation	Line up CC, MLO, and ML views and draw an imaginary line through the lesion Use rolled views to determine whether the mass is upper or lower
Outer breast finding	XCCL, Cleopatra
Inner breast finding	XCCM, cleavage view, spot view
Upper breast finding	Compression from below (or caudal-cranial view), upper-breast-only view
Retroareolar finding	Spot compression with the nipple in profile
Lower inner finding	Superior-inferior oblique
Palpable finding	Spot compression over the mass or a tangential view
Characterization of a mass	Magnification, spot magnification, or calcification views

CC, craniocaudal; ML, mediolateral; MLO, mediolateral oblique; XCCL, laterally exaggerated craniocaudal; XCCM, medially exaggerated craniocaudal.

TABLE 2-7. Mammographic Views and Abbreviations Used to Describe Them

View	Abbreviation
Craniocaudal	CC
Mediolateral oblique	MLO
Mediolateral	ML
Lateral-medial	LM
Laterally exaggerated craniocaudal	XCCL
Medially exaggerated craniocaudal	XCCM
Cleavage view	CV
Rolled view laterally	RL
Rolled view medially	RM
From below	FB

By convention, the side (left or right) precedes the view abbreviation.
From *Mammography quality control manual*, Reston, VA, 1999, American College of Radiology.

by measuring the distance from the nipple to the finding. The breast tissue is scrutinized along a radius of the same distance on the orthogonal view to identify the finding (see Fig. 2-8A). If the finding shows up on the second view, it is considered a true finding and the radiologist then uses additional views to characterize the lesion. If the finding is invisible on the second view, it may represent a true finding hidden on the second view or a fortuitous summation of normal breast tissue.

Many fine-detail mammographic views can be used to determine whether a "one-view" finding is a true lesion or a summation shadow (Box 2-8 and Tables 2-6 and 2-7).

A "one-view" finding often prompts requests for "rolled views." Rolled CC views separate normal fibroglandular elements into their individual components (see Table 2-6). The technologist "rolls" the breast tissue so that the top of the breast is rolled toward the axilla and then recompresses the breast. The bottom of the breast is now directed toward the sternum (Fig. 2-11A). This action rolls the fibroglandular components that form the "fake mass" away from each other. On the rolled view a summation shadow is separated into its normal fibroglandular components and the mass goes away (see Fig. 2-11B to G). On the other hand, true masses retain their shape and size on the rolled view.

Another way to separate true masses from fake ones is to use spot compression. A small compression paddle is used to compress tightly and directly over a finding. This provides greater compression on the area of interest. If used to determine if a finding is a real mass or a superimposition, spot compression separates fake summation shadows into normal fibroglandular components. If the finding is a real mass, the mass should persist within the spot compression field of view (Figs. 2-12 and 2-13). A true mass will retain its shape, size, and density, whereas a summation shadow will disperse into its fibroglandular components. It is important to perform the spot view in the projection in which the finding is best seen or displayed against fat to increase the chance of discovering if it is real (Fig. 2-14).

Step oblique views are mammograms obtained at slightly different oblique angles (i.e., 60, 50, 45 degrees) that throw fibroglandular elements into slight variations of obliquity. As with rolled views, true lesions should persist on multiple-step oblique views. Summation shadows, on the other hand, will separate into their fibroglandular components.

In all cases in which a mass is suspected, ultrasound provides indispensible information. The negative ultrasound confirms findings on "negative" mammograms. If the ultrasound is positive, a mass is confirmed. A repeat mammogram with a marker over the ultrasound-detected mass may show ultrasound findings that correspond to the mammographic findings and show a mass. If they do not correspond, more workup is needed (see Fig. 2-14 G to K).

Text continued on p. 49

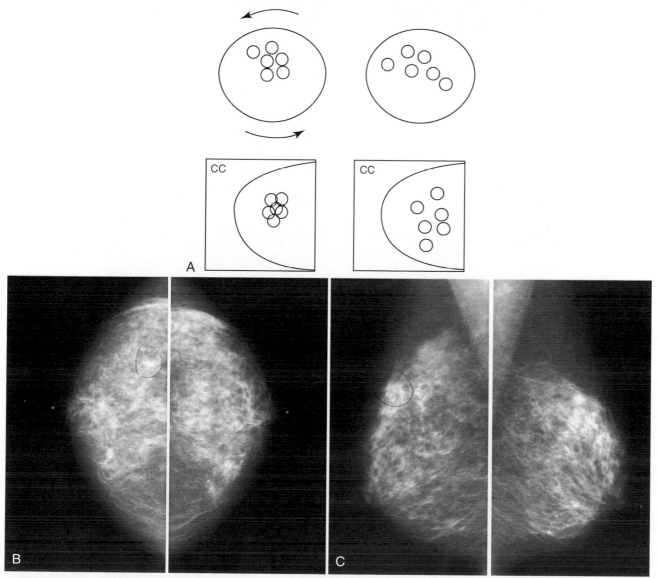

FIGURE 2-11. **A,** Schematic of a rolled view separating summation shadows into their fibroglandular components. The initial craniocaudal (CC) view on the *lower left* shows a "mass" composed of overlapping glandular tissue. The rolled view on the *lower right* shows the fibroglandular components separated into normal structures. In contradistinction, a mass should retain shape, form, and density, as seen on the original mammogram. **B to G,** Rolled views. CC (**B**) and mediolateral oblique (MLO) (**C**) screening mammograms show a possible mass in the outer right breast. (Part A modified from Sickles EA: Practical solutions to common mammographic problems: tailoring the examination, *AJR Am J Roentgenol* 151:31–39, 1988.)

Continued

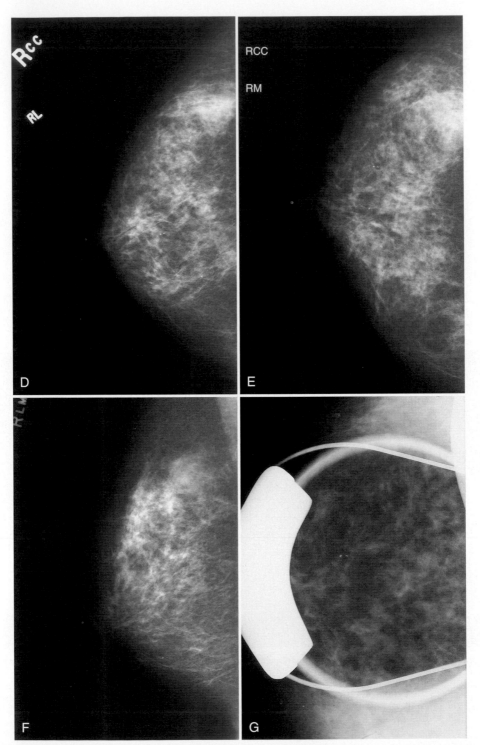

FIGURE 2-11, cont'd. Rolled views laterally (**D**) and medially (**E**) show no focal density. Because no mass is seen on the lateral view (**F**) or on the double spot compression view (**G**), this possible mass actually represents overlapping tissue.

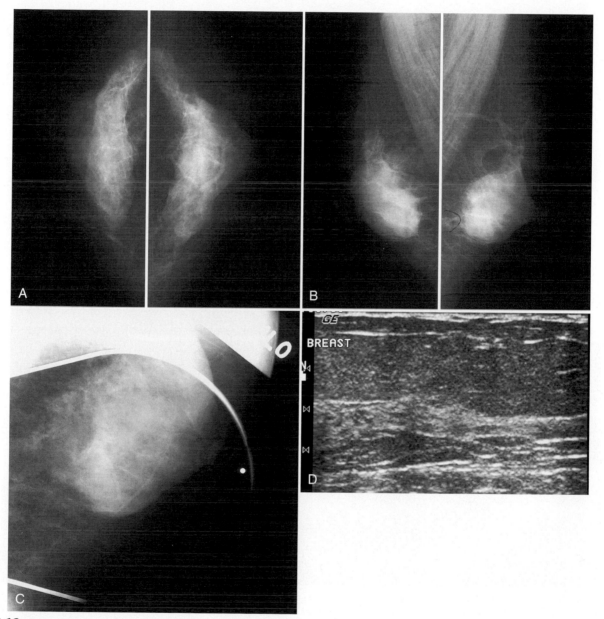

FIGURE 2-12. Spot view workup for a summation shadow. **A,** Craniocaudal (CC) and **B,** mediolateral oblique (MLO) screening mammograms; a possible mass is seen in the lower part of the left breast on the MLO view near the chest wall (*circle*) but not on the CC view. **C,** A spot compression film shows no mass. **D,** Ultrasound in this region shows fatty and scant fibroglandular tissue.

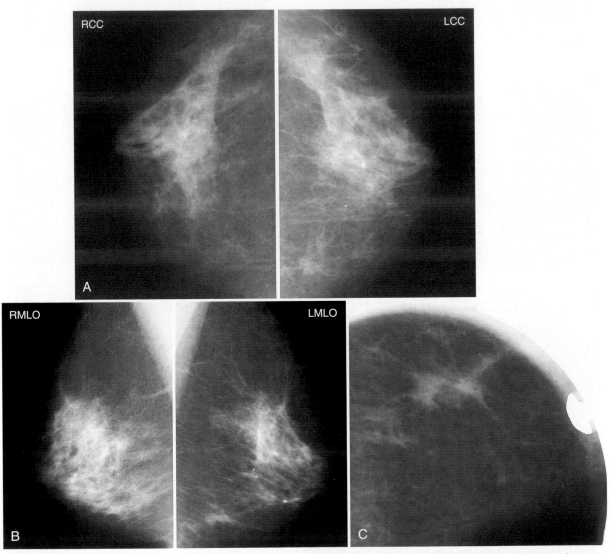

FIGURE 2-13. Spot view workup showing a persistent mass. A mass is seen on craniocaudal (**A**) and mediolateral oblique (**B**) screening mammograms in the lower inner portion of the left breast. A spot compression view (**C**) shows that the density persists and is suggestive of spiculation, representing a mass. Invasive ductal cancer was diagnosed.

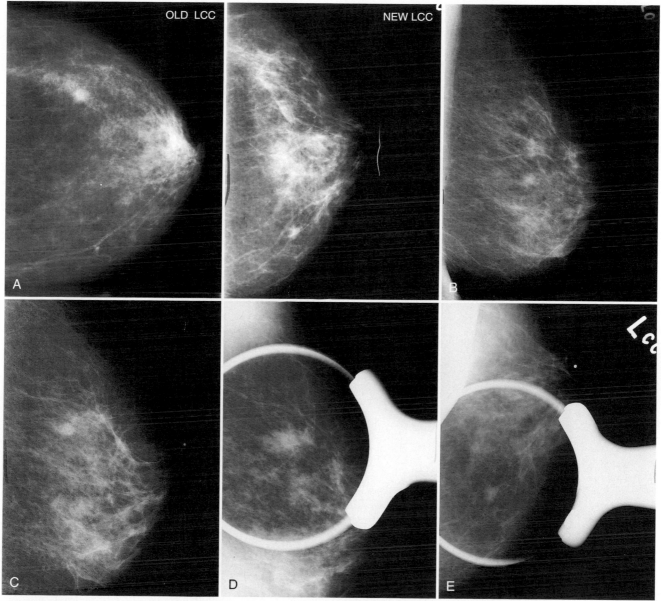

FIGURE 2-14. Importance of using a spot view over an area of fat. Craniocaudal (CC) (**A**) and mediolateral oblique (MLO) (**B**) views; a possible mass in the inner portion of the breast is seen on the CC view only; the mass was new from the previous year. Incidentally, note the linear metallic scar marker over a skin scar in part **A. C,** On the lateral view, the mass is seen in the upper part of the breast. **D,** A spot compression film in the mediolateral view is taken over glandular tissue but shows no mass. **E,** When the spot view is repeated over the fatty area on the CC view, it shows a spiculated mass in the medial breast against the dark fat that was hidden against the glandular tissue on the mediolateral spot view. *Continued*

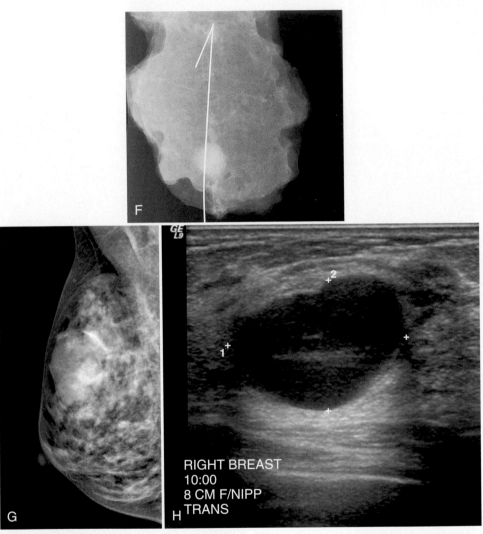

FIGURE 2-14, cont'd. F, The specimen shows the hookwire used for preoperative localization and the mass, which was invasive ductal cancer. **G to K,** Using markers to correlate mammographic findings with ultrasound. Right MLO mammogram (**G**) showed a large equal density mass in the upper right breast. Ultrasound showed two large cysts (**H** and **I**).

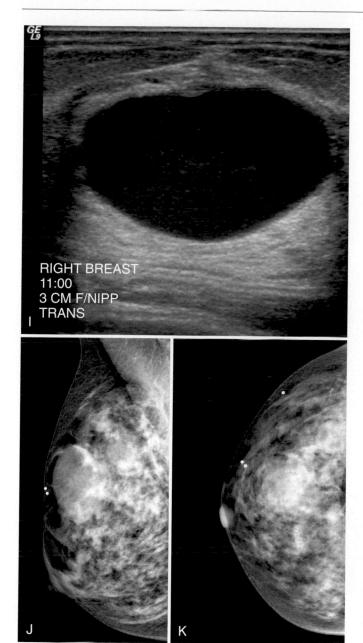

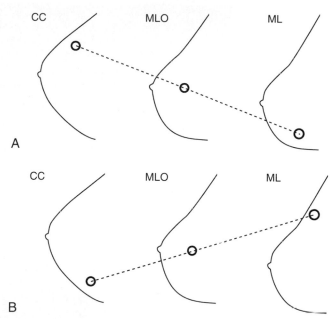

FIGURE 2-15. **A** and **B,** Schematic of how to triangulate findings on the craniocaudal (CC), mediolateral oblique (MLO), and mediolateral (ML) views. Each view area is oriented with the nipples at the same level and the breasts pointing the same way. An imaginary line drawn through the lesions will predict its location on the third view. (Modified from Sickles EA: Practical solutions to common mammographic problems: tailoring the examination, *AJR Am J Roentgenol* 151:31–39, 1988.)

FIGURE 2-14, cont'd. A right MLO (**J**) and CC view (**K**) with BBs placed over the cysts seen at ultrasound show that the masses correlate with the cysts.

TRIANGULATION

Triangulation is the process of localizing a finding within the breast on two orthogonal views. Triangulation provides a clear three-dimensional position of a finding for subsequent imaging or biopsy. Triangulation is commonly used when a finding is seen on only two of the three standard mammographic views (CC, mediolateral [ML], and lateral views). For example, a finding might be seen on both the lateral and MLO views, but not on the CC view, and one has to find the lesion before needle localization. Or there is a finding on CC and MLO screening, and the radiologist needs to see it on the lateral view to guide ultrasound.

To predict a finding's location from the CC and ML screening views, place the CC and MLO views so that the breasts face the same direction and the nipple is at the same level. An imaginary line drawn through the lesion on the CC and MLO views will predict the lesion's location on the ML view. If CC, MLO, and ML views are available, place the MLO between the CC and ML views, with the nipple at the same level on each view (Figs. 2-15 and 2-16). An imaginary line drawn through the lesion on any two of the three views in which it is seen will predict where it will be on the third view.

Sometimes suspicious findings are thought to be true findings but are seen *only* on the CC view and not on either the ML or MLO views. Rolled CC views can show if true masses are located in the upper or lower breast. One does this by comparing the rolled view with the standard CC view. The technologist does a "rolled laterally" view by rolling the top of the breast toward the axilla and the bottom of the breast medially. An upper breast mass should roll laterally with the rolled upper breast tissue. A lower breast mass should roll medially with the lower breast tissue. The radiologist looks at the "regular" CC view and sees how the finding moves on the "rolled laterally" view. If the mass moves toward the axilla, the mass must be in the upper portion of the breast. If the mass moves medially on the "rolled laterally," the mass must be in the lower portion of the breast (Figs. 2-17 and 2-18).

VISUALIZING FINDINGS IN "HARD TO SEE" LOCATIONS

The following section details standard mammographic projections modified to visualize findings in specific "hard to see" locations that are commonly missed by standard CC, MLO, and ML views. It is not uncommon to see a suspicious lesion on one view and not see it on the

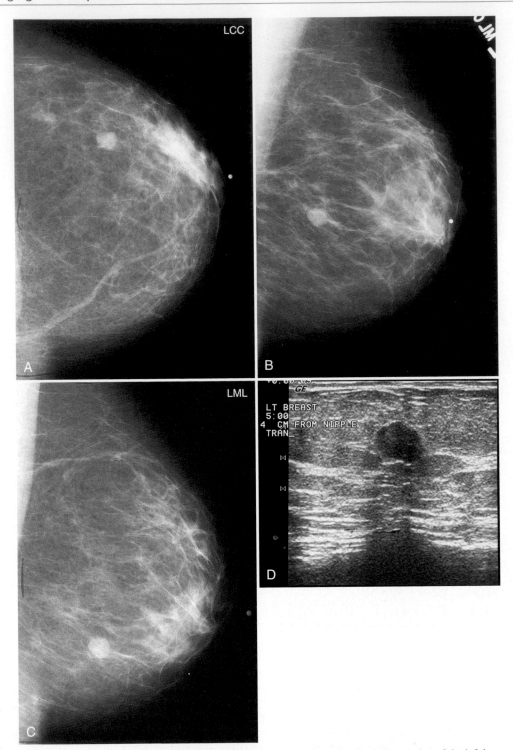

FIGURE 2-16. Triangulation of an outer breast mass to its location on the lateral view. A mass in the outer portion of the left breast on the craniocaudal view (**A**) is lower on the mediolateral oblique (MLO) view (**B**). Putting these two images together and drawing an imaginary line through the masses predicts an even lower position of the mass on the lateral view (**C**). Note that even though the mass is at nipple level on the MLO view, its actual location on the lateral view is at the 5-o'clock position, not the 3-o'clock position. **D,** Ultrasound shows a round microlobulated mass in the lower outer portion of the breast that was diagnosed as invasive ductal cancer.

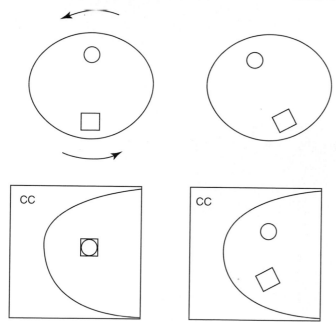

FIGURE 2-17. Schematic showing a rolled craniocaudal (CC) view predicting whether a lesion is located in the upper or lower part of the breast. The initial CC view on the *left* superimposes two lesions on top of each other. When the top of the breast is rolled laterally, the superior lesion rolls with the top of the breast. The inferior lesion moves medially with the lower part of the breast. Comparing whether the lesion moves laterally on the rolled view with respect to the standard view will help predict whether the lesion is in the upper or lower part of the breast. (Modified from Sickles EA: Practical solutions to common mammographic problems: tailoring the examination, *AJR Am J Roentgenol* 151:31–39, 1988.)

orthogonal projection. This can be because of the patient's body configuration or because the location of the finding makes it hard to see on the mammogram.

Some lesions are located in the extreme outer part of the breast not included on the standard CC view. A view that sees more of the outer breast is the CC view exaggerated laterally (XCCL). The technologist obtains an XCCL by modifying a standard CC view. She rotates the patient's body to display more outer breast tissue than is seen on a standard CC view and excludes the medial portion of the breast (Fig. 2-19). This projection sees more outer breast, but doesn't see the inner breast (Fig. 2-20).

The Cleopatra view also includes more outer breast tissue. In this view, the patient rotates laterally, as in the XCCL, but also leans obliquely like Cleopatra reclining on a bed of pillows (see Fig. 2-20E). The Cleopatra view includes much more of the outer part of the breast while excluding inner breast tissue. But unlike the XCCL, which is taken with the patient standing straight up, the Cleopatra view is taken with the patient leaning slightly backward and oblique.

For inner breast lesions, CC views exaggerated medially (XCCM) image the medial portion of the breast while excluding the outer breast tissue (Fig. 2-21A and B). Another view that visualizes the inner breast is the cleavage view (CV), or valley view, which includes the medial portions of both breasts on the image receptor in a modified CC projection. Such views allow visualization of even more of the inner part of the breast than is seen on standard CC views, but also images some of the opposite inner breast (see Fig 2-21C to E).

Some lesions are so close to the chest wall that they are hard to image with normal-sized compression paddles. The small spot compression paddles can get closer to the chest wall. You can use the small spot compression paddles to image extremely inner or deep lesions because they are smaller than the bulky normal compression paddles.

Some lesions in the upper part of the breast are so far back against the chest wall that they can be pushed out of the field of view by the compression paddle (Fig. 2-22). This problem can be solved by the from-below (FB) or caudal-cranial view. For this view, the image receptor is placed on the upper part of the breast. The breast is then compressed from below, excluding the lower part of the breast but including tissue high on the chest wall. In another approach for imaging lesions high on the chest wall, the image receptor is placed on the midportion of the breast with the lower portion excluded; this approach, first described by Sickles and colleagues, incorporates more of the upper portion of the breast because the compression paddle does not have to include lower breast tissue in the field of view.

Another area that is hard to see is the region immediately behind the nipple, which can be hidden by adjacent blood vessels and ducts. Spot compression compresses normal ducts, blood vessels, and tissue while pulling the nipple into profile (Fig. 2-23A and B). The nipple should be in profile on at least one view to see the retroareolar region; otherwise, the nipple may hide a cancer.

Lesions in the lower inner part of the breast are very hard to see. A superior-inferior oblique (SIO), or reverse oblique, view visualizes the lower inner breast. In this view, the technologist places the imaging receptor on the medial part of the breast and the compression plate on the superior breast while the patient leans over the imaging receptor (Fig. 2-24A and B). The compression paddle approaches the breast from the superior axillary side, allowing more of the inner breast tissue to be visualized.

Palpable findings imaged near the periphery of the breast are seen better with spot compression. This type of spot compression tangential to the palpable finding can push the mass against subcutaneous fat, allowing it to be seen. Spot compression directly over the palpable mass, previously known as a *lumpogram*, also can show masses by compressing the surrounding glandular tissue away from the suspicious finding (Fig. 2-25).

ADDITIONAL VIEWS TO CHARACTERIZE TRUE FINDINGS

After the radiologist determines that a mass or cluster of calcifications is a true finding and triangulates its position within the breast, additional mammographic views are used to characterize the finding (Box 2-9). Microfocal spot air-gap magnification views of clustered calcifications

Text continued on p. 58

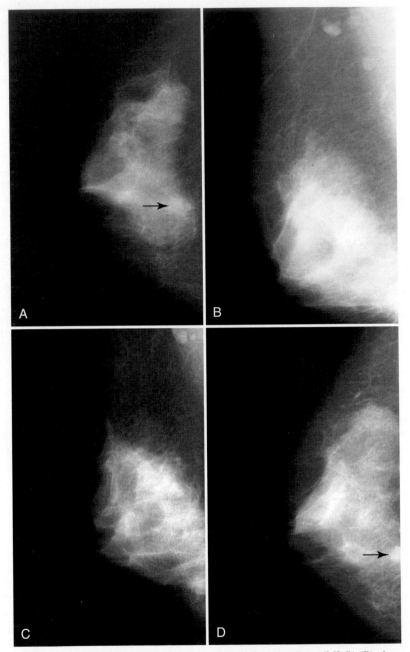

FIGURE 2-18. Rolled craniocaudal (CC) views for triangulation. CC (**A**) and mediolateral oblique (MLO) (**B**) views show a density in the posterior medial aspect of the breast (*arrow*) that was not seen on the MLO view at the time of interpretation. In retrospect, spiculation is seen extending into the lower part of the breast from outside the field of view at the edge of the film. **C**, The mediolateral (ML) view does not show a definite mass at the time of interpretation. **D**, A CC view with the top of the breast rolled laterally shows that the mass is medial in comparison to that seen on the original CC view (*arrow*), thus indicating that it rolled medially with the lower part of the breast.

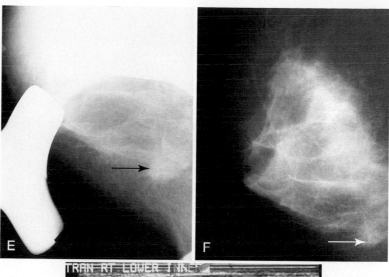

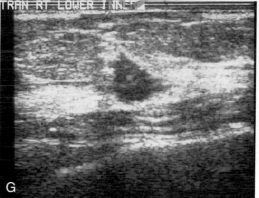

FIGURE 2-18, cont'd. **E,** Spot compression in the lower portion of the breast reveals a spiculated mass (*arrow*); **F,** a repeat ML view with more tissue now shows the mass in the lower part of the breast as a rounded structure (*arrow*). **G,** Ultrasound directed to the lower portion of the breast shows a hypoechoic irregular mass that was diagnosed as invasive ductal cancer.

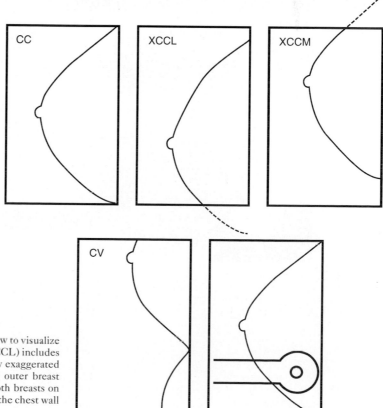

FIGURE 2-19. Schematic of variations of the craniocaudal (CC) view to visualize lesions in specific locations. The CC view exaggerated laterally (XCCL) includes outer breast tissue but excludes medial breast tissue. The CC view exaggerated medially (XCCM) includes medial breast tissue while excluding outer breast tissue. The cleavage view (CV) includes the medial portions of both breasts on the mammogram. Spot compression may visualize findings close to the chest wall that are excluded by a larger compression paddle.

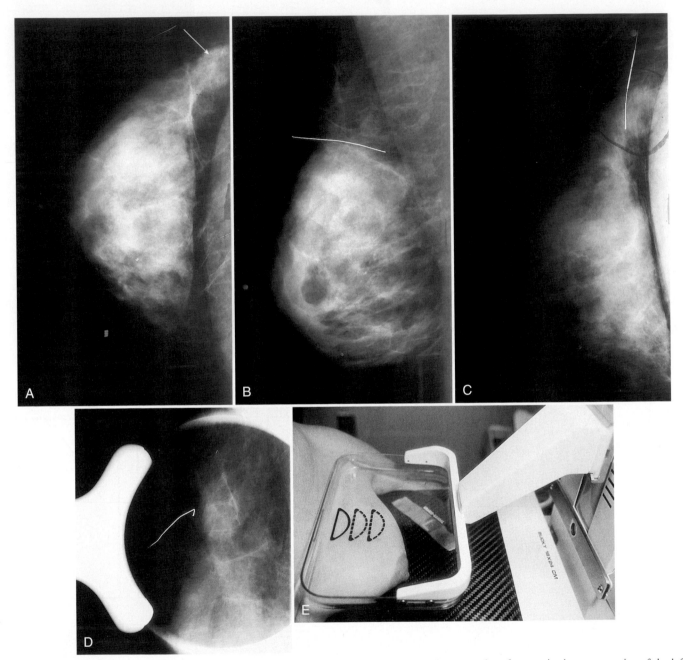

FIGURE 2-20. Outer craniocaudal (CC) view exaggerated laterally (XCCL). **A,** A round density suggestive of a mass in the outer portion of the left breast is seen on the CC view under the scar marker (*arrow*) but is not seen on the mediolateral oblique (MLO) view (**B**). **C,** An XCCL shows the mass better; it is also shown on a spot magnification view (**D**). **E,** Cleopatra view. For this view the patient leans outward and back, essentially performing an XCCL with a degree of obliquity to image more outer tissue. Note the scar marker in parts **B** to **D**.

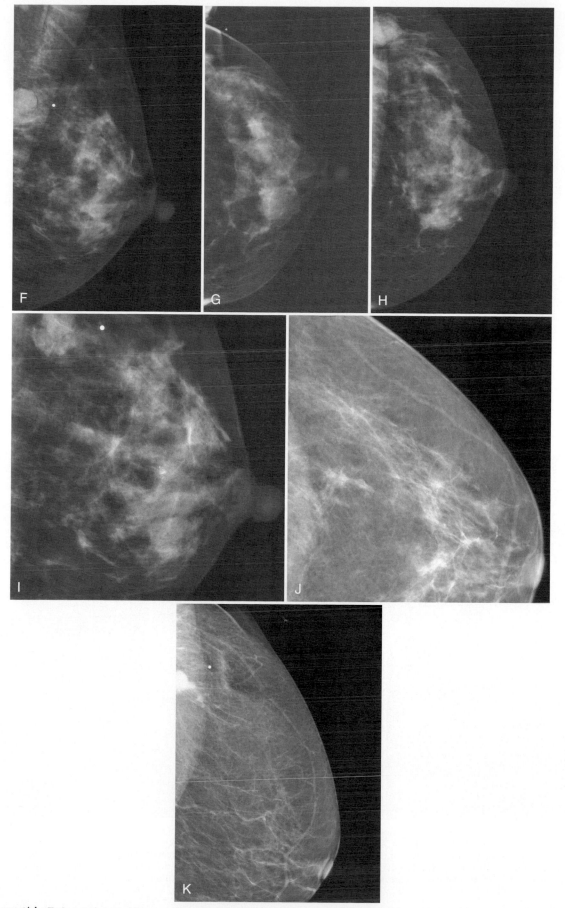

FIGURE 2-20, cont'd. F, A round mass with a marker on it in the upper left breast on the MLO view that is not seen on the CC view (**G**), even though the marker shows the palpable mass. **H,** An exaggerated outer CC now shows the mass by including it in the field of view. **I,** A spot compression MLO view shows the mass—invasive ductal cancer. In another patient the standard CC view shows no mass in the outer breast (**J**), but it is seen clearly on the XCCL view (**K**). Incidentally, note the linear metallic scar marker over a skin scar.

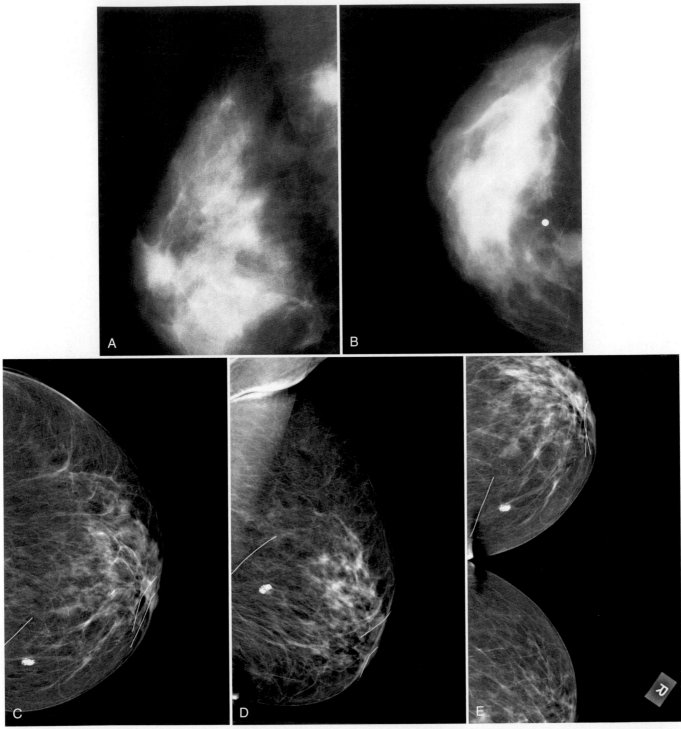

FIGURE 2-21. Craniocaudal view exaggerated medially (XCCM). **A,** A mediolateral oblique (MLO) view shows a round mass near the high chest wall that is excluded on the standard CC view. **B,** An XCCM shows the round inner breast mass, which was diagnosed as invasive ductal cancer. **C** and **E,** Cleavage view (CV) mammogram shows more of the inner breast. A normal CC view shows a degenerating fibroadenoma in the inner left breast (**C**), which is also seen on the MLO view (**D**). The CV mammogram (**E**) shows the fibroadenoma in the inner breast to best advantage and also includes some of the inner portion of the contralateral breast. Incidentally, note the linear metallic scar marker over skin scars in parts **C, D,** and **E.**

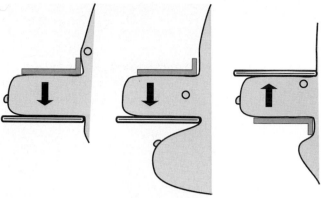

FIGURE 2-22. Methods to visualize high breast lesions. The compression paddle may exclude high breast masses by compressing them out of the field of view (*left image*). The *middle image* shows a view with the cassette holder above the nipple to allow compression of only the upper breast tissue. The *right image* shows a "from below" view, where the image receptor is placed over the upper part of the breast and the compression paddle approaches the receptor from the lower part of the breast. (Modified from Sickles EA: Practical solutions to common mammographic problems: Tailoring the examination, *AJR Am J Roentgenol* 151:31–39, 1988.)

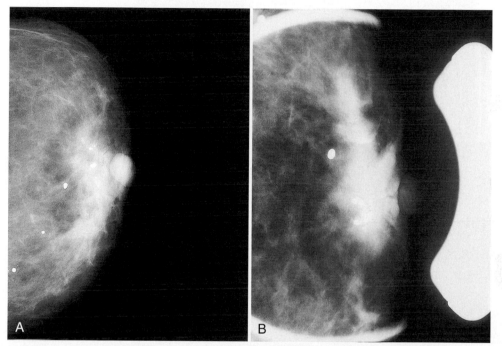

FIGURE 2-23. Spot view showing a mass in the retroareolar region. **A,** A craniocaudal view shows a vague density behind the nipple, but the nipple is not in profile. **B,** A spot view with the nipple in profile shows a spiculated mass that was diagnosed as invasive lobular cancer.

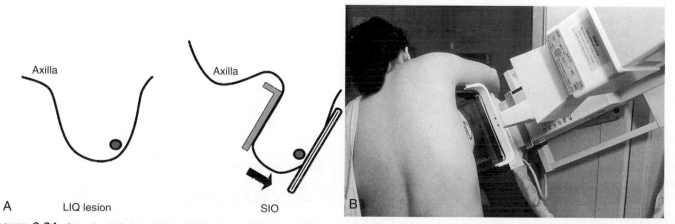

FIGURE 2-24. Superior-inferior oblique (SIO) view. **A,** A schematic shows a lower inner quadrant (LIQ) lesion in the *left image*. The SIO view is obtained with the image receptor next to the inner breast lesion and the compression plate compressing from the superior axillary side. **B,** Model demonstrating positioning for the SIO view.

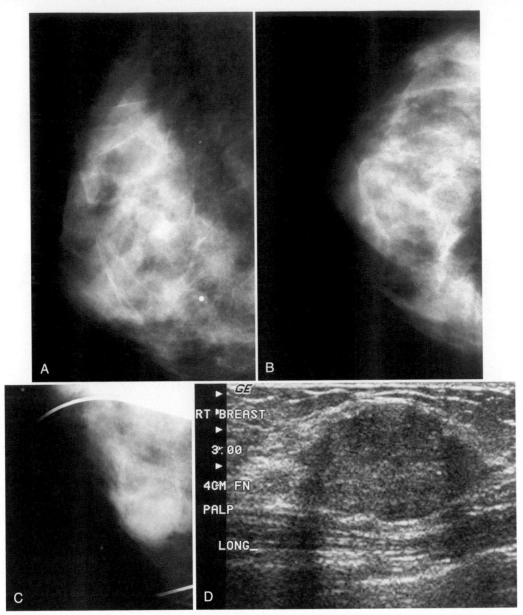

FIGURE 2-25. Spot compression over a palpable mass (the *lumpogram*). Mediolateral oblique (**A**) and craniocaudal (CC) (**B**) views show no defined mass at the 3-o'clock position on the right breast, marked by a BB skin marker. **C,** A spot tangential view over the lump with the marker in the CC projection shows a possible round mass against the dense tissue. **D,** Ultrasound shows an oval smooth mass, representing a fibroadenoma on biopsy.

sharpen and separate calcification forms and display calcifications not detected on nonmagnified studies. Magnification can also depict mass shapes and margins to greater advantage, showing spiculated or irregular margins not discernible at lower resolutions (Fig. 2-26). Spot compression magnification views not only provide greater visualization of the region of interest by pushing fibroglandular tissue away from the finding, but also produce higher resolution of mass margins and calcification shapes. Thus, spot compression magnification mammograms are a mainstay of the radiologist's diagnostic tools to characterize both masses and calcifications.

▬ SUMMARY

This chapter summarizes breast cancer risk factors, describes the signs and symptoms of breast cancer, and outlines a systematic approach to the mammogram to avoid diagnostic mistakes. A standardized, reproducible approach to the mammogram and re-review of mammographic "danger zones" in which cancers are commonly missed helps radiologists to avoid mistakes. After the radiologist discovers a finding, the radiologist has three duties: to determine whether the finding is real, to specify its location within the breast, and to characterize the finding to make a diagnosis. Modifications of standard views and fine-detail mammograms help the radiologist make these determinations.

▬ KEY ELEMENTS

Breast cancer screening in women invited to undergo mammography decreases breast cancer mortality by about 30%.

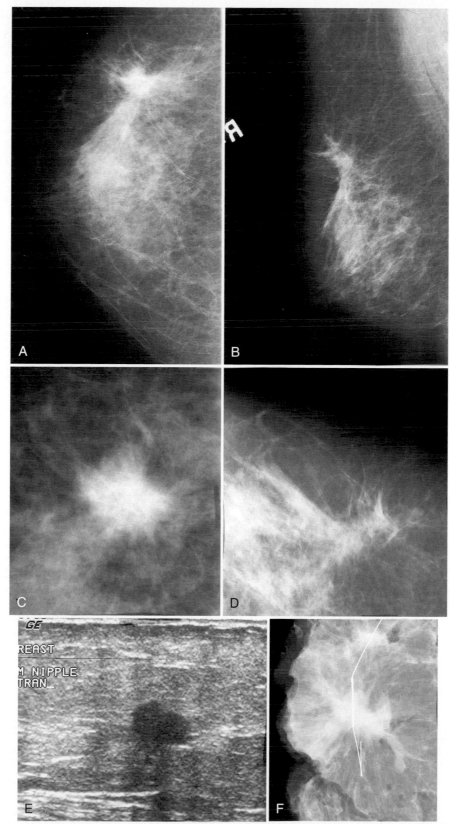

FIGURE 2-26. Use of magnification views. Craniocaudal (CC) (**A**) and mediolateral oblique (MLO) (**B**) mammograms show a spiculated mass, seen better on the CC view than on the MLO view. Distortion and the tent sign are evident in the upper part of the breast. Spot magnification views show the spiculated mass to better advantage on both the CC (**C**) and MLO (**D**) views. **E**, Ultrasound shows an oval, but very hypoechoic mass that has no acoustic spiculation or shadowing, corresponding to the mass on the mammogram. The mass was localized by ultrasound and was removed, as shown by the specimen (**F**). Note the localizing hookwire. Invasive ductal cancer was the diagnosis.

Risk factors for breast cancer include age older than 50 years, personal history of or first-degree relative with breast cancer, nulliparous status, early menarche, late menopause, first birth after age 30, radiation treatment, atypical ductal hyperplasia, lobular carcinoma in situ, and presence of *BRCA1* or *BRCA2* breast cancer susceptibility genes.

Seventy percent of women who have breast cancer have no risk factors other than being female and being older than age 50.

Signs and symptoms of breast cancer include a breast lump, bloody or new spontaneous nipple discharge, new nipple or skin retraction, *peau d'orange*, and symptoms from metastasis.

Signs of breast cancer on mammography include a spiculated mass, pleomorphic calcifications, a round mass, architectural distortion, a developing density, an asymmetric density, a single dilated duct, lymphadenopathy, and breast edema; in some patients, no mammographic signs are present (occult cancer).

A normal mammogram is dense in young women and becomes darker over time as the dense tissue is replaced by fat.

Increasing breast density may be due to pregnancy or hormone replacement therapy.

Unexplained increasing breast density should prompt a workup to exclude breast edema or cancer.

Evaluation of a normal mammogram includes routine inspection for fibroglandular symmetry and examination of the periglandular edges, the skin, retroareolar region and nipple, retroglandular fat, medial part of the breast, chest wall, and axilla.

Normal asymmetric glandular tissue occurs in 3% of women and looks like an asymmetry of normal glandular tissue without a palpable mass, suspicious calcifications or spiculations, a three-dimensional mass, or new findings.

Be alert for findings in the medial part of the breast; the normal sternalis muscle variant is the one normal finding in the medial breast.

To detect developing densities, change, or asymmetries, view films back to back and compare them with old films.

Review both the breast history and the technologist's physical sheet before interpretation of the mammogram to know where previous biopsies were, the meaning of skin markers, and to be aware of patient complaints.

From 10% to 15% of women with breast cancer have normal mammograms.

The skin should normally be 2 to 3 mm thick. Skin thicker than 2 to 3 mm might be breast edema or scarring.

Special mammographic views confirm or exclude questionable findings seen on screening mammography, characterize true lesions, and triangulate the location of a lesion.

Rolled views, compression views, and step oblique views distinguish true lesions from summation shadows.

Magnification spot compression views characterize mass margins and shapes, and see calcification numbers, shapes, and forms better.

Air-gap magnification views resolve the shape and number of calcifications better than standard mammograms.

Laterally exaggerated CC and Cleopatra views display the outer part of the breast.

Medially exaggerated CC and cleavage views display the inner portion of the breast.

"From-below" and upper breast views display the upper part of the breast.

Spot compression and nipple-in-profile images view the nipple and retroareolar region.

Superior-inferior oblique views (reverse oblique) display the lower inner portion of the breast.

The breast location most often excluded by screening mammograms is the upper inner quadrant.

Lesions displayed at the nipple level on the MLO view may be in the upper, lower, or midportion of the breast on the ML view.

Triangulation with the CC and MLO views can be used to predict the location of the lesion on the lateral view.

■ SUGGESTED READINGS

American College of Radiology: ACR BI-RADS®—Mammography. In *ACR Breast Imaging Reporting and Data System, Breast Imaging Atlas*, ed 4, Reston, VA, 2003, American College of Radiology.

Andersson I, Janzon L: Reduced breast cancer mortality in women under age 50: Updated results from the Malmö Mammographic Screening Program, *J Natl Cancer Inst Monogr* 22:63–67, 1997.

Beyer T, Moonka R: Normal mammography and ultrasonography in the setting of palpable breast cancer, *Am J Surg* 185:416–419, 2003.

Birdwell RL, Bandodkar P, Ikeda DM: Computer-aided detection with screening mammography in a university hospital setting, *Radiology* 236(2):451–457, 2005.

Birdwell RL, Ikeda DM, O'Shaughnessy KF, Sickles EA: Mammographic characteristics of 115 missed cancers later detected with screening mammography and the potential utility of computer-aided detection, *Radiology* 219:192–202, 2001.

Bjurstam N, Bjorneld L, Duffy SW, et al: The Gothenburg breast screening trial: First results on mortality, incidence, and mode of detection for women ages 39–49 years at randomization, *Cancer* 80:2091–2099, 1997.

Boyd NF, Guo H, Martin LJ, et al: Mammographic density and the risk and detection of breast cancer, *NEJM* 356(3):227–238, 2007.

Boyd NF, Martin LJ, Rommens JM, et al: Mammographic density: A heritable risk factor for breast cancer, *Methods Mol Biol* 472:343–360, 2009.

Bradley FM, Hoover HC Jr, Hulka CA, et al: The sternalis muscle: An unusual normal finding seen on mammography, *AJR Am J Roentgenol* 166:33–36, 1996.

Brenner RJ, Sickles EA: Acceptability of periodic follow-up as an alternative to biopsy for mammographically detected lesions interpreted as probably benign, *Radiology* 171:645–646, 1989.

Claus EB, Risch N, Thompson WD: Genetic analysis of breast cancer in the cancer and steroid hormone study, *Am J Hum Genet* 48:232–242, 1991.

Claus EB, Risch N, Thompson WD: Autosomal dominant inheritance of early-onset breast cancer. Implications for risk prediction, *Cancer* 73:643–651, 1994.

Colditz GA, Egan KM, Stampfer MJ: Hormone replacement therapy and risk of breast cancer: Results from epidemiologic studies, *Am J Obstet Gynecol* 168:1473–1480, 1993.

Colditz GA, Willett WC, Hunter DJ, et al: Family history, age, and risk of breast cancer. Prospective data from the Nurses' Health Study, *JAMA* 270:338–343, 1993.

Cook KL, Adler DD, Lichter AS, et al: Breast carcinoma in young women previously treated for Hodgkin disease, *AJR Am J Roentgenol* 155:39–42, 1990.

Faulk RM, Sickles EA: Efficacy of spot compression-magnification and tangential views in mammographic evaluation of palpable breast masses, *Radiology* 185:87–90, 1992.

Gail MH, Brinton LA, Byar DP, et al: Projecting individualized probabilities of developing breast cancer for white females who are being examined annually, *J Natl Cancer Inst* 81:1879–1886, 1989.

Goergen SK, Evans J, Cohen GP, MacMillan JH: Characteristics of breast carcinomas missed by screening radiologists, *Radiology* 204:131–135, 1997.

Gunhan-Bilgen I, Bozkaya H, Ustun EE, Memis A: Male breast disease: Clinical, mammographic, and ultrasonographic features, *Eur J Radiol* 43:246–255, 2002.

Hartge P, Struewing JP, Wacholder S, et al: The prevalence of common *BRCA1* and *BRCA2* mutations among Ashkenazi Jews, *Am J Hum Genet* 64:963–970, 1999.

Homer MJ: Proper placement of a metallic marker on an area of concern in the breast, *AJR Am J Roentgenol* 167:390–391, 1996.

Homer MJ, Smith TJ: Asymmetric breast tissue, *Radiology* 173:577–578, 1989.

Ikeda DM, Andersson I, Wattsgard C, et al: Interval carcinomas in the Malmö Mammographic Screening Trial: Radiographic appearance and prognostic considerations, *AJR Am J Roentgenol* 159:287–294, 1992.

Ikeda DM, Birdwell RL, O'Shaughnessy KF, et al: Analysis of 172 subtle findings on prior normal mammograms in women with breast cancer detected at follow-up screening, *Radiology* 226(2):494–503, 2003.

Jonsson H, Bordas P, Wallin H, et al: Service screening with mammography in Northern Sweden: Effects on breast cancer mortality—an update, *J Med Screen* 14(2):87–93, 2007.

Kopans DB: Negative mammographic and US findings do not help exclude breast cancer, *Radiology* 222:857–859, 2002.

Kopans DB, Swann CA, White G, et al: Asymmetric breast tissue, *Radiology* 171:639–643, 1989.

Larsson LG, Andersson I, Bjurstam N, et al: Updated overview of the Swedish Randomized Trials on Breast Cancer Screening with Mammography: Age group 40–49 at randomization, *J Natl Cancer Inst Monogr* 22:57–61, 1997.

Li Y, Baer D, Friedman GD, et al: Wine, liquor, beer and risk of breast cancer in a large population, *Eur J Cancer* 45(5):843–850, 2009.

Logan WW, Janus J: Use of special mammographic views to maximize radiographic information, *Radiol Clin North Am* 25:953–959, 1987.

Lynch HT, Watson P, Conway T, et al: Breast cancer family history as a risk factor for early onset breast cancer, *Breast Cancer Res Treat* 11:263–267, 1988.

Miki Y, Swensen J, Shattuck-Eidens D, et al: A strong candidate for the breast and ovarian cancer susceptibility gene *BRCA1*, *Science* 266:66–71, 1994.

Nystrom L, Andersson I, Bjurstam N, et al: Long-term effects of mammography screening: Updated overview of the Swedish randomised trials, *Lancet* 359:909–919, 2002.

Park JM, Franken EA Jr: Triangulation of breast lesions: Review and clinical applications, *Curr Probl Diagn Radiol*. 37(1):1–14, 2008.

Pearson KL, Sickles EA, Frankel SD, Leung JW: Efficacy of step-oblique mammography for confirmation and localization of densities seen on only one standard mammographic view, *AJR Am J Roentgenol* 174:745–752, 2000.

Ries LAG, Melbert D, Krapcho M, et al, editors: *SEER Cancer Statistics Review 1975–2005*, Bethesda, MD, 2008, National Cancer Institute. http://seer.cancer.gov/csr/1975_2005/, based on November 2007 SEER data submission, posted to the SEER Web site (accessed April 12, 2010).

Rosen EL, Sickles E, Keating D: Ability of mammography to reveal nonpalpable breast cancer in women with palpable breast masses, *AJR Am J Roentgenol* 172:309–312, 1999.

Saslow D, Boetes C, Berke W, et al: American Cancer Society guidelines for breast screening with MRI as an adjunct to mammography, *CA Cancer J Clin* 57(2):75–89, 2007.

Schmidt ME, Steindorf K, Mutschelknauss E, et al: Physical activity and postmenopausal breast cancer: Effect modification by breast cancer subtypes and effective periods in life, *Cancer Epidemiol Biomarkers Prev* 17(12):3402–3410, 2008.

Schubert EL, Mefford HC, Dann JL, et al: *BRCA1* and *BRCA2* mutations in Ashkenazi Jewish families with breast and ovarian cancer, *Genet Test* 1:41–46, 1997.

Shapiro S, Venet W, Strax P, et al: Ten- to fourteen-year effect of screening on breast cancer mortality, *J Natl Cancer Inst* 69:349–355, 1982.

Sickles EA: Mammographic features of 300 consecutive nonpalpable breast cancers, *AJR Am J Roentgenol* 146:661–663, 1986.

Sickles EA: Practical solutions to common mammographic problems: Tailoring the examination, *AJR Am J Roentgenol* 151:31–39, 1988.

Sickles EA: Periodic mammographic follow-up of probably benign lesions: Results in 3,184 consecutive cases, *Radiology* 179:463–468, 1991.

Silvera SA, Jain M, Howe GR, et al: Energy balance and breast cancer risk: A prospective cohort study, *Breast Cancer Res Treat* 97(1):97–106, 2006.

Smith RA, Cokkinides V, Eyre HJ: American Cancer Society guidelines for the early detection of cancer, 2003, *CA Cancer J Clin* 53:27–43, 2003.

Smith RA, Saslow D, Sawyer KA, et al: American Cancer Society guidelines for breast cancer screening: Update 2003, *CA Cancer J Clin* 53:141–169, 2003.

Tabar L, Vitak B, Chen HH, et al: The Swedish Two-County Trial 20 years later. Updated mortality results and new insights from long-term follow-up, *Radiol Clin North Am* 38:625–651, 2000.

Tabar L, Yen MF, Vitak B, et al: Mammography service screening and mortality in breast cancer patients: 20-year follow-up before and after introduction of screening, *Lancet* 361:1405–1410, 2003.

Warren Burhenne LJ, Wood SA, D'Orsi CJ, et al: Potential contribution of computer-aided detection to the sensitivity of screening mammography, *Radiology* 215:554–562, 2000.

Wolverton DE, Sickles EA: Clinical outcome of doubtful mammographic findings, *AJR Am J Roentgenol* 167:1041–1045, 1996.

Wooster R, Neuhausen SL, Mangion J, et al: Localization of a breast cancer susceptibility gene, *BRCA2*, to chromosome 13q12-13, *Science* 265:2088–2090, 1994.

Quiz

Resident Mammography Test

2-1. List findings for cancer and their differential diagnoses.

MAMMOGRAPHIC FINDINGS OF CANCER

1. _____
2. _____
3. _____
4. _____
5. _____
6. _____
7. _____
8. _____
9. _____
10. _____
11. _____

DIFFERENTIAL DIAGNOSIS

1. _____
2. _____
3. _____
4. _____
5. _____
6. _____
7. _____
8. _____
9. _____
10. _____
11. _____

For answers, see Table 2-2.

CHAPTER 3

Mammographic Analysis of Breast Calcifications

Analysis of breast calcifications is important because they may be the only sign of cancer. At histologic examination, 50% to 80% of breast cancers contain calcifications, but only a small percentage of cancers show calcifications on mammography. Calcifications form in breast cancers because of central necrosis of the tumor or from malignant cell secretions. Because cancers grow in breast ducts, the calcifications forming in these tumors often take on the form of the duct, resulting in the typical linear and branching malignant-type calcifications in cancers seen on mammograms.

Most mammograms show calcifications of some type. However, the vast majority of calcifications are due to benign processes. It is tricky to recognize cancer calcifications and distinguish them from the wide variety of common benign calcifications, but it can be done. A careful, systematic approach to the mammogram enables the radiologist to detect cancer-type calcifications. Once the calcification is found, the radiologist looks at the individual forms, the shape and location of the calcification cluster, and any changes over time to see if they point to the presence of cancer. This chapter presents a systematic approach to finding breast calcifications on mammograms, and then covers an approach to classifying breast calcifications into benign, malignant-appearing, or indeterminate categories.

TECHNIQUE FOR FINDING CALCIFICATIONS

The radiologist first makes sure the mammograms are of high quality, which is essential to detect and analyze breast calcifications. Then, the radiologist looks at each standard film using a standard search pattern so that no part of the film is unseen. Some radiologists use a search pattern of parallel lines over the films, like someone mowing a lawn, as described by Dr. Roger J. Jackman, to make sure all parts of the film are covered. With screen-film mammography (SFM), the radiologist uses a bright light to illuminate the darker portions of the film so the calcifications are easier to see. On digital mammography, the radiologist adjusts the windows and levels on the mammography workstation to optimize image contrast and brightness to find calcifications more easily.

After viewing the mammograms at standard magnification, the radiologist then uses a hand-held magnifying lens to examine each film (for analog SFM); this enlarges the mammogram image and makes the calcifications easier to detect. For digital mammography, the radiologist magnifies the mammogram electronically to make calcifications bigger and easier to see. Digital mammogram-viewing protocols usually incorporate electronic magnification of each image as part of the viewing workflow.

If calcifications that need further evaluation are detected, the radiologist orders air-gap magnification mammograms done with a 0.1-mm focal spot. People often mistakenly think that magnifying the SFM with a magnifying glass or electronically magnifying digital mammograms on the workstation is the same as performing air-gap magnification mammograms. It is not the same. Hand-held or electronic magnifiers can enlarge the calcifications that appear on mammogram images, but magnifying the standard images simply makes the image bigger; it does not show more calcifications than were present on the original image nor does it improve image sharpness. These tools simply make whatever was on the original mammogram larger, and if the image was not sharp, they make the nonsharp image larger.

On the other hand, air-gap magnification mammography with a 0.1-mm focal spot actually increases the resolution power of the imaging system by about 1.8 times normal and shows more calcifications than were present on the original image. Air-gap magnification separates closely grouped calcifications into their individual forms, displays faint calcifications not detected at screening, and sharpens the image (see Fig. 1-2). Thus, air-gap magnification mammography is an integral part of calcification analysis and should be obtained on all calcifications requiring further analysis.

ANATOMY

Calcifications form in breast ducts (Fig. 3-1), in lobules (Fig. 3-2A), or within breast tumors. Calcifications forming in the interlobular stroma, in periductal locations, or in blood vessels, fat, or skin are usually benign. Recognizing the location is important because calcifications within the skin, muscle, or nipple are almost invariably benign. Skin calcifications are especially important to recognize because they can easily be mistaken for intraparenchymal calcifications, leading to unnecessary biopsy. Skin calcifications are usually tiny, about the size of the skin pore on the mammogram, and often occur in skin folds where skin touches skin (e.g., axilla, inframammary fold, or in between the breasts). They are classically eggshell-type or contain a lucent center.

In general, clustered intraparenchymal calcifications are more suspicious for cancer than scattered calcifications. To be considered a suspicious intraparenchymal cluster, the

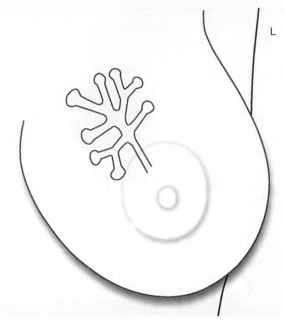

FIGURE 3-1. Schematic of a normal breast duct. The breast has 9 to 22 ducts. Each duct branches into smaller ducts, with the ducts terminating in a terminal ductal lobular unit. Note that the branching duct extends over almost an entire breast quadrant.

finding must represent a true cluster and not simply be scattered calcifications superimposing on one another. The cluster must be tightly grouped on two orthogonal views to prove it is not a fake cluster (see Fig. 3-2B). To prove that clustered calcifications are truly grouped together, the radiologist looks for similar-appearing clustered calcifications over the same volume of tissue on orthogonal views. If the cluster is tightly packed on orthogonal views, it is a true cluster and should be assessed further. If the cluster is tightly packed on one view and scattered on the other view, it represents a superimposition of calcifications, is a fake cluster, and can be dismissed.

BI-RADS® Lexicon for Calcifications and Individual Calcification Shapes

The American College of Radiology (ACR) Breast Imaging Reporting and Data System (BI-RADS®) lexicon has a good section on description and assessment of calcifications. In the mammography report, radiologists use BI-RADS® terms to describe calcification forms, distribution, location, associated findings, and whether any change has occurred since the previous study. BI-RADS® terms are powerful descriptors that help the clinician understand the seriousness of the finding, such as *fine linear branching* in cancers. The BI-RADS® terms also help the radiologist classify calcifications into BI-RADS® assessment categories, which prompt patient management (Boxes 3-1 and 3-2). For example, the BI-RADS® term *pleomorphic*, which is suspicious for cancer, would prompt the radiologist to classify the calcifications into a BI-RADS® category 4, which calls for biopsy to be performed, whereas the term *large rodlike*, which indicates benign secretory disease, would be classified as a BI-RADS® category 2 and would be dismissed.

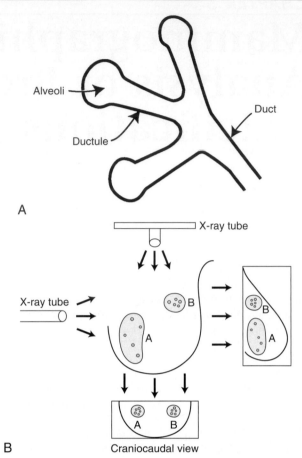

FIGURE 3-2. **A,** Schematic magnification of a terminal ductal lobular unit (TDLU). The ducts branch into smaller ducts, similar to bronchioles and alveoli in the lung, and end in TDLUs. Each duct and lobule are lined by breast epithelium, where breast cancer starts. Cancer grows in the ducts. If the cancer is confined to the duct, it produces linear and branching forms. Cancer can grow from the duct back into the lobule, a process called cancerization of lobules. **B,** Distinguishing clustered versus scattered calcifications on craniocaudal (CC) and lateral views. Both the scattered calcifications (A) and clustered calcifications (B) appear tightly grouped on CC mammograms because the scattered calcifications superimpose on each other, making a fake cluster. The scattered calcifications are dispersed on the lateral view and no longer hang together (A), proving that they are a fake cluster, but the true cluster persists as a tight group (B), distinguishing them from the fake cluster.

Box 3-1. **Calcification Report**

Size of the cluster or calcific group
Location (right or left breast, quadrant or clock position, centimeters from the nipple)
Cluster or group shape
Overall characteristic of the worst-looking individual calcifications in the group
Associated findings
Change, if previous films are compared
BI-RADS® code
Management recommendation

BI-RADS®, Breast Imaging Reporting and Data System.
From American College of Radiology: ACR BI-RADS®—mammography, ed 4, In *ACR Breast Imaging and Reporting and Data System, breast imaging atlas*, Reston, VA, 2003, American College of Radiology.

BI-RADS® terms are based on calcification morphology. Knowing the underlying anatomic structure in which calcific particles form helps the radiologist to understand why some calcific shapes have specific morphologies and why they suggest benign or malignant disease. An example of how anatomic structures influence calcification shapes are the round calcifications that form in round benign terminal breast acini or lobules. These benign calcifications take on the round shape of the acini in which they form, and hence, are round, regular in shape, densely calcified, and sharply marginated (Fig. 3-3A to C). The BI-RADS® term for these calcifications is *punctate;* they are usually benign.

The BI-RADS® term *amorphous or indistinct* describes indeterminate calcifications that are tiny, roundish, flake-shaped particles that are too small and vague to allow further characterization. Both benign and malignant processes produce this type of calcification (Box 3-3). Benign fibrocystic disease and sclerosing adenosis produce blunt duct extension and ductal dilatation that result in indeterminate amorphous or indistinct calcifications (see Fig. 3-3D to F). However, some amorphous or indistinct calcifications can also form in ductal carcinoma in situ (DCIS) (see Fig. 3-3G to J). This overlap between benign- and malignant-appearing calcifications results in "false-positive" biopsies and accounts for up to 75% of benign biopsy results from procedures prompted by calcifications.

Calcifications that develop in DCIS or invasive ductal cancer grow in breast ducts and have classic appearances (Fig. 3-4A and B). The ACR BI-RADS® term for these calcifications is *fine linear or fine linear branching (casting) calcifications.* These calcifications have linear forms because DCIS grows in branching ducts and the calcifications form within the DCIS, making tiny irregular casts of the duct. These calcifications may look like little broken needles with pointy ends or may have a "dot-dash" appearance with both round and linear shapes. Calcific casts of tumors growing in duct branches form X-, Y- or Z-shaped calcifications. Radiologists describe these classic calcifications as fine linear, fine linear branching, casting, or pleomorphic in the report to reflect their concern for cancer. This is in contradistinction to benign-appearing round, punctate calcifications (see Fig. 3-4C to E).

Another suspicious calcification form described by the ACR BI-RADS® lexicon is *pleomorphic or heterogeneous (granular).* This term reflects very tiny, irregularly shaped calcific particles that look like bizarre broken glass shards forming inside pockets of necrotic tumors, such as the micropapillary or cribriform forms of DCIS (Fig. 3-5). The individual calcifications are roughly round in shape but have irregular borders, are faint, smaller than 0.5 mm, and vary in size and density. A cluster containing granular calcifications may not exhibit casting or linear forms but should still be considered suspicious even in their absence. Occasionally, granular calcifications form in a duct and look like sand stuffed in a plastic straw. Unfortunately, benign disease occasionally mimics DCIS and also forms granular calcifications (see Fig. 3-5B to G).

DCIS is classified into high-, intermediate-, and low-grade forms. The description of the histologic architecture of DCIS uses words such as *comedocarcinoma,* which describes the appearance of the comedos of extruded thick tenacious material that resembles a pimple and often calcifies centrally. The terms *micropapillary, solid,* and *cribriform* reflect the DCIS architecture in the duct.

It used to be thought that specific suspicious calcification forms suggested specific DCIS histologies, but this is a myth. Although comedo-type DCIS calcifications are often "casting" and micropapillary and cribriform DCIS calcifications are often "granular," Stomper and Connolly showed that DCIS subtype calcification forms overlap within histologic types. Casting or granular calcifications do not predict a specific DCIS histology, nor do they predict whether cancer is microinvasive or invasive. Casting or granular calcifications can form in DCIS and in microinvasive or invasive ductal cancer. Thus, the radiologist cannot predict if suspicious calcifications are signs of invasive or noninvasive cancers.

Because calcifications can be the only sign of malignancy, is important to analyze all of the individual calcifications in a cluster. Radiologists should not dismiss a calcification cluster simply because it contains a few round benign-appearing calcifications. DCIS may form some benign-appearing round calcifications by spreading into a round lobule, a development called *cancerization of the lobule.* This results in a few round or amorphous calcifications mixed in with pleomorphic calcifications. Thus, the presence of a few round benign-appearing calcifications within a cluster does not exclude a diagnosis of cancer. The radiologist should decide to biopsy a cluster based on the worst-looking calcifications in the group.

Text continued on p. 70

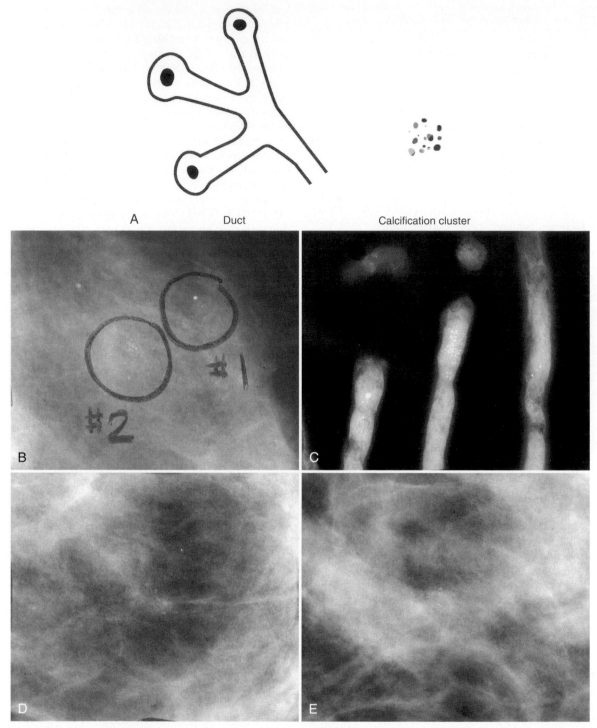

FIGURE 3-3. **A,** Schematic representation of calcifications in benign disease. Calcifications in benign disease form in the acini or lobuli of the duct, so they look round (*left*). On the mammogram, these calcifications will be sharply marginated, round, dense, and punctate because they form in round structures (*right*). These round, benign-appearing calcifications are the result of benign fibrocystic change. Mammogram (**B**) and core biopsy specimen (**C**) of two groups of round calcifications in proliferative fibrocystic change; biopsy was performed because of change in the appearance of the calcifications since the previous screening mammogram. **D** and **E,** Amorphous or indistinct indeterminate calcifications on core biopsy caused by proliferative fibrocystic disease.

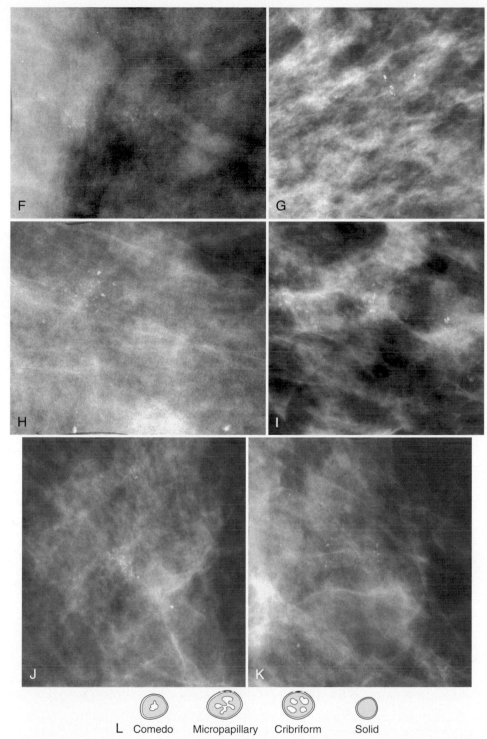

FIGURE 3-3, cont'd. **F,** Amorphous calcifications in fibrocystic change. **G,** Punctate and amorphous calcifications in fibrocystic change. **H** to **K,** Punctate and amorphous calcifications in intermediate-grade ductal carcinoma in situ (DCIS). **L,** Schematic of DCIS in cross-section. Note the spaces in the DCIS tumors, in which the calcifications form.

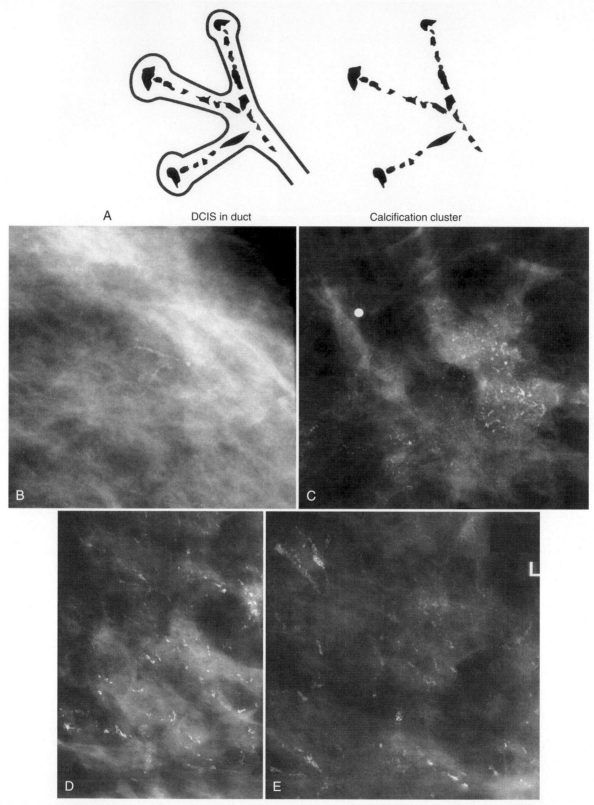

FIGURE 3-4. **A,** Schematic of individual casting calcification forms in ductal carcinoma in situ (DCIS). In DCIS, calcifications form in the middle of necrotic tumors growing in breast ducts (*left*). The ACR BI-RADS® term for suspicious bizarre linear or branching particle-shaped calcifications is *fine linear or fine linear branching (casting) calcifications* because the calcifications are in a line or form a cast of the duct. **B,** Photographic magnification of clustered pleomorphic calcifications in DCIS. Note the branching shape of the calcification in the uppermost part of the cluster. **C** and **D,** Suspicious pleomorphic calcifications in clusters, linear, and linear branching distributions have bizarre and linear individual forms within each cluster. These are typical of DCIS. **E,** Photographic magnification of part **D.**

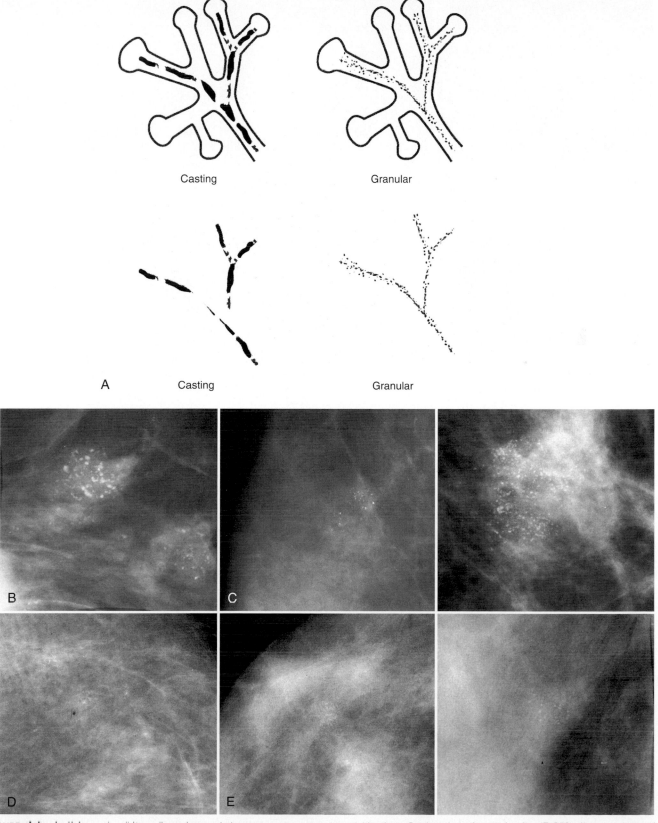

FIGURE 3-5. **A,** Schematic of linear/branching calcifications versus granular calcifications. In ductal carcinoma in situ (DCIS), linear or branching calcifications form if the necrotic center extends along the duct (*left*). Amorphous or granular calcifications in DCIS form in small pockets of DCIS and pack the duct with roundish, but irregular, calcific particles (*right*). Photographic magnification of the granular calcifications in DCIS shows variability in size and density and a "million" tiny calcifications almost too faint to discern in invasive ductal cancer (**B**) and DCIS (**C**). **D,** Clustered, faint granular and amorphous calcification in DCIS. Amorphous or indistinct calcifications also can be present in benign sclerosing adenosis or fibrocystic change. In nonproliferative fibrocystic change, granular calcifications on mammography (**E**) and stereotactic core biopsy (**F**) show the overlap between benign and malignant calcifications.

Continued

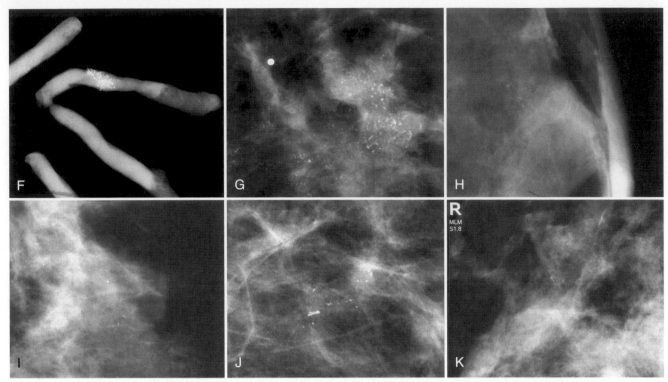

FIGURE 3-5, cont'd. G, Pleomorphic linear calcifications in DCIS. **H,** Amorphous calcifications in DCIS. **I,** Amorphous and pleomorphic calcifications in DCIS. **J,** Amorphous and fine linear calcifications in DCIS. **K,** Granular calcification cluster in DCIS.

Calcification Group Shape or Distribution within the Breasts

Calcification distributions that may represent cancer in the ACR BI-RADS® lexicon are those described as *clustered or grouped*, *linear*, *branching* (calcifications in a line that may show branching) (Fig. 3-6), and *segmental* (Fig. 3-7). Cancer forms in diseased ducts within a breast lobe, or the so-called "sick lobe," as described by Tot and Gere.

Isolated calcification clusters suggest an isolated disease process in a small volume of tissue. This may represent DCIS, invasive cancer, fibrocystic change, papilloma, or sclerosing adenosis. For clusters, one analyzes both the individual calcification forms and the overall cluster shape, which may be a clue to whether the cluster is benign or malignant. Lanyi suggested that the overall cluster shape is especially suspicious if it has a swallowtail, or V, shape, because it suggests cancer in tumor-packed branching ducts. On the other hand, calcifications forming in round clusters may be forming in acini and be benign, especially if the individual calcifications within the cluster are also benign-appearing (see Fig. 3-7E).

The ACR BI-RADS® terms *linear branching* and *segmental* describe suspicious findings because they suggest a process within a duct and its branches. The term *linear* describes calcifications in a line and can represent tumor in a duct or a focal benign process. A segmental distribution is suspicious for cancer because it suggests a process within a branch and its ducts. Segmental calcifications cover slightly less than a quadrant and form in a triangle with its apex pointing at the nipple (see Fig. 3-7F to H).

BI-RADS® terms suggesting benign calcification distributions include *regional* and *diffuse/scattered* (see Fig. 3-7I). This pattern suggests innumerable scattered and occasionally clustered calcifications widely dispersed over the breasts and often reflects benign processes, which are also often spread widely throughout both breasts. Calcifications widely distributed in both breasts are usually due to fibrocystic change. Regional calcifications extend over more than one ductal distribution (Box 3-4). Diffuse extensive benign-appearing calcifications in both breasts rarely represent breast cancer. The decision to biopsy calcifications is based on their distribution within the breasts, the worst features of the individual calcification clusters, change over time, the clinical scenario, and common sense.

Number of Calcifications, Calcification Distribution, and Cluster Shape

The number of calcifications in a cluster is as important as the individual calcification shapes. Sigfusson and colleagues reviewed thousands of calcification clusters on mammograms and showed that clusters containing fewer than five calcifications rarely represented cancer on biopsy. Based on this observation, biopsy of these calcification clusters is unlikely to yield cancer. Biopsy of a cluster containing fewer than five calcifications should be undertaken only if the individual calcification forms are extremely suspicious or if the calcifications present themselves within a suspicious clinical scenario.

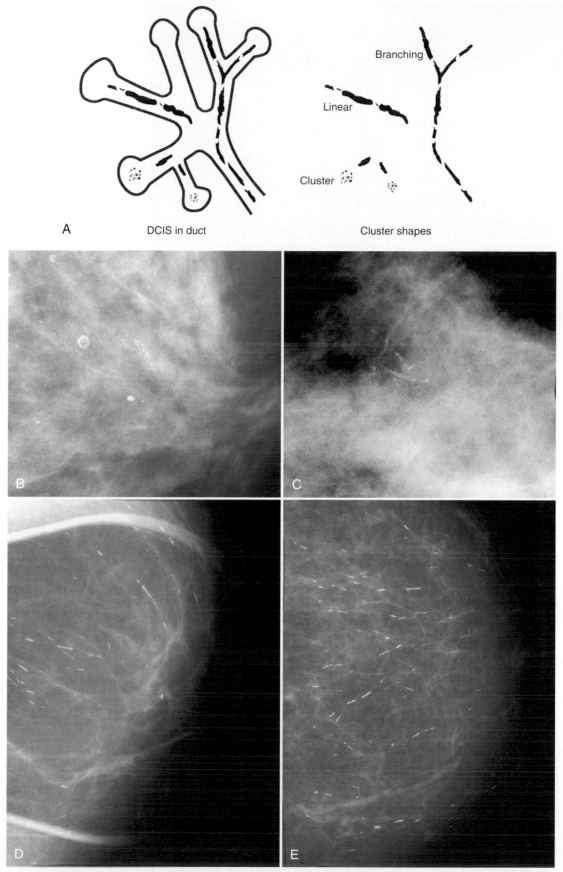

FIGURE 3-6. A, Schematic of the distribution of calcifications in ductal carcinoma in situ (DCIS). In DCIS, individual calcification forms are linear and branching, and the entire cluster can form a linear or branching shape by following the duct (*left*). The resulting calcification distribution forms a cluster or a linear or branching pattern on the mammogram (*right*), depending on where the tumor grows. **B,** Calcifications growing in a V-shaped linear pattern. Note the oil cyst and other nonspecific calcifications near the DCIS. **C,** DCIS calcifications growing in a branching pattern. Linear and branching patterns are seen in benign secretory disease on spot magnification (**D**) and craniocaudal (**E**) mammograms, but the calcifications are larger and rodlike and branch over a wider area than in the DCIS calcifications shown in parts **B** and **C.**

Continued

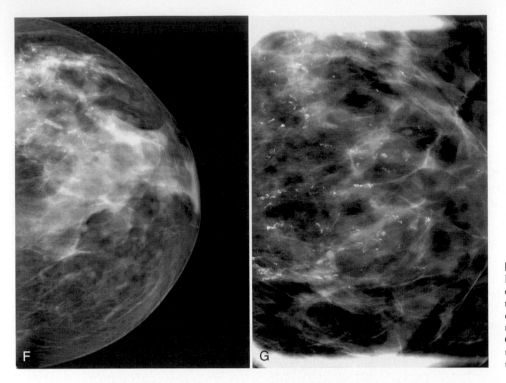

FIGURE 3-6, cont'd. F, Pleomorphic DCIS calcifications in many linear clusters over a segmental distribution. Note that the DCIS calcifications are less sharply defined, smaller, and more tightly packed than the secretory disease calcifications. **G,** Magnification view of part **F** showing the linear and branching cluster shapes of the DCIS calcifications.

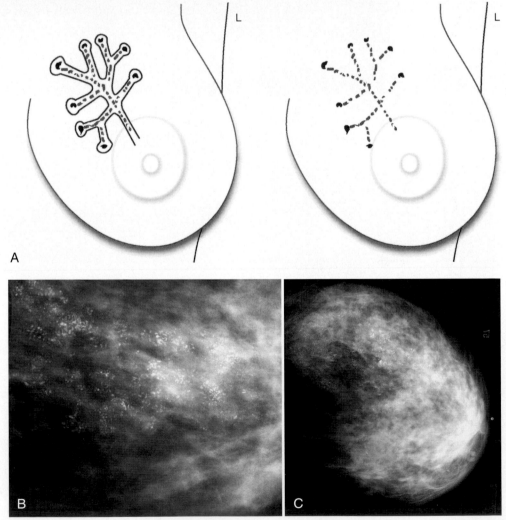

FIGURE 3-7. Segmental calcification and ductal carcinoma in situ (DCIS). **A,** When DCIS grows and calcifies in an entire breast duct (*left*), the resulting calcifications can fill an entire segment (*right*). **B,** A cropped mediolateral mammogram shows pleomorphic calcifications in a segmental distribution, a finding indicative of DCIS growing in a duct and its branches. Note the suggestion of tubular soft tissue in ducts associated with the calcified DCIS. **C,** A craniocaudal mammogram shows DCIS growing in a segmental or regional distribution, a finding indicative of one or two ducts filled with tumor over the entire outer breast quadrant.

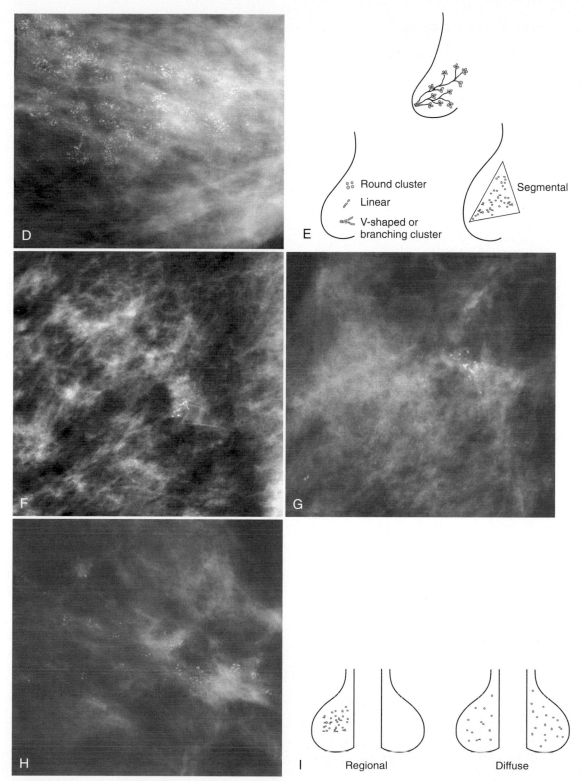

FIGURE 3-7, cont'd. Note the clustered and scattered pleomorphic calcifications in DCIS (**D**). **E,** Schematic of examples of calcification distributions; cluster shapes and segmental calcifications that are usually in cancers versus diffuse or regional calcifications that are usually benign. **F** to **H,** Examples of calcification distributions, all representing DCIS. **F,** Clustered DCIS calcifications with punctate and fine linear forms. **G,** A wide linear cluster of DCIS pleomorphic calcifications. **H,** Segmental pleomorphic DCIS calcifications, similar to part **A** but in a different patient. **I,** Examples of diffuse or regional calcification distributions, which are usually benign.

Sigfusson and colleagues also showed that cancer was more likely with increased numbers of calcifications in the cluster. In clinical practice, calcifications are particularly worrisome if magnification shows many more tiny calcifications than originally suspected on the standard mammogram or if one or more of the calcifications has a linear form.

However, Sigfusson and colleagues also showed that if there were immense numbers of calcifications, and particularly if they were diffusely scattered through the breast, they were most likely benign. Of course, this is true only if the individual calcification shapes are also benign in appearance.

BENIGN CALCIFICATIONS

The specific benign calcifying entities covered in the following subsections require no further workup and should prompt no further action (Box 3-5).

Artifacts Simulating Calcifications

Radiopaque materials on the skin can simulate calcifications. This commonly occurs with deodorant and antiperspirant in the axilla or with radiopaque salves used on dermal skin tags or warts. Sometimes the deodorant or powder will produce dense particles in skin creases, suggesting the diagnosis. If one suspects deodorant artifact, have the patient wash her armpit to remove any deodorant. The deodorant should disappear on repeat films after the armpit has been washed (Fig. 3-8).

Dermal lesions or warts can hide radiopaque salves in their crevices, simulating calcifications in a mass. To distinguish the common dermal lesion from intraparenchymal breast masses, some facilities put radiopaque skin markers on all moles or skin tags. The skin marker on the "mass" distinguishes dermal lesions from masses inside the breast (Fig. 3-9).

To determine whether a calcified "mass" is a skin lesion, the radiologist reviews the patient's breast history sheet to see if a skin lesion is noted on the breast diagram, then correlates the diagram and the image. A physical examination of the patient to see if a skin lesion is located at expected location of the finding on the mammogram will clear up any questions. If there is still uncertainty if a mass is really a skin lesion, the technologist can place a radiopaque marker over the skin lesion, then repeat the mammogram in the view that raised the question. Or a mammogram can be performed tangential to the skin lesion and marker. In either case, the mammogram should show the marker on a superficial "mass" if it is indeed a skin lesion.

Hair artifacts are white, thin, linear, strandlike opacities near the chest wall (Fig. 3-10) that occur when patients with long hair lean forward for their mammogram. Long hair overlaps into the field of view, causing the artifact. A repeat mammogram with the patient's hair pulled away from the field of view will eliminate the strandlike artifacts on the mammogram.

Fingerprints are an artifact seen on SFM. This artifact has a characteristic whorled appearance caused by sticky fingers handling sensitive mammographic films or film-intensifying screens (Fig. 3-11). Sometimes this artifact simulates the linear calcifications in DCIS. A repeat film in the same projection after the screen has been cleaned will have no fingerprints in the same location, thereby resolving the issue.

Round Calcifications (0.5 mm or Less Is Punctate)

Small, 2- to 4-mm round benign intraparenchymal breast calcifications can be seen in any location within the breast. Punctate calcifications form in acini and breast lobules and take on their shape. Punctate calcifications are round, sharply marginated, and densely calcified. Their characteristic appearance suggests a benign diagnosis, and they are often seen in fibrocystic change (Fig. 3-12).

Calcifications with Radiolucent Centers

Rimlike or eggshell-type calcifications with radiolucent centers are virtually always benign. They are usually round

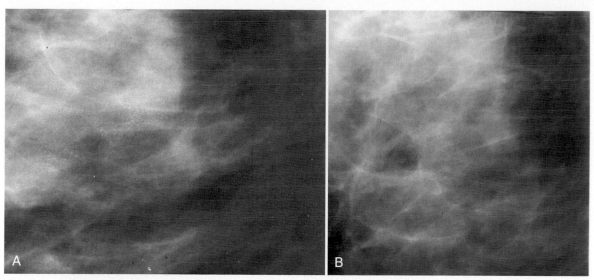

FIGURE 3-8. A, Powder on the skin simulating cancer. A magnification view of the breast shows round tiny calcific particles suggestive of ductal carcinoma in situ, but they were not seen on the orthogonal view. **B,** A repeat mammogram after wiping the patient's skin shows no particles, thereby confirming a skin artifact.

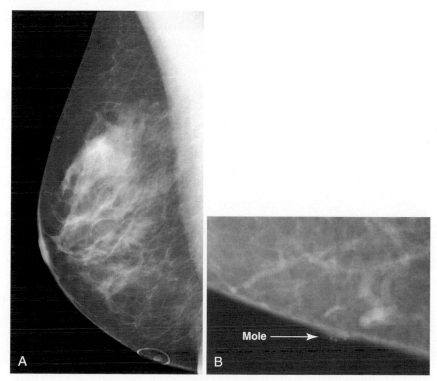

FIGURE 3-9. A, On the mediolateral oblique view, a skin mole covered by a radiopaque ring suggests a nodule. Visual inspection of the patient confirms its dermal location and eliminates the possibility of an intraparenchymal lesion. **B,** Magnification view of another mole in tangent shows calcification as debris in the interstices of a mole, simulating clustered calcifications in the breast.

or oval and calcify along their edges, with the radiolucent center appearing darker than the white calcified rim. Small isolated calcifications with radiolucent centers are benign, can form around debris in ducts, and are scattered in the breast tissue.

Radiolucent oil cysts or fat necrosis can form in patients who have sustained trauma or have undergone surgery. The center of oil cysts or fat necrosis is dark and fatty on the mammogram, and calcifies along its edge from saponi-

fication. Rimlike calcifications surrounding a radiolucent center of a fatty or oil-like substance suggest an oil cyst (Fig. 3-13). On edge, the curvilinear portion of the oil cyst or fat necrosis looks like a long, thin, curved calcification. En face, in the middle of the oil cyst, the calcifications appear amorphous and sheetlike. Calcified oil cysts distributed diagonally across the breast may be caused by blunt trauma from a seat belt or a steering wheel injury from an automobile accident. In any case, when suspecting fat

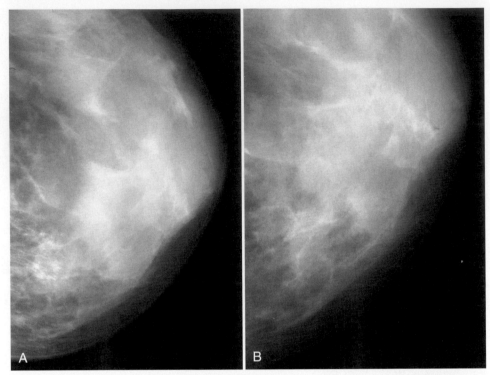

FIGURE 3-10. **A,** A craniocaudal mammogram shows a strandlike, curvilinear hair artifact near the chest wall over the pectoral muscle. **B,** After moving the patient's hair from the field of view, a repeat mammogram shows no hair artifact.

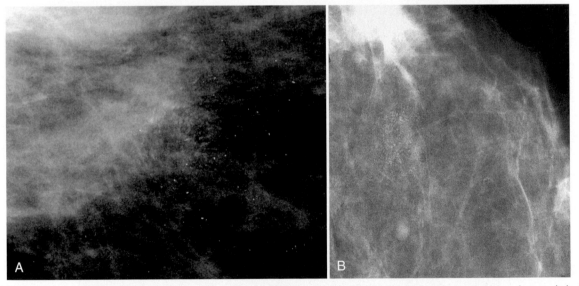

FIGURE 3-11. **A** and **B,** Whorled curvilinear whitish artifacts on two mammograms from two different patients represent characteristic fingerprints caused by sticky fingers lifting the emulsion off sensitive mammography film.

necrosis the radiologist should look at the old mammogram and history to confirm that trauma or surgery has occurred in that area, and that there was fat in the area where the "calcifying fat necrosis" has now formed.

Dermal Calcifications

Skin calcifications are quite small, about the size of skin pores, are single or clustered, and often (but not always) have a calcific rim surrounding a radiolucent center. These eggshell-type skin calcifications are the same size as the skin pores on the mammograms (Fig. 3-14). This entity deserves special attention because dermal calcifications simulate grouped intraparenchymal calcifications when they have no lucent center, prompting biopsy. Any attempt to needle localize dermal calcifications will result in a dismal failure because the hookwire tip will never project onto the calcifications (because the calcifications are in the skin and not in the breast).

The radiologist suspects skin calcifications when the calcifications appear in a peripheral location or close to the skin, when other skin calcifications are present, or when

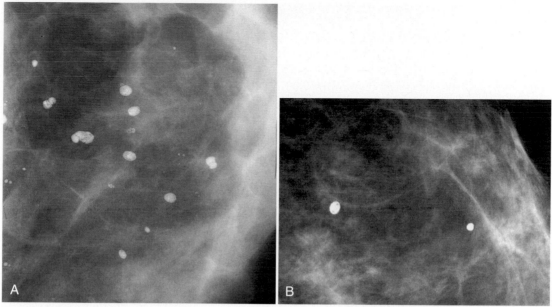

FIGURE 3-12. Craniocaudal mammograms showing large round benign calcifications. **A,** Rounded benign intraparenchymal calcifications scattered in the breast. **B,** Other eggshell-type calcifications may represent calcified dilated ductal structures, clearly uncharacteristic of malignancy.

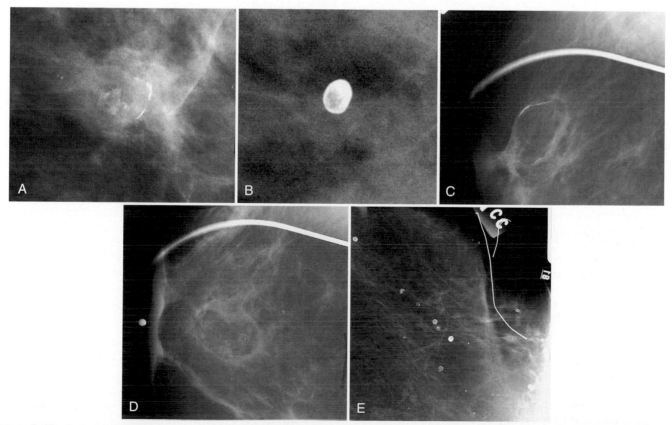

FIGURE 3-13. A, A photographically magnified view of an oil cyst shows partial rim calcification around a radiolucent center, with plaquelike calcifications seen en face in the cyst wall. Normal breast tissue can be seen through the oil cyst. **B,** This oil cyst is more completely calcified along its edge than the example in part **A.** Note that a discernible radiolucent center is still apparent. Lateral-medial (**C**) and craniocaudal (**D**) spot magnification mammograms show a thin rim of calcification around a mostly radiolucent oil cyst. **E,** This patient had previously undergone biopsy, as shown by a linear metallic skin scar marker, and has multiple eggshell-type calcified oil cysts in the biopsy site from surgical trauma. Note the incidental coarse linear secretory calcifications in the lower right corner.

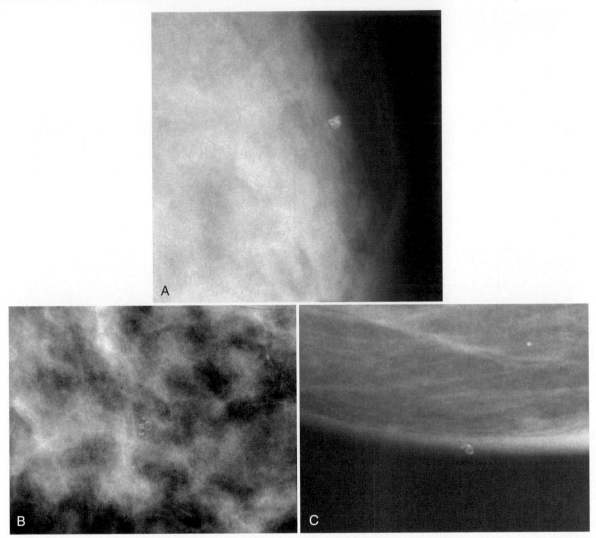

FIGURE 3-14. A, Photographic magnification shows a typical eggshell-type skin calcification around a radiolucent center near the periphery of the breast. B, Other skin calcifications with radiolucent centers. C, A view tangential to the calcifications in part A confirms their dermal origin.

they occur at sites where skin touches skin, such as in the axilla, the inframammary fold, or the medial portion of the breast (Box 3-6).

Special tangential views confirm calcifications within the skin and virtually exclude malignancy. To localize skin calcifications easily, the technologist does a "skin calcification study," which is similar to a needle localization study, but without the needle. To localize the calcifications, the technologist uses a mammographic compression plate that contains perforations or an alphanumeric grid around a hole cut in the compression plate (Fig. 3-15). The technologist positions the breast so that the hole is directly over the skin containing the calcifications; the tangential view will not work if the localizing device is placed over the upper part of the breast in the craniocaudal (CC) view and the calcifications are in the skin on the underside. Therefore, it is important to look at both CC and lateral views to determine which portion of the breast skin contains the calcifications before starting the skin calcification study.

To perform the skin calcification study, the radiologist looks at the mammogram after placing the localizing grid over the calcifications and reads the coordinates of the calcifications. While the patient is still in compression, the technologist places a small radiopaque skin marker at these coordinates to superimpose the marker on the calcifications. She repeats the mammogram to make sure that the

---

BOX 3-6. Reasons to Suspect Skin Calcifications*

Peripheral location in the breast
Location close to the skin surface on one view
Location in the axilla, inframammary fold, or medial part of the breast
Size similar to skin pores
Other skin calcifications present

*A skin calcification study should be performed to exclude calcifications (see text).

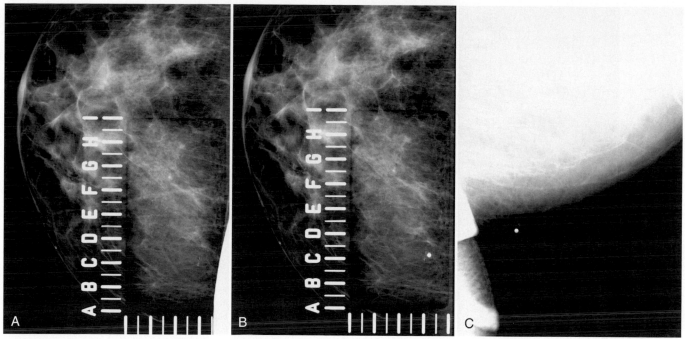

FIGURE 3-15. A skin calcification study. **A,** The technologist places a grid coordinate plate on the skin containing the calcifications and takes a mammogram. **B,** The technologist places a BB at the coordinates identifying the calcifications. **C,** The technologist takes a mammogram tangential to the BB. The calcifications should be in the skin directly under the BB if they are skin calcifications, as in this case.

marker is placed exactly over the calcifications. If the marker is superimposed on the calcifications, it should obscure them on the mammogram and is in the right place. The technologist then takes a mammogram tangential to the skin marker. Dermal calcifications will be in the skin directly under the skin marker. Intraparenchymal calcifications will be within the breast tissue under the marker and not in the skin. This process can take from 10 to 30 minutes, depending on whether the facility performs digital or analog mammography.

Milk of Calcium

Milk of calcium has a classic appearance of sedimented calcifications within tiny benign cysts. Its appearance is pathognomonic on mediolateral and CC mammograms and should be left alone. The calcifications are not fixed to the cyst wall and float around the cyst like fake snow swirling in a snow globe. On the mediolateral mammogram, curvilinear dependently layered milk of calcium settles to the bottom of tiny imperceptible cysts. The layering calcifications are seen as dense, linear, or curvilinear in an upright patient on the lateral view (Fig. 3-16). On the CC projection, the calcifications will have a cloudlike or smudgy appearance like tea leaves in the bottom of a teacup.

The cysts in microcystic milk of calcium are too small to be seen, and only the characteristic linear appearance of calcifications on the lateral view indicates their presence. Microcystic milk of calcium should be suspected when calcifications plainly seen on the lateral or mediolateral oblique view cannot be seen at all on the CC view or just look like a vague smudge (Fig 3-17). Thus, linear calcifications on the lateral view that disappear on the CC view

should suggest milk of calcium, particularly if the calcifications are never found on the CC view after a hard search or even after magnification.

In macrocystic milk of calcium, lateral views with the x-ray beam directed horizontally will show both the typical layering semilunar, linear, or curvilinear calcifications in the bottom of the cyst and the cyst itself.

The differential for linear calcifications includes DCIS, which can mimic milk of calcium; both are linear or curvilinear on the lateral and mediolateral views. DCIS can be distinguished from milk of calcium on the CC mammogram. Milk of calcium is amorphous or smudgy on the CC projection whereas DCIS retains a linear shape (Table 3-1).

Even though milk of calcium is typically benign and should not undergo biopsy, unrecognized milk of calcium may be recommended for biopsy by accident. Because milk of calcium changes its shape in varying projections, the biopsy may be stopped if the condition is recognized in time. Patients undergoing stereotactic core biopsy for unrecognized milk of calcium lie prone on the stereotactic table, and the milk of calcium layers dependently in the prone patient. The "linear" calcifications change their position within the microcysts and are parallel (rather than

TABLE 3-1. Milk of Calcium versus DCIS Calcifications

	Milk of Calcium	DCIS
Lateral-medial mammogram	Linear	Linear
Craniocaudal mammogram	Smudgy	Linear

DCIS, ductal carcinoma in situ.

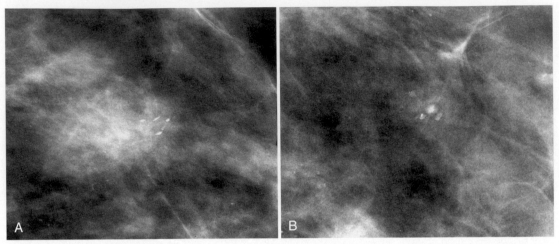

FIGURE 3-16. Milk of calcium in lateral and craniocaudal (CC) views. **A,** The sedimented calcium particles appear linear on the lateral view. **B,** En face the calcifications look smudgy on the CC view.

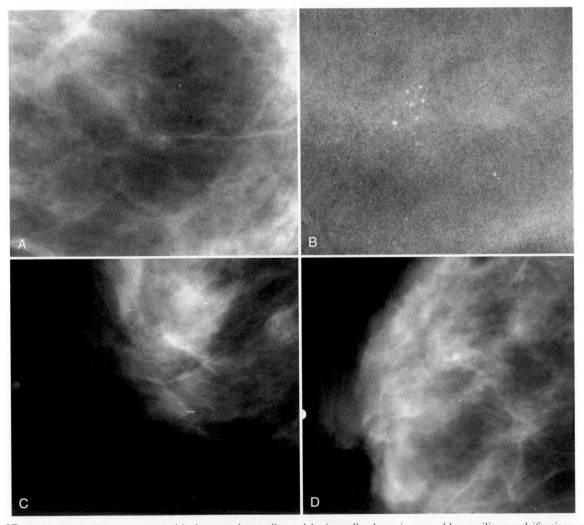

FIGURE 3-17. A, Mediolateral mammogram with the x-ray beam directed horizontally shows innumerable curvilinear calcifications representing calcium layering dependently in a multitude of tiny, invisible cysts. **B,** A craniocaudal (CC) view with the x-ray beam directed vertically shows round calcifications. In another example, milk of calcium is evident in the mediolateral (**C**) and CC (**D**) projections. These clusters could easily be mistaken for ductal carcinoma in situ without the two orthogonal views to confirm the diagnosis of milk of calcium.

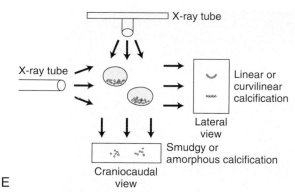

E

FIGURE 3-17, cont'd. **E.** Schematic drawing of milk of calcium in CC and lateral views. The schematic shows the sedimented calcium particles appearing linear or curvilinear on the lateral view. En face the calcifications look smudgy on the CC view.

perpendicular) to the chest wall. Calcifications that appear much different on stereotactic views compared to the pre-biopsy lateral view and layer dependently on the prone view may suggest milk of calcium, thus precluding the need for biopsy (Fig. 3-18).

Large Rodlike Calcifications (Plasma Cell Mastitis, Secretory Disease, Duct Ectasia)

Plasma cell mastitis is a benign asymptomatic inflammation of the breast in older women. The inflammation is periductal or intraductal. Periductal inflammation results in dense, sausage-like calcifications with radiolucent centers oriented along the breast ducts and pointing at the nipple. Intraductal inflammation results in calcifications filling the ducts, producing a solid, large rodlike or a thinner, needle-like calcification (Fig. 3-19) oriented along the ducts and pointing toward the nipple. The calcifications usually are quite dense, have sharp margins, line up along the duct like cars in a train, and may be unilateral or bilateral.

Benign secretory disease, also known as *plasma cell mastitis*, is a DCIS look-alike. Because benign secretory disease forms in ducts, it also forms linear calcifications like those formed in DCIS (see Fig. 3-4C), but unlike DCIS, the calcifications are due to an inflammatory process either within or around the duct. Thus, benign secretory disease calcifications are large, coarse, and "rodlike"; if periductal, they can be sausage-shaped calcifications with a central lucency. Secretory disease calcifications are so big that they

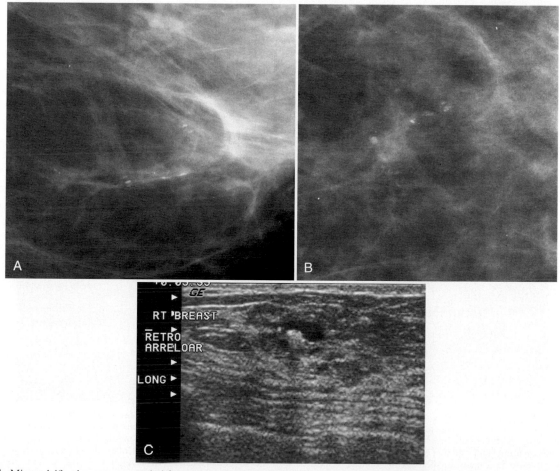

FIGURE 3-18. Microcalcifications recommended for stereotactic biopsy have a curvilinear shape on the mediolateral oblique projection (**A**) and are so smudgy on the craniocaudal view (**B**) that they are not recognized as milk of calcium. A stereotactic core biopsy scout film shows characteristic layering of calcifications in the dependent portion of the breast in a prone patient, which is suggestive of the diagnosis of milk of calcium. If a lateral scout view had been obtained, the true nature of the calcifications might have been detected and no biopsy recommended. **C,** Ultrasound shows milk of calcium in the tiny cysts.

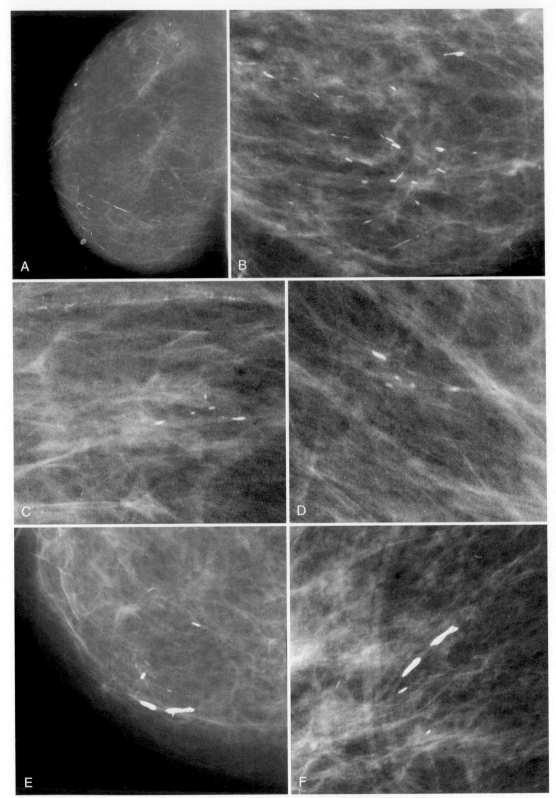

FIGURE 3-19. **A,** A craniocaudal (CC) mammogram demonstrates nonpalpable rodlike or needle-like and occasionally rounded calcifications in a ductal distribution pointing at the nipple, characteristic of plasma cell mastitis or secretory disease. The calcifications are coarse, quite dense, and easily seen and branch over a large portion of the breast. **B,** A magnification view of secretory disease shows typical large rodlike calcifications. CC (**C**) and mediolateral oblique (**D**) mammograms show a linear form and coarse calcifications of early secretory disease. Unlike ductal carcinoma in situ, secretory disease does not usually have many smaller calcific particles associated with the larger calcifications on magnification views. Note the early vascular calcifications in the upper part of image **C**. **E** and **F**, Two views of secretory disease.

can be seen on the mammogram without a magnifier. On the other hand, DCIS calcifications are much smaller, less dense, and finer than those of secretory disease. DCIS calcifications branch quickly and are tightly packed compared to secretory disease calcifications, which branch widely over the breast and can be separated by centimeters (Table 3-2).

Occasionally, secretory disease causes an associated spiculated mass that simulates carcinoma, resulting in biopsy. However, most often, the classic features of plasma cell mastitis or secretory disease calcifications on the mammogram are well-recognized as a benign entity that should be left alone.

Coarse or "Popcorn-like" Calcifications (Calcifying Fibroadenomas)

Fibroadenomas most commonly occur between puberty and age 30. They are benign oval or lobulated solid masses

TABLE 3-2. Plasma Cell Mastitis versus DCIS Calcifications

Plasma Cell Mastitis	DCIS
Lined up along ducts	Lined up along ducts
Point at nipple	Point at nipple
Linear, sometimes branching	Linear, sometimes branching, pleomorphic
Branches over a wide area	Branches many times over 1 cm (ducts are smaller)
No tiny additional calcifications	Magnification shows many more small calcifications
Big calcifications—can be seen without a magnifier	Big and small calcifications
Coarse, rodlike calcifications	Fine, linear calcifications
Sharply marginated	Indefinite margins

DCIS, ductal carcinoma in situ.

equal in density to breast tissue on the mammogram. They occasionally calcify with classic coarse, dense "popcorn-like" features; they should be left alone (Fig. 3-20A). Fibroadenomas are multiple in approximately 10% to 20% of cases and result from epithelial and intraductal proliferation of breast elements. Fibroadenomas have intracanalicular and pericanalicular forms. They are often well-circumscribed, low-density masses that are impossible to distinguish from cysts on the mammogram when they do not calcify.

Calcifications within a fibroadenoma usually start at its periphery. The calcifications are large and dense, although at an early stage they may be somewhat irregular and small (see Fig. 3-20B). Periodic mammography may show slow progression of the calcifications from the tiny irregular forms to the more classic, dense, popcorn-like appearance, occasionally totally replacing the fibroadenoma with calcium (see Fig. 3-20). If the calcifications are not typical of fibroadenoma or if the mass shape or other features are not characteristic, consideration should be given to needle biopsy to establish a histologic diagnosis. However, fibroadenoma with the classic, characteristic mass shape and typical calcifications should be left alone.

Dystrophic Calcifications

After breast biopsy, linear and amorphous calcifications can form in the surgical bed, occasionally accompanied by fat necrosis, causing pleomorphic and bizarre calcifications. A history of previous surgical biopsy or trauma, when correlated with a surgical scar, should reveal the true nature of these calcifications as dystrophic (Fig. 3-21). Some facilities use a metallic linear scar marker directly on the patient's skin scar. This helps radiologists correlate the surface skin scar with underlying postbiopsy scarring

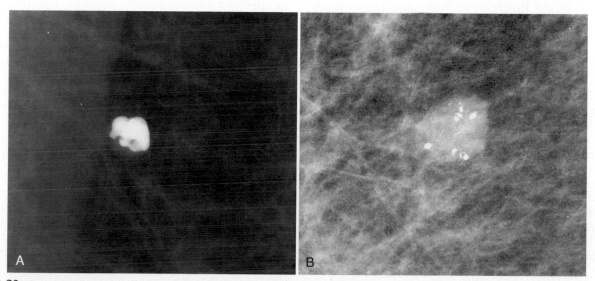

FIGURE 3-20. A, A magnification view shows fibroadenoma with a typical "popcorn-like" appearance. **B,** In another patient, a fibroadenoma appears as dense round calcifications at the edges of the mass. Note the coarse appearance of the calcifications; such an appearance distinguishes fibroadenoma from invasive ductal carcinoma, which would contain fine or pleomorphic calcifications.

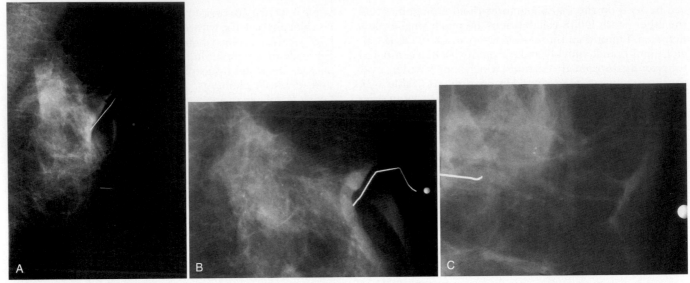

FIGURE 3-21. A, A mediolateral oblique view shows punctate calcifications in the surgical bed after biopsy and radiation therapy for cancer, with a linear metallic marker over the skin (marker also seen in parts **B** and **C**). **B,** Photographic magnification shows round punctate calcifications in the surgical bed, which were benign on biopsy. **C,** Recurrent ductal carcinoma in situ in a biopsy site after radiation therapy is shown as seven new clustered calcifications, similar to the benign calcifications seen in part **B**.

(Box 3-7). Postbiopsy calcifications developing in a cancer biopsy site deserve special consideration because they may be forming in an in-breast tumor recurrence.

Calcifications in an irradiated breast due to calcifying sutures or benign fat necrosis usually develop 2 years or later after surgery and radiation therapy. Dystrophic calcifications in this setting may be difficult to distinguish from cancer (see Fig. 3-21). In the immediate postoperative period, comparing the current study with the prebiopsy, postbiopsy, and specimen mammograms can help determine whether the calcifications represent unresected tumors missed at the initial surgery, residual benign-appearing calcifications, or new calcifications.

The differential diagnosis for new calcifications in an irradiated cancer biopsy site includes fat necrosis and recurrent cancer. Radiation therapy fails at a rate of about 1% per year, thus resulting in failure rates of about 5% at 5 years and 10% after 10 years. If new calcifications are seen at the biopsy site, and if they are fine, innumerable, pleomorphic, and increasing in number over time, biopsy should be performed to exclude recurrent tumor. Because of the problem of recurrent breast cancer in the cancer biopsy site, biopsy may be required more frequently for benign dystrophic calcifications to confirm or exclude cancer recurrence (versus postsurgical calcification).

A special type of calcification forms after accelerated partial breast irradiation (APBI). Unlike whole-breast radiation, APBI or intraoperative radiation therapy uses more intense radiation over a short period of time on only the biopsy site and a small margin of tissue around it. This is because breast cancer recurrences most often occur in or around the biopsy site. APBI can cause typical round, dense dystrophic calcifications in the biopsy bed that are so dense they almost look like metal.

BOX 3-7. Methods to Identify Post-traumatic Dystrophic Calcifications

Metallic scar marker to show the biopsy site
Look for fat on old films in the region where calcifications now project
Look at old films for biopsied lesions; correlate the scar site with the current location of calcifications

Vascular Calcifications

Arterial calcification from atherosclerosis has a characteristic appearance of two parallel calcified lines, representing calcification in the arterial wall (Fig. 3-22). Early arterial calcification along vascular walls may simulate the suspicious linear calcifications of DCIS. Seeing a noncalcified vessel leading to the calcifications may establish that the calcifications are in a calcified part of the blood vessel. Magnification views of vascular calcifications will show arterial tram-track calcifications in two parallel lines, with coarse calcifications en face in the vessel wall between them.

Calcifications from Foreign Bodies (Silicone Injections, Other)

Classically associated with the injection of silicone or a paraffin-like substance into the breast for purposes of augmentation, foreign-body granulomas in the breast have a characteristic eggshell-type appearance (see Fig. 9-9). The eggshell calcifications are innumerable and are packed closely together where the injection occurred. They are usually a few millimeters in size, but occasionally are larger because of fat necrosis or inflammation; they may have

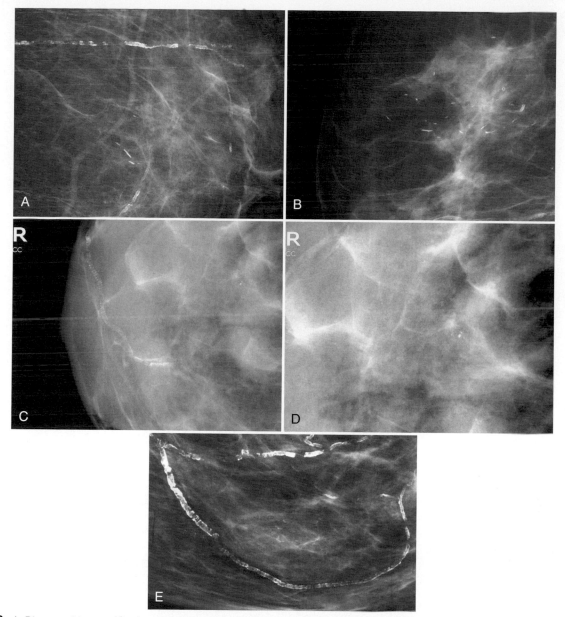

FIGURE 3-22. A, Photographic magnification of easily recognizable dense parallel calcifications along arterial walls. Calcification between the parallel calcific lines represents arterial wall calcifications seen en face. **B,** The tubelike vascular calcification on the right side of the image is easily distinguished from secretory disease and an early oil cyst. **C to E,** Vascular calcifications and ductal carcinoma in situ (DCIS). **C,** Vascular calcifications and five clustered linear calcifications in DCIS. The tram track appearance of the vascular calcifications is easily distinguished from the clustered DCIS calcifications. **D,** Magnification view of DCIS calcifications shown in part **C. E,** Vascular calcifications and linear calcifications in DCIS. The tram track vascular calcifications are hard to distinguish from the linear DCIS calcifications.

surrounding white fibrotic reaction that causes a palpable mass. Silicone injection calcifications obscure the underlying breast on both mammography and ultrasound, making it difficult to evaluate the breast by physical examination or imaging.

Calcifications can also form in the fibrous capsules around breast implants. These are characteristically dense, dystrophic calcifications that parallel the implant (Fig. 3-23).

Objects inserted into the breast cause other foreign-body granulomas or can be seen because they are radiopaque. Foreign objects can be recognized by reading the patient history and by noting the foreign body shape.

CALCIFICATIONS DEVELOPING IN MALIGNANCY

Calcifications that do not fulfill all the criteria for benign entities require further evaluation. Their shapes, location, and distribution must be analyzed carefully to make sure they are not cancer. After establishing that the calcifications are not in the skin, the radiologist finds the calcifications in two orthogonal projections. This establishes their location within the breast and can determine that the finding of a cluster is indeed a cluster (and not a fake cluster caused by the superimposition of dispersed calcific particles) (Box 3-8).

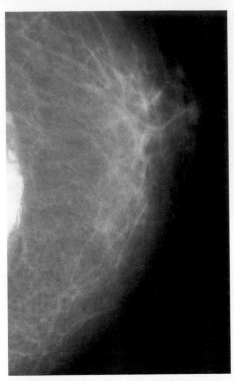

FIGURE 3-23. When a breast implant is removed, the fibrous capsule that forms around the implant is often left in place. The dystrophic calcifications forming in the fibrous capsule are typically seen near the chest wall in the deflated capsule, as shown here. In Figure 9-9, a craniocaudal mammogram shows multiple round tiny eggshell-type calcifications representing calcification around silicone injection granulomas. Silicone and other substances were injected directly into the breast for augmentation in Southeast Asia, but they cause dense calcifications. Direct injections of silicone are easily distinguished from dystrophic calcifications in the implant capsule after implant removal, shown here.

Box 3-8. Benign Calcifications that Simulate Ductal Carcinoma in Situ

Skin calcifications
Scattered calcifications projecting as a group in one projection
Sclerosing adenosis
Fibrocystic change

Calcifications in a localized malignancy are tightly clustered, vary in size and shape, and have bizarre branching irregular or linear forms. A suspicious cluster consists of at least five discrete particles smaller than 0.5 mm distributed over a 1-cm^3 region (Box 3-9). Calcifications that meet these criteria and do not have a characteristic benign appearance should be viewed with suspicion and biopsied (Figs. 3-24 and 3-25).

Calcifications in malignancy are most commonly seen in invasive ductal carcinoma and DCIS. Calcifications are also seen in papillary carcinoma, but this is a more rare form of cancer. The extremely rare osteogenic sarcoma of the breast contains calcifications that look like bone. Calcifications are rarely seen in lobular carcinoma in situ (LCIS) which usually has no mammographic findings and is an

---

Box 3-9. Ductal Carcinoma in Situ

Beware of clusters containing:
  A linear calcification
  Many more calcifications on magnification than initially suspected on the screening mammogram

---

Box 3-10. Cancers Commonly Containing Calcifications*

Invasive ductal cancer
Ductal carcinoma in situ
Papillary carcinoma

*In invasive lobular cancer, calcifications are very rare.

---

incidental finding on a biopsy performed for another radiologic abnormality or patient symptom (Box 3-10). Calcifications are also not usually a feature of invasive lobular carcinoma.

Stability of Pleomorphic Calcifications

In general, stability of calcifications over time on several mammograms indicates that the calcifications are benign. However, the stability of pleomorphic calcifications does not indicate they are benign. Although it is true that calcifications in cancer are usually new or increase over time, suspicious pleomorphic calcifications in cancer can be stable.

A study by Lev-Toaff and colleagues looked at old mammograms of suspicious calcifications that were biopsied and shown to be DCIS or invasive ductal cancer to see how long the calcifications were present and if they had changed at all. They showed that the malignant-appearing calcifications were stable over a 6- to 50-month period. If the calcifications were present previously and changed, they were more likely to be associated with invasive cancer than with DCIS. These findings indicate that suspicious pleomorphic calcifications may represent DCIS or invasive ductal cancer even if they are stable and that biopsy should be performed on any suspicious pleomorphic calcifications.

■ INDETERMINATE CALCIFICATIONS (INCLUDING BI-RADS® CATEGORY 3) AND MANAGEMENT

Even after careful analysis, some calcifications are indeterminate for malignancy (Figs. 3-26 to 3-28). At this point, surgical biopsy, percutaneous biopsy, or periodic short-term mammographic follow-up may be recommended, depending on the clinical history, the desires of the patient, and those of the referring physician.

On the other hand, periodic mammographic follow-up to confirm stability is an accepted method of follow-up for lesions thought to be benign if the calcifications have less than a 2% chance of malignancy. Brenner and Sickles showed that periodic follow-up for lesions thought to be benign is an acceptable management strategy if the

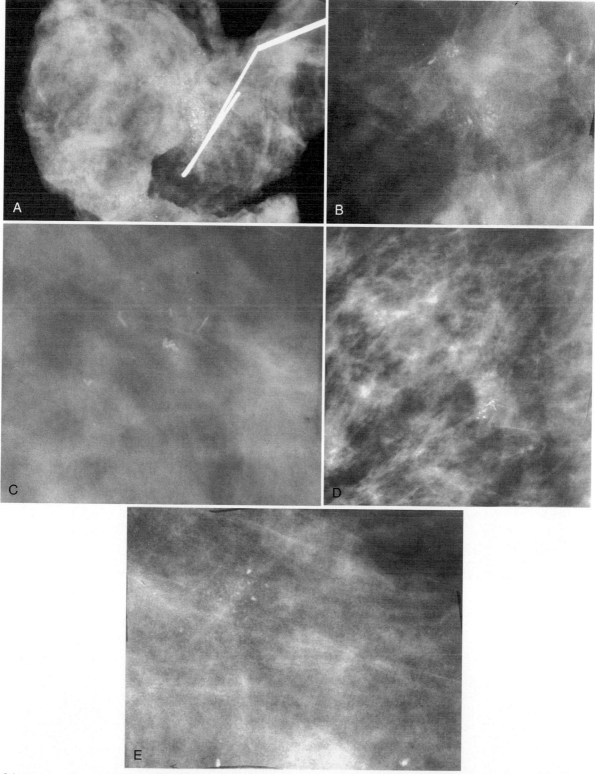

FIGURE 3-24. **A,** A specimen radiograph shows fine calcifications in ductal carcinoma in situ (DCIS), which could also have been fibrocystic change (FCC) based on its radiographic appearance, thus demonstrating the overlap in appearance of DCIS and FCC. Note the hookwire used to localize the calcifications. **B** and **C,** Photographic magnification of the various forms of calcifications seen in DCIS: granular-type DCIS calcifications (**B**) and pleomorphic-type DCIS calcifications (**C**). **D** and **E,** Fine linear suspicious calcification clusters in DCIS.

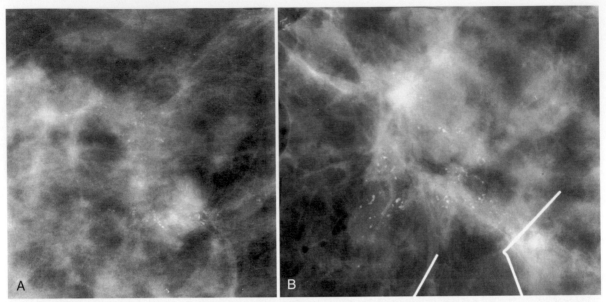

FIGURE 3-25. A, Grouped bizarre calcifications formed within an invasive ductal carcinoma as shown on magnification mammography. **B,** A specimen radiograph shows the hookwire and pleomorphic calcifications to greater advantage. Pleomorphic calcifications without an associated mass may represent invasive ductal cancer or ductal carcinoma in situ and are indistinguishable.

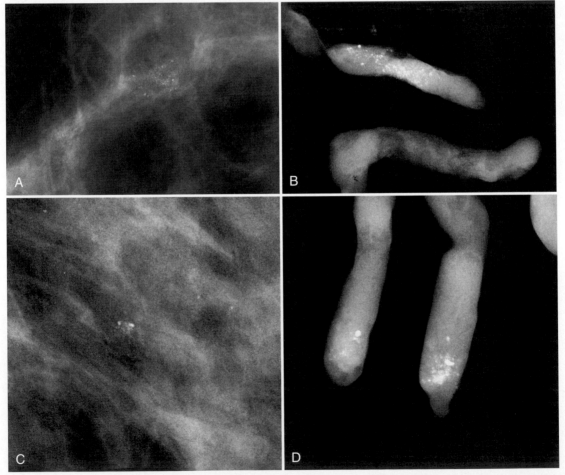

FIGURE 3-26. A, Isolated round punctate and amorphous calcifications grouped in the outer portion of the right breast on the craniocaudal view are of indeterminate suspicion for malignancy (20% to 30% likelihood of cancer). **B,** Calcifications contained within stereotactic core biopsy specimens represent fibrocystic change, sclerosing adenosis, and microcalcifications. **C,** Indeterminate round and amorphous calcifications in another patient. **D,** Stereotactic core biopsy specimens contain the calcifications, which proved to be due to nonproliferative fibrocystic change.

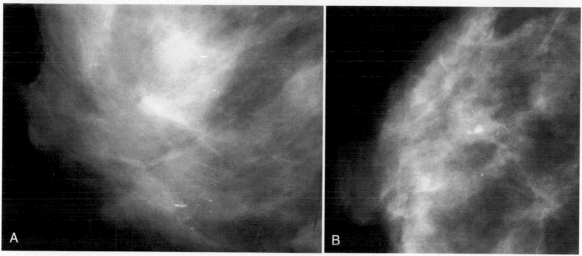

FIGURE 3-27. A and **B,** Nonspecific amorphous or indistinct calcifications grouped over a 20-mm region. Some represent milk of calcium, whereas others are indeterminate for malignancy. Fibrocystic change with calcification was the diagnosis.

findings fulfill all criteria for the probably benign lesion (Box 3-11). Specifically, the finding must be nonpalpable and one of three types: (1) a solitary cluster of round or punctate benign-appearing calcifications, (2) a well-defined round or oval solitary solid mass, or (3) a focal asymmetry without other associated mammographic abnormality. Periodic follow-up at 6 months and then yearly follow-up for 2 to 3 years is standard of care if the calcifications are round or punctate, have no malignant features, and are stable.

New, palpable, increasing, or pleomorphic calcifications do not fulfill criteria for the "probably benign" BI-RADS® category 3 and should be biopsied (Figs. 3-29 and 3-30). In fact two studies, one by Lehman and colleagues and another by Rosen and colleagues, showed that cancers diagnosed in patients sorted to BI-RADS® category 3 were findings that were either suspicious in the first place; calcifications that were new or increasing in number; masses that were suspicious, new, or were growing; findings that were palpable; or asymmetries that had spiculation or calcifications.

Short-term follow-up is an option for calcifications only if the likelihood is high that the calcifications will *not* change. If this alternative is chosen, careful documentation of each follow-up visit is especially important in practices that accept self-referred women; in self-referred cases, the radiologist becomes the "referring physician" and assumes primary care of the woman.

With regard to biopsy of isolated clusters of tiny calcifications, a 20% to 30% true-positive biopsy rate for cancer is acceptable in the United States. It is to be expected that many benign biopsies will be obtained in the search for small carcinomas. Because some calcification clusters considered somewhat suspicious for malignancy ultimately prove to be benign, an audit of one's own practice is the only method to determine the local biopsy yield of cancer.

Box 3-11. Probably Benign Lesions (All Nonpalpable, *Not* New)

Solitary cluster of round or punctate calcifications
Solitary well-defined circumscribed noncalcified solid masses
Single areas of focal asymmetry without accompanying mammographic abnormality

---

Ultrasound in Evaluation of Calcifications

Scientific studies show that high-resolution ultrasound can detect calcifications in the breast or find the masses that have caused the calcifications. Often, however, the normal background speckle of breast parenchyma on ultrasound masks calcifications, if the calcifications alone are the only finding and there is no mass associated with them. Some investigators suggest that ultrasound scans in the region of calcifications are helpful if the scan shows a suspicious mass representing invasive ductal cancer or if it pinpoints the calcifications for percutaneous biopsy or needle localization (Fig. 3-31).

▪ KEY ELEMENTS

Pleomorphic calcifications without a mass are significant because they may represent DCIS or invasive ductal cancer.
Calcifications are not a feature of invasive lobular carcinoma and are rarely a feature of LCIS.
Use a magnifier to seek calcifications on standard mammograms.
Use air-gap magnification views with a 0.1-mm focal spot to work up calcifications.
"Don't touch" calcifications include dermal calcifications, milk of calcium, secretory disease (plasma cell mastitis),

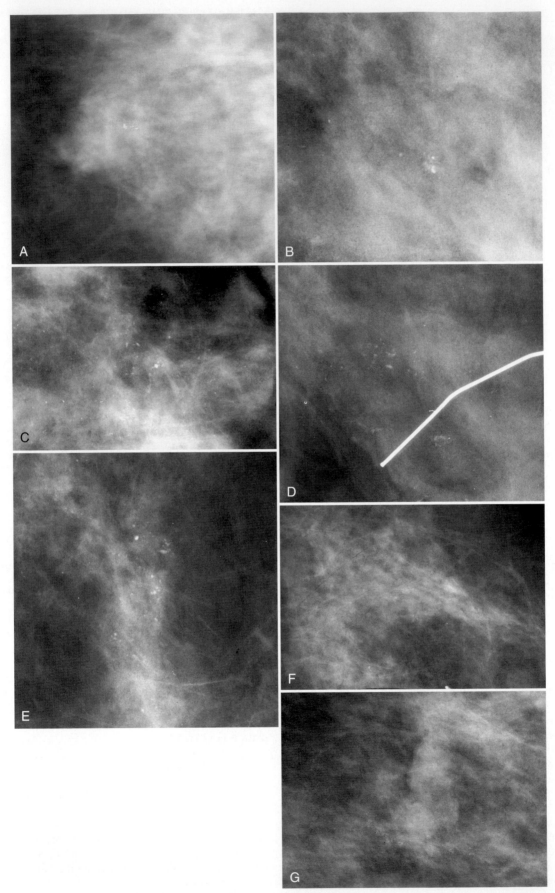

FIGURE 3-28. Examples of indeterminate calcifications with biopsy-proven benign disease. Craniocaudal (CC) (**A**) and photographically magnified (**B**) mammograms show tightly clustered calcifications with one curvilinear shape. Biopsy showed fibrocystic change. In a second patient, nonspecific amorphous and curvilinear calcifications on the mammogram (**C**) prompted biopsy, and the specimen (**D**) showed fibrocystic change and microcalcifications. Note part of a localizing hookwire. **E,** Sclerosing adenosis and calcifications in benign ducts. With sclerosing adenosis and fibrocystic change, the calcifications are so faint that they are almost indiscernible on the CC (**F**) and mediolateral oblique (**G**) views.

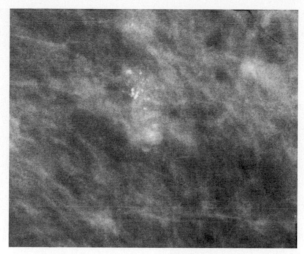

FIGURE 3-29. Round, clustered calcifications variable in size and density. Biopsy showed lobular carcinoma in situ (LCIS) with calcifications, a rare finding because LCIS does not usually have any mammographic features or calcifications.

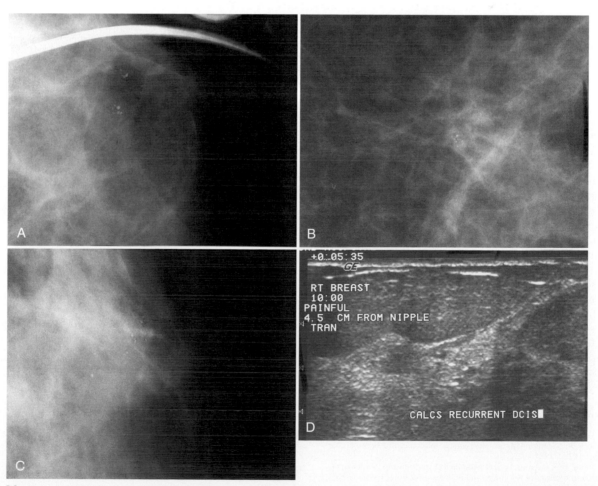

FIGURE 3-30. Ductal carcinoma in situ (DCIS) manifested as benign-appearing, but new calcifications. **A,** A tight cluster of round punctate calcifications was suspicious because they were not evident on the previous screening 12 months earlier. Stereotactic core biopsy showed DCIS. **B,** Faint tight cluster of round and granular calcifications in another patient. **C,** New, loosely grouped granular and amorphous calcifications. **D,** DCIS calcifications from part C shown on ultrasound. Note that although calcifications can be seen, they might be difficult to detect without previous knowledge of their location, masked by the normal speckled appearance of the breast on ultrasound.

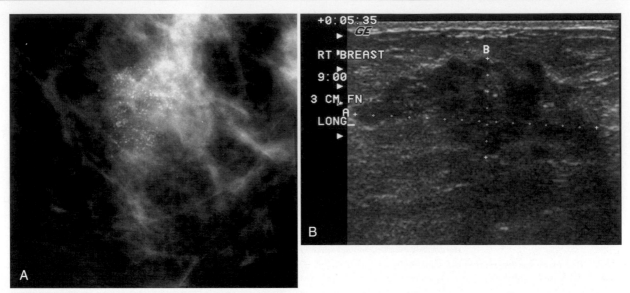

FIGURE 3-31. Calcifications on ultrasound. The role of ultrasound in detecting calcifications is controversial, but it may be helpful if the scan shows a mass in a location known to have calcifications. **A,** Mammography shows suspicious clustered pleomorphic calcifications in a patient with Paget disease of the nipple. **B,** Hypoechoic, irregular mass containing calcifications. Pathologic examination showed invasive lobular and ductal cancer and ductal carcinoma in situ with calcifications.

degenerating fibroadenomas, dystrophic calcifications, vascular calcifications, calcifying implant capsules, and silicone injection calcifications.

Recognize "don't touch" calcifications and leave them alone.

Tangential views identify and diagnose skin calcifications.

Calcifications in malignancy occur in breast parenchyma.

Both the individual calcification forms and the shape/distribution of the overall cluster are clues for finding cancer.

Fine linear, fine linear branching, amorphous, and pleomorphic individual calcification forms are worrisome for malignancy.

Clustered, linear, and segmental calcification distributions are suspicious for cancer, depending on the individual calcification forms within them.

Calcifications that have linear forms within the cluster need biopsy unless they are milk of calcium or secretory disease.

Know the BI-RADS® terms for calcification shapes and distribution.

▪ SUGGESTED READINGS

Adair FE: Plasma cell mastitis—lesion simulating mammary carcinoma: clinical and pathologic study with a report of 10 cases, *Arch Surg* 26:735–749, 1933.

Adair FE, Munzer JT: Fat necrosis of the female breast, *Am J Surg* 74:117–128, 1947.

Bassett LW, Gold RH, Mirra JM: Nonneoplastic breast calcifications in lipid cysts: development after excision and primary irradiation, *AJR Am J Roentgenol* 138:335–338, 1982.

Berkowitz JE, Gatewood OM, Donovan GB, Gayler BW: Dermal breast calcifications: localization with template-guided placement of skin marker, *Radiology* 163:282, 1987.

Black JW, Young B: A radiological and pathological study of the incidence of calcification in diseases of the breast and neoplasms of other tissues, *Br J Radiol* 38:596–598, 1965.

Brenner RJ, Sickles EA: Acceptability of periodic follow-up as an alternative to biopsy for mammographically detected lesions interpreted as probably benign, *Radiology* 171:645–646, 1989.

Coren GS, Libshitz HI, Patchefsky AS: Fat necrosis of the breast: mammographic and thermographic findings, *Br J Radiol* 47:758–762, 1974.

Dershaw DD, Abramson A, Kinne DW: Ductal carcinoma in situ: mammographic findings and clinical implications, *Radiology* 170:411–415, 1989.

Dershaw DD, Chaglassian TA: Mammography after prosthesis placement for augmentation or reconstructive mammoplasty, *Radiology* 170(Pt 1):69–74, 1989.

Dershaw DD, Shank B, Reisinger S: Mammographic findings after breast cancer treatment with local excision and definitive irradiation, *Radiology* 164:455–461, 1987.

DiPiro PJ, Meyer JE, Frenna TH, Denison CM: Seat belt injuries of the breast: findings on mammography and sonography, *AJR Am J Roentgenol* 164:317–320, 1995.

D'Orsi CJ, Feldhaus L, Sonnenfeld M: Unusual lesions of the breast, *Radiol Clin North Am* 21:67–80, 1983.

Egan RL, McSweeney MB, Sewell CW: Intramammary calcifications without an associated mass in benign and malignant diseases, *Radiology* 137(Pt 1):1–7, 1980.

Gershon-Cohen J, Ingleby H, Hermel MB: Calcification in secretory disease of the breast, *AJR Am J Roentgenol* 76:132–135, 1956.

Gunhan-Bilgen I, Oktay A: Management of microcalcifications developing at the lumpectomy bed after conservative surgery and radiation therapy, *AJR Am J Roentgenol* 188(2):393–398, 2007.

Harnist KS, Ikeda DM, Helvie MA: Abnormal mammogram after steering wheel injury, *West J Med* 159:504–506, 1993.

Helvie MA, Rebner M, Sickler EA, Oberman HA: Calcifications in metastatic breast carcinoma in axillary lymph nodes, *AJR Am J Roentgenol* 151:921–922, 1988.

Holland R, Hendriks JH: Microcalcifications associated with ductal carcinoma in situ: mammographic-pathologic correlation, *Semin Diagn Pathol* 11:181–192, 1994.

Hunter TB, Roberts CC, Hunt KR, Fajardo LL: Occurrence of fibroadenomas in postmenopausal women referred for breast biopsy, *J Am Geriatr Soc* 44:61–64, 1996.

Ikeda DM, Sickles EA: Mammographic demonstration of pectoral muscle microcalcifications, *AJR Am J Roentgenol* 151:475–476, 1988.

Kang SS, Ko EY, Han BK, Shin JH: Breast US in patients who had microcalcifications with low concern of malignancy on screening mammography, *Eur J Radiol* 67(2):285–291, 2008.

Kopans DB, Meyer JE, Homer MJ, Grabbe J: Dermal deposits mistaken for breast calcifications, *Radiology* 149:592–594, 1983.

Kopans DB, Nguyen PL, Koerner FC, et al: Mixed form, diffusely scattered calcifications in breast cancer with apocrine features, *Radiology* 177:807–811, 1990.

Krishnamurthy R, Whitman GJ, Stelling CB, Kushwaha AC: Mammographic findings after breast conservation therapy, *Radiographics* 19(Spec No):S53–S63, 1999.

Lanyi M: *Diagnosis and differential diagnosis of breast calcifications*, Berlin, NY, 1988, Springer-Verlag.

Lehman CD, Rutter CM, Eby PR, et al: Lesion and patient characteristics associated with malignancy after a probably benign finding on community practice mammography, *AJR Am J Roentgenol* 190(2):511–515, 2008.

Leung JW, Sickles EA: Developing asymmetry identified on mammography: correlation with imaging outcome and pathologic findings, *AJR Am J Roentgenol* 188(3):667–675, 2007.

Lev-Toaff AS, Feig SA, Saitas VL, et al: Stability of malignant breast microcalcifications, *Radiology* 192(1):153–156, 1994.

Linden SS, Sickles EA: Sedimented calcium in benign breast cysts: the full spectrum of mammographic presentations, *AJR Am J Roentgenol* 152:967–971, 1989.

Mercado CL, Koenigsberg TC, Hamele-Bona D, Smith SJ: Calcifications associated with lactational changes of the breast: mammographic findings with histologic correlation, *AJR Am J Roentgenol* 179:685–689, 2002.

Millis RR, Davis R, Stacey AJ: The detection and significance of calcifications in the breast: a radiological and pathological study, *Br J Radiol* 49:12–26, 1976.

Murphy WA, DeSchryver-Kecskemeti K: Isolated clustered microcalcifications in the breast: radiologic-pathologic correlation, *Radiology* 127:335–341, 1978.

Orson LW, Cigtay OS: Fat necrosis of the breast: characteristic xeromammographic appearance, *Radiology* 146:35–38, 1983.

Pinsky RW, Rebner M, Pierce LJ, et al: Recurrent cancer after breast-conserving surgery with radiation therapy for ductal carcinoma in situ: mammographic features, method of detection, and stage of recurrence, *AJR Am J Roentgenol* 189(1):140–144, 2007.

Rebner M, Pennes DR, Adler DD, et al: Breast microcalcifications after lumpectomy and radiation therapy, *Radiology* 170(Pt 1):691–693, 1989.

Rosen EL, Baker JA, Soo MS: Malignant lesions initially subjected to short-term mammographic follow-up, *Radiology* 223(1):221–228, 2002.

Ross BA, Ikeda DM, Jackman RJ, Nowels KW: Milk of calcium in the breast: appearance on prone stereotactic imaging, *Breast J* 7:53–55, 2001.

Sickles EA: Further experience with microfocal spot magnification mammography in the assessment of clustered breast microcalcifications, *Radiology* 137(Pt 1):9–14, 1980.

Sickles EA: Mammographic detectability of breast microcalcifications, *AJR Am J Roentgenol* 139:913–918, 1982.

Sickles EA: Breast calcifications: mammographic evaluation, *Radiology* 160:289–293, 1986.

Sickles EA: Mammography screening and the self-referred woman, *Radiology* 166(Pt 1):271–273, 1988.

Sickles EA, Abele JS: Milk of calcium within tiny benign breast cysts, *Radiology* 141:655–658, 1981.

Sigfusson BF, Andersson I, Aspegren K, et al: Clustered breast calcifications, *Acta Radiol Diagn* (Stockholm) 24:273–281, 1983.

Spring DB, Kimbrell-Wilmot K: Evaluating the success of mammography at the local level: how to conduct an audit of your practice, *Radiol Clin North Am* 25:983–992, 1987.

Stomper PC, Connolly JL: Ductal carcinoma in situ of the breast: correlation between mammographic calcification and tumor subtype, *AJR Am J Roentgenol* 159:483–485, 1992.

Tot T, Gere M: Radiological-pathological correlation in diagnosing breast carcinoma: the role of pathology in the multimodality era, *Pathol Oncol Res* 14(2):173–178, 2008.

Tse GM, Tan PH, Pang AL, et al: Calcification in breast lesions: pathologists' perspective, *J Clin Pathol* 61(2):145–151, 2008.

Witten D: *The breast. An atlas of tumor radiology*, Chicago, 1969, Year Book.

Quizzes

Resident Calcification Tests

3-1. List "don't touch" calcifications.

_____

_____

_____

_____

_____

_____

_____

_____

_____

_____

_____

_____

_____

_____

_____

_____

_____

_____

For answers, see Box 3-5.

3-2. Name differences between milk of calcium and DCIS on CC and lateral views (linear versus smudgy).

	MILK OF CALCIUM	DCIS
Lateral view	_____	_____
CC view	_____	_____

For answers, see Table 3-1.

3-3. List BI-RADS® terms for suspicious calcifications.

_____

_____

_____

_____

Answers: pleomorphic, fine linear, fine linear-branching, amorphous.

CHAPTER 4

Mammographic and Ultrasound Analysis of Breast Masses

The American College of Radiology (ACR) Breast Imaging Reporting and Data System (BI-RADS®) lexicon defines a breast mass as a three-dimensional space-occupying lesion seen on at least two mammographic projections. Benign masses do not invade surrounding tissue and will usually have pushing or round borders. Malignant masses extend through the basement membrane and invade the surrounding glandular tissue. Because of this, and with few exceptions, cancers produce an irregularly shaped mass with indistinct or spiculated margins. Thus, radiologists look carefully at the shape of a mass and at its margins to determine if it represents cancer.

Ultrasound goes hand in hand with mammography in evaluation of breast masses. Ultrasound shows whether the mass is a cyst or a solid mass, and defines the shape, border, and internal characteristics of solid masses to help determine if the mass is malignant or benign. This chapter reviews mammographic and ultrasound analysis of breast masses.

■ MAMMOGRAPHIC TECHNIQUE AND ANALYSIS

On mammograms, a true mass is a ball-shaped object. The mass should look about the same size, shape, and density in orthogonal mammogram projections because the hard mass is harder than the surrounding glandular tissue. Radiologists often struggle to determine if a focal asymmetry is a mass or if it represents overlapping normal breast tissue. Fine-detail views such as spot compression or spot compression magnification mammograms show the shape and margins of the mass in greater detail. Mass shapes and borders are easiest to assess when displayed against a fatty background; thus, spot magnification views are most optimal in a projection in which the mass overlies fat.

The ACR BI-RADS® lexicon (Table 4-1) defines mass shapes as *round, oval, lobular,* or *irregular.* As the mass shape becomes more irregular, the probability of cancer increases (Fig. 4-1A).

The ACR BI-RADS® lexicon describes mass margins as *circumscribed* (well-defined or sharply defined), *microlobulated, obscured* by surrounding glandular tissue, *indistinct,* or *spiculated* (see Fig. 4-1B to E). As with mass shape, as the mass margin becomes more spiculated the probability of cancer increases. Masses with well-circumscribed borders are likely to be benign, and less than 10% of cancers are smooth. Microlobulated masses have small undulations, like petals on a flower, and are more worrisome for cancer than are smooth masses. An obscured mass

has a border hidden by overlapping adjacent fibroglandular tissue; as a result, that border cannot be assessed. An indistinct mass is worrisome for carcinoma because it suggests that the surrounding glandular tissue is infiltrated by malignancy. Finally, spiculated masses are characterized by thin lines radiating from the central portion of the mass and are especially worrisome for cancer. When caused by cancer, spiculations are due to productive tumor fibrosis or growth of tumor into the surrounding glandular tissue.

Mass density is described by noting how white a mass looks compared to an equal volume of fibroglandular tissue. *High-density* masses are whiter than fibroglandular tissue, and *low-density* masses are blacker than fibroglandular tissue. High-density masses are especially worrisome for cancer, because they may contain cells with a higher atomic number than normal glandular tissue and fat. Low-density masses and masses with density equal to that of surrounding fibroglandular tissue are less worrisome for cancer. However, low-density cancers, such as mucinous cancers, do exist; these cancers are low-density because they contain mucin.

Fat-containing masses are almost always benign, except for the rare liposarcoma. Fat-containing masses include lymph nodes, oil cysts, hamartomas, and fat necrosis.

Masses can have associated findings that can indicate cancer (listed in Box 4-1). Associated findings worrisome for cancer include skin or nipple retraction, skin or trabecular thickening, axillary adenopathy, architectural distortion, and calcifications (see Fig. 4-1F to I).

Associated calcifications in or around a suspicious mass are important for two reasons. If the mass is cancer, calcifications around it may represent ductal carcinoma in situ (DCIS). Subsequent excisional biopsy must remove both the mass and all surrounding suspicious calcifications to excise the entire malignancy (Box 4-2). Knowing the extent of the suspicious calcifications helps the surgeon plan the excision (Fig. 4-2). Second, suspicious calcifications inside a mass may be the only clue that the mass is a cancer.

At histology DCIS constituting more than 25% of an invasive ductal cancer is said to be an *extensive intraductal component* (EIC); such a cancer is called *EIC-positive* (EIC⁺). Because EIC⁺ tumors have an increased risk of local recurrence, breast-conserving surgery is less successful. This is one of the reasons to always look for calcifications when a suspicious mass is present.

Other important associated mammographic findings include skin thickening, which may indicate breast edema or focal tumor invasion; skin retraction or nipple retraction

TABLE 4-1. American College of Radiology BI-RADS® Mass Descriptors

Shape	Margin	Density
Round	Circumscribed	High
Oval	Microlobulated	Equal
Lobular	Obscured	Low
Irregular	Indistinct	Fat containing
	Spiculated	

BI-RADS®, Breast Imaging Reporting and Data System.
From American College of Radiology: ACR BI-RADS®—mammography, ed 4, In *ACR Breast Imaging and Reporting and Data System, breast imaging atlas,* Reston, VA, 2003, American College of Radiology.

BOX 4-1. American College of Radiology BI-RADS® Associated Findings

Skin retraction
Nipple retraction
Skin thickening
Trabecular thickening
Skin lesion
Axillary adenopathy
Architectural distortion
Calcifications

BI-RADS®, Breast Imaging Reporting and Data System.
From American College of Radiology: ACR BI-RADS®—mammography, ed 4, In *ACR Breast Imaging and Reporting and Data System, breast imaging atlas,* Reston, VA, 2003, American College of Radiology.

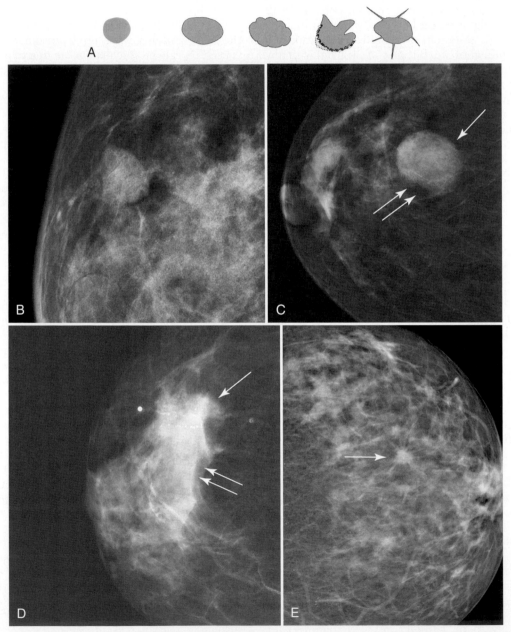

FIGURE 4-1. A, Illustration of American College of Radiology BI-RADS® mass shapes and margins. The probability of cancer increases as mass shape progresses from round to irregular or as mass margin progresses from circumscribed to spiculated. **B to E,** Examples of mass margins in invasive ductal cancer. **B,** Equal-density oval mass with mostly circumscribed borders, representing invasive ductal cancer. **C,** High-density round mass with mostly circumscribed (*arrow*) and partly indistinct (*double arrow*) borders. **D,** A palpable high-density mass in the upper breast marked with a skin marker has partly spiculated and indistinct margins (*arrow*) and obscured borders on its inferior aspect (*double arrows*). **E,** Round mass with spiculated borders in the midbreast (*arrow*) on craniocaudal (CC) view.

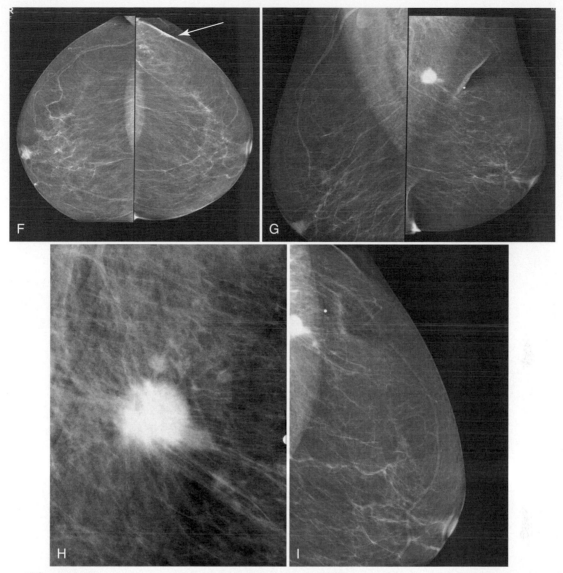

FIGURE 4-1, cont'd. **F** to **I,** Example of skin retraction as an associated finding. **F,** Paired CC mammograms of a fatty breast show skin retraction, seen as a skin fold in the outer left breast (*arrow*). **G,** Paired mediolateral oblique (MLO) views show a marker over a palpable mass in the left axilla on a spiculated high-density mass, with the spiculations extending to the skin, causing the skin retraction. **H,** Magnification MLO view shows the high-density spiculated mass causing the skin tethering. **I,** Exaggerated outer CC mammogram now shows the mass in the field of view. This represents an invasive ductal cancer.

BOX 4-2. **Masses and Microcalcifications**

Beware of pleomorphic calcifications adjacent to a suspicious breast mass. Both the mass and the calcifications should undergo biopsy because the calcifications may represent ductal carcinoma in situ.

---

as a result of focal tumor tethering; axillary lymph node metastases; and architectural distortion.

■ ULTRASOUND TECHNIQUE AND ANALYSIS OF MASSES

The ACR BI-RADS® ultrasound lexicon describes terms and features of breast masses that are key for the diagnosis of cancer (Table 4-2). Stavros and colleagues established another set of terms that are often used in evaluating

breast masses (Box 4-3). Illustrations of these features are shown in Chapter 5.

Evaluation of a breast mass on ultrasound starts with determining whether the mass is cystic or solid. Simple cysts are anechoic (all black inside), round or oval, circumscribed, have an abrupt interface with surrounding tissue, have a thin posterior wall, and are enhanced through sound transmission. Simple cysts can be dismissed. On the other hand, solid breast masses have internal echoes and could be either cancer or a benign mass. Radiologists look at masses to evaluate the mass boundary, internal echo pattern, and acoustic features; its effect on surrounding breast tissue; and the presence and location of calcifications to determine if a solid mass is cancer.

After scanning, the technologist takes representative pictures of the mass and labels the images to clarify the mass's location in the breast. This makes the mass easier to find on repeat ultrasound examinations. Ultrasound

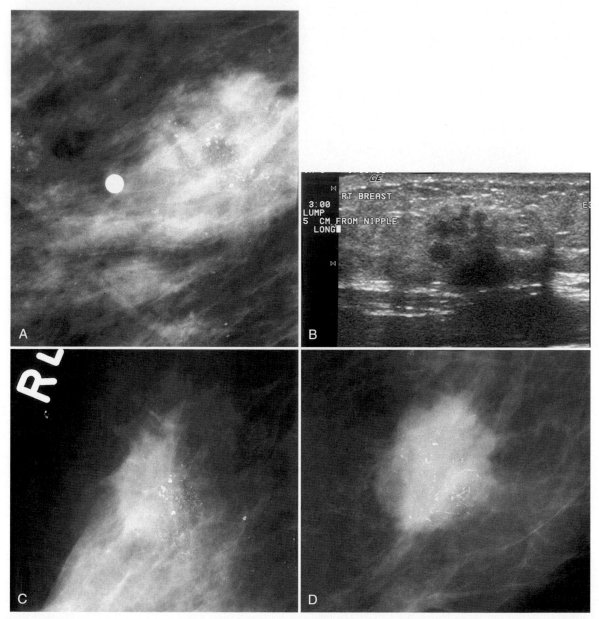

FIGURE 4-2. A to **D,** Relationship of suspicious masses and calcifications. **A,** The mammogram shows a suspicious dense mass containing calcifications, as well as surrounding pleomorphic calcifications that represent invasive ductal cancer (the mass) and ductal carcinoma in situ (DCIS, the calcifications). The radiologist reports both the mass and the extent of calcifications to ensure that all suspicious findings are removed at surgery. **B,** Ultrasound of this mass shows a microlobulated hypoechoic suspicious mass, but the calcifications are hard to see because of the speckles of surrounding normal breast tissue. **C,** A lateral-medial mammogram in another patient shows a spiculated cancer with pleomorphic calcifications and adjacent microcalcifications near but not in the mass; biopsy showed invasive ductal cancer and DCIS with calcifications. **D,** Another patient with grade II invasive ductal cancer and DCIS has a suspicious irregular mass containing pleomorphic calcifications on the mammogram.

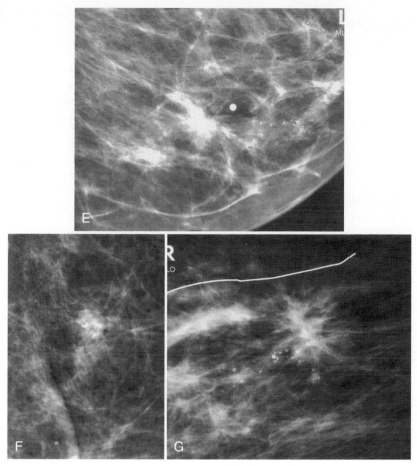

FIGURE 4-2, cont'd. **E** to **G,** Masses representing invasive ductal cancer with adjacent pleomorphic calcifications representing DCIS. **E,** Irregular mass with adjacent pleomorphic calcifications in a linear distribution. **F,** Round mass containing pleomorphic calcifications. **G,** Spiculated mass with fine linear and pleomorphic calcifications within the tumor and extending into the surrounding tissue.

TABLE 4-2. American College of Radiology BI-RADS® Ultrasound Lexicon Descriptors

Shape	Margin	Boundary	Echo Pattern	Posterior Acoustic Features	Effect on Surrounding Tissue	Calcifications
Oval	Circumscribed	Abrupt interface	Anechoic	None	None	None
Round	Angular	Echogenic halo	Hyperechoic	Enhancement	Duct changes	Macrocalcifications
Irregular	Indistinct		Complex	Shadowing	Cooper ligament	(>0.5 mm)
	Microlobulated		Isoechoic	Combined	changes	Microcalcifications
	Spiculated		Hypoechoic		Edema	in or out of a mass
					Architectural distortion	
					Skin thickening	
					Skin retraction/ irregularity	

BI-RADS®, Breast Imaging Reporting and Data System.
From American College of Radiology: ACR BI-RADS®—ultrasound, In *ACR Breast Imaging and Reporting and Data System, breast imaging atlas*, Reston, VA, 2003, American College of Radiology.

labeling includes which breast was scanned (left or right), position of the mass in terms of breast clock face or quadrant, location in centimeters from the nipple, scan angle (radial or antiradial, transverse or longitudinal), and the technologist's initials. The technologist captures the image without and with measuring calipers on the muscle (Box 4-4). It is also helpful to indicate whether the mass is palpable or nonpalpable.

Ultrasound findings suggestive of cancer include an irregular shape, noncircumscribed margins, a thick echogenic rim or halo, duct extension or other effect on surrounding breast tissue, microcalcifications, taller-than-wide configuration, and acoustic spiculation or acoustic shadowing. Benign ultrasound findings include no malignant features, a circumscribed border, intense homogeneous hyperechogenicity, fewer than four gentle lobulations,

---

BOX 4-3. Ultrasound Features of Solid Breast Masses

MALIGNANT
Very hypoechoic
Angulated margins
Acoustic shadowing
Microcalcifications
Duct extension
Taller than wide
Spiculation
Branch pattern

BENIGN
Intense homogeneous hyperechogenicity
Four or fewer gentle lobulations
Thin echogenic pseudocapsule/ellipsoid shape
No malignant characteristics

From Stavros AT, Thickman D, Rapp CL, et al: Solid breast nodules: use of sonography to distinguish between benign and malignant lesions, *Radiology* 196:123–134, 1995.

BOX 4-4. Ultrasound Labeling

Right or left breast
Mass position in terms of clock face or quadrant
Location in centimeters from nipple
Scan angle (radial/antiradial, transverse/long)
Image the lesion without and with measuring
  calipers

---

wider-than-tall configuration, and a thin echogenic capsule. Because benign and malignant features in solid masses overlap, common sense plays a major role in patient management for solid masses, especially if the mass looks benign but the clinical scenario is suspicious (new mass, strong family history).

Correlating Palpable and Nonpalpable Masses on Mammography and Ultrasound

A common problem is correlating palpable masses with ultrasound findings. To do this, the radiologist or technologist places an examining finger or a cotton-tipped swab directly on the palpable mass. The sonographer scans over the finger or cotton-tipped swab on the mass to generate a ring-down shadow. Subsequent removal of the finger or cotton-tipped swab from under the probe produces a scan of the palpable finding. Then the radiologist, technologist, and patient have no doubt that the palpable finding has been scanned because this technique ensures that the transducer is placed directly on the palpable finding.

Sometimes a *palpable* mass on the mammogram has to be correlated to the ultrasound and physical finding. Specifically, the radiologist has to show that the palpable mass, from the ultrasound and from the mammogram, are one and the same. To do this correlation, the radiologist or technologist finds the palpable mass, scans over it, and sees if an ultrasound mass is present. If a mass is present, the

sonographer scans the mass and places a finger or cotton-tipped swab on the mass. The sonographer puts an indelible ink mark on the skin over the mass and places a skin marker over the palpable finding, then repeats the mammogram. If the marker is at or near the mammographic finding, the palpable, mammographic, and ultrasound findings all correlate with each other.

To correlate *nonpalpable* ultrasound findings with mammographic findings, the sonographer identifies the ultrasound finding and places a finger, cotton-tipped swab, or large unwound paper clip under the transducer so that a ring-down shadow is superimposed over the finding. The sonographer removes the transducer and marks this location on the skin with an indelible ink marker. A technologist places a metallic skin marker, such as a BB, on the ink spot and takes orthogonal mammographic views. The skin marker over the ultrasound finding should be in the same location as the mammographic finding on the films. It should be expected that even if the mammogram and ultrasound findings are the same, the mammographic finding might be 1 cm or more away from the skin marker on the films because the skin marker will be compressed away from the mass on the mammogram by the compression paddle.

Sometimes it is still uncertain whether an ultrasound and mammographic finding are one and the same. If the patient agrees to a biopsy of the ultrasound finding, the radiologist places a metallic marker into the mass using an ultrasound-guided, percutaneously placed needle after the biopsy (Fig. 4-3). Repeat mammograms should show the marker in the mass if the two findings are the same. Alternatively, a retractable hookwire may be placed in the mass. A mammogram with the wire in place will show that the ultrasound finding and the mammographic finding represent the same mass. The radiologist can subsequently remove the retractable hookwire.

The mammography and ultrasound report for a breast mass should describe if the mass is palpable; the size, shape, margin, and density of the mass; its location and associated findings; and any change from previous examinations, if known. The report should also include ultrasound finding descriptors and whether it correlates with the mammographic finding. Finally, each report that includes a mammogram should be assigned an ACR BI-RADS® final assessment code indicating the level of suspicion for cancer and follow-up management recommendations (Box 4-5).

BOX 4-5. American College of Radiology BI-RADS® Mass Reporting

Size and location
Mass type and modifiers (shape, margin, density)
Associated calcifications
Associated findings
How changed if previously present
Summary and BI-RADS® code (0 to 6)

BI-RADS®, Breast Imaging Reporting and Data System.
From American College of Radiology: ACR BI-RADS®—mammography, ed 4, In *ACR Breast Imaging and Reporting and Data System, breast imaging atlas*, Reston, VA, 2003, American College of Radiology.

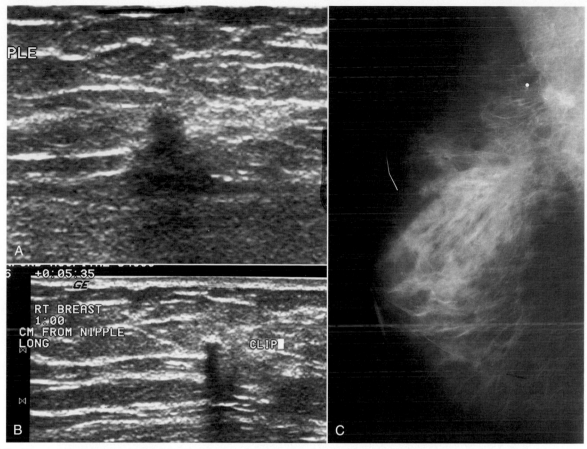

FIGURE 4-3. Ultrasound-guided marker placement to correlate ultrasound and mammography findings. **A,** A patient with a mass seen only on the mediolateral oblique (MLO) view underwent ultrasound, showing an ill-defined round mass with an echogenic rim and acoustic shadowing. **B,** Under ultrasound guidance the patient underwent a core biopsy; a marker was placed in the mass and a BB skin marker was placed over the position where ultrasound detected the mass. **C,** An MLO view shows the marker in the mass and the BB over the mass, thus proving that the ultrasound-detected finding represents the abnormality on mammography. This mass proved to be invasive ductal cancer. Note the metallic linear scar marker on the skin over a previous biopsy.

MASSES WITH SPICULATED BORDERS AND SCLEROSING FEATURES (Box 4-6)

Cancer

Invasive Ductal Cancer

Invasive ductal carcinoma is the most common breast cancer and accounts for approximately 90% of all cancers. Also known as invasive ductal carcinoma not otherwise specified (NOS), invasive ductal cancer usually grows as a hard irregular mass in the breast (Fig. 4-4). The classic appearance of invasive ductal cancer is a dense irregular or spiculated mass, occasionally containing pleomorphic calcifications or having adjacent pleomorphic calcifications representing DCIS. On the mammogram, the mass should be about the same size and density on two orthogonal mammographic views. Spot compression magnification views may show unsuspected calcifications in or around the mass or unsuspected irregular borders.

On ultrasound, spiculated masses shown on mammograms may be round, irregular, or spiculated. Spiculated masses commonly produce acoustic shadowing as a result of either productive fibrosis or tumor extension. When present, acoustic spiculation looks like thin radiating lines extending from the tumor into surrounding breast

Box 4-6. Differential Diagnosis of Spiculated Masses
Invasive ductal carcinoma
Invasive lobular carcinoma
Tubular cancer
Postbiopsy scar
Radial scar
Fat necrosis (atypical)
Sclerosing adenosis

structures. In a dense white breast, the ultrasound spicules are dark against the white glandular tissue. In a fatty breast, the spicules are white against the dark fatty background. On magnetic resonance imaging (MRI), the usual appearance of invasive ductal cancer is a brightly enhancing irregular mass with or without spiculation; enhancement is initially rapid, with a late-phase plateau or washout curve. Rim enhancement, central enhancement, or enhancing internal septations are other worrisome signs for invasive ductal cancer on MRI.

Invasive Lobular Carcinoma

Invasive lobular carcinoma (ILC) is most commonly seen as an equal- or high-density noncalcified mass, occasionally

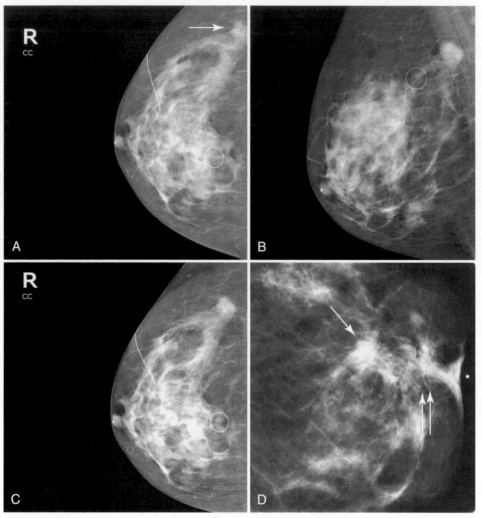

FIGURE 4-4. A to D, Spiculated invasive ductal cancers. **A,** A screening craniocaudal (CC) mammogram with a scar marker and mole marker shows a possible spiculated mass in the outer breast at the edge of the film (*arrow*). A spiculated mass is seen in the axilla on **B,** the mediolateral oblique (MLO) view, and the patient is recalled for a spot view, a lateral view, exaggerated CC, and ultrasound. **C,** On the exaggerated outer right CC view the mass is seen to greater advantage. **D,** In another patient, a spiculated retroareolar invasive ductal cancer (*arrow*) has caused nipple retraction (*double arrow*).

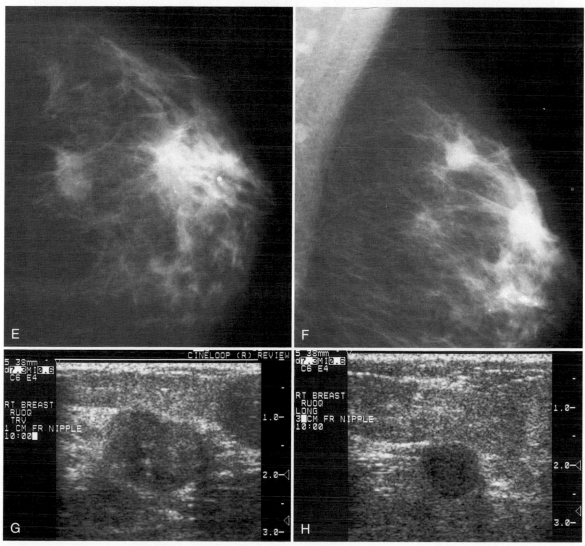

FIGURE 4-4, cont'd. A radiopaque marker has been placed on the nipple. In another patient, two spiculated masses are seen on CC (**E**) and MLO (**F**) views. Ultrasound of the spiculated masses shows an irregular mass (**G**) and a round mass (**H**) without sonographic spiculation.   *Continued*

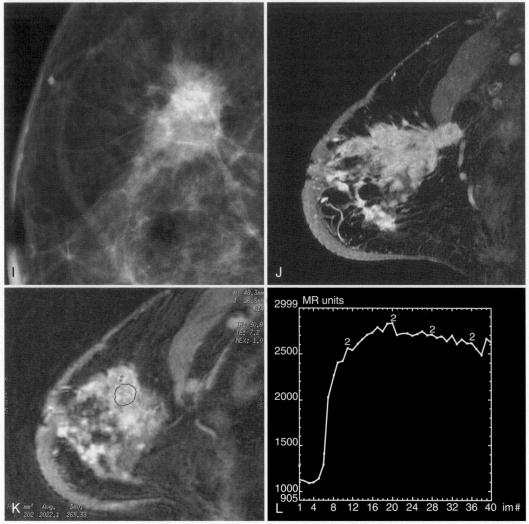

FIGURE 4-4, cont'd. I, Spiculated invasive ductal cancer on magnification view has two benign-appearing calcifications within it. Note that even though the calcifications look benign, the spiculated borders of the mass are so worrisome for cancer that the worst finding overrides the benign look of the calcifications. Biopsy showed invasive ductal cancer. One should judge a mass with calcifications based on the worst characteristics of either the mass or the calcifications. **J to L,** Typical invasive ductal cancer findings on magnetic resonance imaging (MRI). **J,** The MRI shows a large enhancing mass growing through the pectoralis muscle with associated skin thickening. **K,** The ROI over the enhancing portion of the cancer on MRI selects the area in which a kinetic curve will be drawn. **L,** The kinetic curve shows rapid initial enhancement with a late-phase washout. The kinetic curve showing a rapid initial uptake and washout of contrast is very typical of cancer.

showing spiculations or ill-defined borders. ILC has a higher rate of bilaterality and multifocality than does invasive ductal cancer. ILC accounts for less than 10% of all invasive cancers, but historically is the most difficult breast cancer to see on mammograms (Box 4-7). ILC is the cancer that gives radiologists a bad name because it can be missed by mammography, at a rate reported by Brem and colleagues to be as high as 21%. This failure can be partly explained by the growth pattern of the carcinoma. Classically, ILC grows in single lines of tumor cells infiltrating the surrounding glandular tissue and may not produce a mass, making it difficult to see by mammography and difficult to feel by physical examination. ILC usually does *not* contain microcalcifications. It infiltrates the breast, is often seen on only one view, and may cause subtle distortion of the surrounding glandular tissue. When actually seen on the mammogram, ILC masses are often of equal or higher density than fibroglandular tissue and are seen because of the mass itself or its effect on surrounding tissue, such as

Box 4-7. Features of Invasive Lobular Carcinoma

10% of all breast cancers
Grows in single-cell files
Hardest tumor to see on mammography
Often seen on one view
Causes mass or architectural distortion
Calcifications not a feature

architectural distortion and straightening of Cooper ligaments. As with any mass, distortion and tenting of glandular tissue caused by ILC are most easily seen in locations where Cooper ligaments extend out into surrounding fat, such as in the retroglandular fat or along the edge of the normal, scalloped fibroglandular tissue (Fig. 4-5).

On ultrasound, ILC is a hypoechoic, irregular, spiculated, or ill-defined mass that may or may not have acoustic

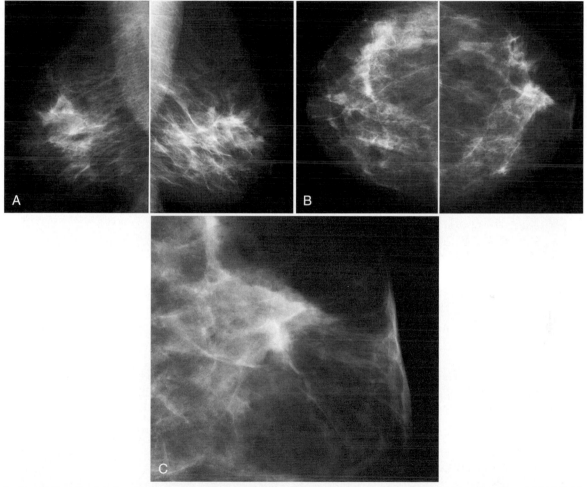

FIGURE 4-5. A to C, Invasive lobular cancer seen on only one view. Screening mediolateral oblique (MLO) (A) and craniocaudal (CC) (B) views; the suggestion of a spiculated mass behind the nipple is seen on the left CC view only. C, A spot compression CC view shows persistent spiculation and distortion caused by the invasive lobular carcinoma (ILC) behind the nipple on the left. The straight lines extending from the tumor into subcutaneous tissue are indicative of its presence.   *Continued*

FIGURE 4-5, cont'd. D, In another patient with ILC, a spiculated mass is seen at the edge of the film in the lower right breast on the right MLO view (*arrow*). The cancer looks very similar to the rest of the breast tissue and is seen only because of the spiculations extending into the fat and because it is a density where there is usually only fat. **E,** The MLO view in this patient shows a density behind the nipple, possibly a mass, but the nipple is not in profile. **F,** The right CC view with the nipple in profile now shows skin thickening and widespread architectural distortion throughout the entire breast tissue. **G and H,** On ultrasound, there is an extensive ILC with marked shadowing throughout the entire upper breast, with cancer in the entire breast on mastectomy. **I and L,** ILC presenting as a focal asymmetry. **I,** MLO paired mammograms show a focal asymmetry near the chest wall of the right breast.

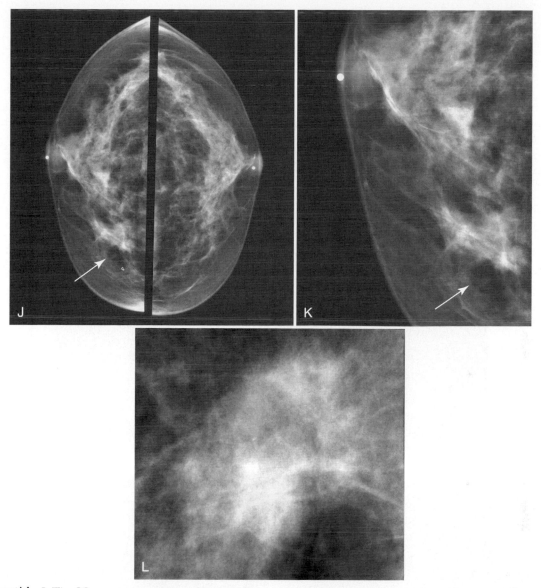

FIGURE 4-5, cont'd. **J,** The CC mammogram shows a focal asymmetry in the medial right breast (*arrow*) roughly corresponding to the mass seen in the MLO view. **K,** Magnification cropped mammogram of the medial right CC study shows the mass that has caused the architectural distortion (*arrow*). **L,** Photographic magnification of the asymmetry shows not only a spiculated mass, but also tiny calcifications. This is invasive lobular cancer. Note that the mass is initially seen only because it is asymmetrically white on the initial mammograms.

shadowing. When ILC becomes very large, only the acoustic shadowing may be apparent; the mass itself can be difficult to see because of its large size. On MRI, invasive lobular cancer looks like a spiculated mass, with some limitations. Unfortunately, ILC has variable enhancing patterns; it can look like a mass, like a distortion of tissue, or like nodular regions connected by strands of tissue. Its enhancement kinetics can be similar to those of normal breast tissue and can thus be a cause of false-negative MRI examinations.

Tubular Cancer

Tubular carcinoma is a generally slow-growing tumor with a bilateral incidence of 12% to 40%. On mammography, tubular cancer is a dense or equal-density spiculated mass with occasional microcalcifications. On occasion it may be apparent on the previous mammogram because of its slow

growth. Although controversial, some pathologists believe that radial scars may be a precursor to tubular carcinoma. In general, tubular carcinoma has a good prognosis and a lower incidence of metastases than does invasive ductal cancer. On ultrasound, tubular cancers are hypoechoic, irregular masses that occasionally produce acoustic shadowing (Fig. 4-6).

Postbiopsy Scar

On mammograms, an old postbiopsy scar looks like a spiculated mass that is impossible to distinguish from cancer. Postbiopsy scars show air and fluid at the biopsy site in the immediate postoperative period. Later, the air and fluid are absorbed and the surrounding glandular tissue is drawn to a central dense nidus of scar tissue. As a result, the mammogram shows a centrally dense spiculated mass (the

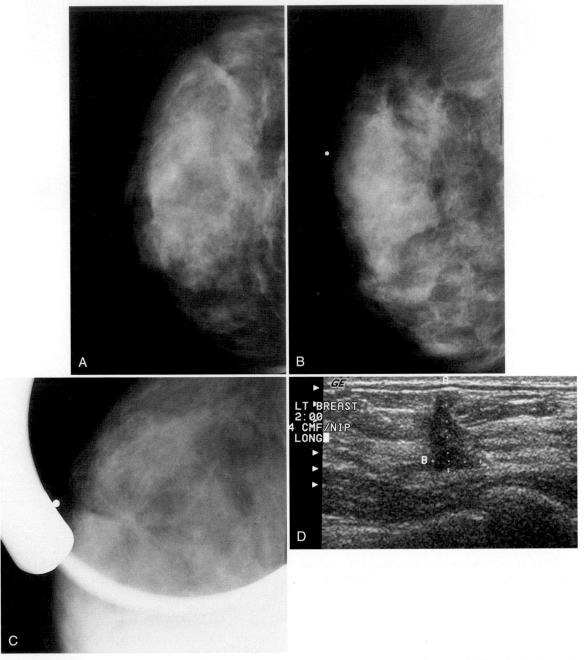

FIGURE 4-6. Spiculated tubular cancer. Craniocaudal (**A**) and mediolateral oblique (**B**) mammograms show a palpable spiculated mass in the upper outer quadrant of the right breast. **C,** Spot compression confirms the presence of the spiculated mass. **D,** Ultrasound shows a spiculated irregular mass that is taller than wide.

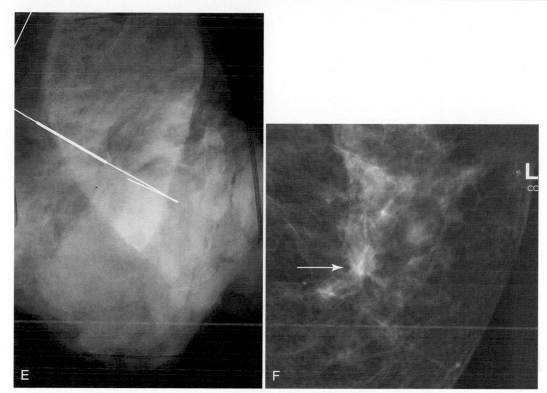

FIGURE 4-6, cont'd. **E,** The specimen shows the tubular cancer and typical spiculations and the localizing hookwire. **F,** Photographic magnification of another spiculated tubular cancer (*arrow*). Note that the tubular cancer is seen only because of the distortion of the surrounding tissue by the cancer and spiculations.

scar) with straightening of the surrounding Cooper ligaments and indrawing of normal glandular tissue, simulating breast cancer. In some patients, no dense central nidus occurs, and the scar appears as a focal architectural distortion. On ultrasound, a postbiopsy scar is a hypoechoic mass with acoustic spiculation and shadowing, similar to cancer. There should be distortion of subcutaneous tissue extending from the scar on the patient's skin down the plane of the incision to the spiculated postbiopsy scar.

The scar is not of concern for cancer if it occupies a surgical site (Box 4-8). To distinguish postbiopsy scars from cancer, the radiologist looks at the previous biopsy locations on the breast history form and reviews older films to see if the "scar" is at the same location. Some facilities place a radiopaque linear metallic scar marker on the patient's skin scar to show the location on the mammogram (Fig. 4-7A to D). The metallic linear scar marker should be on top of the "scar" (see Fig. 4-7E and F). If the "scar" does not correspond to a postbiopsy site, it is not a scar. Because spiculated masses may represent cancer, they should be considered suspicious and should undergo biopsy.

Fat Necrosis, Sclerosing Adenosis, and Other Benign Breast Disease

Fat necrosis is due to saponification of fat from previous trauma, usually from surgery or blunt trauma due to an injury, such as from a steering wheel or seat belt in an automobile accident. On mammography, fat necrosis typically contains a fatty lipid center and is round, but it occasionally has a spiculated appearance. Other appearances

BOX 4-8. How to Confirm Postbiopsy Scans

To determine whether a spiculated mass is a postbiopsy scar, look for a linear scar marker on the skin showing the location of the previous biopsy, or correlate with old prebiopsy mammograms.

include asymmetric opacity, round opacity, and dystrophic or pleomorphic calcifications. The diagnosis may be established by eliciting a history of blunt trauma or previous surgery. On occasion, fat necrosis contains a dense or equal-density central nidus with radiating folds extending from its center, similar to cancer, prompting biopsy. On ultrasound fat necrosis can appear cystic with or without posterior acoustic enhancement or internal echoes in about 30%, showing increased echogenicity in 27% and solid in approximately 14%, as reported by Bilgen and colleagues. With true fat necrosis, follow-up should show a decrease in size of masses; the occasional increasing fat necrosis lesion should undergo biopsy, leading to the diagnosis.

Sclerosing adenosis is a proliferative benign lesion resulting from mammary lobular hyperplasia. It is characterized by the formation of fibrous tissue that distorts and envelops the glandular tissue. The resulting process produces sclerosis of the surrounding tissue. The small duct lumens can contain microcalcifications. This results in spiculations and calcifications that, in mammography, can be difficult to distinguish from invasive cancer, resulting in biopsy.

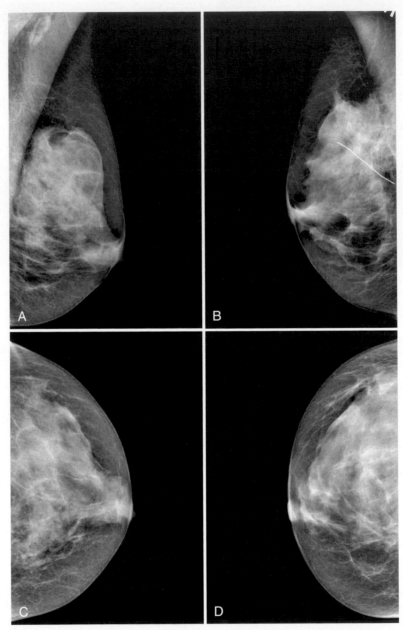

FIGURE 4-7. A to D, Postbiopsy scar versus cancer simulating a scar. Left (**A**) and right (**B**) mediolateral oblique (MLO) and left (**C**) and right (**D**) craniocaudal (CC) views; architectural distortion is seen in the right upper outer quadrant only on the MLO view and not on the CC view in a patient with a history of previous benign surgical biopsy findings. A metallic linear scar marker placed on the patient's scar in the MLO projection (**B**) shows that the distortion lies directly below the skin scar and represents a postbiopsy scar.

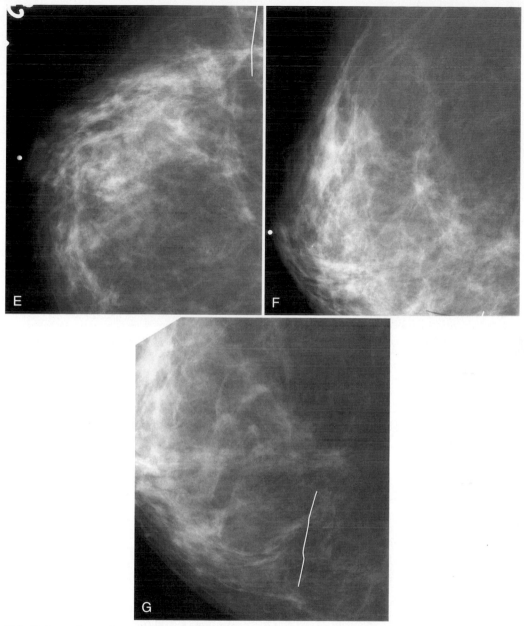

FIGURE 4-7, cont'd. **E,** In another patient, the linear metallic biopsy scar marker lies far from a spiculated mass on the CC view. **F,** A lateral view shows the spiculated mass in the midportion of the breast, above the top of the biopsy scar marker in the lower part of the breast; it is better seen on the MLO view (**G**). Because the spiculated mass was far from the biopsy site, the mass could not represent a postbiopsy scar and was sampled; grade II invasive ductal cancer was diagnosed.

Both sclerosing adenosis and proliferative fibrocystic change may have a slightly spiculated appearance on mammography; they occasionally also contain calcifications and can simulate cancer. When spiculated and associated with calcifications, fat necrosis, sclerosing adenosis and proliferative fibrocystic disease undergo biopsy and are a cause of false-positive biopsies (Fig. 4-8).

Radial Scar

A radial scar is a benign proliferative breast lesion that has nothing to do with a postbiopsy scar but looks like a spiculated mass or postbiopsy scar. Both radial scars and their larger variants, called *complex sclerosing lesions*, may include

adenosis and hyperplasia. In autopsy series, small radial scars are common but often may not be apparent on mammography. The central part of a radial scar undergoes atrophy, thereby resulting in a scarlike formation, with pulling in of the surrounding glandular tissue that produces a spiculated mass. On occasion, because of entrapment of breast ductules, the radial scar may be difficult for pathologists to distinguish from infiltrating ductal carcinoma. However, both epithelial and myoepithelial cells in benign radial scars distinguish them from breast cancer. Radial scars may contain or be associated with atypical ductal hyperplasia, atypical lobular hyperplasia, lobular carcinoma in situ, or cancer. This is one of the rationales for surgical excision. Some pathologists believe

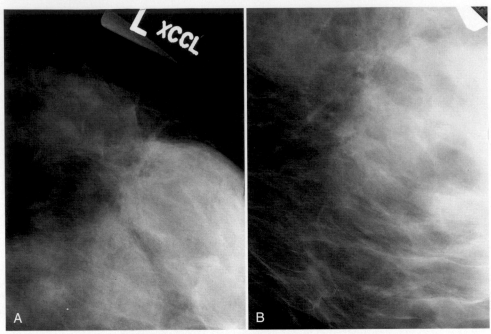

FIGURE 4-8. Proliferative fibrocystic change appearing as architectural distortion. **A,** A magnification exaggerated craniocaudal view shows architectural distortion. **B,** The distortion is very hard to see on the corresponding magnification mediolateral view in the upper outer quadrant of the left breast. Excisional biopsy showed proliferative fibrocystic change and calcifications in benign ducts—a very unusual appearance of proliferative fibrocystic change.

BOX 4-9. Radial Scar versus Cancer

Radial scars cannot be distinguished from cancer on mammography. Spiculated masses not representing postbiopsy scar tissue require a histologic diagnosis.

---

that a radial scar may be a precursor to tubular carcinoma and should be excised, although this position is controversial.

On mammography, a radial scar appears as a spiculated mass with either a dark or white central area that may or may not have associated microcalcifications (Fig. 4-9). It is a myth that radial scars have dark centers in the mass on mammography (Fig. 4-10) and can be distinguished from breast cancers, which have white-centered masses. Scientific studies have shown that radial scars and breast cancer can both have either white or dark centers on mammograms. This means that all spiculated masses not representing a postbiopsy scar should be sampled histologically (Box 4-9). On ultrasound, a radial scar is a hypoechoic mass, with or without acoustic shadowing.

■ SOLID MASSES WITH ROUNDED OR EXPANSILE BORDERS (Box 4-10)

Malignant Tumors

Invasive Ductal Cancer

Invasive ductal cancer is the most common round breast cancer (Fig. 4-11). The "round" invasive ductal cancer is an uncommon form of the most common cancer. Invasive ductal cancer represents approximately 90% of all invasive breast cancers. So even though invasive ductal cancers are

---

BOX 4-10. Differential Diagnosis of Round Masses

Cyst
Fibroadenoma
Invasive ductal cancer not otherwise specified (most common round cancer)
Medullary cancer
Mucinous (colloid) carcinoma
Papillary carcinoma
Intracystic carcinoma
Metastasis
Phyllodes tumor
Papilloma
Lactating adenoma
Adenoid cystic carcinoma
Sebaceous cyst (near skin)
Epidermal inclusion cyst (near skin or in breast after biopsy)

BOX 4-11. Round Breast Cancers

Although medullary and mucinous cancers are often round in form, they are uncommon. The most common round breast cancer is invasive ductal cancer, an uncommon form of the most common cancer.

---

not often "round," there are so many invasive ductal cancers that the uncommon round form of the most frequent breast cancer is the most common histologic type (Box 4-11).

The classic invasive ductal cancer is a dense spiculated or irregular mass on mammography. The much less

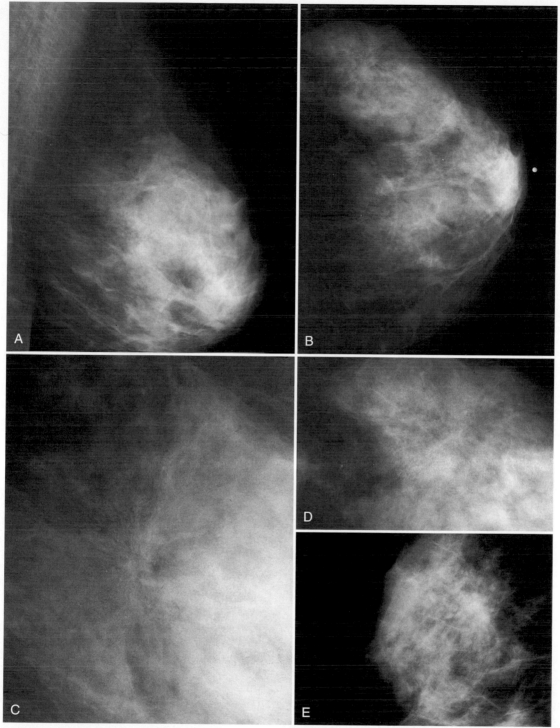

FIGURE 4-9. Radial scar simulating cancer. Mediolateral oblique (MLO) (**A**) and craniocaudal (CC) (**B**) views show the suggestion of a spiculated mass in the upper outer portion of the breast. The presence of a spiculated mass is confirmed on spot magnification MLO (**C**) and CC (**D**) views. Note that a spiculated radial scar is indistinguishable from spiculated cancer. **E,** Another radial scar is seen as a vague spiculated mass with a dense white center in the upper part of the breast, and on ultrasound (**F**) it has characteristics similar to those of cancer, thus showing that radial scars can be indistinguishable from cancer on imaging.

Continued

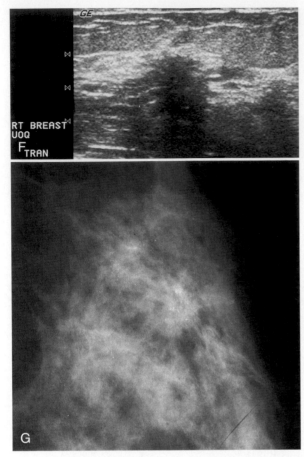

FIGURE 4-9, cont'd. G, A radial scar in a third patient appears as a spiculated mass with associated calcifications and on biopsy contained high-grade ductal carcinoma in situ, fibrocystic change, and calcifications.

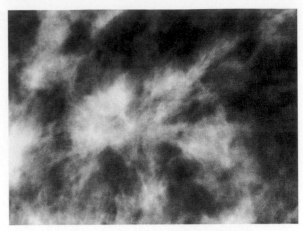

FIGURE 4-10. Radial scar. A craniocaudal mammogram shows a dense spiculated mass suggestive of cancer. Spot compression magnification shows that the central dense portion of the mass is less dense but the architectural distortion remains. Cancer can look exactly the same.

common "round" invasive ductal cancer may grow so rapidly that it does not produce spiculated margins. On screening mammography, round invasive ductal cancer may appear to have a smooth border. However, the borders of the mass may be obscured by surrounding breast tissue, or the standard mammogram may not have the resolution required to reveal abnormal borders. Magnification views may show irregular, microlobulated, or indistinct borders, suggesting invasion of surrounding tissue and the true diagnosis. This is why new round masses on screening mammography are tricky and should be recalled from screening. A new round invasive ductal cancer mimicks benign cysts or fibroadenomas, and the radiologist can mistakenly think the "round" mass is benign until the mass undergoes magnification.

On ultrasound, the round invasive cancer may be smooth-bordered, may show suspicious abnormal findings such as "taller than wide" shape, or may be characterized by a thick echogenic rim. *Taller than wide*, as described by Stavros and colleagues, means a mass that has invaded through the normal horizontal tissue planes as defined by the thin echogenic Cooper ligaments. *Taller* means that the cancer grows up toward the skin and violates normal tissue planes rather than growing horizontally between Cooper ligaments (like benign tumors). The "taller than

wide" ultrasonographic sign is important in the diagnosis of breast cancer.

Medullary Cancer

Medullary cancer is an invasive breast cancer that commonly has a round or pushing border. Medullary cancers occasionally have a surrounding lymphoid infiltrate and have a better prognosis than infiltrating ductal cancer (NOS). They are common in *BRCA1*-associated carcinomas. Atypical medullary cancers have the same prognosis as infiltrating ductal cancer. On screening mammography, medullary cancer is a high- or equal-density round mass whose margins may appear well circumscribed, suggestive of a cyst or fibroadenoma (Fig. 4-12). On ultrasound, medullary cancers are round, solid, and homogeneous. Because they are homogeneous, medullary cancers occasionally cause posterior acoustic enhancement. Because medullary cancers can simulate a breast cyst by their homogeneous nature and posterior acoustic shadowing, it is important to pay careful attention to technical details during scanning to show that the internal features are hypoechoic rather than anechoic. Color or power Doppler ultrasound may show internal vascularity, unlike an anechoic simple cyst. The pushing expansile growth of medullary cancer may produce well-circumscribed mass borders, similar to fibroadenoma, and is a cause for misdiagnosis. This means that a new round solid mass should be biopsied even if it is well-circumscribed.

Mucinous (Colloid) Carcinoma

This rare, round or oval cancer contains malignant tumor cells that float in mucin within a solid tumor rim. The mucinous portion can have fibrovascular bands segregating the mucinous compartments that comprise the tumor and give it its name. On mammography, mucinous cancers with a large volume of mucin show a well-circumscribed low-density round mass that can suggest a cyst or fibroadenoma and can occasionally have lobulated margins. Mixed type mucinous carcinomas may have poorly defined or spiculated margins. On ultrasound, the tumor mass is round and may be isoechoic to fat, occasionally contains fluid-filled

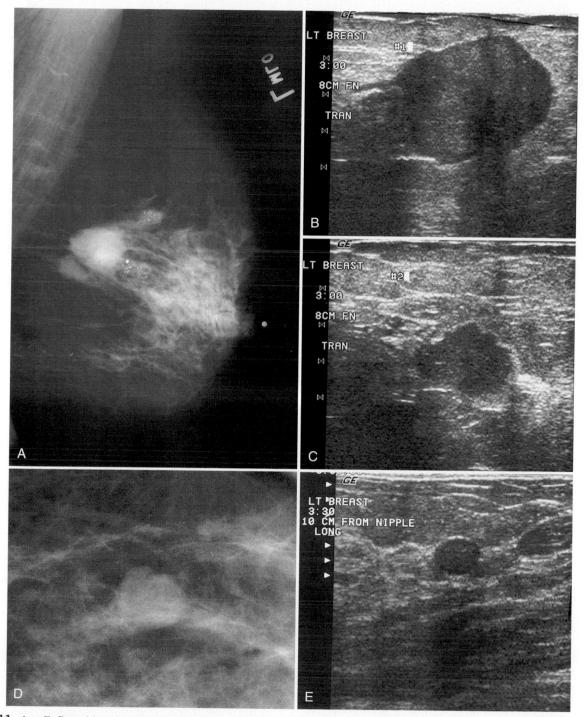

FIGURE 4-11. A to E, Round invasive ductal carcinomas (not otherwise specified). **A,** A mediolateral oblique (MLO) mammogram shows a round dense mass with associated pleomorphic calcifications and a suggestion of smaller round masses adjacent to it. Ultrasound shows an oval hypoechoic irregular mass (**B**) and a multilobulated mass (**C**), both representing invasive ductal cancer. In another patient, a slightly lobulated, circumscribed, round equal-density mass on mammography (**D**) simulates a fibroadenoma; on ultrasound it has a benign circumscribed oval shape (**E**). Biopsy showed invasive ductal cancer.

Continued

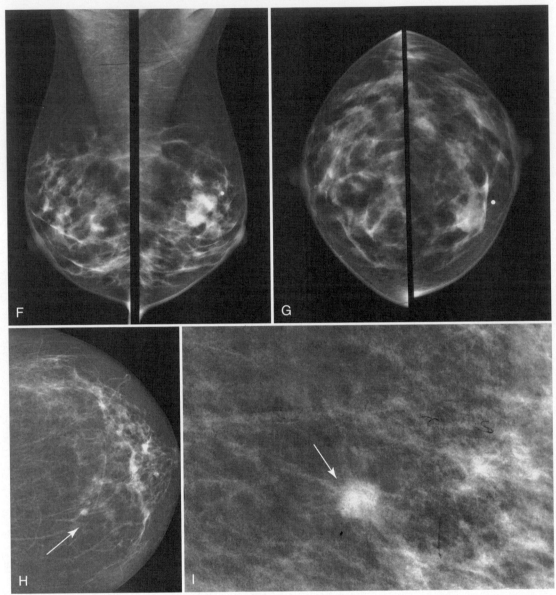

FIGURE 4-11, cont'd. Palpable round mass in left breast representing invasive ductal cancer on MLO (**F**) and craniocaudal (CC) (**G**) views with a marker on the finding. Note that the mass could easily be mistaken for a fibroadenoma or a cyst because of its benign appearance. **H,** CC mammogram shows a vague round mass in the medial left breast, seen because it is against a fatty background and is in a medial location (*arrow*). The differential is a focal area of glandular tissue, a cyst or a solic mass. **I,** Magnification mammogram shows the mass has indistinct borders rather than circumscribed borders (*arrow*). This shows the importance of getting additional views and of being suspicious of medial breast masses. Usually residual fibroglandular tissue is in the upper outer (*not* inner) quadrants. A biopsy showed invasive ductal cancer.

hypoechoic spaces, and may have posterior acoustic enhancement (Fig. 4-13). The mass can simulate a cyst on ultrasound, but unlike the cyst it will not be entirely anechoic. Thus, new round masses on a mammogram that have solid components or do not meet all the specific criteria for a simple cyst on ultrasound should be considered for biopsy.

Papillary Carcinoma

This rare tumor accounts for only 1% to 2% of all cancers and is the malignant form of benign intraductal papilloma. Papillary cancers may be single or multiple (Box 4-12), and DCIS is sometimes seen in surrounding breast tissue. Classically, these masses are round, oval, or lobulated on

---

BOX 4-12. Differential Diagnosis of Multiple Round Masses

Cysts
Fibroadenomas
Multiple round invasive breast cancers
Metastases; vary in size, nonductal growth pattern
Papillomas; may grow in a ductal pattern
False masses: skin lesions

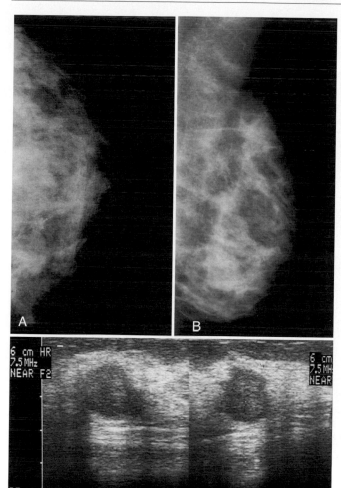

FIGURE 4-12. Medullary cancer. The mammogram shows a round cancer with apparent circumscribed borders when they are not obscured by adjacent dense glandular tissue in the inner portion of the breast on craniocaudal (**A**) and mediolateral oblique (**B**) mammograms. **C,** On ultrasound, the medullary cancer is a round mass with microlobulated and occasionally irregular borders and acoustic enhancement.

mammography, sometimes containing calcifications, and are solid on ultrasound. If associated with nipple discharge and detected by ultrasound, papillary cancers are solid intraductal masses outlined by a fluid-filled structure and are difficult to distinguish from a benign intraductal papilloma (Fig. 4-14).

Intracystic Carcinoma

This extremely rare tumor produces a solid mass in a cyst wall, and the mass looks like a cyst on mammography. Because the tumor is mostly mucin, the mammographic mass is low density unless it has a denser solid component or has bled into the cystic portion to produce a dense mass (Fig. 4-15A). On ultrasound, an intracystic carcinoma is a solid mural mass surrounded by cystic fluid that yields fresh or old blood on aspiration (see Fig. 4-15B). On pneumocystography, the air inside the cyst wall will outline a solid mass along the border of the wall. Intracystic carcinomas must be excised, just as all other cancers are excised. The differential diagnosis for a solid intracystic mass

includes intracystic carcinoma, intracystic papilloma, and a cyst with debris adherent to the cyst wall.

Breast Metastasis

Axillary or intramammary lymph node metastasis from breast cancer, lymphoma, or other malignancy makes the normal benign lymph node change its appearance from a well-defined oval or lobular mass with a central radiolucency to a rounder, bigger, and denser mass with loss of the fatty hilum (Fig. 4-16). This results in a round, dense mass. Metastases can occur from breast cancer, lymphoma, leukemia, melanoma, other adenocarcinomas, and even mesothelioma.

Hematologically spread metastases are single or multiple, round, usually circumscribed, and very dense masses in one or both breasts (see Fig. 4-16). The masses vary in size as a result of the various lengths of time that the metastases have had to grow in breast tissue. Typically, the appearance of multiple new solid masses all over the breast in a nonductal pattern is worrisome for hematogenous spread of cancer from a nonbreast site, similar to pulmonary metastases. Melanoma and renal cell carcinoma were reported to metastasize to the breast in this manner. The differential diagnosis of multiple solid breast masses includes multiple fibroadenomas or papillomas, or metastases when there are no old films for comparison.

Benign Tumors

Fibroadenoma

This most common solid benign tumor in young women is thought to arise from the terminal ductal lobular unit via localized hypertrophy. Fibroadenomas can be single or multiple. A fibroadenoma contains structures suggesting breast ductules and also has stromal tissue, which can be quite cellular in young women. Fibroadenomas may also undergo adenosis or hyperplasia and proliferation and may contain fibrous bands or septations. DuPont and colleagues described fibroadenomas containing such proliferation or cysts with the nomenclature *complex fibroadenomas*. Giant fibroadenomas are 8 cm or larger. Juvenile fibroadenomas occur in adolescents and can grow rapidly, stretch the skin, and become huge. Because juvenile fibroadenomas may grow to such a large size, they may be called giant fibroadenomas, but not all giant fibroadenomas are juvenile fibroadenomas.

On mammograms, the classic fibroadenoma is an oval or lobular equal-density mass with smooth margins. In young patients, fibroadenomas are very cellular. As the fibroadenoma ages, it may become sclerotic and less cellular. Popcornlike calcifications subsequently develop at the periphery of the mass. Eventually, the entire mass may be replaced by dense calcification and look like a "breast rock."

On ultrasound, fibroadenomas are oval, well-circumscribed homogeneous masses, usually wider than tall, with up to four gentle lobulations. They are hypoechoic but may occasionally contain cystic spaces. Posterior acoustic enhancement is increased, equal, or shadowing (Fig. 4-17). Fibroadenomas occasionally display irregular borders or heterogeneous internal characteristics, so biopsy is necessary to distinguish these atypical-appearing fibroadenomas from cancer.

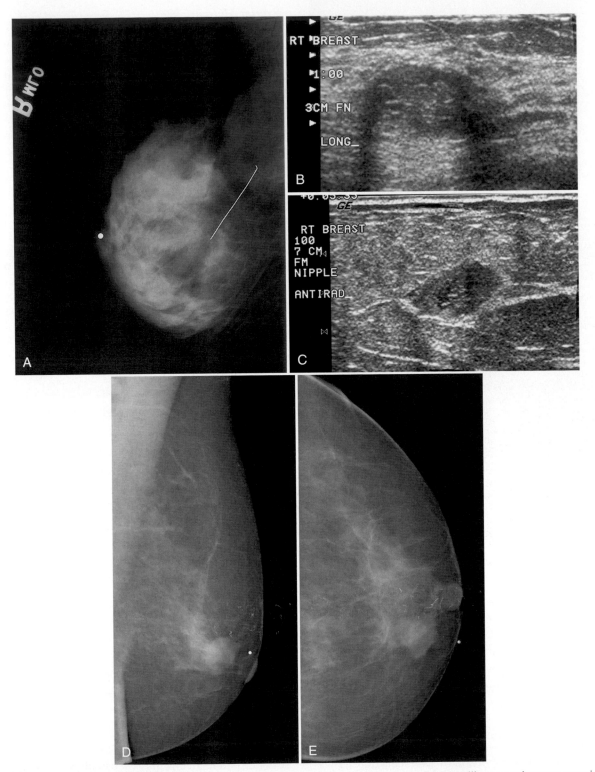

FIGURE 4-13. Mucinous cancer. **A,** A mediolateral oblique (MLO) mammogram shows dense tissue and a metallic scar marker over a previous benign biopsy site; the palpable mass is not seen. **B,** Ultrasound shows an oval solid heterogeneous mass representing the mucinous cancer. **C,** Ultrasound of another patient with mucinous cancer shows an oval heterogeneous mass containing fluid-filled spaces. Left MLO (**D**) and craniocaudal (**E**) mammograms show an equal-density lobulated mass near the nipple with the marker on it.

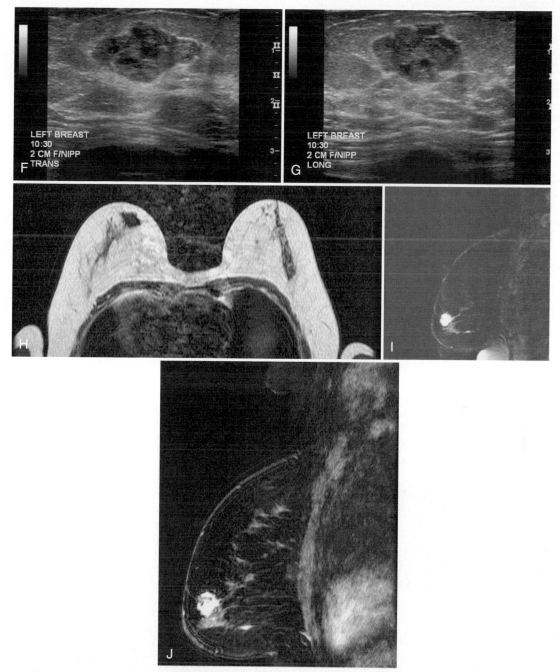

FIGURE 4-13, cont'd. On ultrasound, a microlobulated heterogeneous mass containing cystic structures is seen on transverse (**F**) and longitudinal (**G**) views, worrisome for cancer or a heterogeneous fibroadenoma. Note that the mucinous cancers often contain "cystic" spaces due to the mucin within the tumors. On magnetic resonance imaging (MRI) the axial T1-weighted noncontrast localizer (**H**) shows a low signal intensity mass against the bright fat near the nipple, corresponding to the mass seen on the mammogram and ultrasound. **I**, The unenhanced T2-weighted sagittal MRI shows a high signal intensity mass with dark septations within the mass, suggesting either fibroadenoma or mucinous cancer. **J**, The contrast-enhanced 3-D spectral-spatial excitation magnetization transfer (SSMT) sagittal image shows an irregular round mass with either dark septations or central necrosis. The irregular mass margin and thick irregular internal dark septations suggest cancer instead of fibroadenoma (in fibroadenoma the septations are thinner and regular, and the mass border is usually smooth). Core biopsy showed mucinous cancer.

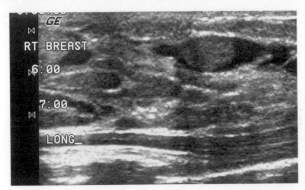

FIGURE 4-14. Papillary carcinoma. Ultrasound of a papillary cancer shows a fluid-filled dilated duct with a solid oval intraductal mass that cannot be distinguished from a benign intraductal papilloma on the scan.

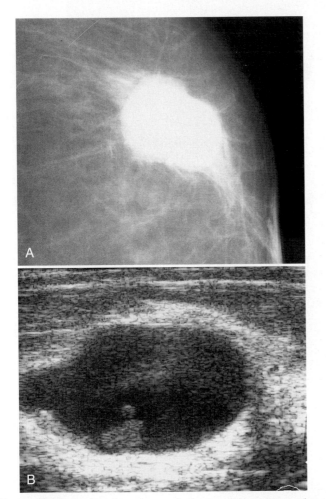

FIGURE 4-15. Intracystic carcinoma. **A,** A mammogram shows a dense oval mass. **B,** Ultrasound shows a fluid-filled cyst with an irregular mural mass. Although this mass was an intracystic carcinoma, the differential diagnosis includes papilloma or debris in a benign cyst.

Because fibroadenomas contain ductal elements, ductal or lobular carcinoma in situ occurs in fibroadenomas rarely. Any suspicious change in a fibroadenoma should prompt biopsy for this reason.

On MRI, fibroadenomas have the classic appearance of an enhancing oval or lobulated mass with well-circumscribed borders. In 20% they contain dark internal septations. Kinetic data shows a gradual initial enhancement rate and a late persistent enhancement curve. The initial enhancement rate in fibroadenomas can change from slow to rapid, depending on the phase of the woman's menstrual cycle. In premenopausal women, the initial enhancement changes from slow to rapid, as rapid as cancer, just before menses. But unlike cancer, which shows late plateau or washout curves, the late enhancement curve of a fibroadenoma is persistent. In the week or two after the onset of menses, the initial enhancement curves in fibroadenoma revert back to a gradual initial enhancement curve.

Phyllodes Tumor

Phyllodes tumors used to be called *cystosarcoma phyllodes*, which is a misnomer because most of these uncommon tumors are benign. Classically, the phyllodes tumor occurs in women in their fifth decade, with a median age of 45 years, and can be quite large, up to 5 cm in size when first detected. In the clinic, most often women with a phyllodes tumor seek advice for a rapidly growing palpable mass. Because the phyllodes tumor can have a biphasic growth pattern, some women report growth of a mass that has been stable for many years. A phyllodes tumor has both stromal and epithelial elements, in contrast to fibroadenoma. The phyllodes tumor also has fluidlike spaces containing solid growth of cellular stroma and epithelium in a leaflike configuration, from which the tumor gets its name. The preferred treatment is wide surgical excision. Incomplete excision of either benign or malignant phyllodes tumors may result in local recurrence in 15% of cases, and they may be excised again and again, only to grow back. About 25% of phyllodes tumors are malignant; 20% of the malignant subtype may metastasize. No distinguishing imaging features can be used to differentiate malignant phyllodes tumors from the more common benign form.

On mammography, a phyllodes tumor is a dense round, oval, or lobulated noncalcified mass with smooth borders. On ultrasound, a phyllodes tumor is a smoothly marginated inhomogeneous mass that occasionally contains cystic spaces producing acoustic posterior enhancement, and it can be mistaken for a fibroadenoma or circumscribed cancer (Fig. 4-18). The goal of imaging is to identify the tumor for wide excision and to search for recurrence in the biopsy bed after surgery when the patient returns for routine follow-up.

Papilloma

Papillomas are either solitary or multiple. In young patients, papillomas are called *juvenile papillomas*. Solitary papillomas are either central or peripheral, originate in the ductal epithelium, and are often seen in the subareolar region or in subareolar ducts. Tumors starting in the terminal ducts further from the nipple are called *peripheral papillomas* and are considered a risk factor for breast cancer. Multiple papillomas are usually in a more peripheral location in younger women. Juvenile papillomatosis occurs in young women, but multiple papillomas can also be seen in much older women. Papillomas grow on fibrovascular stalks, which can twist and lead to ischemia, necrosis, and blood extending into the duct. The bleeding papilloma results in the classic symptom of bloody nipple discharge, similar to a symptom of DCIS, causing patients to seek advice.

Text continued on p. 127

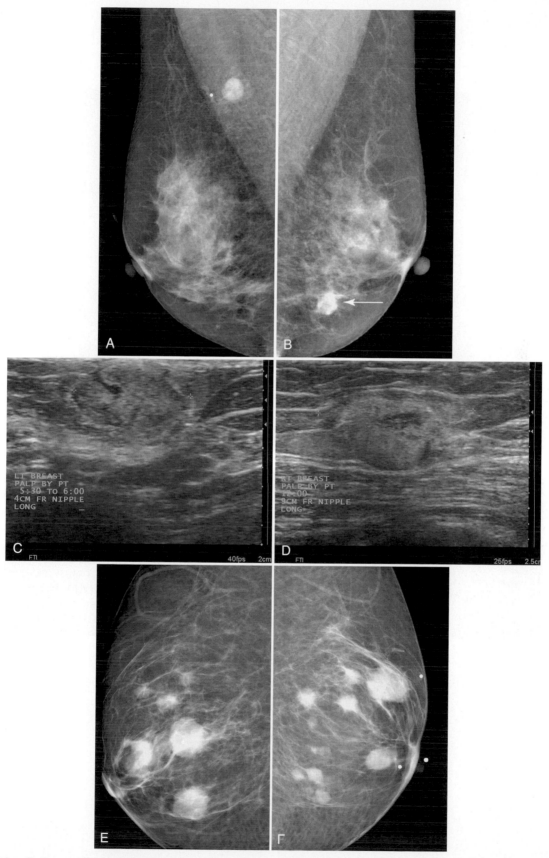

FIGURE 4-16. **A** to **D**, Breast metastases. Bilateral right (**A**) and left (**B**) mediolateral oblique (MLO) views in a patient with colon cancer show a palpable round dense mass in the right axilla with a marker on it (**A**) and a palpable round mass in the lower left breast (*arrow*) (**B**). Ultrasound on the left (**C**) and right (**D**) masses shows round echogenic but heterogeneous masses. The differential diagnosis is metastasis, primary breast cancer, or fibroadenoma. Biopsy showed metastatic colon carcinoma. Bilateral right (**E**) and left (**F**) MLO views in a patient with neuroendocrine cervical cancer show multiple dense masses in the retroareolar regions.

Continued

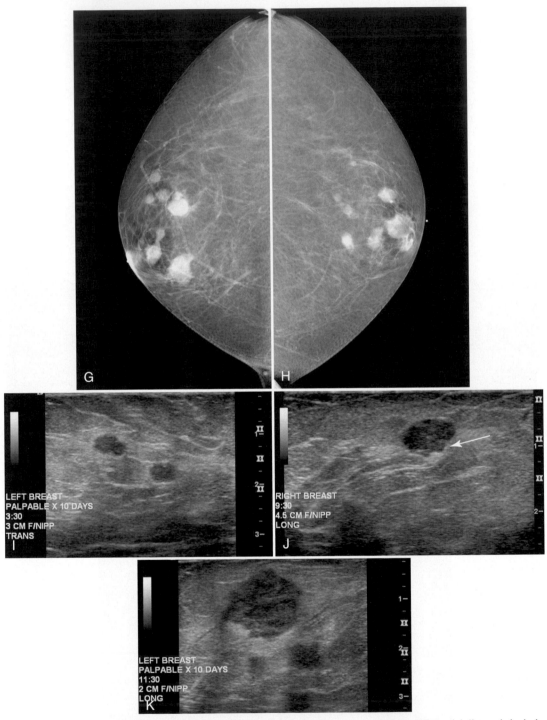

FIGURE 4-16, cont'd. The masses are also seen on the right (**G**) and left (**H**) craniocaudal views. The differential diagnosis includes multiple cysts, fibroadenomas, cancers, papillomas, and metastases. On breast ultrasound, the masses are solid; some are round or oval (**I**), but others have at least one microlobulated border (*arrow*) (**J**) or irregular borders (**K**), excluding the diagnosis of cysts or fibroadenomas. Core biopsy showed bilateral breast metastases.

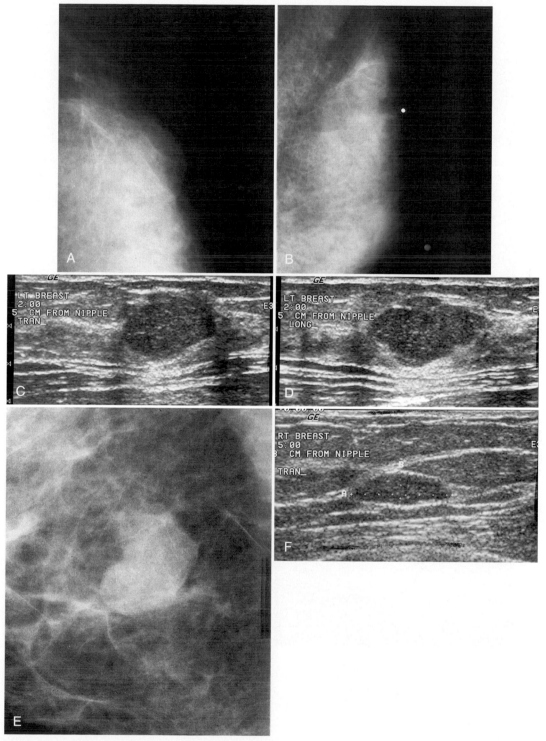

FIGURE 4-17. **A** to **F**, Biopsy-proven fibroadenomas. Magnification craniocaudal (**A**) and mediolateral oblique (**B**) views in a young woman show an equal-density, circumscribed oval mass that is hard to see against the dense tissue. Ultrasound shows an oval, lobulated, well-circumscribed homogeneous mass on transverse (**C**) and longitudinal (**D**) scans. **E**, In another patient, the mammogram shows a lobular well-circumscribed mass whose borders are partly obscured. **F**, Ultrasound shows an oval well-circumscribed homogeneous mass.

Continued

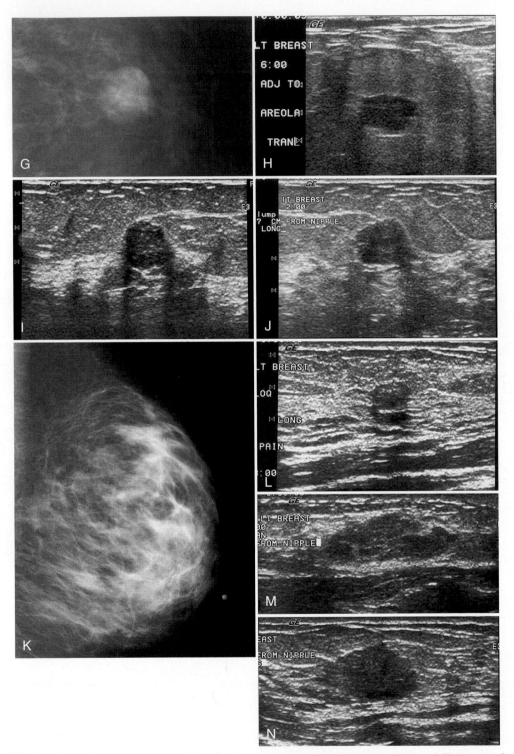

FIGURE 4-17, cont'd. Another patient has a round equal-density mass on mammogram (**G**), but on ultrasound (**H**) the mass is multilobulated and very hypoechoic, similar to cancer. **I** and **J**, Ultrasound of another atypical biopsy-proven fibroadenoma shows a taller than wide multilobulated mass with internal speckles. Another atypical palpable biopsy-proven microlobulated fibroadenoma, seen on the mammogram in the lower part of the breast (**K**) and on ultrasound (**L**). **M** and **N**, Other atypical appearances of biopsy-proven fibroadenoma on ultrasound.

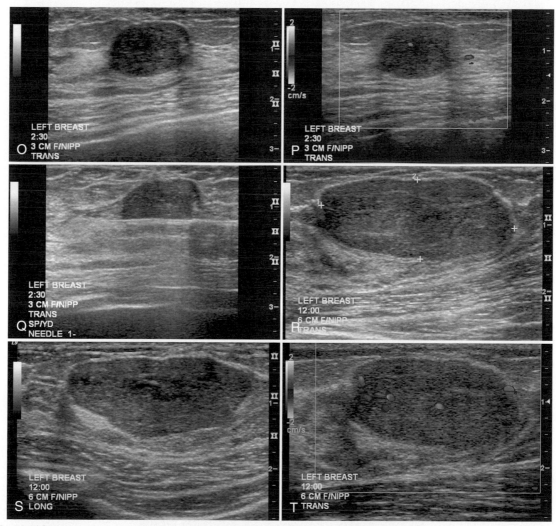

FIGURE 4-17, cont'd. **O** to **Q,** Ultrasound of a typical fibroadenoma. **O,** Ultrasound of a palpable mass in a young woman shows a typical well-circumscribed homogeneous mass suggestive of fibroadenoma. **P,** Doppler ultrasound shows vascularity within the fibroadenoma. **Q,** Image of the needle during ultrasound-guided core biopsy. Pathology showed fibroadenoma. **R** to **T,** Ultrasound of a complex fibroadenoma. Ultrasound of a palpable mass in a young patient shows a well-circumscribed oval solid mass with bright linear septa and a slightly hypoechoic central area in transverse (**R**) and longitudinal (**S**) images. The mass has five gentle lobulations on the longitudinal scan and an area of central hypoechogenicity. **T,** Color Doppler ultrasound shows flow within the mass. Biopsy was done because of the central hypoechogenicity and five lobulations. Biopsy showed fibroadenoma.

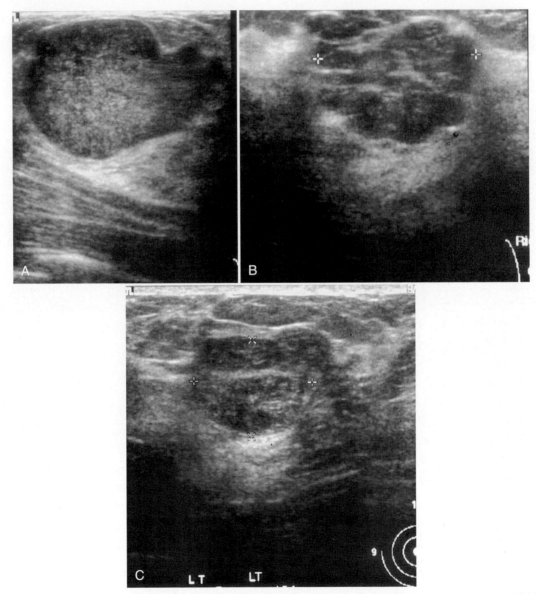

FIGURE 4-18. Phyllodes tumors. A to C, Ultrasound of three separate phyllodes tumors in a young woman shows palpable solid lobulated masses, two of which are circumscribed and lobulated. One is heterogeneous and slightly suggestive of cancer.

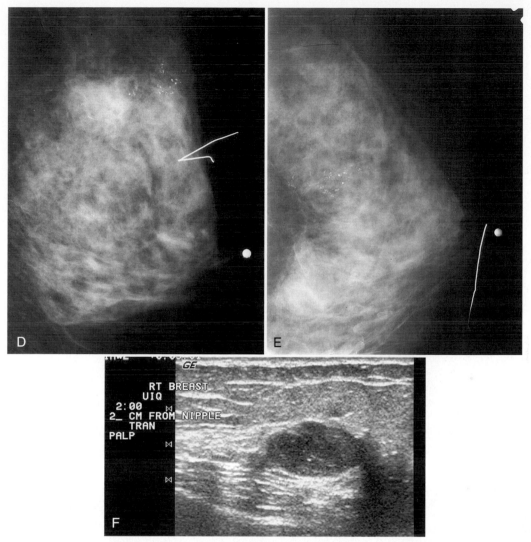

FIGURE 4-18, cont'd. In another patient with a phyllodes tumor, lateral (**D**) and craniocaudal (**E**) mammograms show a dense circumscribed mass and a separate cluster of pleomorphic calcifications. Note metallic scar markers showing a previous biopsy site. **F,** Ultrasound reveals a lobulated circumscribed hypoechoic mass that was removed by excisional biopsy; examination of the specimen showed a phyllodes tumor and calcifications in benign ducts.

Clinically, papillomas can also cause new, spontaneous clear or serous nipple discharge. Papillomas are usually excised to exclude DCIS or papillary cancer.

On mammography, papillomas are round, well-circumscribed, equal-density masses that occasionally contain calcifications. They are usually located in the subareolar region. In papillomatosis, papillomas can be multiple and peripherally located (Fig. 4-19). Occasionally, papillomas are not seen on mammography or ultrasound at all despite the symptom of bloody or clear nipple discharge. On ultrasound, papillomas are solid round, oval, or microlobulated hypoechoic masses. Small internal cystic spaces are seen occasionally in juvenile papillomatosis. In patients with nipple discharge, ultrasound may show papilloma as a solid mass in a fluid-filled subareolar duct. On galactography, the papilloma produces an intraductal filling defect.

On MRI, papillomas are round enhancing masses, with a rapid initial rise and a late plateau as washout on kinetic curves, indistinguishable from invasive ductal cancers. Bright T2-weighted signal in ducts on precontrast studies,

when seen, represents fluid-filled ducts. If a papilloma is present, the high signal in the duct may obscure an enhancing papilloma within it.

The finding of a round solid mass suspected to be papilloma requires a histologic diagnosis. Follow-up for papillomas diagnosed by core biopsy is controversial. However, surgical excisional biopsy is universally advised for papillomas with papillary carcinoma, atypia, or nonconcordant imaging findings. Surgical excisional biopsy for papillomas without atypia or malignancy diagnosed by core biopsy is variable, but many investigators recommend excision.

Lactating Adenoma

Occurring in young pregnant patients in the second or third trimester, lactating adenomas are solid well-circumscribed masses that can enlarge rapidly during pregnancy. Patients seek clinical evaluation because of a growing palpable mass not previously felt. On ultrasound, a lactating adenoma is oval or lobular, smoothly marginated, and can contain cystic or necrotic spaces; biopsy by

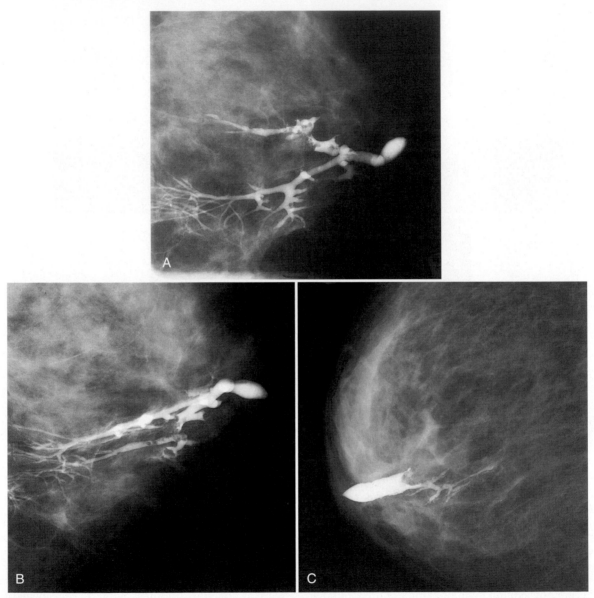

FIGURE 4-19. Papillomas. Craniocaudal (CC) (**A**) and mediolateral (**B**) magnification views of a galactogram show an irregular microlobulated filling defect from a papilloma. **C,** A galactogram in another patient shows a papilloma as a smooth filling defect obstructing a dilated duct.

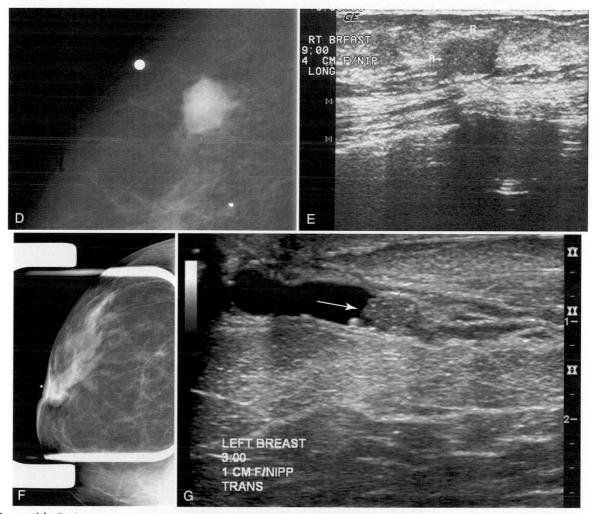

FIGURE 4-19, cont'd. **D,** A mammogram in another patient shows a palpable round irregular mass with calcifications. **E,** Ultrasound shows a circumscribed oval homogeneous mass. Biopsy revealed intraductal papilloma with apocrine atypia. **F,** In another patient with nipple discharge and a marker on the nipple, CC spot mammogram shows dilated ducts, a possible mass in the retroareolar region, and scattered benign-appearing calcifications. Ultrasound shows an intraductal mass in a fluid-filled duct in transverse **(G)** and longitudinal **(H)** images (*arrows*). The differential diagnosis includes papilloma, papillary cancer, and ductal carcinoma in situ. Biopsy showed papilloma.   *Continued*

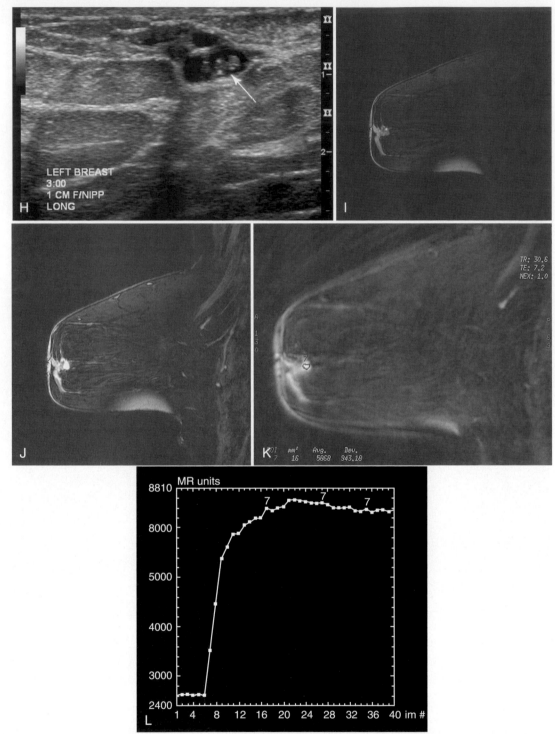

FIGURE 4-19, cont'd. I to L, Papilloma on magnetic resonance imaging (MRI). **I,** Noncontrast T1-weighted fat-suppressed sagittal MRI of the mass seen in parts **F** to **H** shows high precontrast signal intensity in a dot in the retroareolar region on the right, which may represent debris in the fluid-filled duct. **J,** Postcontrast 3-D spectral-spatial excitation magnetization transfer (SSMT) sagittal MRI shows an enhancing mass in the retroareolar region. **K,** Spiral dynamic sagittal MRI with an ROI over the enhancing mass; the corresponding kinetic curve (**L**) shows that the mass has a rapid initial enhancement curve and washout. The MRI findings are compatible with either invasive ductal cancer or a papilloma. Biopsy showed papilloma.

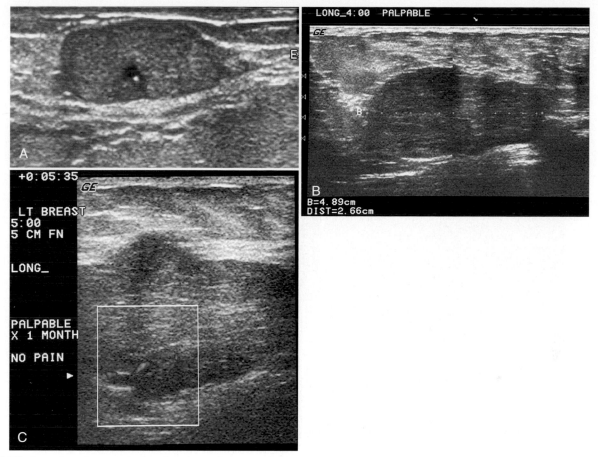

FIGURE 4-20. Lactating adenoma. **A,** A periareolar, well-circumscribed mass containing one calcification in a 7-month-pregnant woman grew in the previous few weeks and was confirmed to be a lactating adenoma on biopsy. **B,** A 4.8-cm heterogeneous lobulated oval mass in another pregnant patient. **C,** It is seen to contain blood vessels within the lactating adenoma on Doppler ultrasonography.

either fine-needle aspiration or core needle biopsy is used to evaluate it (Fig. 4-20). The mass may regress in size in the postpartum period.

Adenoid Cystic Carcinoma

A very rare tumor that clinically manifests as a palpable firm mass, the adenoid cystic carcinoma has a mixture of glandular and stromal elements that infiltrate the normal fibroglandular tissue in approximately 50% of cases. The tumor has a good prognosis if completely resected; however, recurrence is possible if the mass is not entirely excised. Imaging characteristics vary because of the rarity of reported cases and range from a well-circumscribed lobulated mass to ill-defined masses or focal asymmetric densities.

■ SOLID MASSES WITH INDISTINCT MARGINS (Box 4-13)

Invasive Ductal Cancer

On mammography, the indistinct margins of invasive ductal cancer are due to infiltration of the surrounding glandular tissue by tumor. The mass margin can appear unsharp or smudged, similar to a line partially erased by a pencil eraser. The indistinct margin is best seen on spot magnification views against a fatty background. On ultra-

---

BOX 4-13. Solid Masses with Indistinct Margins

Invasive ductal cancer
Invasive lobular carcinoma
Primary or secondary non-Hodgkin lymphoma
Breast sarcoma
Squamous cell carcinoma
Focal fibrosis
Pseudoangiomatous stromal hyperplasia

---

sound, the indistinct tumor mass occasionally has an echogenic rim or halo that suggests the diagnosis (Fig. 4-21).

Invasive Lobular Carcinoma

Often seen on only one view, lobular carcinoma may appear as an indistinct mass without microcalcifications. A more typical appearance of invasive lobular carcinoma is a spiculated mass or architectural distortion without calcifications.

Sarcoma

Breast sarcomas are rare. Typically, they contain malignant stromal elements but, on occasion, may contain fibrous

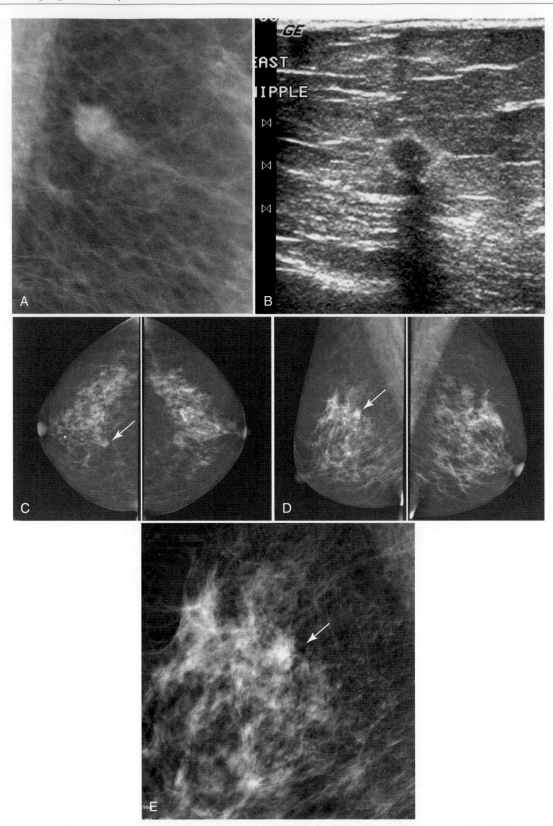

FIGURE 4-21. **A** and **B,** Indistinct invasive ductal cancer. **A,** Mammography shows a round mass with indistinct margins and an upper partly spiculated border displayed against a fatty background. **B,** Ultrasound shows a round, irregular mass with a thick echogenic halo. **C** to **E,** Indistinct invasive ductal cancer. **C,** Craniocaudal (CC) paired mammograms show a focal asymmetry in the medial right breast (*arrow*). **D,** Paired mediolateral oblique mammograms show a focal asymmetry in the upper right breast corresponding to the finding on the CC mammogram (*arrow*). **E,** Photographic magnification shows an indistinct mass representing invasive ductal cancer (*arrow*).

elements, seen in the rare fibrosarcoma. Even more rarely, a breast sarcoma contains osseous elements and bone. As in invasive ductal cancer, these tumors are usually solid masses with ill-defined margins on both mammography and ultrasound.

Lymphoma

Lymphoma can involve breast lymph nodes or can occur as a primary or secondary site in the breast parenchyma. Lymphadenopathy is the most common appearance of lymphoma involving the breast and is seen on the mammogram as large dense lymph nodes in the axilla that have

lost their fatty hila and become bigger and rounder (Fig. 4-22A). Primary or secondary breast lymphoma is usually caused by non-Hodgkin lymphomatous infiltration into breast tissue and not into a lymph node. It is a rare cause of an ill-defined mass that looks just like invasive ductal cancer on mammography (see Fig. 4-22B to F). The borders of the mass are indistinct because of lymphomatous infiltration into the surrounding glandular tissue, but it can occasionally be well-circumscribed or lobulated. On ultrasound, primary or secondary breast lymphomas in the breast tissue appear as hypoechoic masses.

Without a diagnosis of lymphoma elsewhere in the body, the diagnosis of primary breast lymphoma is often

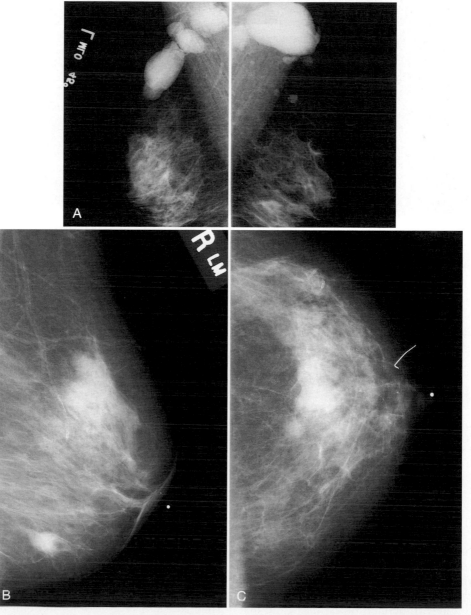

FIGURE 4-22. Breast lymphoma involving the axillary lymph nodes. **A,** Bilateral mediolateral oblique mammograms show large dense masses in each axilla representing lymphadenopathy from lymphoma. Bilateral lymphadenopathy suggests systemic disease, such as lymphoma, leukemia, metastatic disease, systemic infection, or collagen vascular disease. Primary breast lymphoma in another patient appears as an equal-density, ill-defined mass in the lower part of the breast on lateral medial (**B**) and craniocaudal (CC) (**C**) mammograms in breast tissue that is indistinguishable from breast cancer. Note the linear scar marker showing a previous biopsy site.

Continued

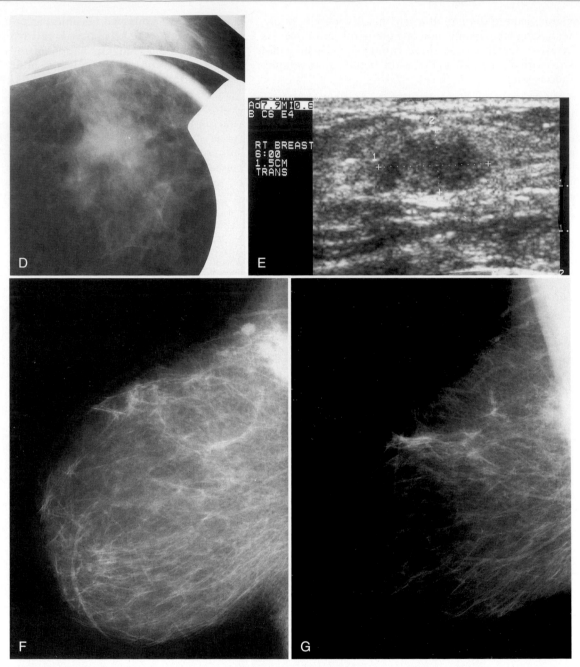

FIGURE 4-22, cont'd. D, Craniocaudal spot compression shows that the mass persists. **E,** Ultrasound reveals a hypoechoic mass. Primary breast lymphoma in another patient appearing as an ill-defined mass near the chest wall on craniocaudal (**F**) and mediolateral (**G**) mammograms is less distinct and less dense than the lymphoma that appears more mas7slike in parts **B** to **D.**

unsuspected until percutaneous biopsy is performed on the breast mass prompting the investigation. Primary breast lymphoma is treated by chemotherapy and radiation therapy, not by surgical excisional biopsy, thus distinguishing its treatment from that of breast cancer. If a patient has a primary diagnosis of lymphoma elsewhere in the body and presents with a new ill-defined breast mass, the first and foremost diagnosis for the breast mass should be primary breast cancer, with a secondary but important differential diagnosis of breast lymphoma. Because breast cancer and lymphoma of the breast are treated differently,

fine-needle or core biopsy should be done to establish a diagnosis and determine patient management.

Pseudoangiomatous Stromal Hyperplasia

Pseudoangiomatous stromal hyperplasia (PASH) is a rare benign cause of a growing ill-defined noncalcified round or oval mass. It occurs in premenopausal women or in postmenopausal women receiving exogenous hormone therapy (Fig. 4-23). Occasionally, the mass may be well-circumscribed. This entity is of unknown etiology and is

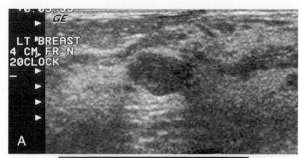

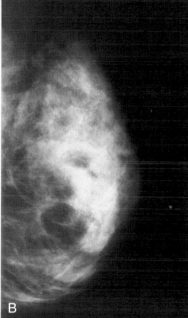

FIGURE 4-23. Pseudoangiomatous stromal hyperplasia (PASH). **A,** This solid oval mass on ultrasound in an older woman looks like fibroadenoma or cancer but proved to be PASH on biopsy. **B,** In another patient, biopsy-proven PASH was discovered on the mammogram as a dense, partly obscured mass in the midportion of the breast, and a biopsy of the mass was performed.

composed of stromal and epithelial proliferation; it occasionally shows rapid growth on mammography and requires biopsy. On ultrasound, PASH is a mixed or hypoechoic mass with ill-defined borders in 62%, as reported by Wieman and colleagues. It is thought that there is a hormonal influence on its development, and PASH is more often seen in premenopausal women or postmenopausal women receiving hormone therapy. Fine-needle aspiration can be inconclusive, as can core needle biopsy. Because low-grade angiosarcoma can mimic PASH on core biopsy, excisional biopsy is recommended if the mass grows.

Squamous Cell Carcinoma

Squamous cell tumors are even rarer than adenoid cystic carcinoma and produce a large, round, noncalcified, ill-defined mass. Other reports describe well-defined masses. On ultrasound, the masses are hypoechoic, with some reports describing central cystic spaces. They are located in breast tissue and are not found near the skin. The diagnosis of a primary squamous cell carcinoma should be established after the exclusion of the possibility of

metastasis from another site, such as either a primary skin cancer or cancer at a distant site such as cervical carcinoma.

■ MASSES CONTAINING FAT
(Box 4-14)

Lymph Nodes

The lymph nodes are typically seen in the axilla. They are round or oval and contain a radiolucent fatty center. Benign lymph nodes may be of any size, have a smooth solid cortex, and contain a fatty hilum (Fig. 4-24). An intramammary lymph node has the same appearance as lymph nodes in the axilla; it is often located in the upper outer quadrant of the breast along blood vessels and should not be mistaken for a malignancy. In questionable cases, spot magnification views demonstrate a well-circumscribed oval or lobulated mass and, importantly, its fatty hilum. On breast ultrasound, the lymph node is hypoechoic and bean-shaped and contains a fatty center. On color Doppler ultrasound, the lymph node hilum or fatty center will contain a pulsating blood vessel (see Fig. 4-24D). On MRI, the lymph node kinetics show rapid initial enhancement with late washout, similar to cancer, due to its central blood vessel. However, its typical appearance on MRI, which shows a solid mass with the fatty hilum and high signal on T2-weighted images, should distinguish it from cancer, which has no fatty hilum and commonly has low signal on T2-weighted images.

Hamartoma

This entity, also known as a *fibroadenolipoma*, is a benign mass that contains fat and other elements found in the breast. On physical examination, a hamartoma may not be felt distinctly if it contains mostly fat and glandular tissue. The classic appearance is that of an oval mass containing fat and fibroglandular tissue with a thin capsule or rim, the "breast within a breast" appearance (Fig. 4-25). Breast hamartomas have a variable appearance, depending on the amount of fat and stromal elements that they contain. On occasion, a hamartoma may have mostly stromal and glandular elements and appear as a dense mass rather than one containing mostly fat and glandular elements (Fig. 4-26). Because cancer can develop in breast elements and ducts, cancer can develop in hamartomas. Biopsy should be performed on hamartomas if suspicious microcalcifications are

---

BOX 4-14. Differential Diagnosis of Masses Containing Fat

Lymph node
Hamartoma
Oil cyst
Lipoma
Liposarcoma
Steatocystoma multiplex
Galactocele (rarely seen fat/fluid level on upright mammogram)

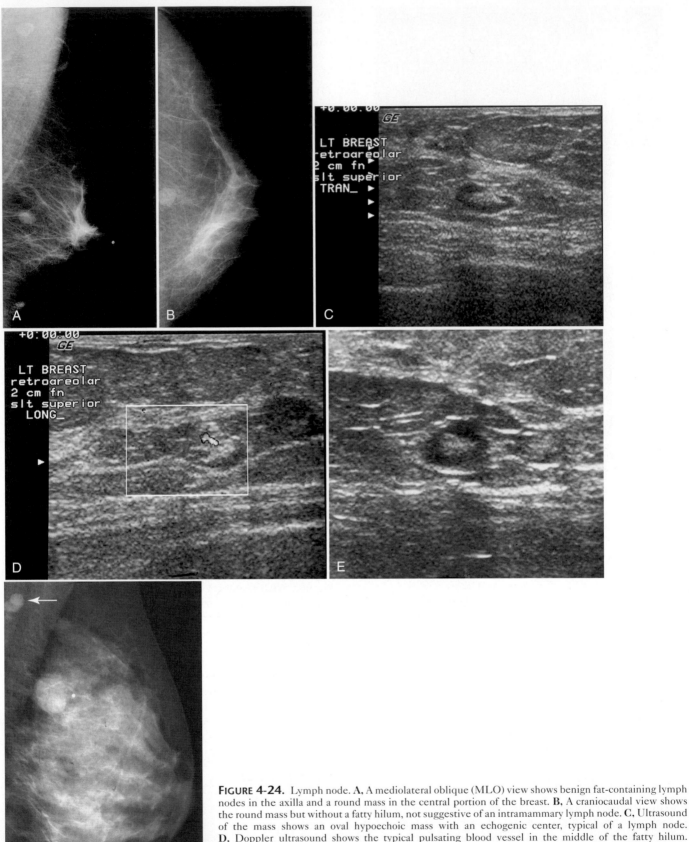

FIGURE 4-24. Lymph node. **A,** A mediolateral oblique (MLO) view shows benign fat-containing lymph nodes in the axilla and a round mass in the central portion of the breast. **B,** A craniocaudal view shows the round mass but without a fatty hilum, not suggestive of an intramammary lymph node. **C,** Ultrasound of the mass shows an oval hypoechoic mass with an echogenic center, typical of a lymph node. **D,** Doppler ultrasound shows the typical pulsating blood vessel in the middle of the fatty hilum. **E,** Ultrasound shows a typical lymph node in the axilla of the same breast. **F,** Lymphadenopathy and cancer. MLO mammogram with the marker on a round cancer in the upper left breast shows an abnormal round, dense lymph node in the axilla overlying the pectoralis muscle (*arrow*). Note the abnormal lymph node that has lost most of its fatty hilum, compared to the normal axillary lymph node overlying the pectoralis muscle in the same location in part **A.**

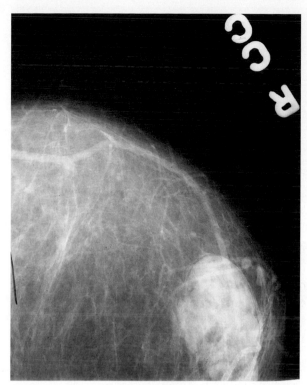

FIGURE 4-25. Typical hamartoma. A mammogram shows an oval mass containing fat and fibroglandular elements typical of a hamartoma. On breast physical examination, the mass was difficult to feel despite its large size.

developing within it. Otherwise, a classic "breast within a breast" hamartoma is benign and should be left alone.

Oil Cyst

An oil cyst is a sequela of fat necrosis after blunt trauma or surgery. A benign oil cyst is a radiolucent oval or round mass containing fatty fluid with a thin radiodense rim (Fig. 4-27). Oil cysts may subsequently calcify and result in eggshell-type calcifications. On ultrasound, oil cysts are round or oval and contain liquefied fat that is usually hypoechoic or isoechoic. The oil cyst is benign and is one of the "don't touch" lesions that should be left alone.

Lipoma

Breast lipomas are similar to lipomas elsewhere in the body. They produce a soft mass or a mass that may not be felt at all. On mammography, a lipoma is a fatty mass containing a radiolucent center that may have a distinguishable thin discrete rim separating it from the surrounding glandular tissue. Unlike a post-traumatic oil cyst, a lipoma never calcifies. Typically, a lipoma is discovered because the patient feels a mass. If a technologist places a skin marker over the palpable lipoma, a spot compression view of the mass shows only fat (Fig. 4-28). Ultrasound of a lipoma shows only fatty tissue in a well-circumscribed oval or round mass. Lipomas are benign and should be left alone.

Liposarcoma

Liposarcoma is the only fat-containing malignancy and is extremely rare. A fat-containing, but rapidly growing mass should raise suspicion of the rare liposarcoma.

Steatocystoma Multiplex

This is a rare, autosomal dominantly inherited condition that is characterized by multiple and extensive intradermal oil cysts bilaterally. The oil cysts may be palpable or non-palpable. Mammography shows extensive bilateral well-circumscribed radiolucent masses with a typical appearance of oil cysts, but unlike post-traumatic intraparenchymal oil cysts, the oil cysts in steatocystoma multiplex are intradermal in location, innumerable, and bilateral without a history of trauma. In 40% of affected patients, a typical family history of steatocystoma multiplex confirms the diagnosis.

■ FLUID-CONTAINING MASSES
(Box 4-15)

Cyst

A simple cyst occurs in 10% of all women and is frequently seen in women receiving exogenous hormone replacement therapy. Caused by obstruction and dilatation of the terminal ducts with fluid trapped within them, a cyst can enlarge with the patient's menstrual cycle and decrease after the onset of menses. Cysts may be asymptomatic or may become painful and produce a palpable lump. They may be single or multiple, and they can regress or grow spontaneously and rapidly.

Because cysts often produce a palpable mass, they are a frequent cause of symptoms for which patients seek advice. On mammography, cysts are round or oval, well-circumscribed, and are low-density or equal in density to fibroglandular tissue. Spot compression magnification will show an equal-density or low-density mass with a sharply marginated border where they are not obscured by adjacent dense glandular tissue.

Breast ultrasound shows an anechoic mass with imperceptible walls, a sharp back wall, and enhanced posterior transmission of sound (Fig. 4-29). Cysts may have internal echoes as a result of debris. Cysts may be left alone (Box 4-16) or can be aspirated by palpation or under ultrasound guidance if symptomatic, but they have no malignant potential. If a cyst is causing a palpable mass, the palpable finding should resolve after cyst aspiration. On MRI cysts

---

BOX 4-15. Differential Diagnosis of Fluid-Containing Masses

Cyst
Necrotic cancer
Hematoma
Intracystic carcinoma
Intracystic papilloma
Abscess
Galactocele
Seroma

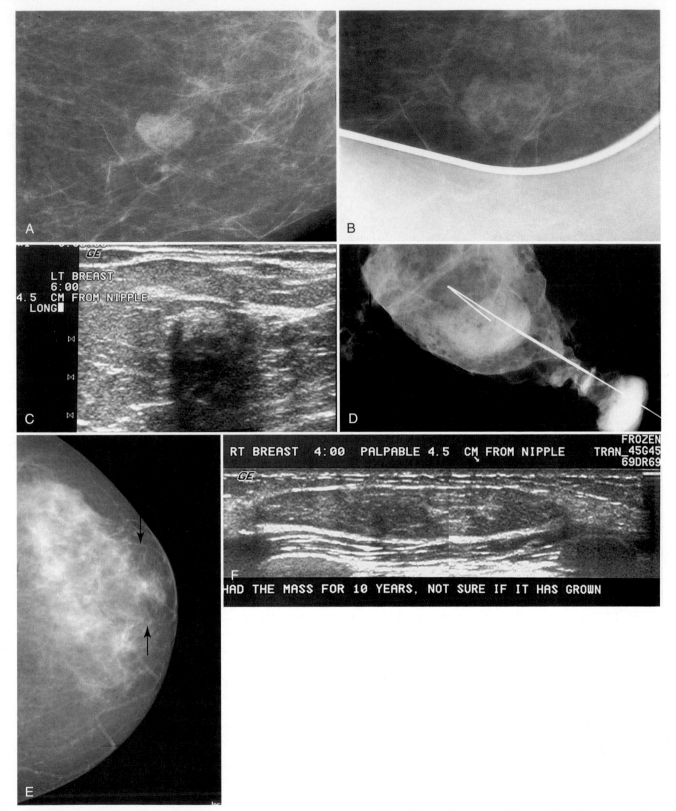

FIGURE 4-26. Typical hamartomas. Hamartomas may have a variable appearance, depending on the amount of fat and glandular elements that they contain. **A,** A mammogram reveals a lobular, partly circumscribed, partly indistinct mass that may contain fat. **B,** A spot magnification view shows the mass to better advantage. **C,** Ultrasound shows a partly echogenic, partly hypoechoic shadowing mass. **D,** A specimen radiograph confirms that the hamartoma contains fat. Note the localizing hookwire. **E,** In another patient, the hamartoma is an oval mass containing fat and fibroglandular elements with a thin capsule near the anterior portion of the breast (*arrows*); it has an oval shape on ultrasound (**F**).

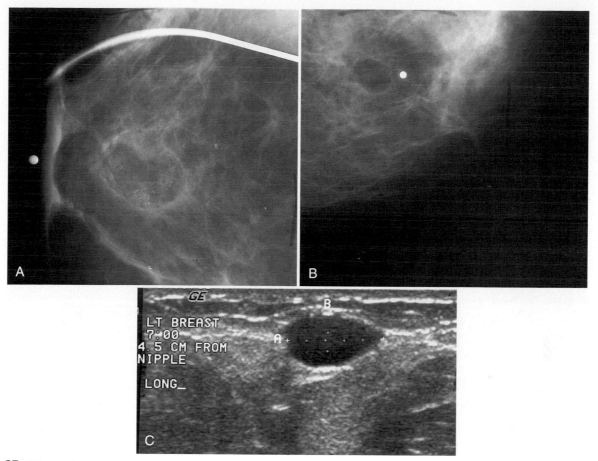

FIGURE 4-27. Oil cyst. **A,** A spot compression magnification view shows a thin-walled mass with a radiolucent center and faint calcifications along its rim in the area of a previous biopsy. **B,** In another patient, a palpable oil cyst is marked by a skin marker and is seen as a fat-containing thin-walled mass. **C,** Ultrasound shows a hypoechoic, oval, well-circumscribed mass.

BOX 4-16. Benign Masses That Should be Left Alone

Simple cyst
Benign postbiopsy scar
Lymph node
Hamartoma
Oil cyst
Lipoma
Hematoma
Seroma
Sebaceous cysts
Galactocele

---

have a high T2-weighted signal and show no enhancement. Occasionally inflamed cysts show rim enhancement and can be a cause of a false-positive MRI. However, the bright T2-weighted signal, no enhancement after contrast injection, and a thin rim should differentiate the inflamed cyst from cancer.

Hematoma/Seroma

Breast hematomas and seromas occur after biopsy or trauma, and their diagnosis is established by correlating the hematoma/seroma to the clinical history. On mammography, a hematoma has an irregular or ill-defined border and may be high-density or equal density (Fig. 4-30). In the acute phase, surrounding hemorrhage may obscure hematomas. A hematoma will become smaller with time as the blood resorbs. Initially on ultrasound, a hematoma is a fluid-filled mass. Later, as the hematoma evolves, ultrasound shows that the previously hypoechoic blood-filled mass changes to serous fluid. Subsequently, the seroma may contain thin movable septa that move on real-time ultrasound, or it may contain debris or fluid/fluid levels.

Necrotic Cancer

Cancers with central necrosis may contain fluid. In general, necrotic tumors usually have a thick, irregular solid rim, thus distinguishing it from a thin-walled simple or complex cyst.

Intracystic Carcinoma

See the section "Solid Masses with Rounded or Expansile Borders" in this chapter.

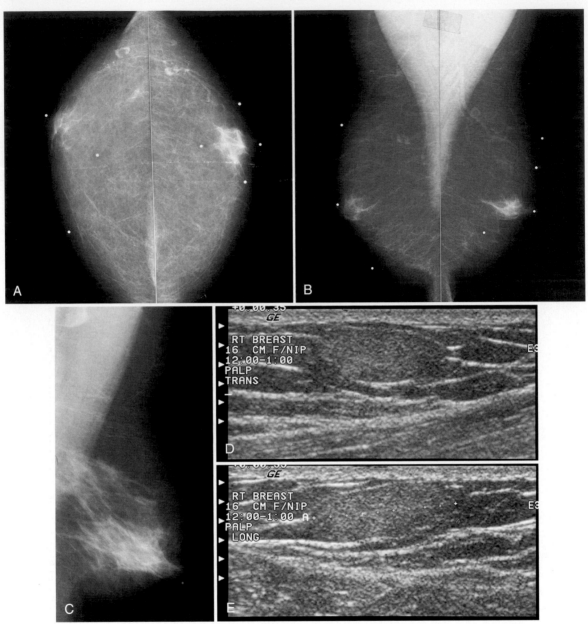

FIGURE 4-28. Lipomas. **A,** Craniocaudal and **B,** mediolateral oblique (MLO) mammograms show markers over palpable masses where only fat is present. **C,** In another patient, the palpable lipoma is not seen high in the breast on the MLO view where only fat is present, but ultrasound (**D** and **E**) shows a hypoechoic fatty mass corresponding to the palpable finding that proved to be a lipoma on excisional biopsy. Note that the lipoma blends into the surrounding fat and is seen only with the calipers.

Intracystic Papilloma

This tumor is also rare and appears as a round mass on mammography. On ultrasound, an intracystic papilloma is a solid mural nodule or mass in a round fluid-filled mass, with a similar appearance to that of the rare intracystic carcinoma.

Abscess

A breast abscess occurs after mastitis. *Staphylococcus aureus* or *Streptococcus* is the usual pathogen in abscess. In a nursing mother, the infection develops as a result of bacterial entry through a cracked nipple. In teenagers, infection may occur during sexual contact. In older women, those who are diabetic or immunocompromised are especially at risk for mastitis and abscess. Typically, an abscess is a painful hard mass that is tender to touch, with overlying red, edematous skin and surrounding cellulitis.

On mammography, an abscess is usually subareolar, appears as a dense or equal-density noncalcified irregular mass with focal or diffuse skin thickening, and may be obscured by surrounding breast edema.

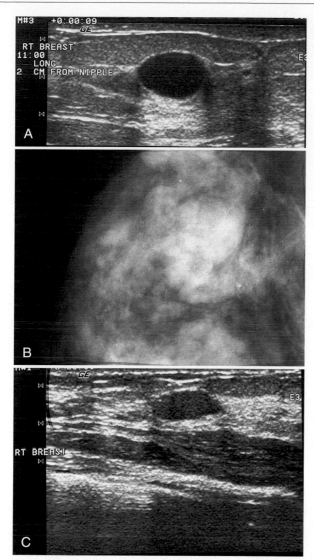

FIGURE 4-29. Cyst on ultrasound. **A,** A well-circumscribed anechoic mass with an imperceptible back wall and enhanced transmission of sound is a simple cyst and needs no further follow-up unless it is symptomatic. **B,** In another patient, a mammogram shows multiple round circumscribed, partly obscured, equal-density masses representing cysts. **C,** Notice that on the ultrasound this complex cyst had debris within it and could not be distinguished from a solid mass until aspiration.

On ultrasound, an abscess is an irregular fluid-filled mass occasionally containing debris or septations (Fig. 4-31). The surrounding edema blurs the normal adjacent breast structures, makes the adjacent fat gray, and causes skin thickening. A breast abscess usually does not contain air. Bright echoes or specular reflectors may represent air in the abscess after attempted drainage.

Treatment involves antibiotic therapy and drainage of the abscess by either percutaneous or surgical methods. Surgery usually involves incision and debridement, leaving the abscess cavity open to heal by granulomatous formation by second intention. Percutaneous needle aspiration without catheter placement is usually unsuccessful as the only method of drainage if the abscess is large (>2.4 to 3 cm) or septated, or if incompletely drained pockets are left in the surrounding breast tissue. In these cases,

percutaneous needle drainage without an indwelling catheter may be palliative. Women with a chronic subareolar abscess caused by chronic duct obstruction are in a special category and require duct excision as well as abscess treatment. The chronic subareolar abscess may have an adjacent skin fistula. The abscess requires excision of the fistula as well as incision and debridement of the abscess.

Sebaceous and Epidermal Inclusion Cysts

Sebaceous cysts are not cysts at all, but result from keratin accumulation in plugged ducts. Sebaceous cysts have an epithelial cell lining from the sebaceous gland, whereas epidermal cysts have a true epidermal cell lining and no sebaceous glands. Because they have almost no malignant potential, biopsy is not required unless the patient desires removal.

Clinically, sebaceous cysts can produce a palpable mass, a "blackhead" that when squeezed will yield cheesy yellow or white material. On mammography, sebaceous and epidermal inclusion cysts are identical, with subcutaneous oval or round well-defined masses that are often overexposed because of their location near the skin surface; they occasionally contain calcifications (Fig. 4-32A to C). Ultrasound shows an oval, well-circumscribed, hypoechoic or anechoic mass in a subcutaneous location with a little tail extending into the skin, representing the dilated hair follicle (see Fig. 4-32D to F).

Displacement of epidermal fragments from the skin surface to locations deep within the breast parenchyma cause epidermal inclusion cysts after percutaneous biopsy or surgery. The epidermal inclusion cyst produces a round or oval mass located within breast tissue far away from the skin surface. Because epidermal inclusion cysts have an epithelial lining, they can produce a growing mass on the mammogram as a result of accumulating inspissated material within them. Because they cause a growing solid mass, the epidermal inclusion cyst often requires biopsy to exclude cancer.

Galactocele

Typically seen in lactating women, a galactocele represents a focal collection of breast milk that occasionally causes a palpable mass. On mammography, a galactocele is a low- or equal-density, oval or round, well-circumscribed mass (Fig. 4-33A and C), but it can be of higher density, depending on resorption of its fluid contents and the residual solid component. On an upright mammogram, a classic, but rarely seen finding of a fat/fluid level in the mass represents fat rising to the top of the galactocele while the other milk components layer dependently below. On ultrasound, a galactocele may look like a well-defined hypoechoic cyst-like mass. Galactoceles containing more solid elements simulate a solid mass that occasionally displays posterior acoustic shadowing (see Fig. 4-33B and D). On aspiration, milky fluid will be obtained. Atypical galactoceles with a round or irregular shape, nonparallel orientation, indistinct or microlobulated noncircumscribed margin, but with a relatively sharp convex anterior or posterior echogenic rim, requiring biopsy, have been reported by Kim and colleagues.

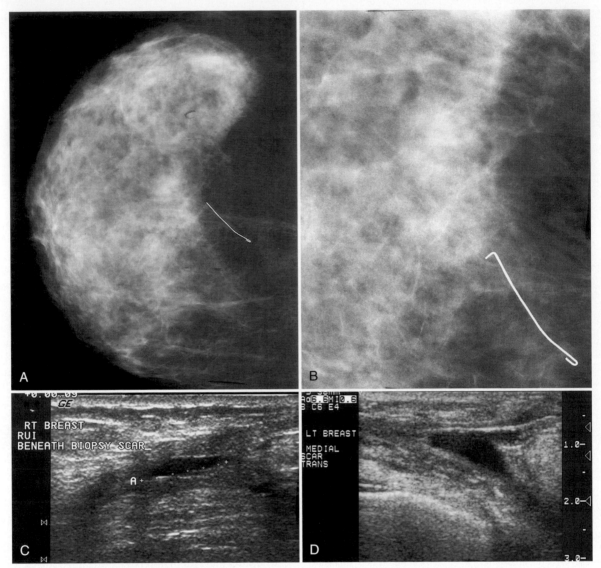

FIGURE 4-30. Hematoma/seroma. A mammogram shows a density near a linear metallic scar marker 5 months after biopsy of a benign tumor that is hard to see on the craniocaudal mammogram (**A**) but easier to see on the magnification view (**B**). **C,** Ultrasound shows a fluid-filled biopsy cavity with healing hypoechoic breast tissue surrounding it. **D,** Ultrasound of another biopsy cavity shows a V-shaped fluid-filled cavity, with the upper portion of the V representing fluid tracking along the incision toward the skin.

▬ KEY ELEMENTS

A mass is a three-dimensional object seen on at least two mammographic projections.

On mammography, the mass repeat includes a description of the shape, margins, density, location, the mass's associated findings, and how it has changed if previously present.

Mass shapes are round, oval, lobular, and irregular, with the probability of cancer increasing with increasing irregularity of the shape.

Mass margins are circumscribed, microlobulated, obscured, indistinct, or spiculated, with the probability of cancer increasing with increasing spiculation of the margin.

Fat-containing masses are almost never malignant.

Mass density is lower, equal to, or higher than an equal amount of fibroglandular tissue. High-density masses are suspicious for cancer.

The differential diagnosis for spiculated masses includes invasive ductal cancer, invasive lobular cancer, tubular cancer, postbiopsy scar, radial scar, fat necrosis, and sclerosing adenosis.

To determine whether a spiculated mass represents a postbiopsy scar, correlate the postbiopsy mammogram with the prebiopsy study showing where the finding was removed.

Spiculated masses that do not represent postbiopsy scars should undergo biopsy to exclude cancer.

Radial scars cannot be distinguished from spiculated breast cancer on mammography.

Invasive lobular cancer accounts for approximately 10% of all cancers but is one of the hardest to see on mammography because of its single-file cellular growth pattern.

The differential diagnosis for solid masses with round or expansile borders includes fibroadenoma, cancer, phyllodes tumor, papilloma, lactating adenoma, tubular

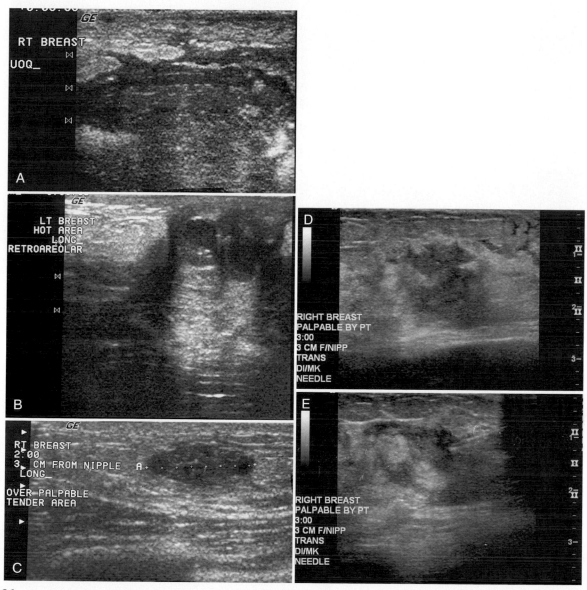

Figure 4-31. A to C, Abscesses. **A,** Ultrasound shows an irregular heterogeneous mass with extensions of fluid into tissue. Notice the thickened skin and indistinctness of the surrounding breast tissue structures from cellulitis. **B,** In another patient, two hot retroareolar, painful, round, well-organized fluid-filled abscesses were surrounded by a less well-organized infection. **C,** In a third patient, the abscess is well-formed and encapsulated and appears as an oval mass with septated fluid collections within it. **D and E,** Abscess drainage. **D,** Ultrasound shows a hypoechoic irregular indistinct mass representing a breast abscess. The surrounding fat has turned gray (instead of the normal black color), indicating breast edema, and there are dilated subdermal lymphatics in the upper right corner of the image. There is a needle within the abscess. **E,** Another view shows solid clumped debris within the fluid-filled abscess and a needle during attempted drainage. Because the pus was too thick to be drained through a needle, a percutaneous drainage catheter was placed in the interventional radiology department.

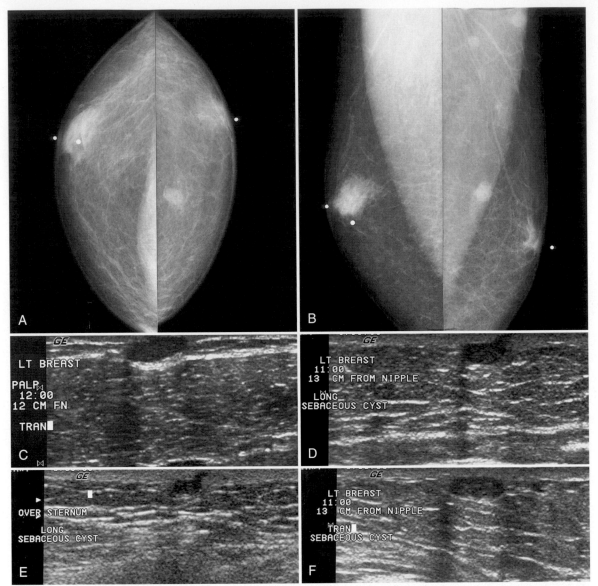

FIGURE 4-32. Sebaceous cyst. In a patient with gynecomastia and a palpable mass, craniocaudal (**A**) and mediolateral oblique (**B**) views show bilateral subareolar breast tissue that is palpable on the left and marked by a skin marker, as well as a separate discrete upper inner quadrant mass that was detected in the skin on physical examination. **C,** Ultrasound of the sebaceous cyst shows an oval, hypoechoic, well-circumscribed mass in the skin that correlates with the physical finding. **D** and **E,** In another patient, ultrasound scans of two sebaceous cysts show oval hypoechoic sebaceous cysts at the junction of the skin surface and subcutaneous fat, with the typical thin tail extending into the skin from the cyst. Note that on the transverse scan (**F**), the sebaceous cyst in part **D** is seen as an oval mass without the "tail." The tail is seen only with careful scanning and attention to the skin surface in masses suspected of being a sebaceous cyst.

adenoma, metastases, sebaceous cyst, and epidermal inclusion cyst.

The most common round cancer is invasive ductal cancer, an uncommon form of the most common breast cancer.

Medullary and mucinous breast cancers are commonly round in shape, but they are much rarer than invasive ductal cancer.

Fat-containing masses include lymph nodes, hamartoma, oil cyst, lipoma, and the rare liposarcoma.

Normal lymph nodes are oval, have an echogenic fatty hilum, and may contain a central pulsating blood vessel on color or power Doppler ultrasound in the fatty hilum.

Abnormal lymph nodes lose their fatty hilum and become larger and rounder than previously.

Fluid-containing masses include cysts, hematoma/seroma, necrotic cancer, intracystic carcinoma, intracystic papilloma, abscess, and galactocele.

Hamartomas look like a "breast within a breast" and should be left alone.

Galactoceles may rarely show a fat/fluid level on upright mammographic views.

Know the typical appearance of "don't touch" benign lymph nodes, hamartomas, oil cysts, lipomas, galactoceles, cysts, and postbiopsy scars.

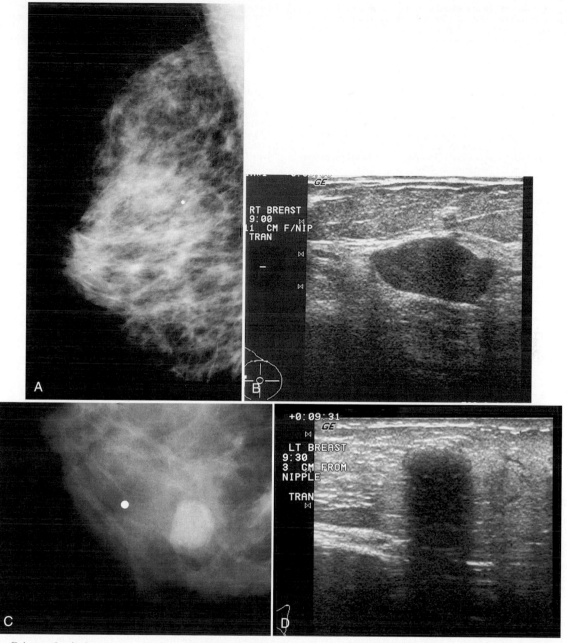

FIGURE 4-33. Galactocele. **A,** A mammogram shows a palpable equal-density mass marked by a skin marker that is difficult to see against the dense fibroglandular tissue. **B,** On ultrasound, the galactocele is oval and hypoechoic and yielded milk on aspiration. **C,** In another patient, the galactocele is a dense round mass on the mammogram. **D,** Ultrasound of the galactocele in this patient shows an oval, shadowing mass. Excisional biopsy revealed a galactocele.

SUGGESTED READINGS

Adler DD, Helvie MA, Oberman HA, et al: Radial sclerosing lesion of the breast: mammographic features, *Radiology* 176:737–740, 1990.

Adler DD, Hyde DL, Ikeda DM: Quantitative sonographic parameters as a means of distinguishing breast cancers from benign solid breast masses, *J Ultrasound Med* 10:505–508, 1991.

American College of Radiology: *Illustrated Breast Imaging Reporting and Data System (BI-RADS®)*, ed 3, Reston, VA, 1998, American College of Radiology.

Baker JA, Soo MS: Breast US: assessment of technical quality and image interpretation, *Radiology* 223:229–238, 2002.

Baker TP, Lenert JT, Parker J, et al: Lactating adenoma: a diagnosis of exclusion, *Breast J* 7:354–735, 2001.

Bilgen IG, Ustun EE, Memis A: Fat necrosis of the breast: clinical, mammographic and sonographic features, *Eur J Radiol* 39:92–99, 2001.

Brem RF, Ioffe M, Rapelyea JA, et al: Invasive lobular carcinoma: detection with mammography, sonography, MRI, and breast-specific gamma imaging, *AJR Am J Roentgenol* 192:379–383, 2009.

Brookes MJ, Bourke AG: Radiological appearances of papillary breast lesions, *Clin Radiol* 63:1265–1273, 2008.

Cardenosa G, Doudna C, Eklund GW: Mucinous (colloid) breast cancer: clinical and mammographic findings in 10 patients, *AJR Am J Roentgenol* 162:1077–1079, 1994.

Castro CY, Whitman GJ, Sahin AA: Pseudoangiomatous stromal hyperplasia of the breast, *Am J Clin Oncol* 25:213–216, 2002.

Cawson JN, Law EM, Kavanagh AM: Invasive lobular carcinoma: sonographic features of cancers detected in a BreastScreen Program, *Australas Radiol* 45:25–30, 2001.

Chao TC, Lo YF, Chen SC, Chen MF: Sonographic features of phyllodes tumors of the breast, *Ultrasound Obstet Gynecol* 20:64–71, 2002.

Chapellier C, Balu-Maestro C, Bleuse A, et al: Ultrasonography of invasive lobular carcinoma of the breast: sonographic patterns and diagnostic value: report of 102 cases, *Clin Imaging* 24:333–336, 2000.

Cheung YC, Wan YL, Chen SC, et al: Sonographic evaluation of mammographically detected microcalcifications without a mass prior to stereotactic core needle biopsy, *J Clin Ultrasound* 30:323–331, 2002.

Chopra S, Evans AJ, Pinder SE, et al: Pure mucinous breast cancer—mammographic and ultrasound findings, *Clin Radiol* 51:421–424, 1996.

Cohen MA, Morris EA, Rosen PP, et al: Pseudoangiomatous stromal hyperplasia: mammographic, sonographic, and clinical patterns, *Radiology* 198:117–120, 1996.

Cole-Beuglet C, Soriano RZ, Kurtz AB, Goldberg BB: Fibroadenoma of the breast: sonomammography correlated with pathology in 122 patients, *AJR Am J Roentgenol* 140:369–375, 1983.

Conant EF, Dillon RL, Palazzo J, et al: Imaging findings in mucin-containing carcinomas of the breast: correlation with pathologic features, *AJR Am J Roentgenol* 163:821–824, 1994.

Darling ML, Smith DN, Rhei E, et al: Lactating adenoma: sonographic features, *Breast J* 6:252–256, 2000.

Denison CM, Ward VL, Lester SC, et al: Epidermal inclusion cysts of the breast: three lesions with calcifications, *Radiology* 204:493–496, 1997.

Domchek SM, Hecht JL, Fleming MD, et al: Lymphomas of the breast: primary and secondary involvement, *Cancer* 94:6–13, 2002.

Doyle EM, Banville N, Quinn CM, et al:. Radial scars/complex sclerosing lesions and malignancy in a screening programme: incidence and histological features revisited, *Histopathology* 50:607–614, 2007.

Dupont WD, Page DL, Pari FF, et al: Long-term risk of breast cancer in women with fibroadenoma, *N Engl J Med* 351(1):10–15, 1994.

Eisinger F, Nogues C, Birnbaum D, et al: *BRCA1* and medullary breast cancer, *JAMA* 280:1227–1228, 1998.

Elson BC, Helvie MA, Frank TS, et al: Tubular carcinoma of the breast: mode of presentation, mammographic appearance, and frequency of nodal metastases, *AJR Am J Roentgenol* 161:1173–1176, 1993.

Elson BC, Ikeda DM, Andersson I, Wattsgard C: Fibrosarcoma of the breast: mammographic findings in five cases, *AJR Am J Roentgenol* 158:993–995, 1992.

Estabrook A, Asch T, Gump F, et al: Mammographic features of intracystic papillary lesions, *Surg Gynecol Obstet* 170:113–116, 1990.

Fornage BD, Lorigan JG, Andry E: Fibroadenoma of the breast: sonographic appearance, *Radiology* 172:671–675, 1989.

Gordon PB, Goldenberg SL: Malignant breast masses detected only by ultrasound. A retrospective review, *Cancer* 76:626–630, 1995.

Gunhan-Bilgen I, Memis A, Ustun EE: Metastatic intramammary lymph nodes: mammographic and ultrasonographic features, *Eur J Radiol* 40:24–29, 2001.

Gunhan-Bilgen I, Zekioglu O, Ustun EE, et al: Invasive micropapillary carcinoma of the breast: clinical, mammographic, and sonographic findings with histopathologic correlation, *AJR Am J Roentgenol* 179:927–931, 2002.

Harnist KS, Ikeda DM, Helvie MA: Abnormal mammogram after steering wheel injury, *West J Med* 159:504–506, 1993.

Harvey JA, Moran RE, Maurer EJ, DeAngelis GA: Sonographic features of mammary oil cysts, *J Ultrasound Med* 16:719–724, 1997.

Hashimoto BE, Kramer DJ, Picozzi VJ: High detection rate of breast ductal carcinoma in situ calcifications on mammographically directed high-resolution sonography, *J Ultrasound Med* 20:501–508, 2001.

Hilton SV, Leopold GR, Olson LK, Willson SA: Real-time breast sonography: application in 300 consecutive patients, *AJR Am J Roentgenol* 147:479–486, 1986.

Homer MJ: Proper placement of a metallic marker on an area of concern in the breast, *AJR Am J Roentgenol* 167:390–391, 1996.

Jorge Blanco A, Vargas Serrano B, Rodriguez Romero R, Martinez Cendejas E: Phyllodes tumors of the breast, *Eur Radiol* 9:356–360, 1999.

Kim MJ, Kim EK, Park SY, et al: Galactoceles mimicking suspicious solid masses on sonography, *J Ultrasound Med* 25:145–151, 2006.

Lee CH, Giurescu ME, Philpotts LE, et al: Clinical importance of unilaterally enlarging lymph nodes on otherwise normal mammograms, *Radiology* 203:329–334, 1997.

Levrini G, Mori CA, Vacondio R, et al: MRI patterns of invasive lobular cancer: T1 and T2 features, *Radiol Med* 113:1110–1125, 2008.

Lindfors KK, Kopans DB, Googe PB, et al: Breast cancer metastasis to intramammary lymph nodes, *AJR Am J Roentgenol* 146:133–136, 1986.

Memis A, Ozdemir N, Parildar M, et al: Mucinous (colloid) breast cancer: mammographic and US features with histologic correlation, *Eur J Radiol* 35:39–43, 2000.

Meyer JE, Amin E, Lindfors KK, et al: Medullary carcinoma of the breast: mammographic and US appearance, *Radiology* 170:79–82, 1989.

Ohlinger R, Frese H, Schwesinger G, et al: Papillary intracystic carcinoma of the female breast—role of ultrasonography, *Ultraschall Med* 26:325–328, 2005.

Paramagul CP, Helvie MA, Adler DD: Invasive lobular carcinoma: sonographic appearance and role of sonography in improving diagnostic sensitivity, *Radiology* 195:231–234, 1995.

Ribeiro-Silva A, Mendes CF, Costa IS, et al: Metastases to the breast from extramammary malignancies: a clinicopathologic study of 12 cases, *Pol J Pathol* 57:161–165, 2006.

Rodriguez-Pinilla SM, Rodriguez-Gil Y, Moreno-Bueno G, et al: Sporadic invasive breast carcinomas with medullary features display a basal-like phenotype: an immunohistochemical and gene amplification study, *Am J Surg Pathol* 31:501–508, 2007.

Rosen EL, Soo MS, Bentley RC: Focal fibrosis: a common breast lesion diagnosed at imaging-guided core biopsy, *AJR Am J Roentgenol* 173:1657–1662, 1999.

Salvador R, Salvador M, Jimenez JA, et al: Galactocele of the breast: radiologic and ultrasonographic findings, *Br J Radiol* 63:140–142, 1990.

Samardar P, de Paredes ES, Grimes MM, Wilson JD: Focal asymmetric densities seen at mammography: US and pathologic correlation, *Radiographics* 22:19–33, 2002.

Schneider JA: Invasive papillary breast carcinoma: mammographic and sonographic appearance, *Radiology* 171:377–379, 1989.

Schrading S, Kuhl CK: Mammographic, US, and MR imaging phenotypes of familial breast cancer, *Radiology* 246:58–70, 2008.

Sheppard DG, Whitman GJ, Huynh PT, et al: Tubular carcinoma of the breast: mammographic and sonographic features, *AJR Am J Roentgenol* 174:253–257, 2000.

Sickles EA: Mammographic features of 300 consecutive nonpalpable breast cancers, *AJR Am J Roentgenol* 146:661–663, 1986.

Sickles E: Practical solutions to common mammographic problems: tailoring the examination, *AJR Am J Roentgenol* 151:31–39, 1988.

Sickles EA, Herzog KA: Intramammary scar tissue: a mimic of the mammographic appearance of carcinoma, *AJR Am J Roentgenol* 135:349–352, 1980.

Soo MS, Dash N, Bentley R, et al: Tubular adenomas of the breast: imaging findings with histologic correlation, *AJR Am J Roentgenol* 174:757–761, 2000.

Sperber F, Blank A, Metser U: Adenoid cystic carcinoma of the breast: mammographic, sonographic, and pathological correlation, *Breast J* 8:53–54, 2002.

Stavros AT, Thickman D, Rapp CL, et al: Solid breast nodules: use of sonography to distinguish between benign and malignant lesions, *Radiology* 196:123–134, 1995.

Sumkin JH, Perrone AM, Harris KM, et al: Lactating adenoma: US features and literature review, *Radiology* 206:271–274, 1998.

Tabar L, Pentek Z, Dean PB: The diagnostic and therapeutic value of breast cyst puncture and pneumocystography, *Radiology* 141:659–663, 1981.

Venta LA, Wiley EL, Gabriel H, Adler YT: Imaging features of focal breast fibrosis: mammographic-pathologic correlation of noncalcified breast lesions, *AJR Am J Roentgenol* 173:309–316, 1999.

Vo T, Xing Y, Meric-Bernstam F, et al: Long-term outcomes in patients with mucinous, medullary, tubular, and invasive ductal carcinomas after lumpectomy, *Am J Surg* 194:527–531, 2007.

Wahner-Roedler DL, Sebo TJ, Gisvold JJ: Hamartomas of the breast: clinical, radiologic, and pathologic manifestations, *Breast J* 7:101–105, 2001.

Walsh R, Kornguth PJ, Soo MS, et al: Axillary lymph nodes: mammographic, pathologic, and clinical correlation, *AJR Am J Roentgenol* 168:33–38, 1997.

Weigel RJ, Ikeda DM, Nowels KW: Primary squamous cell carcinoma of the breast, *South Med J* 89:511–515, 1996.

Wieman SM, Landercasper J, Johnson JM, et al: Tumoral pseudoangiomatous stromal hyperplasia of the breast, *Am Surg* 74:1211–1214, 2008.

Woods ER, Helvie MA, Ikeda DM, et al: Solitary breast papilloma: comparison of mammographic, galactographic, and pathologic findings, *AJR Am J Roentgenol* 159:487–491, 1992.

Quizzes

4-1. Name the differential diagnosis for fat-containing masses.

1. _____

2. _____

3. _____

4. _____

5. _____

6. _____

7. _____

For answers, see Box 4-14.

4-2. Name the differential diagnosis for fluid-containing masses.

1. _____

2. _____

3. _____

4. _____

5. _____

6. _____

7. _____

8. _____

For answers, see Box 4-15.

4-3. Name "don't touch" benign masses that should be left alone.

1. _____

2. _____

3. _____

4. _____

5. _____

6. _____

7. _____

8. _____

9. _____

10. _____

For answers, see Box 4-16.

4-4. Name ultrasound features of solid breast masses.

MALIGNANT	BENIGN
1. _____	1. _____
2. _____	2. _____
3. _____	3. _____
4. _____	4. _____
5. _____	
6. _____	
7. _____	
8. _____	

For answers, see Box 4-3.

4-5. Name the differential diagnosis for spiculated masses.

1. _____

2. _____

3. _____

4. _____

5. _____

6. _____

7. _____

For answers, see Box 4-6.

4-6. Name the elements of ultrasound image labeling.

1. _____

2. _____

3. _____

4. _____

5. _____

For answers, see Box 4-4.

4-7. Name the differential diagnosis for round masses.

1. _____

2. _____

3. _____

4. _____

5. _____

6. _____

7. _____

8. _____

9. _____

10. _____

11. _____

12. _____

13. _____

14. _____

For answers, see Box 4-10.

4-8. Name the differential diagnosis for multiple round masses.

1. _____

2. _____

3. _____

4. _____

5. _____

6. _____

For answers, see Box 4-12.

4-9. Name the differential diagnosis for solid indistinct masses.

1. _____

2. _____

3. _____

4. _____

5. _____

6. _____

7. _____

For answers, see Box 4-13.

CHAPTER 5

Breast Ultrasound

Ultrasound is a useful adjunct to mammography for the diagnosis and management of benign and malignant breast disease. Technical advances have resulted in consistent, reproducible, high-resolution clinical ultrasound images. Although whole-breast automated scanners are now available, most practices use high-resolution hand-held transducers. Scientific evidence and clinical experience support the use of hand-held real-time breast ultrasound to distinguish cysts from solid masses, determine the sonographic characteristics of solid masses, evaluate palpable lumps in young women, and provide guidance for percutaneous biopsy. Given improvements in image quality and data processing, studies suggest roles for breast ultrasound in breast cancer screening and evaluation of breast calcifications identified on mammography, with specific caveats on the technologic limitations of ultrasound for these indications. This chapter explores these and other indications for breast ultrasound.

▪ TECHNICAL CONSIDERATIONS

Real-time hand-held scanners provide easy and rapid direct visualization of breast lesions for diagnosis or ultrasound-directed breast biopsy. Hand-held units should include a linear array, high-frequency transducer operating at a frequency of 7.5 to 10 MHz or greater, which provides good tissue penetration to 4 or 5 cm. All scanners should also include a marking system to document and annotate ultrasound images.

Technical issues must be overcome to obtain good sonographic image quality. Superficial lesions in the near field of the transducer may be distorted, but they can be imaged by using a high-frequency transducer or a soft fluid offset. The heterogeneity of breast tissue results in absorption of the ultrasound beam with increasing distance from the transducer. Extensive diffraction of the ultrasound beam leads to beam defocusing and poor image quality the further the lesion is from the transducer. Thus, accurate diagnosis of cysts and deep lesions depends on appropriate power, gain, and focal zone settings. Improper adjustments of any of these parameters can result in misdiagnosis by producing suboptimal images or artifactual echoes within simple cysts. Routine calibration of the unit and evaluation of the unit's performance with a breast phantom help prevent these technical errors.

The amount of shadowing at normal breast tissue interfaces depends on the transducer's diameter and the distance of the tissue from the transducer. Artificial shadowing can be caused by Cooper ligaments and normal breast structures, which usually angle up toward the skin and the transducer.

Flattening or compressing the breast tissue decreases the amount of tissue penetrated by the ultrasound beam and diminishes edge artifacts by straightening Cooper ligaments parallel to the transducer. To flatten the breast tissue in the upper outer quadrant, the patient is scanned supine with her hand behind her head in a posterior oblique position, with her back supported by a wedge. Facilities often use the sponge wedges used for positioning posterior oblique lumbar spine radiographs to help the patient achieve this position. For medial lesions, the patient lies flat on her back, which flattens the medial breast tissue. Sonographers use moderate compression during scanning by lightly but firmly pressing the breast with the transducer. This decreases the thickness of the tissue to be scanned, reduces beam absorption and defocusing, allows better penetration, and decreases shadowing from ligaments and glandular elements.

To ensure that the field of view includes all the breast tissue from the skin surface to the chest wall, the sonographer makes sure that the image includes the pectoralis muscle and chest wall at the bottom of the screen. The time-compensated gain (TCG) curve should be adjusted so that fat is uniformly gray from the subcutaneous tissues to the chest wall. This adjustment enables accurate evaluation of masses as cystic or solid at any depth in the breast. Incorrect settings that make the fat look anechoic may also make a solid mass look like an anechoic cyst.

Once the sonographer identifies an area of interest or a mass, he or she magnifies the finding to fill the monitor or screen appropriately because it is hard to see and analyze a lesion if it is too small on the screen. The sonographer then resets the focal zone, TCG curve, and depth-compensated gain (DCG) curves on the lesion to evaluate the finding's shape, margins, and internal characteristics.

When scanning a breast with palpable findings, the sonographer asks the patient to point out the mass or symptomatic area to ensure evaluation of the area prompting investigation. This ensures that the patient's area of concern is addressed and that the patient is more confident that her questioned area was investigated (because she pointed it out). If the patient is unsure of the location of the mass, the sonographer scans the quadrant or area requested by the referring physician on the order or requisition.

To scan palpable masses, the sonographer scans the palpable finding, then places a finger over the mass. The sonographer scans over the finger on the mass, and then removes the finger to scan only the palpable finding. This ensures that the palpable finding is in the field of view. Alternatively, the palpable finding can be trapped between two fingers. The sonographer scans the trapped mass between two fingers so that the mass does not roll out of the field of view from under the transducer.

The American College of Radiology (ACR) has made specific recommendations for ultrasound labeling. The sonographer labels each finding according to its location in right or left breast, quadrant or clock position, scan plane (radial or antiradial, longitudinal or transverse), and number of centimeters from the nipple, along with the sonographer's initials (Box 5-1). The sonographer takes images of the mass with and without measuring calipers. Any other

pertinent clinical information, such as whether the lesion
is palpable, may also be helpful to note.

NORMAL SONOGRAPHIC BREAST ANATOMY

The breast is composed of fibrous connective tissue
(Cooper ligaments) arranged in a honeycomb-like structure surrounding the breast ducts and fat (Fig. 5-1A and
B). The proportion of supporting stroma to glandular tissue
varies widely in the normal population and depends on the
patient's age, parity, and hormonal status. In young women,
breast tissue is composed of mostly dense fibroglandular
tissue. In later years, dense tissue involutes into fat in
varying degrees, producing a mixed fatty and dense breast
or an all-fatty breast (see Fig. 5-1C to F).

Breast tissues are either echogenic (white) or hypoechoic
(black) on ultrasound. The skin is an echogenic line immediately under the transducer in the near field. It is normally
about 2 to 3 mm thick and has a hypoechoic layer of dark
subcutaneous fat immediately beneath it (Box 5-2). Unlike
echogenic or white-appearing fat around the superior mes-
enteric artery in the abdomen, fat in the breast appears
dark or hypoechoic. The only exception to hypoechoic fat
in the breast is the echogenic fat in the middle of a lymph
node. The normal lymph node is an oval, well-circumscribed
mass with a hypoechoic cortex and fatty echogenic hilum,
often seen in the upper outer quadrant and axilla, and
often near an artery (see Fig. 5-1G and H).

Breast glandular tissue and connective tissue are echogenic or white. Connective tissue has the highest acoustic
impedance, fat has the lowest, and glandular parenchyma

is of intermediate echogenicity. The Cooper ligaments are
thin, sharply defined linear structures that support the surrounding fat and glandular elements (see Fig. 5-1I and J).
Cooper ligaments in a fatty breast look like thin, white,
gently curving lines surrounding hypoechoic fat. Normally,
Cooper ligaments are thin and sharply demarcated. In
breast edema, the fat becomes gray and the normally sharp
Cooper ligaments become blurred.

Subareolar ducts are dark, hypoechoic, tubular structures leading to the nipple. The glandular tissue elements
are echogenic (white), so normal hypoechoic ducts appear
like dark tubes against the normal white background when
imaged along their long axis. In cross-section, the ducts are
dark, hypoechoic, round or oval circles seen against the
white echogenic normal glandular tissue.

The pectoralis muscle is a hypoechoic structure of
varying thickness that contains thin lines of supporting
stroma coursing along its long axis at the chest wall near
the bottom of the image. The pectoralis muscle abuts the
intercostal muscles and fascia of the chest wall (see Fig.
5-1K and L). Ribs in between the intercostal muscles are
round or oval in cross-section, shadow intensely, and are
seen at regular intervals along the chest wall. High-
resolution transducers may display calcifications in the
anterior portions of the cartilaginous elements of the ribs.
Newcomers to breast ultrasound may mistake the ribs for
masses, but their periodicity along the chest wall and the
fact that one can palpate the ribs along their course will
help prevent newcomers from making this mistake.

The nipple is a hypoechoic structure at the skin surface
that occasionally produces an intense acoustic shadow as a
result of the dense connective tissue within it (Fig. 5-2A
and B). Because of the presence of retroareolar ducts and
blood vessels, there may be marked vascularity in the retroareolar region on color or power Doppler imaging. Newcomers to breast ultrasound may mistake the nipple for a
breast mass because of its hypoechoic appearance, shadowing, and the intense vascularity beneath it. However,
knowledge of the shadowing, vascularity, and the ability
to correlate the mass with the nipple on physical examination will help prevent newcomers from making this
mistake.

In children, the breast bud that develops into the adult
breast is right underneath the nipple. The breast bud
may produce an asymmetric lump under the nipple
that may be mistaken for a mass rather than a normal
developing structure (see Fig. 5-2C and D). This normal
structure should be left alone because surgical removal
of the breast bud results in no breast formation on the
ipsilateral side.

ULTRASOUND EVALUATION OF MAMMOGRAPHICALLY DETECTED FINDINGS

The ACR Breast Imaging Reporting and Data System (BI-
RADS®) committee developed an ultrasound lexicon to
provide descriptors for findings seen by ultrasound and
recommended specific descriptors for breast masses (Table
5-1). Use of the words in the ACR BI-RADS® lexicon
helps clarify one's impression of the finding, improves
communication between the radiologist and referring

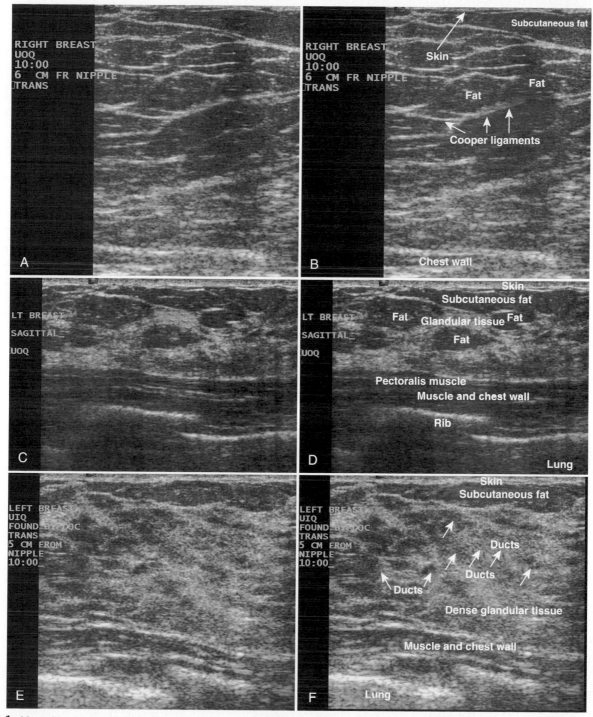

FIGURE 5-1. Normal breast ultrasound images. **A** and **B,** Normal breast ultrasound scans in fatty, mixed, and dense breasts. Unlabeled (**A**) and labeled (**B**) ultrasounds of a normal fatty breast show the thin, white, superficial skin line (*arrow*); dark subcutaneous fat; dark fatty lobules separated by sharp thin Cooper ligaments; and the muscle and chest wall at the posterior aspect of the image. Note that the fat is uniformly gray throughout the image, and multiple fatty lobules are interspersed between the thin, linear Cooper ligaments. Unlabeled (**C**) and labeled (**D**) normal breast ultrasounds of fibroglandular and fatty breast tissue show the thin, white, superficial skin line; dark subcutaneous fat; and white glandular tissue interspersed by dark hypoechoic fatty lobules. Note how the white glandular tissue is thicker than the Cooper ligaments seen in **A** and how the fatty islands might be mistaken for breast masses. Unlabeled (**E**) and labeled (**F**) ultrasounds of a normal dense breast show mostly white glandular tissue with scant amounts of fat and hypoechoic ducts over an area of thickening in a young patient. Note how the ducts appear as small, round, dark structures interspersed in the dense glandular tissue when caught in cross section and appear like long tubes when caught in longitudinal section. *Continued*

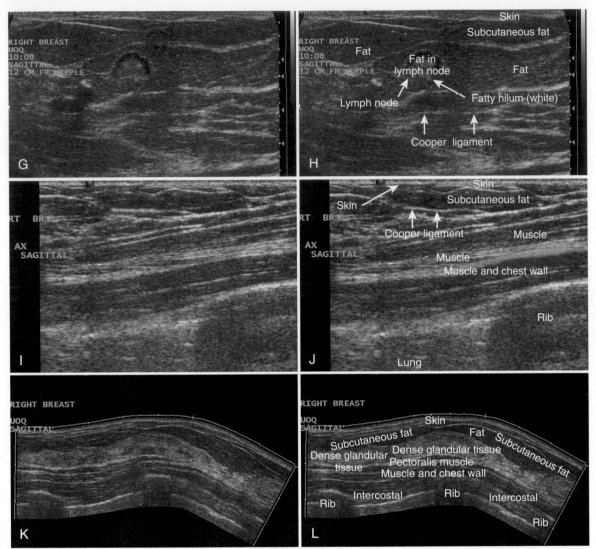

FIGURE 5-1, cont'd. Unlabeled (**G**) and labeled (**H**) ultrasounds of a normal lymph node show a lobulated hypoechoic mass with an echogenic center that represents the fatty hilum. Note that the fat outside the lymph node in the adjacent breast tissue is hypoechoic (dark), whereas fat inside the lymph node is echogenic (white). This is the typical appearance of a normal lymph node. **I** and **J,** Cooper ligaments and normal fatty tissue in a thin fatty breast. Unlabeled (**I**) and labeled (**J**) normal breast ultrasounds show the thin echogenic skin line at the top of the image; dark hypoechoic sub-cutaneous fat; thin, gently curving Cooper ligaments coursing through the fat; and the thin, parallel, tightly packed lines of muscle just above the chest wall and the rib. **K** and **L,** Landscape ultrasound view of normal dense tissue in a thin dense breast. Unlabeled (**K**) and labeled (**L**) landscape ultra-sounds over a thin dense breast show the echogenic skin line, dark subcutaneous fat, dense white glandular tissue, and the pectoralis muscle and chest wall overlying the periodic round shadows of the ribs and intercostal muscles. The ribs cause acoustic shadowing. However, the ribs should not be mistaken for breast masses because they are located behind the muscle and chest wall just above the lung and are not within the breast.

TABLE 5-1. American College of Radiology BI-RADS® Ultrasound Lexicon Descriptors

Shape	Margin	Boundary	Echo Pattern	Posterior Acoustic Features	Effect on Surrounding Tissue	Calcifications
Oval	Circumscribed	Abrupt interface	Anechoic	No posterior acoustic features	No effect	None
Round	Angular	Echogenic halo	Hyperechoic	Enhancement	Duct changes	Macrocalcifications (>0.5 mm)
Irregular	Indistinct		Complex	Shadowing	Cooper ligament changes	Microcalcifications in or out of a mass
	Microlobulated		Isoechoic	Combined	Edema	
			Hypoechoic		Architectural distortion	
					Skin thickening	
					Skin retraction/ irregularity	

Modified from American College of Radiology: ACR BI-RADS®—ultrasound, In *ACR Breast Imaging and Reporting and Data System, breast imaging atlas*, Reston, VA, 2003, American College of Radiology.

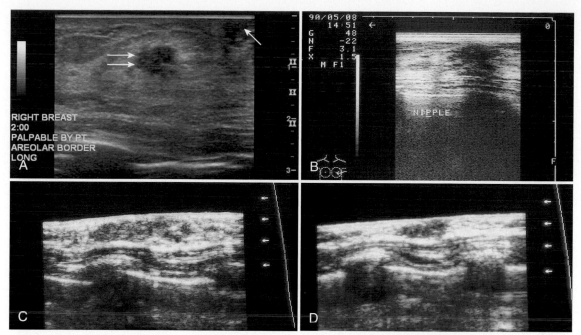

FIGURE 5-2. The nipple and adjacent breast mass. **A,** Ultrasound shows a hypoechoic, shadowing nipple in the near field *(arrow)* separated from an irregular hypoechoic mass *(double arrows)*. Note that the nipple is at the skin surface and can be easily distinguished from a breast mass once the normal nipple appearance is recognized. The mass was an invasive ductal cancer. **B,** Ultrasound of a normal nipple shows that the flattened nipple appears as a hypoechoic mass, sometimes with intense shadowing. **C,** This 5-year-old girl had a breast lump under the nipple, representing the normal breast bud, that was asymmetric on the right side. **D,** Breast ultrasound shows the normal hypoechoic nipple–breast bud complex on the enlarged side and the smaller nipple–breast bud complex on the normal side.

TABLE 5-2. Ultrasound Features of Cancer, Cysts, and Fibroadenomas*

Feature	Cancer	Cyst	Fibroadenoma	Benign Ultrasound Features
Shape	Irregular Round	Oval Round	Oval	Oval
Margin	Microlobulated Indistinct Angular Spiculated	Circumscribed	Circumscribed 3–4 gentle lobulations	Circumscribed
Boundary	Echogenic halo	Abrupt	Abrupt	Abrupt
Orientation	Not parallel "Taller than wide"	Parallel** "Wider than tall"	Parallel** "Wider than tall"	Parallel
Internal Echoes	Heterogeneous Complex	Anechoic	Hypoechoic Homogeneous	Hypoechoic Homogeneous Echogenic
Posterior Acoustic Features	Shadowing Combined	Enhancement	Can be anything	
Other	Duct extension Very hypoechoic	No malignant features	No malignant features	No malignant features

*As with any generalities, there are exceptions to every descriptor in every category.
**Parallel ("wider than tall") means the mass does not disrupt tissue planes and displaces them or grows between them rather than invading or growing through them (nonparallel or "taller than wide"). Parallel is more often associated with benign lesions. Nonparallel or "taller than wide" is more often associated with malignancies. Data from Stavros AT, Thickman D, Rapp CL, et al: Solid breast nodules: use of sonography to distinguish between benign and malignant lesions, *Radiology* 196: 123 134, 1995, and Hong AS, Rosen EL, Soo MS, Baker JA: BI-RADS for sonography: positive and negative predictive values of sonographic features. AJR Am J Roentgenol 184(4):1260–1265, 2005.

physician, and may trigger specific patient managements. This is because specific ultrasound features described by the lexicon suggest either benign masses or cancer. Although there is some overlap in benign versus malignant ultrasound features, the radiologist can use the lexicon to be reminded of what features should be searched for on the image (Table 5-2).

The BI-RADS® ultrasound lexicon descriptors for breast masses and their effect on the surrounding breast tissue are illustrated in Figures 5-3 to 5-6. Mass shapes are reported as *oval, round,* or *irregular.* Mass margins are *circumscribed, angular, indistinct, microlobulated,* or *spiculated.* The internal echo pattern is described as *anechoic* (all black inside), *hyperechoic* (white), *complex* (mixed black and

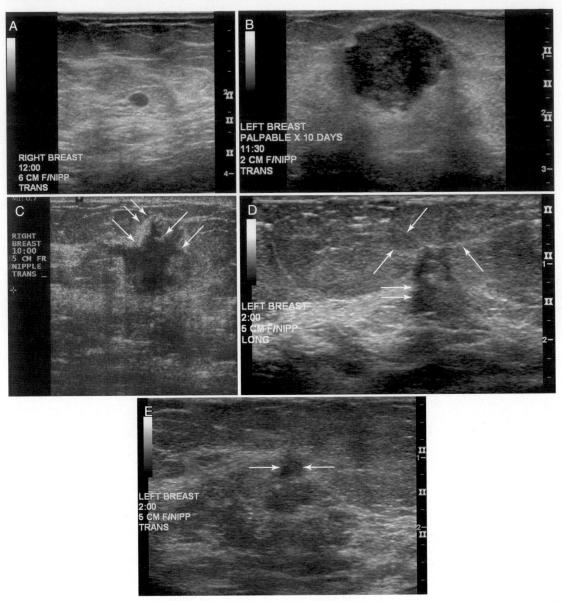

FIGURE 5-3. Examples of BI-RADS® ultrasound lexicon descriptors for mass shape and margins. **A,** An oval, deeply situated, well-circumscribed mass has homogeneous internal characteristics and no posterior acoustic enhancement. This was a complicated cyst at biopsy. **B,** A suspicious, round, microlobulated mass with well-circumscribed borders has complex hypoechoic internal characteristics and acoustic enhancement; this is an unusual appearance of a breast metastasis. **C,** Irregularly shaped invasive ductal cancer with angular margins *(arrows)* and an echogenic halo *(double arrows)* in its anterior surface. **D,** Round, irregular, hypoechoic invasive ductal cancer *(double arrows)* with acoustic spiculations at its anterior surface *(arrows)*. Note that when the mass is spiculated and displayed against the dark fat, the acoustic spiculations are white. **E,** Round mass displayed against the white glandular tissue with indistinct margins *(arrows)*. Contrast the indistinct margins to the well-circumscribed margins in part **A**; part **E** represents invasive ductal cancer.

white), *isoechoic* (equal), or *hypoechoic* (dark). Posterior acoustic features are described as *no posterior acoustic features*, *enhancement* (white), *shadowing* (dark), or a combined pattern. The boundary between the mass and the surrounding tissue is described as having an *abrupt interface* or as containing an *echogenic halo* (a white blurry band surrounding the mass). Calcifications are described as *no calcifications*, *macrocalcifications* (>0.5 mm), *microcalcifications within the mass*, or *microcalcifications outside the mass*. Effects of the mass on surrounding breast tissue are described using the terms *no effect, duct changes, changes in Cooper ligaments, edema, architectural distortion, skin thickening, skin retraction,* and *skin irregularity.*

The terms *parallel* or *not parallel* relate to tumor growth patterns with respect to normal tissue planes. They are important because they indicate if the mass is growing along or in between tissue planes versus growing through them. A parallel growth pattern indicates a benign finding (*wider than tall*, as described by Stavros and colleagues) because it indicates a growth pattern along tissue planes. *Not parallel* or *taller than wide* indicates that the mass is growing through the normal tissue planes, which is not normal and indicates cancer (see Fig. 5-6E).

Finally, the ultrasound BI-RADS® lexicon suggests standard reporting for masses, as in Box 5-3.

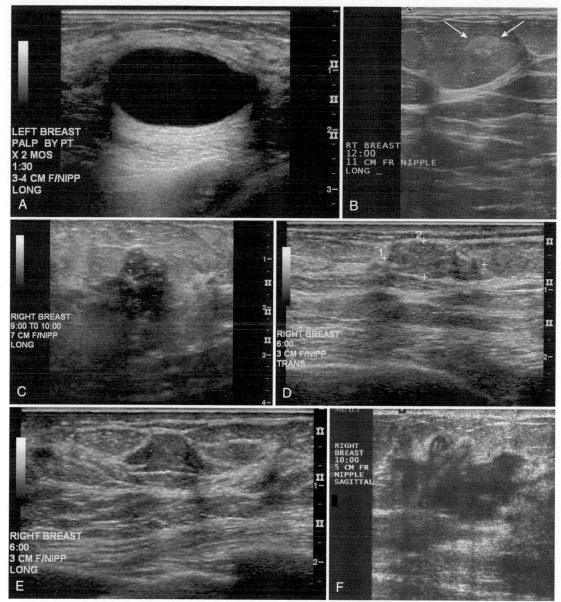

FIGURE 5-4. Examples of BI-RADS® ultrasound lexicon descriptors for internal echo pattern. **A,** This cyst is anechoic, or completely black inside, and has the typical appearance of a cyst; that is, it is well-circumscribed, oval, and has an imperceptible back wall and enhanced through-sound transmission. **B,** Oval, well-circumscribed, hyperechoic mass in the near field *(arrows)* is whiter than the surrounding dark hypoechoic fat. Biopsy showed angiolipoma. **C,** A taller than wide, irregularly shaped invasive ductal cancer has a well-circumscribed superficial border; the lateral and posterior borders are indistinct. Internally there are bright and dark shadows compatible with a complex internal echo pattern. **D** and **E,** An oval, wider than tall, isoechoic breast mass has well-circumscribed borders with a tapering lateral margin; note that the internal echogenicity is the same as the surrounding breast tissue, making this mass isoechoic. Biopsy showed fibroadenoma. **F,** This hypoechoic invasive ductal cancer has mixed internal echogenicity within it, angulated anterior margins, and a combined posterior acoustic pattern comprised of both acoustic shadowing and enhancement.

Breast Cysts, Intracystic Tumors, and Cystic-Appearing Masses

The most frequent clinical application of breast ultrasonography is to characterize masses initially detected by mammography as cystic or solid. Cysts are the most common breast mass and occur in an estimated 7% to 10% of all women. Cysts are lined by apocrine cells that actively secrete material, predisposing these types of cysts to recur after aspiration. Sometimes, cysts are lined by a flat epithelial lining that is less active. The accuracy of ultrasound in distinguishing cystic from solid masses can be as high as 98% to 100%, as reported by Hilton and colleagues.

Strict ultrasound criteria for a simple cyst include a mass with well-circumscribed margins, sharp imperceptible anterior and posterior walls, a round or oval contour, absence of internal echoes, and posterior acoustic enhancement (Box 5-4 and Fig. 5-7A). Cysts may be single or multiple, gathered into small clusters, or contain thin septations (see Fig. 5-7B to D). Cysts are not malignant or premalignant, but examination of them is important because they may cause lumps that mimic round cancer

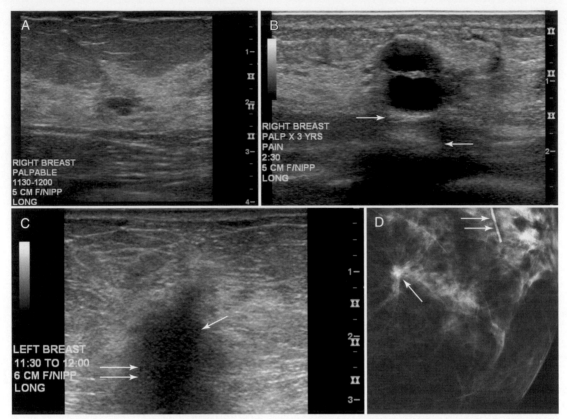

FIGURE 5-5. Examples of BI-RADS® ultrasound lexicon descriptors for posterior acoustic features. **A,** An oval, lobular, hypoechoic mass with thin septations deep within the breast has no posterior acoustic features. This was a cyst at aspiration. **B,** Two cysts adjacent to each other with a thick septation between them have posterior acoustic enhancement, which is the white enhancement of sound deep to the cysts *(arrows)*. **C,** A taller than wide, not parallel, hypoechoic invasive ductal cancer shows as a mass *(arrow)* that has an irregular shape, indistinct margins, an echogenic halo, and marked acoustic shadowing *(double arrows)*. Note that the mass itself is difficult to distinguish from the acoustic shadowing because both are so dark. Note also that the acoustic shadowing, which is the dark, black band posterior to the mass, can be caused by productive fibrosis from the tumor, and is often seen in masses that appear spiculated on the mammogram. **D,** Magnified craniocaudal mammogram shows a spiculated mass *(arrow)* corresponding to the hypoechoic shadowing cancer. Note that the cancer is far from the linear scar marker *(double arrows)* and cannot represent a postbiopsy scar.

BOX 5-3. Ultrasound Mass Reporting

Size and location (with centimeters from nipple)
Mass shape, margin, boundary (abrupt vs. echogenic halo)
Orientation
    Parallel; "wider than tall"
    Nonparallel; "taller than wide"
Internal echo patterns
Posterior acoustic features
Effect on surrounding tissue
Calcifications (if present)
Important vascularity features
How changed, if previously present
Correlation to physical findings and other imaging
BI-RADS® summary code
Management recommendation

BOX 5-4. Simple Cyst Criteria

Oval or round shape with circumscribed margins
Anechoic
Imperceptible back wall
Enhanced transmission of sound

---

on physical examination or mammography. When palpable, a cyst is a smooth, mobile mass on physical examination. Occasionally cysts appear as a visible mass if the patient is supine and the cyst is large. Cysts may be painful and may wax and wane with the patient's menstrual cycle.

If a mass is proven to be a cyst by ultrasound, the patient can be monitored by screening mammography because cysts are not cancer. Symptomatic cysts that are painful or cause a lump that disturbs the patient can be treated by aspiration. Cysts may be simple or "complicated," meaning that the cyst contains sloughed debris. These complicated cysts contain material within them rather than being anechoic. Some complicated cysts require aspiration to confirm that they are cysts rather than solid masses (see Fig. 5-7E).

Attention to technical detail is especially important because increasing the TCG curve may produce artifactual echoes in benign cysts that suggest a solid mass. An improperly set DCG curve may inaccurately evaluate the internal matrix of the mass and make a cyst look solid and

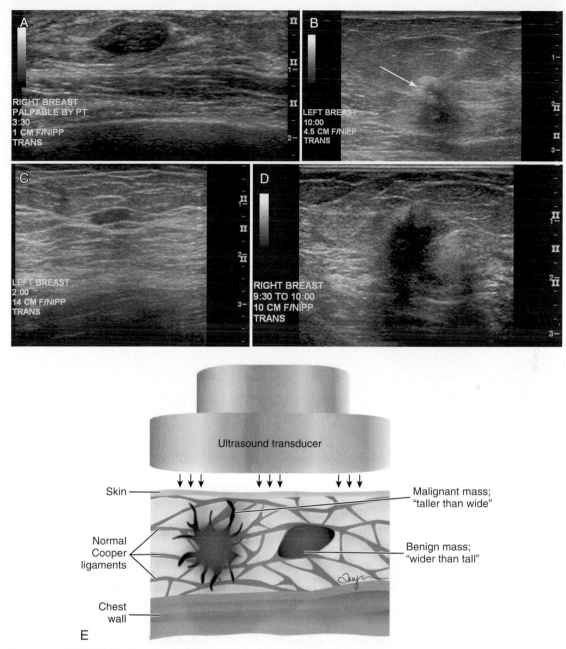

FIGURE 5-6. Examples of BI-RADS® ultrasound lexicon descriptors for tissue interface and growth pattern. **A,** Benign masses usually have an abrupt interface with the surrounding tissue. This benign fibroadenoma is oval, well-circumscribed, and fairly homogeneous. It is parallel, wider than tall, and has an abrupt interface with the surrounding glandular tissue. Note the sharp margins compared to part **B. B,** An indistinct white band surrounding a mass is an *echogenic halo* in the BI-RADS® lexicon and is a sign of cancer. There is an echogenic halo in the superior portion of this invasive ductal cancer *(arrow).* The cancer itself is hypoechoic, taller than wide, and has indistinct margins. **C,** This fibroadenoma is a well circumscribed, oval, parallel (wider than tall) mass and has homogeneous internal characteristics. Note that the parallel mass respects adjacent tissue planes and does not cross Cooper ligaments, which is typical for benign masses. **D,** This hypoechoic, spiculated invasive ductal cancer with an echogenic halo is taller than wide (not parallel), meaning that it is growing through Cooper ligaments perpendicular to the transducer surface. The mass is most likely malignant because it is growing through tissue planes. The *not parallel* or *taller than wide* sign on ultrasound is always worrisome for cancer. **E,** Schematic of taller than wide malignant versus wider than tall benign mass growth patterns on ultrasound.

may make a solid mass appear to be a cyst. On real-time imaging, cyst contours may be flattened with compression, whereas solid masses are less compressible. Alternatively, small, clustered, or deeply located cysts may be at the technical limits of ultrasound to distinguish the usually anechoic cyst from a solid mass.

Deeply located cysts may not show enhanced through-sound transmission because of their location close to the chest wall, and lateral cyst walls may be obscured by refractive shadows (see Fig. 5-7F). These problems may be resolved by repositioning the patient or the transducer to scan from a different angle. This permits visualization of distal acoustic enhancement or eliminates the refractive shadows obscuring the sharp cyst walls. Acorn cysts contain a fluid/fluid level, with the dark dependent portion of the cyst representing clear fluid (the acorn) and the lighter top

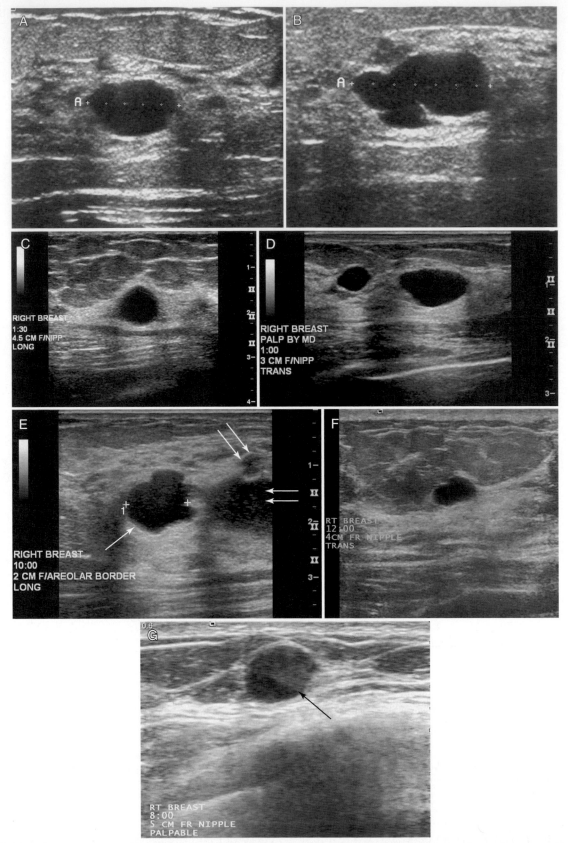

FIGURE 5-7. Examples of breast cysts. **A,** This simple cyst has an anechoic interior, an imperceptible wall, sharply marginated smooth borders, and enhanced transmission of sound. **B,** This simple cyst is lobulated and contains thin septations and imperceptible walls. **C,** A typical anechoic simple cyst with imperceptible walls and enhanced through-sound transmission. **D,** Two typical anechoic simple cysts that are sharply marginated with imperceptible walls and enhanced through-sound transmission. **E,** Two cysts adjacent to each other include a simple cyst *(arrow)* with lobulated borders that is anechoic and has an imperceptible wall and enhanced through-sound transmission. Adjacent to the simple cyst are complicated cysts *(double arrows)* that contain debris and have indistinct margins and enhanced through-sound transmission; needle aspiration showed simple cyst fluid. **F,** This simple cyst does not show enhanced through-sound transmission because of focal zones that are located too deep for proper evaluation of the cyst. **G,** Acorn cyst. An oval, well-circumscribed mass has a lower cystic component and a possible solid upper component, comprising the "acorn cyst," which has a fluid/fluid level *(arrow)*. Aspiration showed a cyst with debris in it.

representing layering fluid above it (the acorn cap) (see Fig. 5-7G). Changing the patient's position may cause the layer to move dependently, clinching the diagnosis of an acorn cyst.

The internal characteristics of cysts must be analyzed to exclude mural masses or irregular thick walls, which indicate complex masses. Complex masses contain cystic and solid components; intracystic tumors and necrotic neoplasms are in the differential diagnosis. Complex masses are different from complicated cysts, which contain debris. Complex masses might be cancer, but complicated cysts are benign (Table 5-3 and Boxes 5-5 and 5-6).

Real-time ultrasound imaging can help distinguish speckle artifact from debris in cyst fluid from a solid mass. Real-time ultrasound can show particulate matter slowly moving inside the cyst. On real-time imaging, the debris causes speckle artifact, which swirls in the cyst like fake snow in a snow globe (Fig. 5-8A to C). Placing the patient in the decubitus position can cause a difference in the sedimentation pattern in the complicated cyst, but not always. Color Doppler or power Doppler ultrasound can detect movement of particulate matter within complicated breast cysts or blood vessels in solid masses (see Fig. 5-8D and E). Doppler imaging will show no blood vessels in breast cysts. Unfortunately, the absence of blood flow in a mass is not diagnostic of a cyst because Doppler imaging does not always detect blood flow in solid masses or even in cancers.

In everyday clinical practice, cysts do not always fulfill all the strict sonographic criteria for cysts because of a variety of technical factors, or they may contain echoes from debris within the fluid. Posterior enhanced through-transmission of sound was not seen on all images in 25% of 80 cysts reported by Hilton and colleagues. Internal cyst echoes may be produced by reverberation artifacts, although the near-field reverberations may be reduced by scanning through an offset. However, Berg and colleagues (2003, 2005) and other researchers have shown that complicated cysts with low-level internal echoes, no mural masses, thin walls, and thin septations rarely represent cancer and can either be monitored or aspirated with little or no morbidity.

Differentiation of complicated cysts from benign or malignant cystic masses can be tricky (see Table 5-3). Some cysts contain true internal echoes as a result of thick tenacious fluid or hemorrhage from previous aspirations. Some cysts have thick walls as a result of inflammation from cyst fluid leaking into the surrounding tissues. In cases in which all the sonographic criteria of a simple cyst have not been met, fine-needle aspiration may obviate the need for core needle biopsy or surgical biopsy. Once the needle is within the mass, the presence of cyst fluid rather than solid tissue can be confirmed by moving the needle, as suggested by Stavros and colleagues (Fig. 5-9). Cysts that do not fulfill all criteria for simple cysts, in the right clinical setting, require aspiration (see Fig. 5-9C to E). Cyst fluid should be sent for cytologic analysis if it is bloody, if there is an intracystic mass on ultrasound or pneumocystography, or if the patient has had prior intracystic carcinoma. Clear cyst fluid can be discarded if there are no clinical factors that would require cytologic examination.

On the other hand, complex cystic masses (i.e., fluid-filled masses with thick walls or mural projections) require biopsy to exclude the rare intracystic papilloma, intracystic carcinoma, phyllodes tumor with a marked cystic component, or solid cancers with central necrosis. Other complex masses include hematoma, abscess, galactocele, and seroma; management of these masses is based on their appearance and the clinical situation (Fig. 5-10).

Intracystic carcinomas are a rare subgroup of tumors that arise from the walls of a cyst; they represent 0.5% to 1.3% of all breast cancers (Fig. 5-11A). These tumors have a better prognosis than other malignant breast neoplasms do. On ultrasound, intracystic carcinomas often appear as solid mural excrescences projecting into the cyst fluid. Differentiation of intracystic carcinoma from benign intracystic papilloma is not possible, and surgical biopsy is thus necessary. The finding of a mural nodule within a cyst has the differential of an intracystic carcinoma, papilloma, a cyst

TABLE 5-3. BI-RADS® Ultrasound Special Cases (Cystic)

Cystic Mass Type	Description	Differential Diagnosis
Clustered microcysts	2- to 3-mm cysts Thin (<0.5 mm) septations No solid component	Benign
Complicated cysts	Cyst with debris or fluid/debris level Debris may shift at real-time Not pus or blood	Benign
Complex mass	Has cystic and solid components	Cancer Hematoma/seroma Abscess Phyllodes tumor Intracystic papilloma or cancer Galactocele

Modified from American College of Radiology: ACR BI-RADS®—ultrasound, In *ACR Breast Imaging and Reporting and Data System, breast imaging atlas*, Reston, VA, 2003, American College of Radiology.

BOX 5-5. Complicated Cysts

A complicated cyst is different from a complex mass. A complicated cyst has an imperceptible wall and cyst fluid with debris. A complex mass has cystic and *solid* components and might be cancer.

BOX 5-6. Differential Diagnosis for Cystic or Fluid-Containing Masses

Simple cyst
Complicated cyst
Intracystic papilloma
Intracystic carcinoma
Necrotic cancer
Hematoma
Abscess
Galactocele
Seroma/postsurgical scar (early)

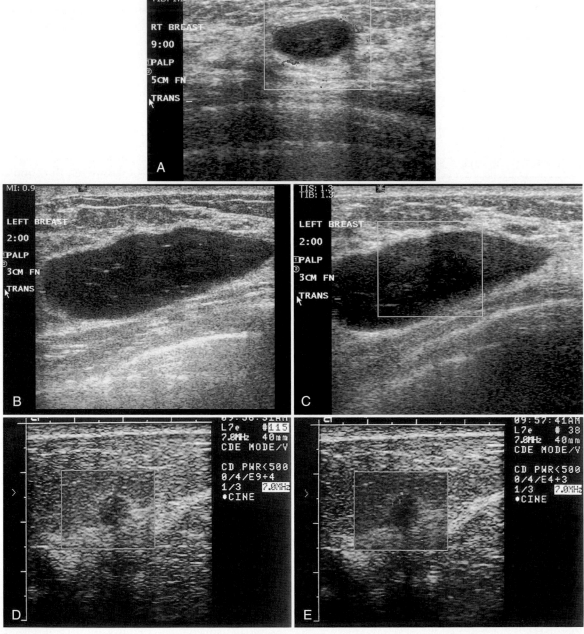

FIGURE 5-8. Complicated cysts and Doppler ultrasound. **A,** This complicated cyst had debris within it that did not move at real-time imaging. Color Doppler ultrasound shows pulsating blood vessels around the cyst but not within it. Aspiration yielded cloudy fluid. **B,** Ultrasound of a palpable mass showed speckle artifact within a complicated cyst that moved at real-time imaging. **C,** Color Doppler ultrasound detected movement of the debris in real time. In contradistinction, color Doppler (**D**) and power Doppler (**E**) imaging show a pulsating vessel flowing into a round cancer, thus differentiating it from complicated cysts.

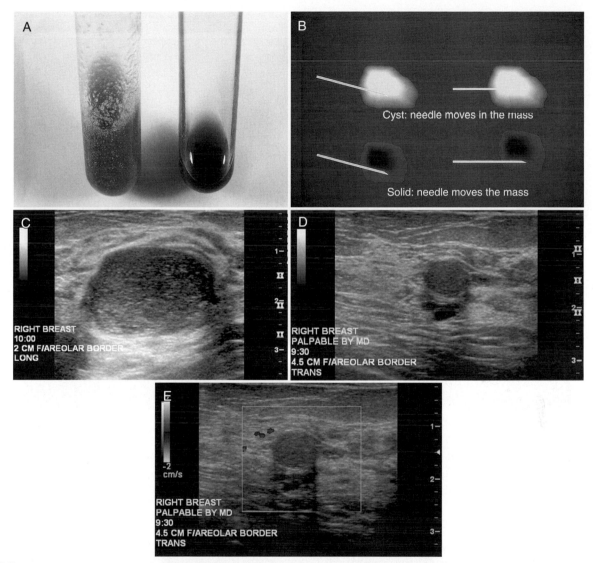

FIGURE 5-9. Simple cyst fluid compared with cyst fluid containing debris. **A,** The complicated cyst fluid in the left test tube, which contains debris consisting of particulate matter, causes speckles within the cyst on ultrasound. The simple cyst fluid in the right test tube is clear and contains no debris. Both fluids are normal and may be discarded after aspiration. **B,** A simple way to tell whether a mass is cystic at needle biopsy is to move the needle tip within the mass. In a complicated cyst, the needle will move within the mass. In a solid mass, the needle will move the mass up and down. **C,** Complicated cyst. This patient felt a palpable mass; ultrasound shows an oval, hypoechoic mass with sharp walls and enhanced through-sound transmission, suggesting cystic or solid material. Doppler ultrasound showed no flow. Aspiration showed yellow fluid with debris within it compatible with a cyst. **D** and **E,** Deeply located complicated cyst and simple cyst. Ultrasound shows an oval, well circumscribed hypoechoic mass with an imperceptible wall anterior to a simple cyst near the chest wall. Despite scanning from several angles, the hypoechoic mass could not be shown to be a simple cyst and Doppler imaging showed no flow. Fine-needle aspiration under ultrasound guidance showed cystic fluid from both masses. The anterior mass represented a complicated cyst and the deeper mass represented a simple cyst.

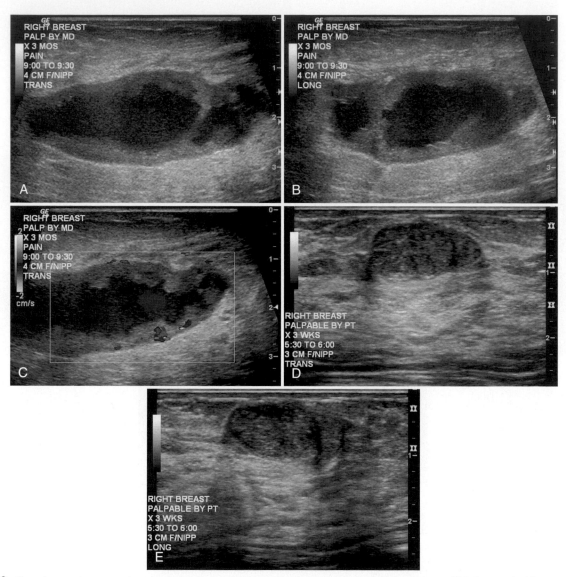

FIGURE 5-10. Complex cystic masses that contain both anechoic (cystic) and echogenic (solid) components. This large palpable mass, in a patient with diabetes, has an anechoic center and a solid, irregular rim in transverse (**A**) and longitudinal (**B**) scans. **C,** Doppler ultrasound showed pulsation in the rim. Another complex cystic mass is oval and has small cystic structures with some solid components on transverse (**D**) and longitudinal (**E**) scans. This was a phyllodes tumor. Phyllodes tumors have solid leaflike components floating in small cystic structures, which give the tumor its name and account for the cystic and solid appearance in this image. The cystic versus solid components vary according to each tumor.

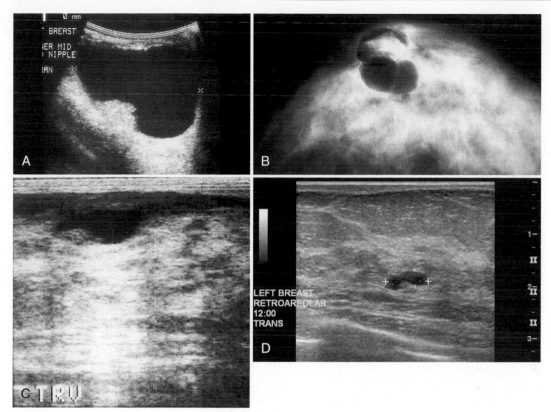

FIGURE 5-11. Intracystic tumors. **A,** An intracystic carcinoma is shown as a mural mass projecting into the fluid-filled center of a cyst on ultrasound. **B,** In another patient, an intracystic papilloma is shown as a mass surrounded by air after fluid aspiration and pneumocystography. **C,** In a third patient, an apparent intracystic mass was shown to represent debris stuck to the side wall of a complicated cyst at aspiration. **D,** This oval, well-circumscribed cystic mass has a round, solid mural nodule. Because it is not completely anechoic, it cannot be considered a simple cyst and is a complex mass; the differential is intracystic cancer papilloma or debris in a cyst. Aspiration was performed, showing cystic fluid and debris without atypia or cancer on cytology.

with debris, and reverberations in a simple cyst produced by high gain settings (see Fig. 5-11B to D). Color or power Doppler imaging may be helpful if a blood vessel can be identified in the intracystic mass.

Benign Solid Masses: Fibroadenoma and Fatty Pseudolesions

Fibroadenomas arise from breast lobules and are the most common solid benign masses in women younger than age 30 years. Once diagnosed, fibroadenomas may remain stable in 80% of cases, regress in about 15%, and grow in 5% to 10%. Fibroadenomas are benign, although cancer can occur within a fibroadenoma. Women with a specific histologic diagnosis of *complex fibroadenomas* have cysts or histologic elements other than the fibroadenoma and have a small increased risk of future breast cancer, as described by DuPont and colleagues. Fibroadenomas may be single or multiple and are called *giant fibroadenomas* if larger than 8 cm.

On ultrasound, Cole-Beuglet and colleagues describe typical fibroadenomas as solid masses with well-circumscribed, round or oval borders and containing weak low-level homogeneous internal echoes with enhanced, decreased, or unchanged sound transmission. Stavros and colleagues and Fornage and colleagues have described fibroadenomas as smooth, wider than tall solid masses. Stavros and colleagues further characterize fibroadenomas

> **BOX 5-7. Benign Mass Characteristics**
>
> Ellipsoid shape (wider than tall)
> Four or fewer gentle lobulations
> Intense homogeneous hyperechogenicity (in comparison to fat)
> Thin, echogenic capsule
> No malignant sonographic criteria

From Stavros AT, Thickman D, Rapp CL, et al: Solid breast nodules: use of sonography to distinguish between benign and malignant lesions, *Radiology* 196:123–134, 1995.

as having at most four gentle lobulations and homogeneous internal echo texture (Box 5-7 and Fig. 5-12A to C).

Fibroadenoma appearances, however, can be highly variable (see Fig. 5-12D and E). Fibroadenomas may occasionally display irregular margins, inhomogeneous echo texture, lobulated borders, or posterior acoustic shadowing. These atypical features result in biopsy of the fibroadenoma to exclude cancer.

Stavros and colleagues also described specific ultrasound features of benign solid masses (see Box 5-7): smooth margins with fewer than four gentle lobulations, intense homogeneous hyperechogenicity, thin echogenic pseudocapsule, wider than tall elongated appearance, and no malignant sonographic signs. Suspicious ultrasound findings include acoustic shadowing, microlobulation, microcalcifications, ductal extension, angulated margins, or a very hypoechoic pattern (Box 5-8). In their 1995 study, Stavros and colleagues compared large-core needle or surgical biopsy pathology to prospectively determined ultrasound features of solid breast masses to see if the ultrasound criteria could predict malignancy. When the sonographic findings were benign by their criteria, the results yielded 424 true negatives and 2 false negatives. The negative predictive value was 99.5% and the sensitivity was 98.4%

with strict adherence to their benign ultrasound features. However, it is also known that some well-circumscribed carcinomas may simulate fibroadenomas and should undergo biopsy if new or in the appropriate clinical setting (see Fig. 5-12H to J) because not all round or oval solid masses are benign (Box 5-9).

After finding a mass by ultrasound, it is important to re-evaluate the mammogram to make sure the ultrasound findings represent the mammographic findings on the film. The mammogram may provide important clues to the

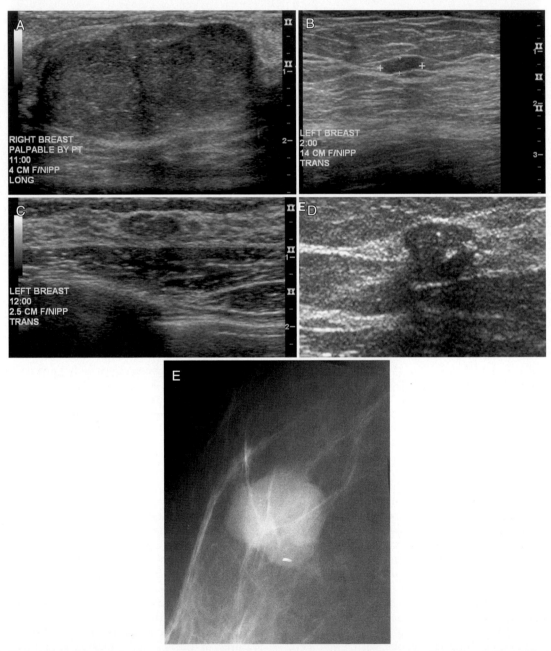

FIGURE 5-12. Typical fibroadenomas. **A,** Ultrasound of a typical fibroadenoma shows a mass that is wider than tall, smooth, and homogeneous with edge refraction. **B,** Nonpalpable, oval, homogeneous, sharply defined typical fibroadenoma. **C,** Oval, homogeneous, well-circumscribed fibroadenoma in a third patient is well-displayed against the echogenic glandular tissue. **D,** Ultrasound of another fibroadenoma shows an atypical round shape containing calcifications. **E,** The corresponding mammogram shows a well-circumscribed, dense smooth mass with peripheral coarse calcifications. Biopsy revealed fibroadenoma.

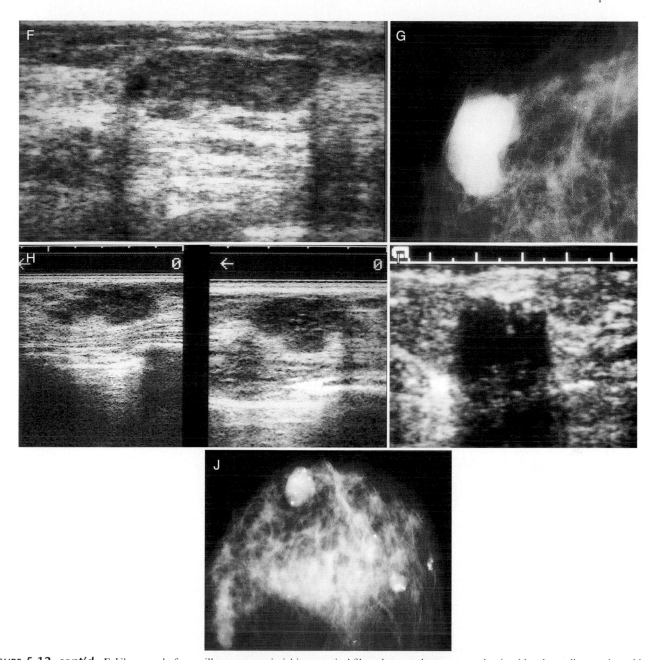

FIGURE 5-12, cont'd. **F,** Ultrasound of a papillary cancer mimicking a typical fibroadenoma shows a mass that is wider than tall, smooth, and homogeneous with a few gentle lobulations. **G,** The corresponding mammogram shows the cancer as a dense, well-circumscribed, lobulated mass. **H,** Ultrasound of another papillary cancer shows a wider than tall homogeneous mass with more than three gentle lobulations, findings suggestive of cancer and not easily mistaken for fibroadenoma. **I,** Importance of correlating ultrasound with the mammogram. Ultrasound of a calcified fibroadenoma mimicking a typical cancer shows a calcified, intensely shadowing mass that is suspicious for carcinoma. **J,** The corresponding mammogram shows that the mass in **I** has typical peripheral popcorn-like calcifications in a well-circumscribed lobulated fibroadenoma, among other typical calcifying fibroadenomas in the same breast, and biopsy was avoided. *Continued*

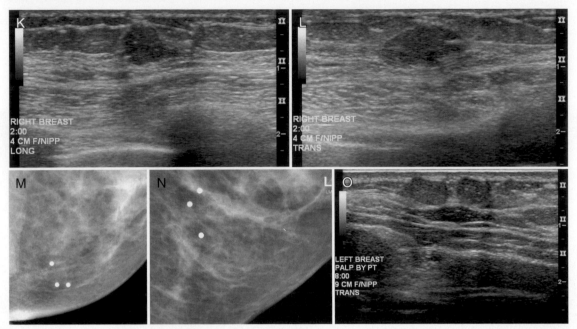

FIGURE 5-12, cont'd. **K** and **L**, Importance of evaluating a mass in orthogonal planes. A longitudinal ultrasound (**K**) shows a mostly round, well-circumscribed mass. However, note that on the transverse image (**L**), the mass is oval, wider than tall, and well-circumscribed. Biopsy showed fibroadenoma. **M** to **O**, Lipomas on mammography and ultrasound. **M**, Cropped craniocaudal mammogram shows markers over fatty palpable masses that have thin rims. **N**, Magnified cropped mammogram shows the masses to greater advantage. **O**, Ultrasound shows round, well-circumscribed masses with an abrupt interface and fatty echogenicity compatible with lipomas.

BOX 5-8. Suspicious Ultrasound Characteristics of Solid Breast Masses

Taller than wide
Acoustic shadowing
Spiculation
Microlobulation
Microcalcifications
Duct extension
Branch pattern
Angular margins
Markedly hypoechoic (in comparison to fat)

From Stavros AT, Thickman D, Rapp CL, et al: Solid breast nodules: use of sonography to distinguish between benign and malignant lesions, *Radiology* 196:123–134, 1995.

BOX 5-9. Differential Diagnosis of Round or Oval Solid Breast Masses

Fibroadenoma
Invasive ductal cancer, not otherwise specified
Medullary cancer
Mucinous (colloid) carcinoma
Papillary carcinoma
Metastasis
Phyllodes tumor
Papilloma

---

correct diagnosis. For example, if there are calcifications in a mass on ultrasound, the mass may be a typical calcifying fibroadenoma, benign fat necrosis, or calcifying cancer. By placing a skin marker over the ultrasound finding and retaking a mammogram, one can analyze the calcifications further and make a diagnosis. This is especially true if the calcifications found by ultrasound show up on the mammogram as typical for fibroadenoma (popcorn-type) or cancer (pleomorphic) (see Fig 5-9K and L).

It is also important to scan masses in orthogonal planes and at multiple angles to see all the borders. A mass that appears round in one plane might actually be the cross-section of an oval mass (see Fig 5-9M and N). Scanning carefully in multiple planes allows the sonographer to evaluate both the true mass shape and all the margins of the mass.

Palpable pseudolesions can be produced by fatty deposits or oil cysts in the breast. A mammogram taken with a skin marker on the palpable mass should clarify that the mass is actually a fatty deposit or an oil cyst by showing only fat under the marker. When a fatty pseudomass is scanned from various projections, the masslike appearance of the fatty lobule should blend into the surrounding tissue and lack three-dimensional features. Oil cysts are well-circumscribed cystic or fat echogenic masses on ultrasound. If unsure if an ultrasound finding represents a fatty lobule, the sonographer can place a skin marker over the ultrasound finding and repeat the mammogram (see Fig. 5-9O to Q). If the finding is a fatty mass, there should be only fat under the skin marker.

Other benign solid breast masses include papillomas, hamartomas, lymph nodes, and healed postsurgical scars. In these various benign conditions, the clinical setting and mammographic appearance usually help identify the true nature of the lesion because sonographic features alone are rarely diagnostic (except in the case of lymph nodes). Examples of these masses are shown in Chapter 4.

Malignant Solid Masses

Cancers are generally hypoechoic relative to the brightly echogenic normal fibroglandular tissue. They often have irregular or round shapes and angulated or spiculated margins. Cancers often can show invasion by extending through normal breast planes ("taller than wide") and may have an echogenic halo. They can show posterior acoustic shadowing, which is a dark band posterior to the mass that is reported to occur in 60% to 97% of spiculated carcinomas. Posterior acoustic shadowing is extremely suspicious for cancer and is thought to relate to fibrosis or collagen associated with the tumor. Acoustic shadowing is different from edge shadowing, which is an artifact caused by the edge of the mass against normal breast tissue. To distinguish edge shadowing from true acoustic shadowing, the sonographer scans from different planes. Edge shadowing will not persist in all planes, but true acoustic shadowing will persist. Examples of breast cancers on ultrasound are shown in Figures 5-13 to 5-15.

The ACR BI-RADS® ultrasound lexicon and terms developed by Stavros and colleagues include features that suggest cancer, such as margins that are angulated, indistinct, microlobulated, or spiculated; acoustic shadowing; microcalcifications; ductal extension; an echogenic halo; and a taller than wide configuration (see Box 5-8 and Table 5-2).

However, one cannot always be sure that round, well-circumscribed masses are benign. Unfortunately, round circumscribed solid cancers simulate benign breast masses on ultrasound. The most common round breast cancer is invasive ductal cancer (Box 5-10). The round form of invasive ductal cancer is an uncommon form of the most common cancer. Although the round, circumscribed form is uncommon for invasive ductal cancer, invasive ductal

---

BOX 5-10. Round Breast Cancer

The most common round breast malignancy is invasive ductal cancer. It is an uncommon form of a very common tumor.

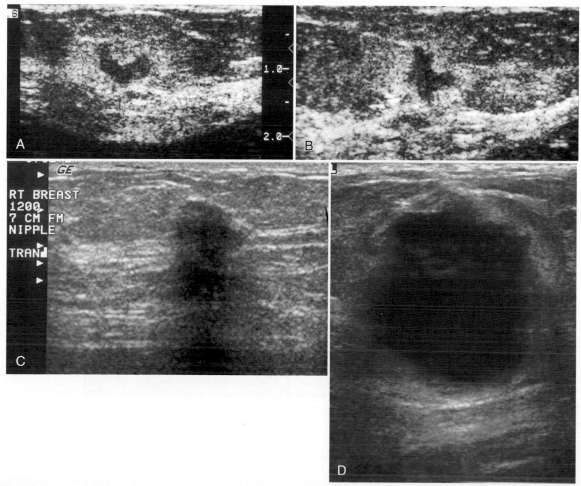

FIGURE 5-13. Typical breast cancers on ultrasound. Transverse (**A**) and longitudinal (**B**) scans show a typical invasive ductal cancer: very hypoechoic relative to normal breast tissue and surrounded by a fuzzy echogenic halo. The irregular shape, angulated margins, invasive growth through normal tissue planes, and taller than wide configuration are all suspicious for cancer. Note that acoustic shadowing is absent in this cancer and that shadowing is not necessary to make the diagnosis. **C,** Ultrasound of a grade II invasive ductal carcinoma shows a very hypoechoic indistinct irregular mass with marked acoustic shadowing. **D,** Invasive ductal carcinoma as irregular hypoechoic mass with enhanced through-sound transmission.

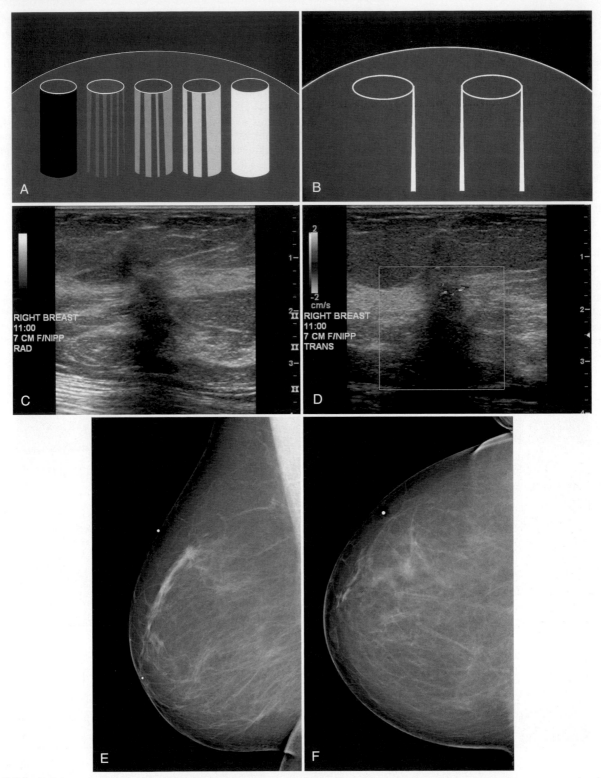

FIGURE 5-14. **A,** Schematic drawing of acoustic shadowing on the left with variations of shadowing and acoustic enhancement on the right. **B,** In comparison, the artifact of edge refraction will be seen only at the edge of a mass, where it meets the surrounding breast tissue, and not in the middle of the mass. **C to F,** Acoustic shadowing in cancer. **C,** Radio ultrasound shows a taller than wide, very hypoechoic, spiculated mass with acoustic shadowing, representing invasive ductal cancer. D, Doppler ultrasound shows a pulsating vessel within the cancer. To correlate the ultrasound mass with mammographic findings, the technologist placed a metallic marker over the mass and repeated the mammogram. Right digital mammograms show the marker in close proximity to a spiculated mass in an otherwise fatty breast on the lateral view (**E**), but it is at least 2 cm away from the mass on the craniocaudal view (**F**). This is because the skin containing the BB compressed away from mass in a projection, which is not uncommon when using skin markers to correlate mammograms to ultrasound findings. The mass was invasive ductal cancer.

cancers are so common that a round cancer is statistically likely to be invasive ductal cancer (Fig. 5-16A). Other round, circumscribed malignancies include medullary, solid papillary, and colloid (mucinous) carcinoma. These cancers can simulate benign fibroadenomas on ultrasound by appearing round or oval in shape with enhanced transmission of sound (see Fig. 5-16B and C).

Careful attention to the margins of a mass may prompt biopsy and suggest cancer when, at first glance, the margins appear to be circumscribed. The borders of some tumors may appear circumscribed in one scan plane but irregular in another plane, so it is important to scan in multiple planes to evaluate all mass borders for margin irregularity (see Fig. 5-16D).

Necrosis or mucin within cancers may produce anechoic regions, resulting in posterior acoustic enhancement of sound, thereby mimicking the enhanced transmission of sound seen in cysts. Thus, some benign sonographic features of fibroadenomas and benign complex cystic lesions can also be seen in round malignancies (Table 5-4).

Some of the larger calcifications in breast cancer may be seen by ultrasonography, but this important diagnostic sign is not generally visualized with regularity by ultrasound (Fig. 5-17A and B).

TABLE 5-4. Unfortunate Ultrasound Look-Alikes

Finding	Look-Alikes
Fibroadenoma	Well-circumscribed cancer
	Papillary cancer
Solid benign mass	Complicated cyst with no swirling debris
	Well-circumscribed cancer
Complex benign mass	Cystic/solid cancer

Abnormal lymph nodes in the axilla are hypoechoic oval masses without a fatty hilum (see Fig. 5-17C to E). Lobulated or irregular abnormal lymph node borders or a thickened lymph node cortex can also indicate metastatic disease. Benign reactive lymph nodes cannot be reliably differentiated from lymph nodes containing metastases or lymphoma (see Fig. 5-17F and G). On the other hand, one cannot tell if a normal-appearing lymph node contains occult metastases. In the setting of known cancer, referring physicians may request needle biopsy of lymph nodes to make a diagnosis of metastatic disease before surgery or neoadjuvant chemotherapy.

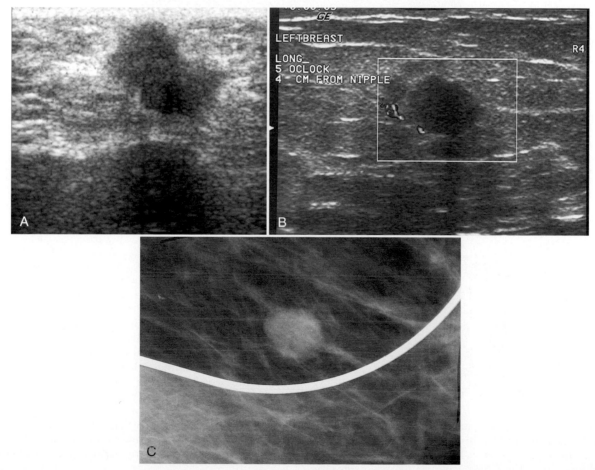

FIGURE 5-15. Features of breast cancers without acoustic shadowing on ultrasound. **A,** Ultrasound of an invasive ductal carcinoma shows a very hypoechoic irregular mass with an echogenic halo near an implant. **B,** Ultrasound of a grade II invasive ductal cancer shows a very hypoechoic microlobulated mass with a small blood vessel adjacent to it. **C,** The corresponding mammogram shows a round mass, perhaps with microlobulations.

Continued

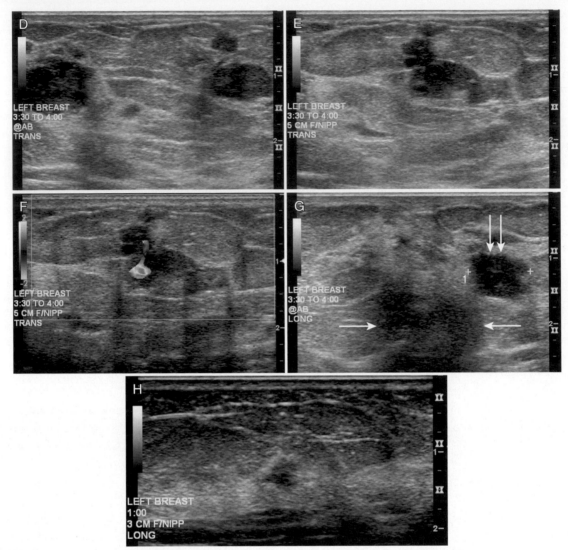

FIGURE 5-15, cont'd. **D,** Ultrasound of an extensive breast cancer, shown as multiple nodules on the mammogram, reveals an irregular, hypoechoic, oval mass corresponding to an extensive multifocal invasive ductal cancer without acoustic shadowing. **E,** In the same patient, another irregular, hypoechoic mass without acoustic shadowing represents a different invasive ductal cancer. **F,** Doppler ultrasound shows a large pulsating artery within the cancer. **G,** Contrast two foci of invasive ductal cancer on the same image; one is an irregular mass without acoustic shadowing *(double arrows)* and the other is shown only as acoustic shadowing *(arrows)*. **H,** Suspicious mass on longitudinal scan shows a tiny irregular mass with an echogenic halo and no acoustic shadowing; this was invasive ductal cancer.

BOX 5-11. Secondary Signs of Breast Cancer on Ultrasound

Calcifications
Lymphadenopathy
Skin thickening
Architectural distortion
Breast edema
Retraction of Cooper ligaments

Secondary signs of breast cancer include skin thickening, architectural distortion, breast edema, and retraction of Cooper ligaments (Box 5-11; see also Fig. 5-17H). Inflammatory carcinomas may have all of these signs, as well as marked attenuation of the sound beam due to breast edema (see Fig. 5-17I to K).

Breast Calcifications

Breast calcifications may be the only indication of breast cancer on mammography and therefore it is important to understand them. Calcifications are often seen in ductal carcinoma in situ (DCIS) but may also be the only indication of invasive ductal cancer. If ultrasound is done in the region of the abnormal calcifications, ultrasound may show an associated mass that was obscured or hidden by dense breast tissue on the mammogram. The purpose of detecting these associated masses is to further analyze the finding and direct subsequent ultrasound-guided biopsy. If no suspicious mass or calcifications are discovered on targeted ultrasound, the decision to biopsy the calcifications is based solely on mammographic analysis of the calcifications.

Although mammography effectively detects calcifications in DCIS, ultrasound is limited in finding calcifications

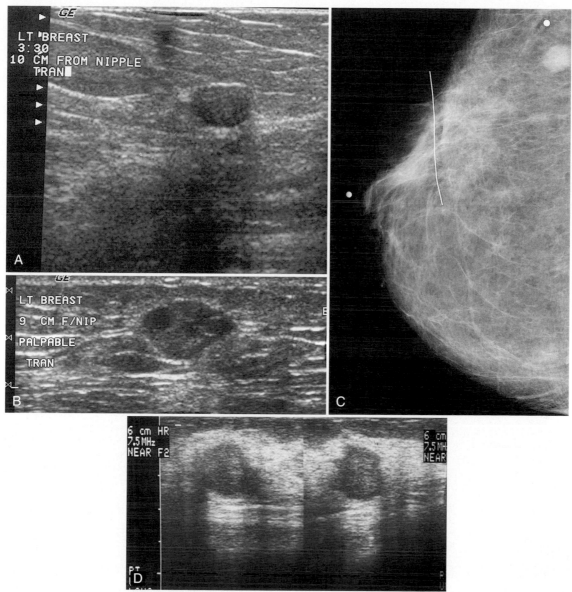

FIGURE 5-16. Breast cancer mimicking benign masses on ultrasound. A, A well-circumscribed, oval, hypoechoic mass on ultrasound is an invasive ductal cancer that was new on the mammogram from the previous year. Although medullary and mucinous cancers are often round, invasive ductal cancer is more common (accounting for about 90% of all breast cancers) and is the most common round cancer. B, Mucinous cancer mimicking a complicated cyst on ultrasound. Ultrasound of a palpable mass shows an oval, circumscribed, complex cystic mass with rather thick septa. Correlation with the mammogram (C) shows a dense, slightly irregular mass that would be unusual for a multilobulated cyst. Biopsy revealed mucinous cancer. D, Medullary cancer. Ultrasound of a palpable mass in a young woman shows a round mass with acoustic enhancement. Note that some of the borders are circumscribed on one scan plane, but one side of the mass has three spiculations, thus demonstrating the importance of scanning all the margins of the mass in more than one plane.

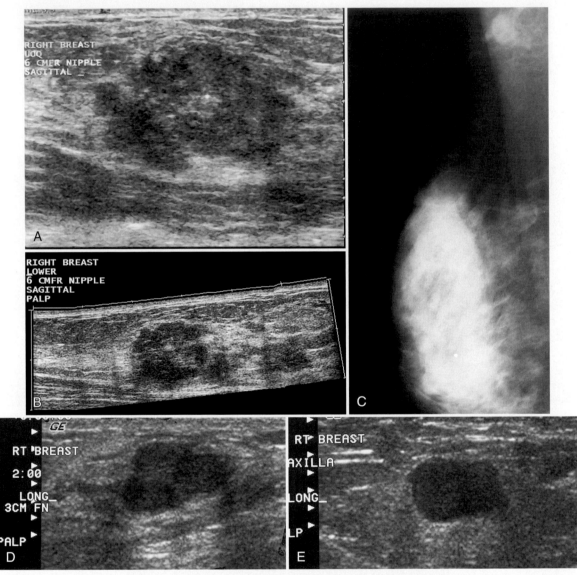

FIGURE 5-17. Features of malignancy on ultrasound. **A,** This invasive ductal cancer has microlobulated borders and bright internal echoes, representing calcifications within the tumor. **B,** A landscape overview shows the invasive ductal cancer of part **A** with its internal calcifications and a smaller second tumor slightly inferior and lateral to it. **C to G,** Axillary metastasis. **C,** A mediolateral oblique (MLO) mammogram shows a dense breast with an abnormal dense lymph node in the axilla. **D,** Ultrasound of a palpable mass in the breast tissue on the ipsilateral side, not seen on the mammogram, shows a circumscribed lobulated mass with enhanced transmission of sound that represents an invasive ductal cancer. **E,** Ultrasound of the abnormal lymph node in the axilla shows a hypoechoic mass without a fatty hilum that represents lymphadenopathy from the metastasis. Contrast the abnormal lymph node with the normal lymph node shown in Figure 5-1G.

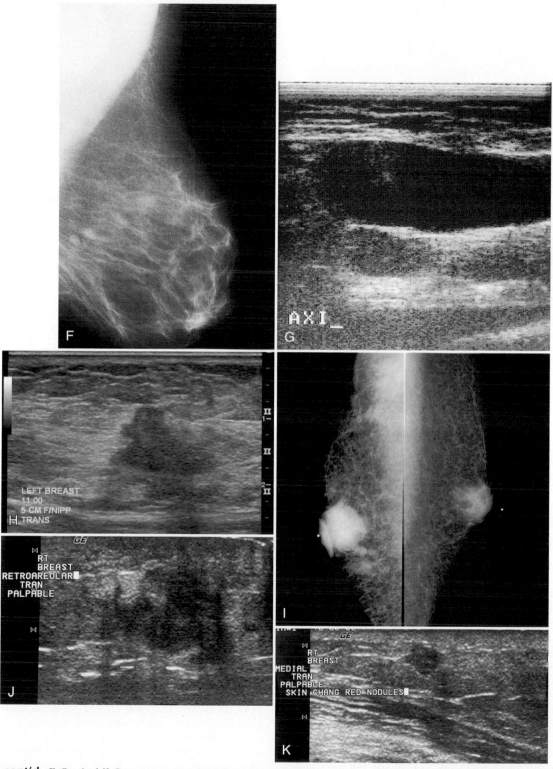

FIGURE 5-17, cont'd. F, On the MLO mammogram, a huge dense abnormal lymph node is evident in the axilla. **G,** Ultrasound shows a hypoechoic mass so homogeneous that it almost looks like a cyst. Biopsy findings were consistent with lymphoma. **H,** A hypoechoic, irregular invasive ductal cancer with angulated margins is not parallel and has indistinct borders. **I** to **K,** Inflammatory cancer in a male with red skin nodules. **I,** MLO mammograms show bilateral gynecomastia with an irregular right retroareolar mass, skin and nipple thickening, and a second mass in the axilla. **J,** Ultrasound shows a hypoechoic spiculated and angulated retroareolar mass with acoustic shadowing and thickening of the areola–nipple complex. **K,** Ultrasound of the skin changes and red nodules shows marked skin thickening and a hypoechoic mass in the skin from inflammatory cancer.

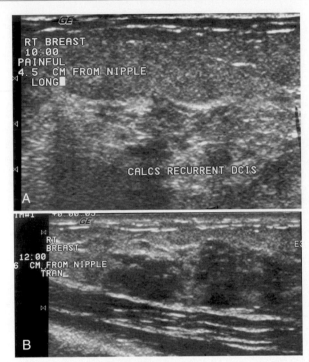

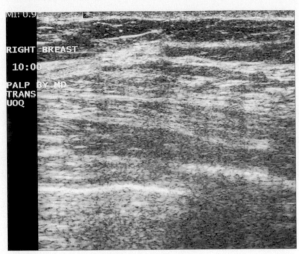

FIGURE 5-19. Ultrasound of a palpable mass felt by the patient's physician shows normal breast tissue and no discrete mass. This image was taken after the patient pointed out the mass prompting this examination; the mass was palpated by the sonographer who scanned over it. With a negative mammogram and ultrasound, management of the palpable finding is based on clinical grounds alone, and the patient is encouraged to follow up with her referring physician for the palpable finding. In this case, an image of the normal breast tissue was obtained; however, some facilities take no images of normal breast tissue and only take an image of specific areas described by breast side, clock or quadrant position of the finding, number of centimeters from the nipple, and "palpable finding."

FIGURE 5-18. **A,** Ultrasound of recurrent ductal carcinoma in situ (DCIS) shows a few calcifications as bright echoes near hypoechoic dilated ducts, but they might easily be lost in the normal speckled background of breast tissue. **B,** Ultrasound of DCIS in another patient shows clumped hypoechoic nodular ducts on the chest wall and a few bright echoes within ducts, possibly representing the microcalcifications easily seen on mammography.

because the calcifications may be lost in the normal speckle artifact of normal breast tissue (Fig. 5-18A). On ultrasound, DCIS looks like multiple dark hypoechoic nodules or enlarged knobby ducts that may conglomerate into a mass. This is because DCIS expands normal ducts. Ultrasound is much better at finding invasive breast cancer as breast masses than in detecting breast calcifications, unless the calcifications are associated with a mass. In a 2004 study of 111 women with breast cancer by Berg, mammography was compared with ultrasound for detection of invasive and noninvasive breast cancer. Ultrasound showed 12% (129/139) of invasive breast cancers and 47% (18/38) of DCIS, whereas mammography depicted 71% (99/139) of invasive cancers and 55% (21/38) of DCIS. Thus, mammography is better at showing calcifications than ultrasound.

On occasion, highly aggressive DCIS shows up on ultrasound as hypoechoic masses, as reported by Soo and colleagues, Huang and colleagues, and Moon and colleagues (see Fig. 5-18B). Nondetection of DCIS calcifications is reported by others when ultrasound is used as a primary and stand-alone method of breast cancer screening. The nondetection of calcifications alone may limit ultrasound's use as a stand-alone screening modality, discussed in this chapter in the section, "Breast Cancer Screening with Ultrasound."

PALPABLE OR MAMMOGRAPHICALLY DETECTED FINDINGS UNDETECTED BY ULTRASOUND

Benign fibrofatty nodules, areas of dense glandular tissue, benign breast tissue, or breast cancer all may be felt as a mass or lump by the patient or her physician. Ultrasound can be normal when scanning directly over the palpable finding (Fig. 5-19). If the mammogram is normal, the patient is directed back to her referring physician for management of the palpable mass. In these cases, management of the palpable mass is based on clinical grounds alone. The decision may be made to perform biopsy based solely on the physical examination because some cancers are missed by both mammography and ultrasound, and the only indication of cancer is the palpable breast lump.

For patients with suspicious physical findings and both a normal mammogram and ultrasound, the decision to perform biopsy is based on the physical findings and the clinical situation alone. Invasive lobular cancer is especially notorious for producing extremely subtle or no mammographic findings and yet still producing a palpable mass that causes the patient to seek advice. Invasive lobular cancer also may be missed by ultrasound.

Some breast cancers and solid benign breast masses discovered by mammography are ultrasonographically "invisible." In the setting of a mammographically suspicious lesion and a "normal" ultrasound examination, further investigation or biopsy should be based on the mammogram. If the suspicious mammographic finding is not found by targeted ultrasound, the mass is presumed to be composed of solid tissue and could be benign or malignant. In these cases, the decision to perform biopsy is based solely on the mammographic impression, clinical situation, and physical findings.

YOUNG PATIENTS AND PALPABLE FINDINGS IN DENSE BREASTS

Ultrasound is commonly used as the first modality to evaluate palpable findings in young patients. This is particularly true in women younger than age 30 because breasts in younger women are composed of mostly glandular tissue, which may hide a cancer. Similarly, ultrasound may be used to evaluate palpable masses in women with radiographically dense breasts on mammography at any age.

Invasive cancers can hide in the dense breast tissue on some views and may initially be seen as a "one-view-only" finding. Some invasive cancers may be palpable but not seen at all by mammography. Ultrasound can be extremely helpful when one suspects a mass that can be seen on only one view or if it is palpable and suspicious. However, ultrasound should be used only after the full mammographic workup is complete (Fig. 5-20).

Ultrasound may confirm that a suspicious finding on one view only is actually overlapping breast tissue rather than a real mass (see Fig. 5-20H). If no mass is seen on breast ultrasound, the decision for biopsy of the palpable finding is based on clinical grounds alone because some cancers are "invisible" to ultrasound.

CORRELATING MAMMOGRAPHIC FINDINGS WITH ULTRASOUND FINDINGS

When ultrasound finds a mass that was initially discovered by mammography, the next step is to determine whether the ultrasound finding and the mammographic finding represent the same thing. To accomplish this, the sonographer places a metallic skin marker over the ultrasound finding and repeats the mammogram. To determine where to place the skin marker, the sonographer scans directly over the finding and slides a finger, jumbo paper clip, or cotton-tipped swab under the transducer so that it overlies the ultrasound finding (Fig. 5-21A). This produces a ring-down shadow over the finding (see Fig. 5-21B). Once the ring-down shadow overlies the finding, the sonographer removes the transducer, leaving the fingertip, paper clip, or cotton-tipped swab on top of the skin over the mass. The sonographer marks that spot on the skin with a permanent ink marker, then places a radiopaque skin marker on the ink spot and takes a craniocaudal and mediolateral mammogram. The skin marker should correlate with the mammographic finding if the ultrasound and mammography findings are one and the same. Because the lesion may be deep in the breast, the skin marker may be compressed a few centimeters away from the lesion on the follow-up mammogram (see Fig. 5-21C to E).

If the radiologist is still unsure if the findings correlate, the radiologist can place a radiopaque marker in the finding through a needle under ultrasound guidance. Follow-up

Box 5-12. Differential Diagnosis of Breast Edema

UNILATERAL
Mastitis
Inflammatory cancer
Radiation therapy
Unilateral lymphadenopathy
Trauma (focal)

BILATERAL (SYSTEMIC PROBLEMS)
Anasarca
Congestive heart failure
Bilateral lymphadenopathy
Renal failure

orthogonal mammograms will determine whether the marker lies in the mammographic finding, showing whether the mammographic finding and the ultrasound findings are one and the same.

BREAST EDEMA

Breast edema occurs in women with mastitis, inflammatory cancer, radiation therapy, postbiopsy trauma, or blockage of lymphatic drainage by various etiologies (Box 5-12). On physical examination an edematous breast is heavy and boggy. The skin may show *peau d'orange*, or orange-peel skin, in which skin pitting occurs where hair follicles hold the skin down and the surrounding tissues rise up with edema. On ultrasound, breast edema shows skin thickening greater than 2 to 3 mm. When compared with the contralateral breast, the edematous subcutaneous fat is gray as a result of fluid leakage, the normally sharp Cooper ligaments are less well defined, and breast tissue loses the sharp clarity of individual structures because the edema blurs normal breast landmarks. On occasion, dermal and subdermal lymphatics may become engorged and filled with fluid, producing fluid-filled branching tubules simulating blood vessels or ducts (Fig. 5-22A). Fluid-filled lymphatics can be distinguished from blood vessels by Doppler ultrasound; blood vessels will show pulsation, but fluid-filled lymphatics will show no flow (see Fig. 5-22B). Fluid-filled lymphatics will parallel the skin surface and branch quickly along the superficial layers of the breast. Fluid-filled lymphatics are easily distinguished from normal fluid-filled breast because breast ducts are larger than lymphatics and should branch and converge on the nipple.

The key to identifying breast edema is to look for fat that is grayer and skin that is thicker in comparison to the normal contralateral breast (see Fig. 5-22C and D). In a normal breast the fat is dark, and Cooper ligaments and breast structures are sharply demarcated. In an edematous breast the fat is gray, and normal breast structures are less well defined.

Breast edema in inflammatory breast cancer can cause tremendous skin thickening and breast enlargement that attenuates both the x-ray and ultrasound beams because of the enlarged, dense breast tissue filled with fluid and tumor (see Fig. 5-22 E to G).

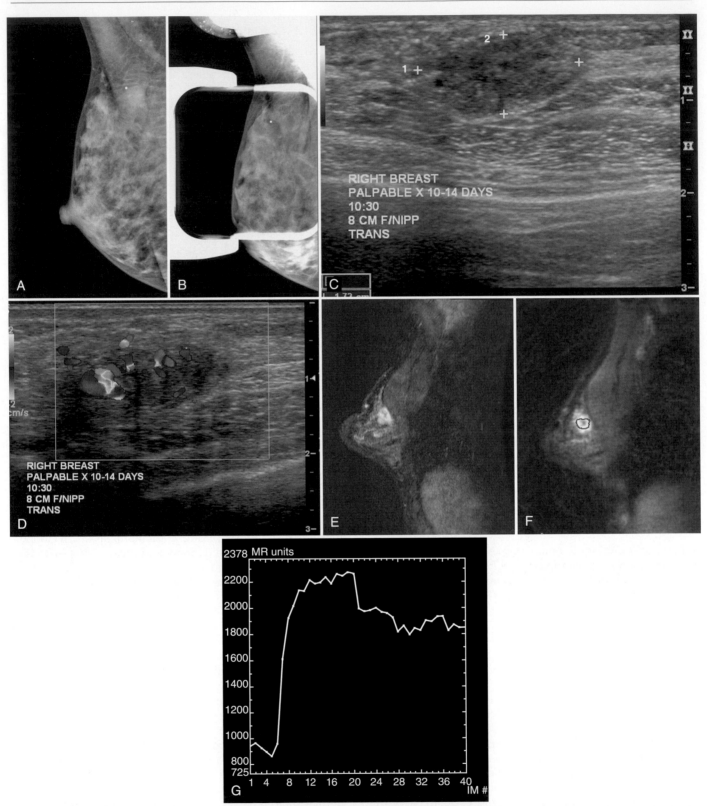

FIGURE 5-20. Correlating a palpable finding to mammograms. **A,** Right mediolateral oblique mammogram in a dense breast shows a marker in the upper right over the palpable mass. **B,** Spot compression in the right mammogram does not show the mass, which is obscured by adjacent glandular tissue. **C,** Ultrasound shows an oval, well-circumscribed complex mass corresponding to the palpable finding. **D,** Color Doppler ultrasound shows marked vascularity in the mass. **E,** Sagittal 3-D spectral-spatial excitation magnetization transfer (3DSSMT) postcontrast breast magnetic resonance imaging (MRI) shows an enhancing upper right breast mass with a small satellite lesion inferiorly. **F,** Sagittal ROI over the mass under spiral dynamic postcontrast MRI shows a rapid initial rise in signal intensity and late washout (**G**). Biopsy showed invasive ductal cancer.

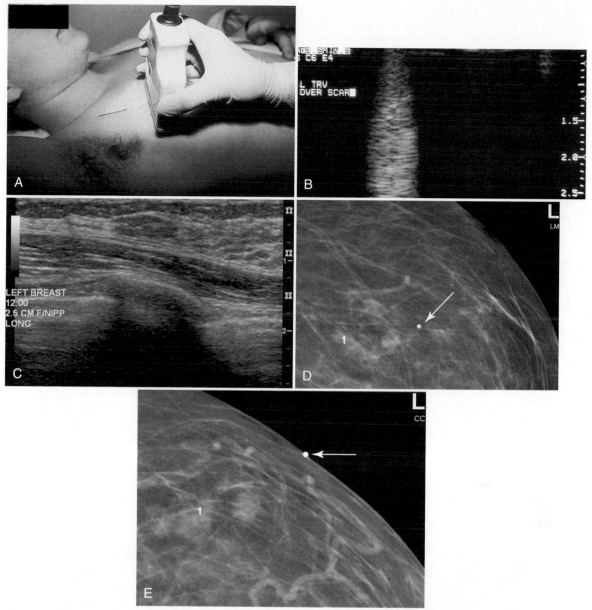

FIGURE 5-21. Correlating the ultrasound finding with the mammogram. **A,** A large open paper clip is placed under the transducer over a finding. **B,** The ring-down shadow from the paper clip produces a bright shadow on the image. Superimposing this ring-down shadow over the lesion triangulates its location directly under the skin. **C,** Ultrasound shows a palpable, well-circumscribed, homogeneous mass in the outer right breast. Using the ring-down shadow technique, a metallic BB was placed on the skin directly over the mass. Cropped magnified lateral (**D**) and craniocaudal (**E**) mammograms show the BB *(arrows)* directly over a well-circumscribed, equal-density round mass, showing that the ultrasound finding corresponds to the mammographic finding. Biopsy showed fibroadenoma.

■ MASTITIS AND BREAST ABSCESS

Mastitis is a breast infection commonly caused by *Staphylococcus aureus* or *Streptococcus*. It is common in nursing mothers, in whom the pathogen enters the breast through a cracked nipple. Mastitis also occurs de novo in adolescents from sexual contact and in diabetics and other immunocompromised patients. Mastitis also can occur in the postoperative period or after percutaneous biopsy.

Mastitis can be hard to scan because the breast is painful and enlarged. On physical examination the skin may be reddened, with focal *peau d'orange*. On ultrasound the

normally black fat turns gray, the skin becomes thick, and the normal breast structures are blurred.

Mastitis is treated with antibiotics. As the breast responds to treatment, it becomes less red, less painful, and less swollen. The object of ultrasound scanning of mastitis in the acute phase is to search for an abscess (focal collection of pus) within the affected breast because an abscess needs immediate intervention by image-guided or surgical drainage to prevent continuing infection and complications from that infection. Thus, the sonographer carefully searches the breast for a focal, well-defined fluid abscess collection that can be drained by a needle. This can be

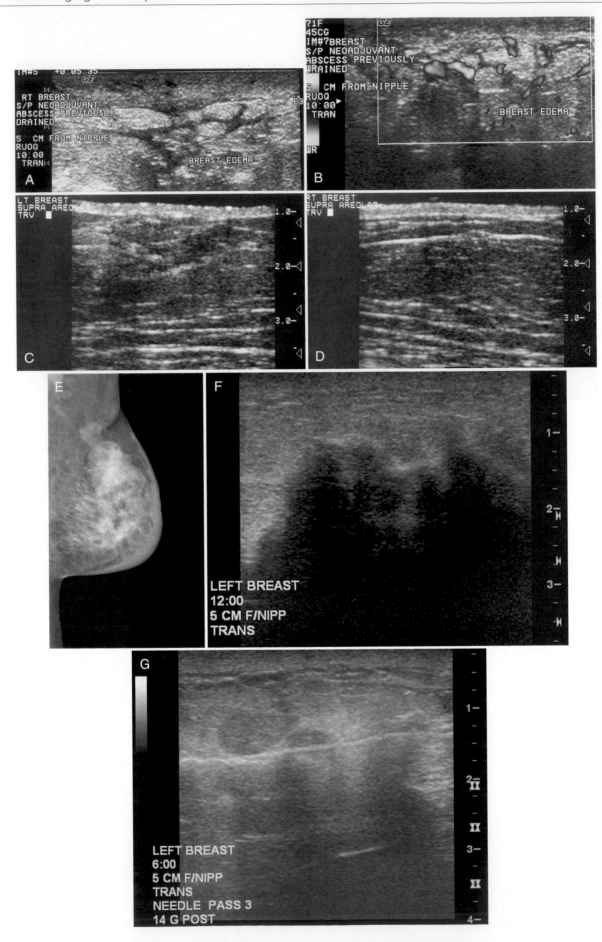

FIGURE 5-22. Breast edema. **A,** Ultrasound shows marked skin thickening and a gray tinge to the normally markedly hypoechoic subcutaneous fat in this patient with marked breast edema. Just below the skin surface are numerous tubular fluid-filled structures representing blood vessels and fluid-filled lymphatics. Cooper ligaments are not seen distinctly. **B,** Power Doppler ultrasound shows that some of the structures represent blood vessels from hyperemia, whereas others show no flow and represent fluid-filled dilated lymphatics. **C,** Breast edema in another patient shows gray-appearing fat, a marked hypoechoic streak through the normal breast tissue, and loss of the usual speckled appearance of Cooper ligaments. In this case, there is no skin thickening or dermal lymphatic engorgement. **D,** For comparison, the normal opposite side shows normal dark hypoechoic fat, the normal thin lines of Cooper ligaments, and a thinner breast. **E,** Left mediolateral oblique view shows marked skin thickening and an extensible breast cancer and axillary adenopathy. Note the marked skin thickening and breast edema. **F,** Left breast ultrasound shows the marked skin thickening in the near field and a markedly shadowing spiculated invasive ductal cancer. **G,** Image during a core biopsy of a lower invasive ductal cancer in the same patient shows the skin thickening in the near field to greater advantage. The fat is gray, compatible with breast edema.

difficult to do because fluid percolates through the infected area. The goal is to find a focal well-defined abscess collection, not percolating fluid. The other goal is to exclude inflammatory cancer, which can present just like mastitis but will persist despite antibiotics.

If untreated, mastitis can give rise to an abscess, which is a pus collection that forms a thick wall. When an abscess forms, the patient may feel a mass, and the patient's breast will become even more painful to touch, hot, erythematous, and edematous. The patient may develop a fever and have an elevated white blood cell count. Focal abscesses are frequently subareolar because the infection is often introduced through the nipple. Antibiotics, though indi-

cated for treatment, cannot penetrate the thick walls around abscesses. To allow the antibiotics to treat the infection, the abscess must be percutaneously or surgically drained to remove the pus.

On ultrasound, an abscess is an irregular but focal fluid collection that is ill-defined along its edges in the early phases and may be either irregular or well encapsulated in later phases (Fig. 5-23A). A breast abscess usually does not contain air (unlike abscesses in other parts of the body). The abscess can be hard to see because surrounding breast edema obscures normal breast structures. An abscess may contain only one pocket of pus that can be drained by a needle (see Fig. 5-23B); at other

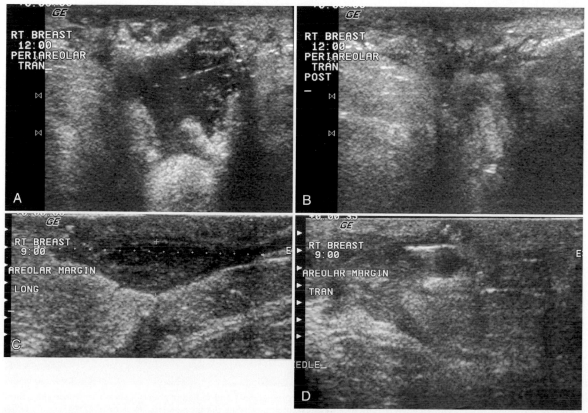

FIGURE 5-23. **A,** Ultrasound shows breast edema surrounding an irregular fluid collection with enhanced transmission of sound characteristic of a retroareolar abscess. Note the needle used to drain the abscess. **B,** After drainage of the pus, a postaspiration ultrasound shows skin thickening and persistent edema, with less fluid in the abscess cavity. **C,** In another patient with an abscess, the fluid collection is just below the skin at the areolar margin, with marked skin thickening and surrounding edema. **D,** Unlike the patient in parts **A** and **B,** even though the fluid collection was in only one pocket, a 19-gauge needle could not drain the collection shown in part **C** because of its thick tenacious nature, and the ultrasound image with the needle tip in the superior lateral portion of the collection shows no change in its size. This collection was drained surgically (in some facilities a catheter might be placed percutaneously into the collection).

times, they may have multiple septae, contain debris or thick pus that cannot be drained without using a larger needle or leaving a catheter in place (see Fig. 5-23C and D). In larger abscesses, percutaneous drainage may help palliate the patient until surgery can be arranged. Although air does not usually occur in breast abscess, percutaneous abscess drainage can introduce air into the biopsy cavity.

Large abscesses are drained surgically, with irrigation of the abscess cavity and manual description of the septa, and the abscess is packed and left open to the air to heal by granulation.

■ BREAST BIOPSY SCARS

In patients undergoing lumpectomy for cancer, the surgeon excises the tumor and closes only the subcutaneous tissues and the skin above the cavity. The lumpectomy cavity fills with fluid afterward. Right after surgery, the biopsy bed is a fluid-filled pocket on ultrasound, is hypoechoic, and may have a sharp or ill-defined edematous rim with or without shadowing. Careful scanning over the skin biopsy scar shows the thickened skin at the incision and distortion of breast tissue along the incision from the skin surface to the biopsy scar (Fig. 5-24A). Later, serous fluid in the biopsy

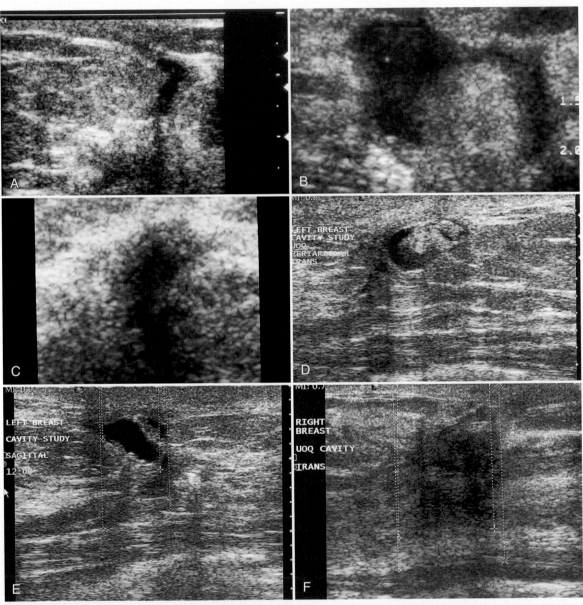

FIGURE 5-24. Postbiopsy scars. **A,** Ultrasound of a postbiopsy scar after lumpectomy and radiation therapy shows a crescent-like fluid collection, representing fluid in the biopsy cavity, with an edge trailing toward the skin, representing the incision site. **B,** A postbiopsy scar in another patient is associated with an irregular fluid-filled mass and an echogenic ball within it, representing fibrin and debris after biopsy. **C,** Ultrasound of the postbiopsy scar months later shows a hypoechoic irregular spiculated mass corresponding to the biopsy site. Without the correct history, the scar could easily be mistaken for breast cancer. **D,** Postbiopsy cavities before radiation therapy. Ultrasound for planning of electron beam boost shows a fluid-filled biopsy cavity with echogenic solid debris within it. **E,** Imaging of a biopsy cavity in another patient shows the fluid-filled cavity with a thick septation and hypoechoic breast edema around the biopsy site. The measurements show the distance from the skin surface to the bottom of the cavity and from the skin surface to the chest wall for planning of electron beam boost. **F,** In a third patient, ultrasound shows the cavity as a hypoechoic, spiculated mass with very little fluid within it.

cavity may be totally clear or may contain solid debris or fibrous septa that move during real-time scanning (see Fig. 5-24B). Subsequently, the biopsy scar fills in with granulation tissue and becomes fibrotic, forming a hypoechoic spiculated mass with or without acoustic shadowing that mimics a spiculated breast cancer (see Fig. 5-24C to F).

Breast cancers occurring near the biopsy site will have the same malignant characteristics and appearance of other breast cancers on ultrasound, but they are separated from the scar by normal breast parenchyma. The separation of a mass from the scar can help distinguish breast cancer from the biopsy scar. Admittedly, it is hard to distinguish breast cancer recurrences directly in the biopsy bed from the scar itself. Clues to the presence of cancer in a postbiopsy scar include the scar growing larger or more rounded like a mass.

CANCERS UNDERGOING NEOADJUVANT CHEMOTHERAPY

The term *locally advanced breast cancer* includes inflammatory breast cancer and tumors larger than 5 cm. Locally advanced breast cancer accounts for a small fraction of all breast cancer in the United States. Locally advanced cancers may have bulky or matted lymph nodes containing metastatic disease. In past times, these women usually underwent mastectomy with poor local control and poor 5-year survival rates.

Investigators have reported that preoperative neoadjuvant chemotherapy improves disease-free and overall survival for women. Preoperative neoadjuvant chemotherapy is defined as combination chemotherapy given *before* definitive surgical treatment (lumpectomy and mastectomy). It is usually given to breast cancer patients who have large tumor masses (stage T3 or T4) or regional lymph node involvement. Neoadjuvant chemotherapy provides tumor shrinkage, decreases tumor burden, and allows some patients to undergo lumpectomy and radiation for local control, rather than mastectomy. After surgery for local control, patients usually have chemotherapy again. There is about a 50% 5-year survival after neoadjuvant chemotherapy. Poor outcomes in these patients are usually due to distant micrometastatic disease at the time of diagnosis.

In the setting of neoadjuvant chemotherapy, ultrasound can guide percutaneous biopsy to establish a histologic diagnosis as needed, determine initial tumor size and extent, document treatment response, and evaluate for residual tumor after chemotherapy (Fig. 5-25). Magnetic resonance imaging is another tool used for detecting both disease extent and chemotherapy response. After neoadjuvant chemotherapy, the original tumor site is often resected to establish the type and extent of residual tumor. This information is important for predicting prognosis. A complete pathologic response (no residual cancer in the original tumor bed by histology) is a good prognostic indicator. Surgical lumpectomy with negative margins also helps to determine whether breast-conserving therapy is an option.

On occasion, neoadjuvant chemotherapy may produce a complete clinical response and the tumor is undetectable by both physical examination and imaging. This is a dilemma because how can the surgeon resect the original tumor bed if no residual tumor exists?

Because some tumors become undetectable by both clinical examination and imaging after neoadjuvant chemotherapy, the radiologist may place a metallic marker in the tumor under imaging guidance before the patient undergoes chemotherapy (Fig. 5-26). Then, if all traces of the tumor fade with chemotherapy, the marker will show the location of the original tumor site and can be used for subsequent preoperative needle localization to excise the now-invisible tumor bed.

POSTBIOPSY BREAST MARKERS AND CORE BIOPSY SITES

Ultrasound-guided vacuum-assisted biopsy methods may actually remove an entire lesion. Usually, air or fluid is present in the biopsy track, in the biopsy site, or in a hematoma immediately after vacuum-assisted core biopsy. Air and fluid are absorbed relatively quickly after biopsy. After hematoma resorption, the only ultrasound findings are often residua of the original mass, if any remains (Fig. 5-27A to C). This is a problem if the entire lesion is removed and shows cancer, requiring surgical excisional biopsy. Fluid, air, or blood accumulating in the biopsy cavity may resorb before the surgery date and cannot be relied on to guide the surgeon. To solve this problem, tiny permanent metallic markers were developed to place in the biopsy site during percutaneous needle biopsy. The metallic marker provides a landmark in the biopsy cavity to guide subsequent mammographic or ultrasonographic preoperative needle localization.

On ultrasound, the metallic markers look like tiny bright echogenic lines, but the metallic marker echo can be lost in the speckle artifact of normal breast tissue (see Fig. 5-27D). To overcome problems in imaging the metallic markers by ultrasound, some manufacturers encase the markers in echogenic pledgets composed of various materials. The radiologist places the pledgets and their encased metallic markers through a vacuum-assisted biopsy probe or directly through a separate needle deployment device under ultrasound guidance. The pledgets are radiolucent and invisible to mammography, but they are detectable as echogenic lines or plugs on ultrasound (see Fig. 5-27E). These pledgets are absorbed by the body at a slower rate than blood or seromas and were developed primarily to be targets for subsequent ultrasound-guided preoperative needle localization. If using these pledgets, the radiologist should be familiar with the pledget resorption rate for the specific manufacturer.

COLOR DOPPLER, POWER DOPPLER, ULTRASOUND CONTRAST AGENTS, THREE-DIMENSIONAL IMAGING, AND ELASTOGRAPHY

Color Doppler and power Doppler ultrasound depict the location of blood vessels when planning the trajectory of a percutaneous breast biopsy needle (Fig. 5-28). As a diagnostic tool, color and power Doppler imaging may show swirling debris in cysts or pulsating blood vessels within breast masses (Fig. 5-29).

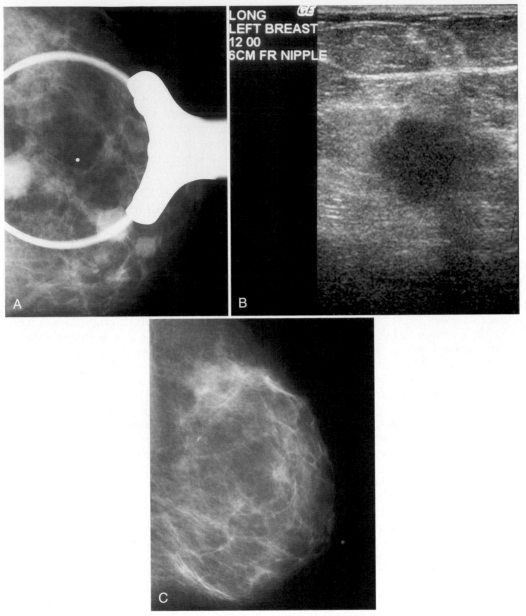

FIGURE 5-25. Response to neoadjuvant chemotherapy. **A,** A spot mammogram shows multiple dense round masses in the left breast, some of which were palpable and marked with a skin marker. **B,** Ultrasound of the mass in the 12-o'clock position shows an ill-defined hypoechoic round mass that was biopsied under ultrasound guidance; invasive ductal cancer was diagnosed, and a marker was placed in the mass under ultrasound control. **C,** After neoadjuvant chemotherapy, the mass has disappeared, but the metallic marker remains in the initial tumor site, which was localized under mammographic guidance to establish a pathologic response.

It was hoped that color Doppler imaging would distinguish cancer from benign breast lesions by showing increased blood flow in breast malignancies. The increased flow was thought to arise from tumor angiogenesis. However, color Doppler imaging does not always detect increased flow in breast cancer, and there is overlap between benign and malignant blood flow patterns. Attempts to increase the sensitivity of ultrasound for detecting blood flow with power Doppler improved these results, but not enough to advocate its use as a screening mechanism for breast cancer or to influence the decision to monitor a mass in lieu of biopsy. The use of contrast agents has been proposed as a means of increasing the

ability of ultrasound vascular imaging techniques to detect small increases in vascular density. Three-dimensional gray-scale ultrasound, though promising, is also still being developed.

Elastography uses Hook's law to determine the relative stiffness of breast tissues on ultrasound. Using ultrasound, elastography shows cancers, which are generally stiffer than normal soft breast tissue, as darker and larger than on the B-mode gray-scale ultrasound. Benign masses are soft and less stiff than cancers. The elastogram shows benign masses as smaller on elastography than on B-mode gray-scale images. Cysts are not stiff, and on the elastogram, cysts are smaller than on B-mode gray-scale ultrasound and

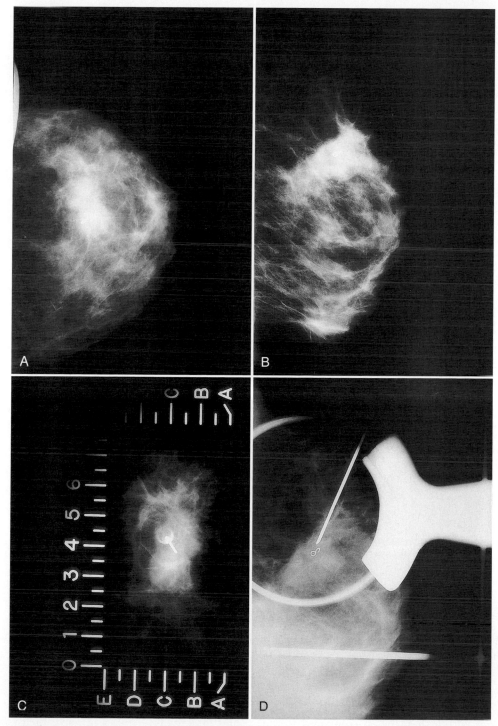

FIGURE 5-26. Placement of a marker under x-ray guidance. Craniocaudal (**A**) and mediolateral (**B**) mammograms show a 3-cm invasive ductal cancer in the 12-o'clock position on the breast. Because the patient was to undergo neoadjuvant chemotherapy, a marker was placed in the mass under x-ray guidance. **C,** An alphanumeric grid is placed over the tumor and a needle inserted into the tumor. **D,** An orthogonal view shows the tip of the needle in the middle of the tumor; the marker is deployed through the needle, and the needle is removed.

Continued

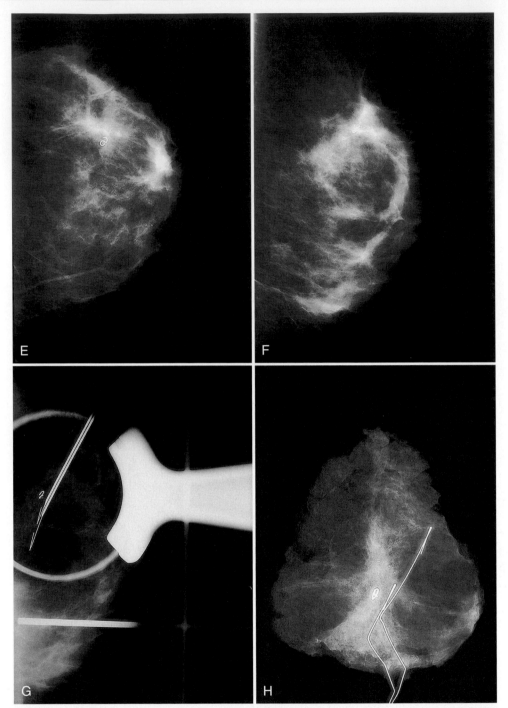

FIGURE 5-26, cont'd. After neoadjuvant chemotherapy, the tumor is much smaller and the marker is still in place on craniocaudal (**E**) and mediolateral (**F**) mammograms. **G,** Preoperative needle localization bracket wires are placed around the marker and residual tumor, which is resected in toto, as shown on the specimen (**H**).

have a bright target within them when compared to the B-mode ultrasound. Elastography is not in widespread use in the United States.

▬ BREAST CANCER SCREENING WITH ULTRASOUND

X-ray mammography is the gold standard for breast cancer screening and diagnosis. It depicts calcifications in DCIS and effectively displays invasive breast cancer masses in fatty breasts, but its limitations in dense breast tissue are well-known. On mammograms, Stomper and colleagues showed that dense breast tissue exists in about one third of women over age 50, but in only about half of women under age 50.

Because breast ultrasound is not limited by dense breast tissue, is relatively easy to use, requires only moderate breast compression, does not use ionizing radiation, and is

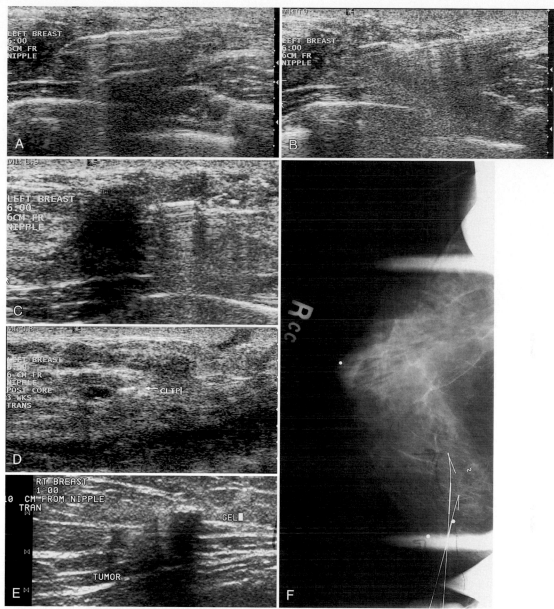

FIGURE 5-27. **A,** Ultrasound shows a core biopsy needle in the post-fire position in an irregular hypoechoic invasive ductal cancer. **B,** After biopsy, a second needle was placed in the mass and a marker deployed to a position near the biopsied mass. The marker is the thin, bright echogenic line just beyond the needle tip. **C,** Ultrasound after marker placement shows the mass and the bright echogenic linear clip, easily seen adjacent to the hypoechoic irregular mass, which is the residua after biopsy. In this case, either the clip or the mass would be used as a target for preoperative needle localization for subsequent excisional biopsy. **D,** Another portion of the same breast shown in parts **A** to **C** had undergone stereotactic vacuum-assisted biopsy 3 weeks before. Ultrasound shows a small oval fluid-filled cavity, and the marker was placed adjacent to the fluid collection by stereotaxis. The clip is a thin, bright echogenic line that might subsequently be lost in the speckle artifact of normal breast tissue once the fluid collection is resorbed. **E,** In another patient, an echogenic pledget with a metallic marker is placed near a tumor close to the chest wall. The marker is the thick echogenic line to the left of the word *gel*. In this case, the tumor was difficult to see on the craniocaudal mammogram because of its position in the high inner aspect of the breast, and the residual tumor and the clip were used for bracket localization, as shown in the craniocaudal postlocalization mammogram (**F**).

widely available; there was great hope that screening for breast cancer with ultrasound would replace mammography.

The initial clinical investigations of screening breast ultrasound from the early 1980s were disappointing. An automated whole-breast ultrasound screening study by Kopans and colleagues depicted only 64% of 127 breast cancers in a study of 1140 women; in contrast, mammography detected 94% of the cancers. Another study with a similar number of patients by Sickles and colleagues resulted in sonographic detection of 58% (37 of 64) of cancers and mammographic detection of 97% (62 of 64). Only 8% of the ultrasound-detected tumors were smaller than 1 cm, but mammography detected all tumors less than 1 cm in size. Breast ultrasound had very poor visualization of microcalcifications, which were lost in the normal speckled breast tissue background. Furthermore, the limitations of ultrasound in fatty breasts resulted in an early recommendation that ultrasound not be used for breast cancer screening.

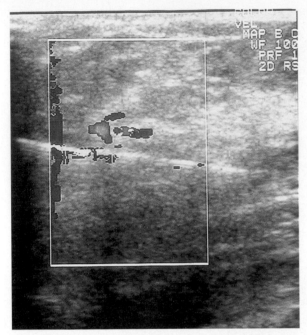

FIGURE 5-28. Color Doppler ultrasound shows a blood vessel that was avoided during biopsy of a mass deep in the breast tissue. Because the vessel's location was known, the needle was guided below it to approach the mass, which proved to be a cyst.

Subsequent improvements in transducer and ultrasound technology resulted in more optimistic results. Hand-held whole-breast ultrasound screening studies found small invasive cancers undetected by mammography in asymptomatic women. A 2002 study of 11,130 asymptomatic dense-breasted women undergoing screening mammography and whole-breast ultrasound screening by Kolb and colleagues showed 246 cancers in 221 women (1.98% of the 11,130 women). Mammography had a sensitivity and specificity of 77.6% and 98.8% versus 75.3% and 96.8%, respectively, for ultrasound. A 1995 study by Gordon and colleagues showed 1575 solid nonpalpable masses invisible by mammography but visualized by ultrasound in 12,706 women. Of these, 279 ultrasound-detected masses underwent biopsy, with 44 cancers found (16% of 279, 2.8% of the 1575 solid masses, 0.35% of 12,706 women).

The early promise and enthusiasm for whole-breast ultrasound screening was dampened by limited availability of trained sonographers, unreliable reproducibility, nondetection of calcifications in DCIS, and lack of specificity, resulting in unnecessary biopsies of incidentally detected benign breast lesions. A follow-up large-scale trial of breast cancer screening with ultrasound was then done under the American College of Radiology Imaging Network (ACRIN) to determine whether the sensitivity and specificity of screening breast ultrasound could be reproduced across multiple facilities.

In her review article on screening breast ultrasound, Berg reviewed mammography screening supplemented

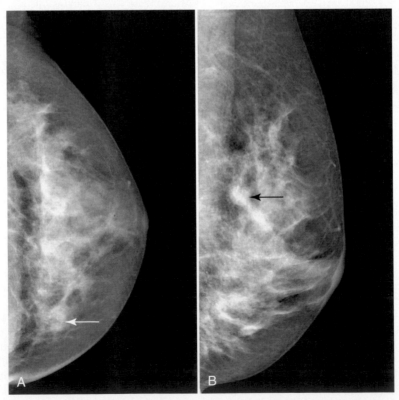

FIGURE 5-29. **A,** The craniocaudal mammogram shows a possible round mass in the inner breast *(arrow).* **B,** The left mediolateral oblique (MLO) view shows the possible mass in the upper left breast *(arrow).*

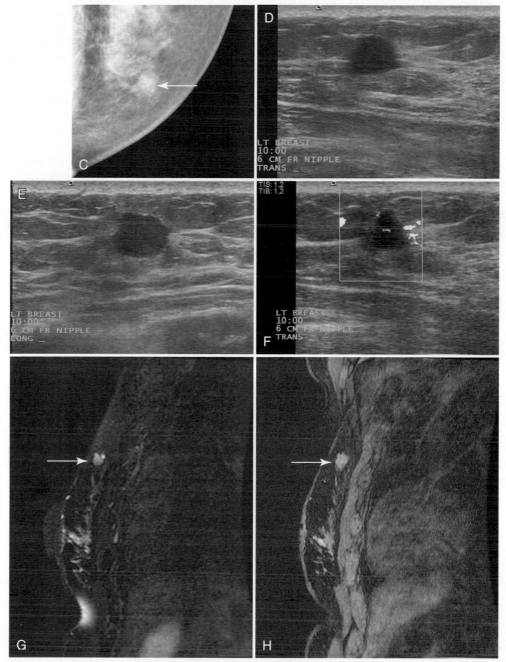

FIGURE 5-29, cont'd. C, Spot compression mammogram shows the round mass *(arrow)* to better advantage. The transverse **(D)** and longitudinal **(E)** scans show a hypoechoic round mass with slightly microlobulated borders. **F,** Color Doppler ultrasound shows that the mass is not a cyst and has a pulsating blood vessel within it; it is invasive ductal cancer. **G,** Sagittal noncontrast T2-weighted magnetic resonance imaging (MRI) shows a high signal intensity mass in the upper breast *(arrow)*. **H,** MRI shows a mass in the upper breast *(arrow)* on the noncontrast 3-D spectral-spatial excitation magnetization transfer (3DSSMT).   *Continued*

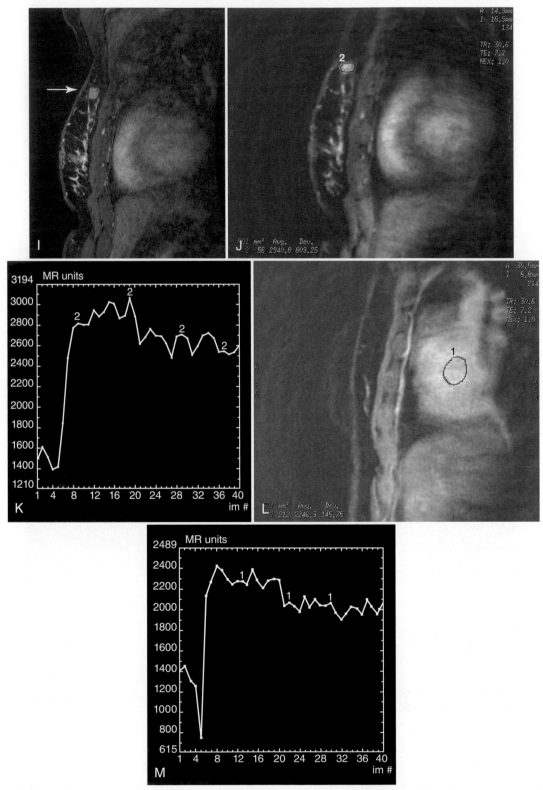

FIGURE 5-29, cont'd. I, The mass enhances with contrast and is slightly heterogeneous *(arrow)*. The ROI over the mass **(J)** and spiral dynamic image **(K)** shows rapid enhancement and washout of the enhancement curve. This was just as rapid as the ROI over the heart **(L)**. **M,** Contrast enhancement of invasive ductal cancer usually has a rapid initial upstroke, with either a late plateau or washout phase, as seen in this case.

with ultrasound compared to mammography screening alone. Berg noted that in seven single institutional trials, the trial conducted by Corsetti and coworkers in Italy, two multicenter trials, and the ACRIN Protocol 6666, supplemental screening ultrasound showed additional breast cancers at a rate of between 2.7 and 4.6 cancers per 1000 women. In the ACRIN trial, most of the cancers were invasive, with a median size of 9 to 11 mm, and were node-negative. However, Berg also noted that false-positive ultrasound findings were common in the ACRIN study, yielding only an 8.8% cancer rate in sonographically prompted biopsies. This limits the applicability of breast ultrasound in the United States, where there are not enough trained sonographers to perform screening ultrasound and where reimbursement does not cover the examination costs. Her recommendation in this 2009 review article is to retain mammography with digital technique as the mainstay of screening for women with dense breasts in the United States, with the supplement of MRI in high-risk women. In the United States, for high-risk women with dense breasts unable to tolerate MRI, she suggests that ultrasound screening "is an option at facilities with availability of qualified personnel."

Additional research on women undergoing screening ultrasound is ongoing both in the United States and overseas, particularly in Asia, where women have mostly dense breast tissue.

▬ KEY ELEMENTS

Breast ultrasound is a useful adjunct to mammography and clinical examination, particularly for the diagnosis of cysts and in certain other limited settings.

Ultrasound results should be considered in conjunction with mammographic and clinical findings to avoid misdiagnosis.

Cysts are anechoic, round or oval, well-circumscribed masses with imperceptible walls and enhanced transmission of sound.

Fibroadenomas are classically described as ellipsoid, well-circumscribed masses with fewer than four gentle lobulations, and they are wider than tall.

Overlap is noted in the ultrasound appearance of benign fibroadenomas and well-circumscribed breast cancers.

Suspicious ultrasound findings in solid masses include acoustic spiculation; shadowing; taller than wide configuration; angulated, indistinct, microlobulated, or spiculated margins; irregular shape; and an echogenic halo.

Secondary signs of breast cancer on ultrasound are changes in Cooper ligaments, breast edema, architectural distortion, skin thickening, skin retraction or irregularity, and suspicious microcalcifications.

Cystic breast masses include breast cysts, complex breast cysts, intracystic carcinoma or papilloma, mucinous cancer, necrotic cancer, abscess, seroma, hematoma, and galactocele.

Solid round or oval masses include fibroadenoma, papilloma, cancer (invasive ductal, medullary, mucinous, papillary), metastasis, and phyllodes tumor.

The most common round cancer is invasive ductal cancer, an uncommon form of a very common tumor.

Multiple solid masses include fibroadenomas, papillomas, multiple breast cancers, and metastases.

Breast edema is characterized by skin thickening, gray fat, loss of crisply defined breast structures, increased breast thickness when compared with the contralateral side and, occasionally, fluid-filled lymphatics.

Breast abscesses are usually caused by *Staphylococcus aureus* or *Streptococcus*, are generally subareolar, and cause a hot, painful hypoechoic pus-filled mass with surrounding breast edema.

Breast biopsy scars look just like cancer on ultrasound after the seroma is resorbed, and correlation with the skin scar and surgical history is necessary.

Metallic markers may be placed in breast biopsy cavities or in tumors before neoadjuvant chemotherapy to guide subsequent preoperative needle localization.

Mammography is the gold standard for breast cancer screening, and supplemental screening by MRI produces the highest cancer sensitivity.

Mammography with ultrasound as a supplemental study might be an option for women with dense breasts who cannot undergo MRI, but there is a shortage of trained sonographers and no insurance reimbursement for screening ultrasound in the United States.

▬ SUGGESTED READINGS

Abe H, Schmidt RA, Kulkarni K, et al: Axillary lymph nodes suspicious for breast cancer metastasis: sampling with US-guided 14-gauge core-needle biopsy—clinical experience in 100 patients, *Radiology* 250:41–49, 2009.

American College of Radiology: *American College of Radiology Standards*. Reston, VA, 2002, American College of Radiology, pp 593–595.

American College of Radiology. *Illustrated Breast Imaging Reporting and Data System (BI-RADS®)*, ed 4. Reston, VA, American College of Radiology (in press).

Baker JA, Soo MS: Breast US: Assessment of technical quality and image interpretation, *Radiology* 223:229–238, 2002.

Bedi DG, Krishnamurthy R, Krishnamurthy S, et al: Cortical morphologic features of axillary lymph nodes as a predictor of metastasis in breast cancer: in vitro sonographic study, *AJR* 191:646–652, 2008.

Berg WA: Rationale for a trial of screening breast ultrasound: American College of Radiology Imaging Network (ACRIN) 6666, *AJR* 180:1225–1228, 2003.

Berg WA: Sonographically depicted breast clustered microcysts: is follow-up appropriate? *AJR* 185:952–959, 2005.

Berg WA: Tailored supplemental screening for breast cancer: what now and what next? *AJR* 192:390–399, 2009.

Berg WA, Blume JD, Cormack JB, et al: Lesion detection and characterization in a breast US phantom: results of the ACRIN 6666 Investigators, *Radiology* 239:693–702, 2006.

Berg WA, Blume JD, Cormack JB, Mendelson EB: Operator dependence of physician-performed whole-breast US: lesion detection and characterization, *Radiology* 241:355–365, 2006.

Berg WA, Blume JD, Cormack JB, et al: Combined screening with ultrasound and mammography vs. mammography alone in women at elevated risk of breast cancer, *JAMA* 299:2151–2163, 2008.

Berg WA, Campassi CI, Ioffe OB: Cystic lesions of the breast: sonographic-pathologic correlation, *Radiology* 227:183–191, 2003.

Berg WA, Gutierrez L, Ness Aiver MS, et al: Diagnostic accuracy of mammography, clinical examination, US, and MR imaging in preoperative assessment of breast cancer, *Radiology* 233:830–849, 2004.

Birdwell RL, Ikeda DM, Jeffrey SS, et al: Preliminary experience with power Doppler imaging of solid breast masses, *AJR* 169:703–707, 1997.

Brookes MJ, Bourke AG: Radiological appearances of papillary breast lesions, *Clin Radiol* 63:1265–1273, 2008.

Buchberger W, DeKoekkoek-Doll P, Springer P, et al: Incidental findings on sonography of the breast: clinical significance and diagnostic workup, *AJR* 173:921–927, 1999.

Burnside ES, Hall TJ, Sommer AM, et al: Differentiating benign from malignant solid breast masses with US strain imaging, *Radiology* 245:401–410, 2007.

Chao TC, Chao HH, Chen MF: Sonographic features of breast hamartomas, *J Ultrasound Med* 26(4):447–453, 2007.

Chopra S, Evans AJ, Pinder SE, et al: Pure mucinous breast cancer—mammographic and ultrasound findings, *Clin Radiol* 51:421–424, 1996.

Cole-Beuglet C, Soriano RZ, Kurtz AB, Goldberg BB: Ultrasound analysis of 104 primary breast carcinomas classified according to histologic type, *Radiology* 147:191–196, 1983.

Cole-Beuglet C, Soriano RZ, Kurtz AB, Goldberg BB: Fibroadenoma of the breast: sonomammography correlated with pathology in 122 patients, *AJR* 140:369–375, 1983.

Corsetti V, Ferrari A, Ghirardi M, et al: Role of ultrasonography in detecting mammographically occult breast carcinoma in women with dense breasts, *Radiol Med (Torino)* 111:440–448, 2006.

Corsetti V, Houssami N, Ferrari A, et al: Breast screening with ultrasound in women with mammography-negative dense breasts: evidence on incremental cancer detection and false positives, and associated cost, *Eur J Cancer* 44:539–544, 2008.

Dennis MA, Parker SH, Klaus AJ, et al: Breast biopsy avoidance: the value of normal mammograms and normal sonograms in the setting of a palpable lump, *Radiology* 219:186–191, 2001.

Doshi DJ, March DE, Crisi GM, Coughlin BF: Complex cystic breast masses: diagnostic approach and imaging—pathologic correlation, *Radiographics* 27(Suppl 1):S53–S64, 2007.

DuPont WD, Page DL, Pari FF, et al: Long-term risk of breast cancer in women with fibroadenoma, *N Engl J Med* 351:10–15, 1994.

Fornage BD, Lorigan JG, Andry E: Fibroadenoma of the breast: sonographic appearance, *Radiology* 172:671–675, 1989.

Gordon PB: Ultrasound for breast cancer screening and staging, *Radiol Clin North Am* 40:431–441, 2002.

Gordon PB, Goldenberg SL: Malignant breast masses detected only by ultrasound. A retrospective review, *Cancer* 76:626–630, 1995.

Graf O, Helbich TH, Hopf G, et al: Probably benign breast masses at US: is follow-up an acceptable alternative to biopsy? *Radiology* 244:87–93, 2007.

Hashimoto BE, Kramer DJ, Picozzi VJ: High detection rate of breast ductal carcinoma in situ calcifications on mammographically directed high-resolution sonography, *J Ultrasound Med* 20:501–508, 2001.

Hilton SW, Leopold GR, Olson LK, Wilson SA: Real time breast sonography: application in 300 consecutive patients, *AJR* 147:479–486, 1986.

Huang CS, Wu CY, Chu JS, et al: Microcalcifications of nonpalpable breast lesions detected by ultrasonography: correlation with mammography and histopathology, *Ultrasound Obstet Gynecol* 13:431–436, 1999.

Jain A, Haisfield-Wolfe ME, Lange J, et al: The role of ultrasound-guided fine-needle aspiration of axillary nodes in the staging of breast cancer, *Ann Surg Oncol* 15:462–471, 2008.

Kaplan SS: Clinical utility of bilateral whole-breast US in the evaluation of women with dense breast tissue, *Radiology* 221:641–649, 2001.

Kim EK, Ko KH, Oh KK, et al: Clinical application of the BI-RADS final assessment to breast sonography in conjunction with mammography, *AJR* 190:1209–1215, 2008.

Kolb TM, Lichy J, Newhouse JH: Occult cancer in women with dense breasts: detection with screening US—diagnostic yield and tumor characteristics, *Radiology* 207:191–199, 1998.

Kolb TM, Lichy J, Newhouse JH: Comparison of the performance of screening mammography, physical examination, and breast US and evaluation of factors that influence them: an analysis of 27,825 patient evaluations, *Radiology* 225:165–175, 2002.

Kopans DB, Meyer JE, Lindfors KK, et al: Breast sonography to guide cyst aspiration and wire localization of occult solid lesions, *AJR* 143:489–492, 1984.

Kopans DB, Meyer JE, Lindfors KK: Whole-breast US imaging: four year follow-up, *Radiology* 157:505–507, 1985.

Lee E, Wylie E, Metcalf C: Ultrasound imaging features of radial scars of the breast, *Australas Radiol* 51:240–245, 2007.

Lee JW, Han W, Ko E, et al: Sonographic lesion size of ductal carcinoma in situ as a preoperative predictor for the presence of an invasive focus, *J Surg Oncol* 98:15–20, 2008.

Lehman CD, Isaacs C, Schnall MD, et al: Cancer yield of mammography, MR, and US in high-risk women: prospective multi-institution breast cancer screening study, *Radiology* 244:381–388, 2007.

Liberman L, Feng TL, Dershaw DD, et al: US-guided core breast biopsy: use and cost-effectiveness, *Radiology* 208:717–723, 1998.

Mendelson EB, Berg WA, Merritt CR: Toward a standardized breast ultrasound lexicon, BI-RADS: ultrasound, *Semin Roentgenol* 36:17–25, 2001.

Mercado CL, Guth AA, Toth HK, et al: Sonographically guided marker placement for confirmation of removal of mammographically occult lesions after localization, *AJR* 191:1216–1219, 2008.

Meyer JE, Amin E, Lindfors KK: Medullary carcinoma of the breast: mammographic and US appearance, *Radiology* 170:79–82, 1989.

Moon WK, Im JG, Koh YH, et al: US of mammographically detected clustered microcalcifications, *Radiology* 217:849–854, 2000.

Moon WK, Myung JS, Lee YJ, et al: US of ductal carcinoma in situ, *Radiographics* 22:269–280, 2002.

Moon WK, Noh DY, Im JG: Multifocal, multicentric, and contralateral breast cancers: bilateral whole-breast US in the preoperative evaluation of patients, *Radiology* 224:569–576, 2002.

Murphy IG, Dillon MF, Doherty AO, et al: Analysis of patients with false negative mammography and symptomatic breast carcinoma, *J Surg Oncol* 96:457–463, 2007.

Nicholson BT, Harvey JA, Cohen MA: Nipple–areolar complex: normal anatomy and benign and malignant processes, *Radiographics* 29:509–523, 2009.

Parker SH, Jobe WE, Dennis MA, et al: US-guided automated large-core breast biopsy, *Radiology* 187:507–511, 1993.

Raza S, Chikarmane SA, Neilsen SS, et al: BI-RADS 3, 4, and 5 lesions: value of US in management—follow-up and outcome, *Radiology* 248:773–781, 2008.

Reuter K, D'Orsi CJH, Reale F: Intracystic carcinoma of the breast: the role of ultrasonography, *Radiology* 153:233–234, 1984.

Rizzo M, Lund MJ, Oprea G, et al: Surgical follow-up and clinical presentation of 142 breast papillary lesions diagnosed by ultrasound-guided core-needle biopsy, *Ann Surg Oncol* 15:1040–1047, 2008.

Saslow D, Boetes C, Burke W, et al: American Cancer Society guidelines for breast screening with MRI as an adjunct to mammography, *CA Cancer J Clin* 57:75–89, 2007.

Schneck CD, Lehman DA: Sonographic anatomy of the breast, *Semin Ultrasound* 3:13–33, 1982.

Schrading S, Kuhl CK: Mammographic, US, and MR imaging phenotypes of familial breast cancer, *Radiology* 246:58–70, 2008.

Sickles EA: Sonographic detectability of breast calcifications, *SPIE* 419:51–52, 1983.

Sickles EA, Filly RA, Callen RW: Breast cancer detection with sonography and mammography: comparison using state-of-the-art equipment, *AJR* 140:843–845, 1983.

Sickles EA, Filly RA, Callen PW: Benign breast lesions: ultrasound detection and diagnosis, *Radiology* 151:467–470, 1984.

Skaane P, Sauer T: Ultrasonography of malignant breast neoplasms. Analysis of carcinomas missed as tumor, *Acta Radiol* 40:376–382, 1999.

Soo MS, Baker JA, Rosen EL, et al: Sonographically guided biopsy of suspicious microcalcifications of the breast: a pilot study, *AJR* 178:1007–1015, 2002.

Stavros AT, Thickman D, Rapp CL, et al: Solid breast nodules: use of sonography to distinguish between benign and malignant lesions, *Radiology* 196:123–134, 1995.

Stomper PC, D'Souza DJ, DiNitto PA, Arredondo MA: Analysis of parenchymal density on mammograms in 1353 women 25–79 years old, *AJR* 167:1261–1265, 1996.

Tabár L, Péntek Z, Dena PB: The diagnostic and therapeutic value of breast cyst puncture and pneumocystography, *Radiology* 141:659–663, 1981.

The WL, Wilson AR, Evan AJ, et al: Ultrasound guided core biopsy of suspicious mammographic calcifications using high frequency and power Doppler ultrasound, *Clin Radiol* 55:390–394, 2000.

Thomas A, Warm M, Hoopmann M, et al: Tissue Doppler and strain imaging for evaluating tissue elasticity of breast lesions, *Acad Radiol* 14:522–529, 2007.

Vade A, Lafita VS, Ward KA, et al: Role of breast sonography in imaging of adolescents with palpable solid breast masses, *AJR* 191:659–663, 2008.

Weind KL, Maier CF, Rutt BK, Moussa M: Invasive carcinomas and fibroadenomas of the breast: comparison of microvessel distributions—implications for imaging modalities, *Radiology* 208:477–483, 1998.

Zhi H, Ou B, Luo BM, et al: Comparison of ultrasound elastography, mammography, and sonography in the diagnosis of solid breast lesions, *J Ultrasound Med* 26:807–815, 2007.

Quizzes

5-1. Fill in the elements for ultrasound labeling.

_____

_____

_____

_____

_____

For answers, see Box 5-1.

5-2. Fill in echogenic versus hypoechoic appearances of a normal ultrasound image of breast tissue.

Skin: _____

Fat: _____

Glandular tissue: _____

Breast ducts: _____

Nipple: _____

Cooper ligaments: _____

Ribs: _____

For answers, see Box 5-2.

5-3. Fill in the simple cyst criteria.

_____

_____

_____

_____

For answers, see Box 5-4.

5-4. Fill in the differential diagnosis for cystic or fluid-containing masses.

_____

_____

_____

_____

_____

_____

_____

_____

_____

_____

For answers, see Box 5-6.

5-5. Fill in the benign mass characteristics.

_____

_____

_____

_____

_____

For answers, see Box 5-7.

5-6. Fill in the suspicious ultrasound characteristics of solid breast masses.

_____

_____

_____

_____

_____

_____

_____

For answers, see Box 5-8.

5-7. Fill in the differential diagnosis of round or oval solid breast masses.

_____

_____

_____

_____

_____

_____

_____

_____

For answers, see Box 5-9.

5-8. Fill in the secondary signs of breast cancer seen on ultrasound.

_____

_____

_____

_____

_____

_____

For answers, see Box 5-11.

5-9. Fill in the differential diagnosis of breast edema.

UNILATERAL	BILATERAL (SYSTEMIC PROBLEMS)
_____	_____
_____	_____
_____	_____
_____	_____
_____	

For answers, see Box 5-12.

5-10. Fill in the descriptors for the ACR BI-RADS® ultrasound lexicon.

Shape   _____   _____

               _____

Margin   _____   _____

               _____   _____

Boundary   _____   _____

Echo pattern   _____   _____

               _____   _____

               _____

Posterior   _____   _____
acoustic
features   _____   _____

For answers, see Table 5-1.

5-11. Fill in the unfortunate ultrasound look-alikes.

FINDING	LOOK-ALIKES
Fibroadenoma	_____
Solid benign mass	_____
Complex benign mass	_____

For answers, see Table 5-4.

5-12. Fill in the ultrasound features of cancer, cysts, and fibroadenomas.

	CANCER	CYST	FIBROADENOMA	BENIGN ULTRASOUND FEATURES
Shape	_____	_____	_____	_____
	_____	_____		
Margin	_____	_____	_____	_____
	_____		_____	
	_____			
Boundary	_____	_____	_____	_____
Orientation	_____	_____	_____	_____
	_____	_____	_____	_____
Internal echos	_____	_____	_____	_____
	_____		_____	_____
				_____
Posterior acoustic features	_____	_____	_____	
	_____			
Other	_____	_____	_____	_____
	_____			

For answers, see Table 5-2.

5-13. Fill in the description and differential diagnosis for BI-RADS® ultrasound special cases (cystic).

CYSTIC MASS TYPE	DESCRIPTION	DIFFERENTIAL DIAGNOSIS
Clustered microcysts	_____	_____
Complicated cysts	_____	_____
Complex mass	_____	_____

For answers, see Table 5-3.

CHAPTER 6

Mammographic and Ultrasound-Guided Breast Biopsy Procedures

Biopsy of nonpalpable imaging-detected breast lesions is an important part of the breast imaging service. The advantage of percutaneous biopsy is that it can provide a diagnosis with a minimum of patient trauma, and the diagnosis can guide appropriate follow-up, including definitive surgery. If the diagnosis is cancer, the patient can decide on lumpectomy versus mastectomy. Furthermore, patients with invasive cancer can have both tumor excision and axillary lymph node biopsy at the first surgery. This chapter describes percutaneous x-ray– and ultrasound-guided breast needle biopsy techniques, preoperative needle localization, and imaging–pathology correlation. Magnetic resonance imaging (MRI)-guided breast procedures are covered in Chapter 7.

▬ PREBIOPSY PATIENT WORKUP

Nonpalpable, imaging-detected breast lesions are amenable to preoperative localization and surgical or percutaneous needle biopsy. The decision whether to operate or do a needle biopsy to make a diagnosis requires communication between the surgeon, patient, and radiologist to determine the correct approach. There is a strong progressive trend toward using needle biopsy to diagnose nonpalpable breast lesions whenever possible, reserving breast surgery for therapy.

Nothing substitutes for complete imaging workup of nonpalpable breast lesions. The radiologist must have the lesion's location within the breast firmly entrenched in his or her mind to plan an approach that will be successful in biopsying the lesion with safety and accuracy. For mammography, this means visualization of the lesion in craniocaudal and mediolateral orthogonal views (Box 6-1). When the finding is not seen definitively in craniocaudal (CC) and mediolateral views, the radiologist locates the lesion with fine-detail mammographic views, views with skin markers, triangulation, stereotactic targeting, ultrasound, and physical examination. This is to make sure the lesion is real and to determine its location in the breast. For ultrasound, this means the lesion is visualized on orthogonal scans. *Do not attempt to biopsy a breast lesion if you do not know whether it is real or if you do not know its location in the breast!*

Suboptimal workup results in procedure cancellation. Philpotts and colleagues reported various reasons for cancellation of stereotactic biopsy in 16% of cases examined (89/572). Canceled procedures and lost time would have been avoided by a full workup or accurate clinical history in most of these cases. With improved workup and advanced biopsy technique, Jackman and Marzoni reported cancellation of stereotactic biopsy in only 2% (29/1809) of cases.

Some calcifications prompting biopsy may be within the skin and not require biopsy at all. Peripheral location of calcifications and radiolucent calcification centers may be clues to a skin location for calcifications. Tangential views can then identify dermal calcifications, and the procedure can be canceled.

For a nonpalpable lesion to be biopsied with safety and accuracy, the patient must be able to cooperate and hold still during the procedure, have no allergies to medications used during the procedure, be able to follow postbiopsy instructions to diminish bleeding and other complications, and be compliant with postbiopsy follow-up (see Box 6-1).

▬ INFORMED CONSENT

Informed consent is an important part of any procedure (Box 6-2). For percutaneous needle biopsy, the radiologist informs the patient of the risks, benefits, and alternatives to percutaneous biopsy (e.g., surgical biopsy), as well as the risks and benefits of any alternatives. The most common complication after core or vacuum needle biopsy is hematoma formation, but it is rarely significant. Other rare complications include untoward bleeding (very rarely requiring surgical intervention), infection (with mastitis very rare), pneumothorax, pseudoaneurysm formation, implant rupture, milk fistula (if the patient is pregnant or nursing), and vasovagal reactions (see Box 6-2). The patient is told that later surgical excision will be needed if the biopsy reveals a malignancy, high-risk lesion, or discordant benign lesion, or if the needle biopsy cannot be completed because of technical limitations (see Box 6-2). She is told that the postbiopsy metallic marker may end up in a suboptimal location. The patient is informed about wound management after the biopsy and about when and how to obtain biopsy results.

For preoperative needle localization, the surgeon obtains informed consent for both the needle localization and surgical excision. The radiologist confirms that the patient is properly informed about the needle localization part of the procedure.

SKIN STERILIZATION, LOCAL ANESTHESIA, AND SKIN NICKS

The breast skin is sterilized with a cleansing agent, usually alcohol- or iodine based, before anesthetic needle insertion. Most facilities routinely use local anesthesia for percutaneous needle biopsy and preoperative needle localization. A common local anesthetic for breast biopsies is 1% lidocaine buffered with 8.4% sodium bicarbonate in a 10:1 ratio. The lidocaine is given without epinephrine in the skin and subcutaneous tissue (to avoid skin necrosis) and with 1:100,000 epinephrine in the deeper tissue (to increase hemostasis and prolong the anesthetic effect). To avoid mix-ups, the two solutions may be drawn up in different-sized syringes, with a 25-gauge skin injection needle placed only on the syringe containing plain lidocaine, and each syringe is labeled with its contents. The maximum dose of 1% lidocaine with epinephrine is 7 mg/kg (3.5 mg/pound) body weight, not to exceed 500 mg. This translates to 50 mL in a 70-kg patient. The maximum dose of 1% lidocaine without epinephrine is 4.5 mg/kg (2 mg/pound), not to exceed 300 mg. This translates to 30 mL in a 70-kg patient.

A small skin nick is usually made with a scalpel to facilitate insertion of the larger needles used for needle biopsy; however, it is usually not needed for insertion of a small biopsy needle or localizing needle used to guide surgical excision.

PREOPERATIVE NEEDLE LOCALIZATION

Preoperative needle localization can be guided by orthogonal radiographic, stereotactic, and ultrasound techniques; these are discussed in this section, along with specimen radiography and pathology correlation.

The intent of preoperative localization is to give the surgeon a "road map" to find the lesion inside the breast and excise it. Because the surgeon sees only breast skin on the patient in the operating room, the surgeon cannot find nonpalpable masses or calcifications that were detected by x-ray or ultrasound. To guide the surgeon to the lesion, the radiologist places a needle into the middle of the lesion under imaging guidance. In some facilities, the radiologist injects a small amount of sterile blue dye through the needle to stain the tissue around the lesion for the surgeon to find in the operating room. The radiologist places a hookwire through the needle and removes the needle, with the hooked end of the wire left near or in the lesion and the other end of the wire sticking out of the skin. The technologist takes orthogonal mammograms for both x-ray— and ultrasound-guided needle localizations with the wire in place to show the relationship of the lesion and the hookwire tip. The radiologist then labels the films for the surgeon, and the patient is sent to the operating room with the films. Various ways can be used to guide the needle into the lesion for this type of procedure, as discussed here.

The surgeon uses the wire and mammograms to guide him or her to the lesion and excises the lesion and hookwire. The excised tissue is called a *breast specimen*. The technologist radiographs the breast specimen. The radiologist reviews the specimen radiograph to see if the lesion and the entire hookwire (with an intact hook) are included (Fig. 6-1A to G).

A special scenario regarding needle localizations occurs when surgeons use "bracketing" wires to remove a large area of breast tissue (Fig. 6-2), a scenario that happens when the mass or calcifications extend over too wide an area to be localized by one wire. In this situation, the radiologist places two wires in the breast, with one wire at one end of the lesion and the other wire at the other end of the lesion. The "brackets" help the surgeon remove the lesion between the two wires in toto. These "bracketed" breast specimens should include the two wires and the mass or calcifications between them.

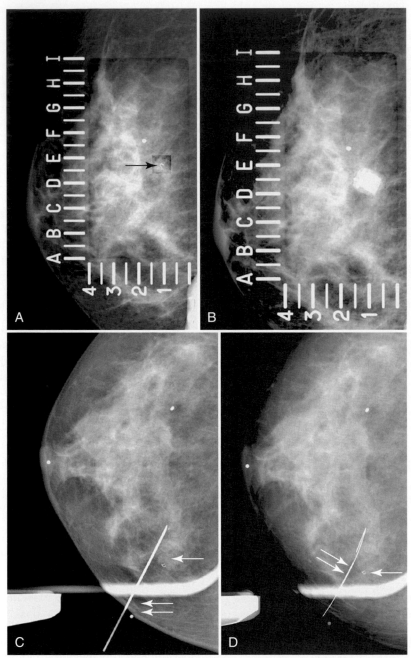

FIGURE 6-1. X-ray–guided needle localization with specimen radiography. Mammograms had shown a marker in the left upper inner quadrant where core biopsy showed ductal carcinoma in situ (DCIS). The patient presented for preoperative needle localization to excise the marker and the DCIS site. **A,** Enhanced digital lateral mammogram shows an alphanumeric plate placed over the skin closest to the marker (*arrow*). The marker is at coordinates 1.0/D.5. **B,** After needle placement, the needle hub overlies the marker at coordinates 1.0/D.5. Because the needle hub overlies the marker and the needle shaft, the needle is traveling straight to the marker. **C,** A craniocaudal (CC) view with the needle in place shows that the needle shaft is adjacent to the marker (*arrow*) and the needle tip is lateral to it. A BB was placed at the skin entry site (*double arrows*). **D,** The radiologist places a wire through the needle and subsequently removes it, leaving only the hookwire in the breast. The CC mammogram shows the marker (*arrow*) and the hookwire tip 1 cm lateral to the marker. The stiffened part of the wire shaft (which is thicker than the rest of the wire) (*double arrows*) is right next to the marker. The surgeon can feel this stiffened part of the wire more easily than the rest of the wire.

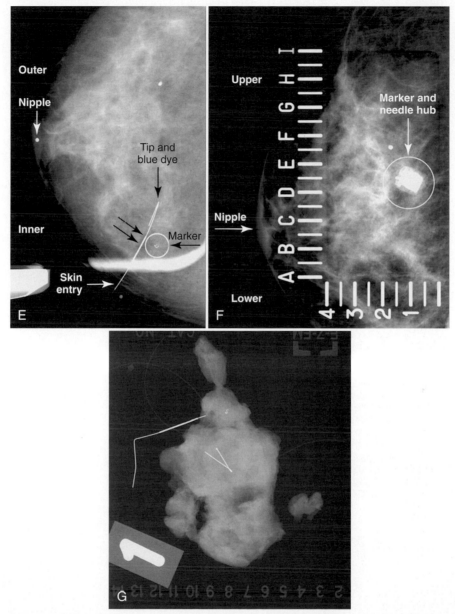

FIGURE 6-1, cont'd. E, Annotated CC mammogram shows the relative positions of the nipple, wire, hookwire tip 1 cm lateral to the marker, and injected dye. **F,** Annotated lateral view with the needle in place. Some facilities also obtain a lateral view with the wire in the lateral projection. The surgeon uses the annotated CC and mediolateral mammograms and the wire as a "road map" to the marker in the operating room. **G,** A specimen radiograph shows inclusion of the hookwire, a transected hookwire tip, the marker, and one calcification. During the operation the surgeon transected the hookwire but sent the hookwire shaft and its tip for radiography. It is essential that the hookwire tip is removed during surgery, because if left in the breast the hookwire tip can travel to other body parts. These findings were reported to the surgeon in the operating room. Pathology showed residual high-grade DCIS despite only one calcification remaining. This demonstrates that DCIS can be present in the postbiopsy site even when all the calcifications are removed by stereotactic biopsy, because DCIS does not always calcify.

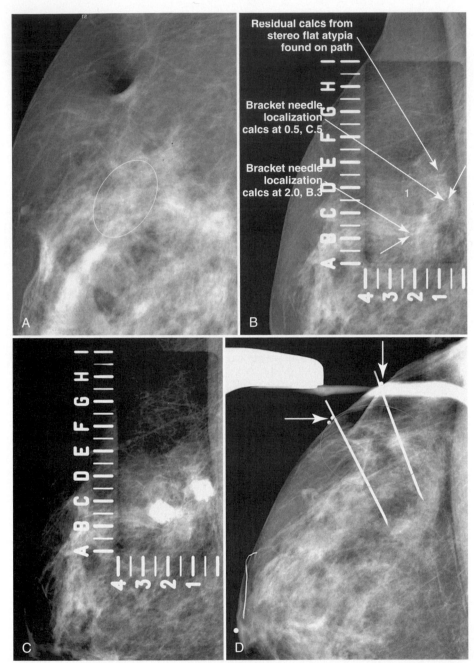

FIGURE 6-2. Bracket localization for a large area of calcifications. **A,** Suspicious area of calcifications in the left upper outer quadrant (*circle*) underwent stereotactic core biopsy and showed flat epithelial atypia. No marker was placed after stereotactic biopsy at the outside facility. To remove all of the suspicious calcifications, the surgeon requests a bracket localization, in which wires are placed at the extreme ends of the calcifications to remove all of the tissue between the wire tips. **B,** Scout mediolateral digital mammogram with an alphanumeric plate shows that the calcifications are at 0.5/C.5 and 2.0/B.3 (*arrows*). **C,** Mediolateral mammogram shows the needles in place. **D,** Craniocaudal (CC) spot mammogram shows the needles on either side of the suspicious calcifications (*circled*) in the outer aspect of the right breast. Note the BBs at the skin entry of the needles.

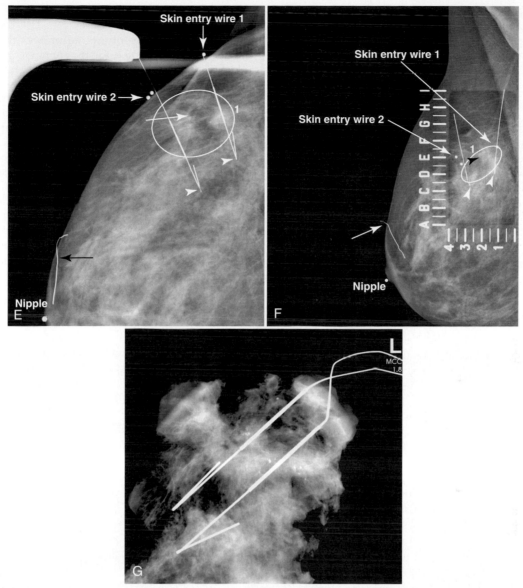

FIGURE 6-2, cont'd. E, Annotated spot CC mammogram after the wire placement shows the residual calcifications (*white arrow*), the wire skin entry sites marked by BBs, the location of the hookwire tips and blue dye (*arrowheads*), a linear wire marker on the areolar border (*black arrow*), and a marker on the nipple. **F,** Annotated mediolateral mammogram shows the two wires around the calcifications. Hookwire tips and blue dye are marked by *white arrowheads* residual calcifications between the wires at the stiffeners are marked by a *black arrowhead* the linear wire on the areolar border is marked with an *arrow*. **G,** The magnified cropped specimen radiograph shows the hookwires, hookwire tips, and the calcifications. This is ductal carcinoma in situ.

Orthogonal Radiographic Guidance (X-Ray–Guided Needle Localization)

One guidance method uses an upright mammographic unit with a compression plate that has an open aperture with an alphanumeric grid or that contains a series of holes. To perform needle localization, the radiologist reviews the original orthogonal mammograms to identify the shortest distance to the lesion from the skin surface. The technologist places the aperture over the skin closest to the lesion, places permanent ink marks at the edges of the aperture at its contact with skin to make sure the patient has not moved, takes a single mammogram image, and leaves the breast in compression. The mammogram should show the lesion within the open aperture. The

radiologist determines the coordinates of the lesion on the mammogram and, with the patient still in compression, marks this location in ink on the patient's skin, cleans the skin, and injects a local anesthetic on the ink mark.

The radiologist then passes a needle parallel to the chest wall into and through the lesion. To ensure that the needle path is straight, the radiologist should check that the shadow from the needle hub lies directly over the needle shaft during insertion. After the radiologist passes the needle deep enough into the breast to pass through the lesion, the technologist takes a mammogram to ensure that the needle shaft projects over the lesion.

Once the radiologist confirms that the needle is through the lesion, he or she holds the needle deep in the breast; the technologist releases compression and takes an orthogonal mammogram with the needle still in place. The radiologist reviews the orthogonal mammogram and adjusts the needle depth so that the needle tip is just through the lesion. Blue dye, if used, and a hookwire are inserted.

Stereotactic Guidance

With this technique, the radiologist localizes the lesion under stereotactic guidance, as described for stereotactic core biopsy later in this chapter. The radiologist places a needle into the breast, obtains stereotactic views to make sure the needle is in the middle of the lesion, may inject blue dye, and inserts the hookwire. The patient is removed from the stereotactic device and undergoes standard orthogonal mammograms. The usual problem with stereotactic wire placements is adjusting the depth of the needle in the z-axis.

Ultrasound Guidance

Real-time hand-held ultrasound units with a small transducer provide guidance for preoperative needle localization for ultrasonographically detected breast lesions (Fig. 6-3). To do the localization, the patient is placed in the supine position and the radiologist plans the needle path to the lesion. The radiologist rolls or angles the patient on the table until the needle path is directed safely away from the chest wall to prevent pneumothorax. Using sterile technique and under direct ultrasound visualization, the radiologist anesthetizes the skin and inserts a longer needle for deep anesthesia, keeping the entire shaft of the needle, the needle tip, and the target in the same plane. The anesthesia needle can be used as a "trial run" to judge the safety of the needle path and the difficulty of needle insertion. Then the radiologist inserts the preoperative localization needle into the lesion under real-time

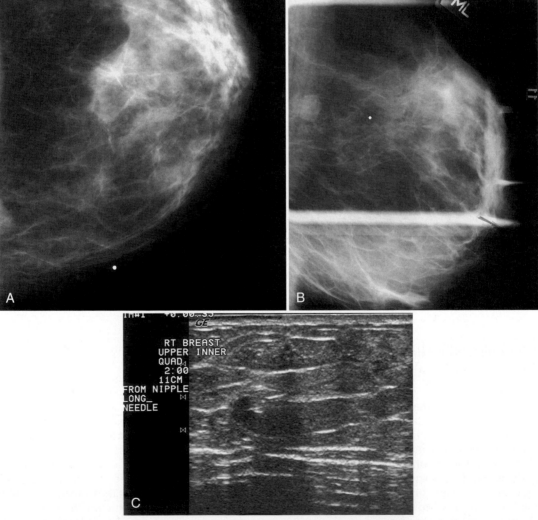

FIGURE 6-3. Ultrasound-guided needle localization. Craniocaudal (CC) (**A**) and spot compression mediolateral (ML) (**B**) mammograms show a mass in the medial portion of the breast that was solid on ultrasound, and excisional biopsy was requested by the patient. **C,** Ultrasound was used to guide a needle into the mass for preoperative localization; the image shows the needle tip in the middle of the mass.

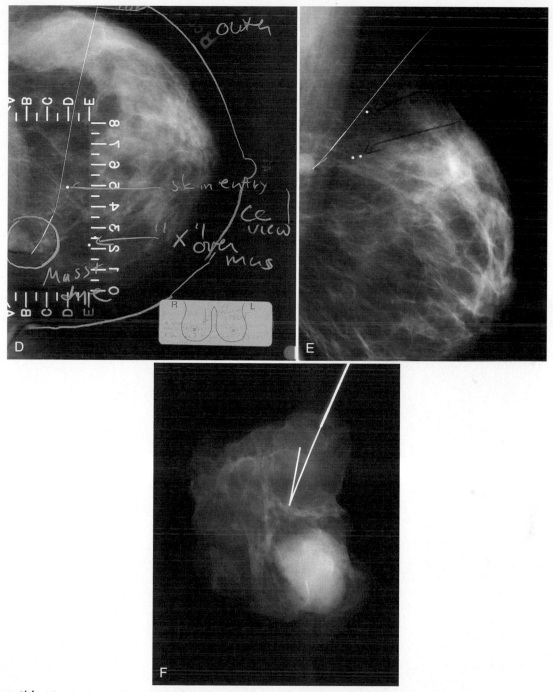

FIGURE 6-3, cont'd. After hookwire deployment, CC (**D**) and ML (**E**) mammograms show the hookwire tip in the mass. The films were marked with a white grease pen to show the skin outline and skin entry, and an X was placed on the skin over the mass marked with two BBs. **F,** The specimen radiograph shows inclusion of the mass and the hookwire. Histologic examination revealed a fibroadenoma.

ultrasound guidance. Blue dye, if used, and a hookwire are inserted.

At this point, some facilities place skin BBs before the postwire localization mammogram is obtained. A skin BB may be placed at the wire skin entry site. In addition, the radiologist may place two skin BBs and an indelible ink X over the skin where the lesion lies for the surgeon to see when the patient arrives in the operating room. The technologist then takes a mammogram with the ultrasound-placed wire within the breast.

In some facilities, radiologists or surgeons perform intraoperative ultrasound to direct the breast biopsy.

Specimen Radiography

The needle localization procedure is not over until the specimen radiograph is taken by the technologist and reviewed by the radiologist. The radiologist reports whether the specimen contains the entire lesion, how far the lesion is away from the specimen edge, if the lesion was transected, and whether the hookwire, hookwire tip, and any markers are included (Box 6-3). The radiologist then calls these findings to the surgeon in the operating room. If the lesion is not in the specimen, the radiologist directs the surgeon to the expected location by using landmarks in the excised tissue and on the mammogram and waits for a second specimen (Fig. 6-4). If subsequent specimen radiographs still do not contain the lesion, the surgeon may close the breast and obtain a mammogram to determine whether the targeted lesion is still in the breast. The mammogram is usually done a few weeks after the biopsy.

Tissue excised at ultrasound-guided preoperative localizations also undergoes specimen radiography, even if the finding cannot be seen on mammogram. The specimen radiograph may or may not show the ultrasound-localized finding, but will show if the entire hookwire or its tip, as well as any metallic markers, was excised. If the specimen radiograph does not show the ultrasound-localized finding, the radiologist can perform specimen ultrasound to see if the tissue contains the mass (Figs. 6-5 and 6-6).

BOX 6-3. Surgical Breast Specimen Reporting

Specimen includes lesion and any associated markers
Hookwire included
Hookwire tip included
Lesion is at or away from the specimen edge, or is transected

---

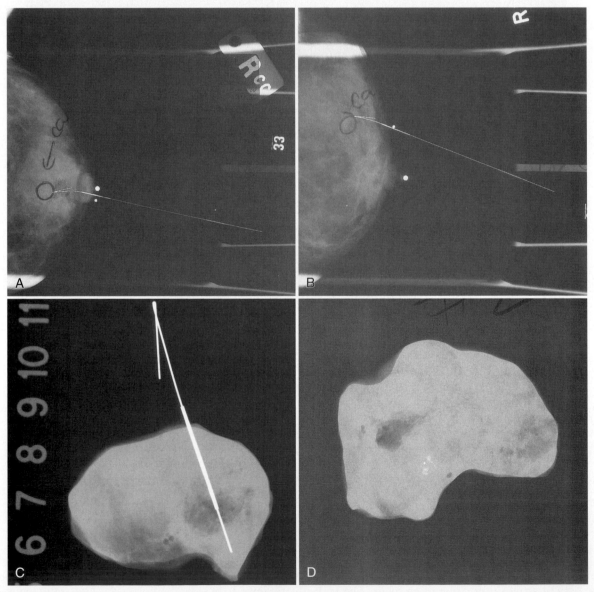

FIGURE 6-4. Importance of specimen radiography. The hookwire films from a freehand localization show the tip of the hookwire in microcalcifications on the craniocaudal (**A**) and mediolateral (**B**) views. **C,** The first specimen shows the hookwire but no calcifications. These findings were reported to the surgeon in the operating room. **D,** Calcifications are seen in the second specimen.

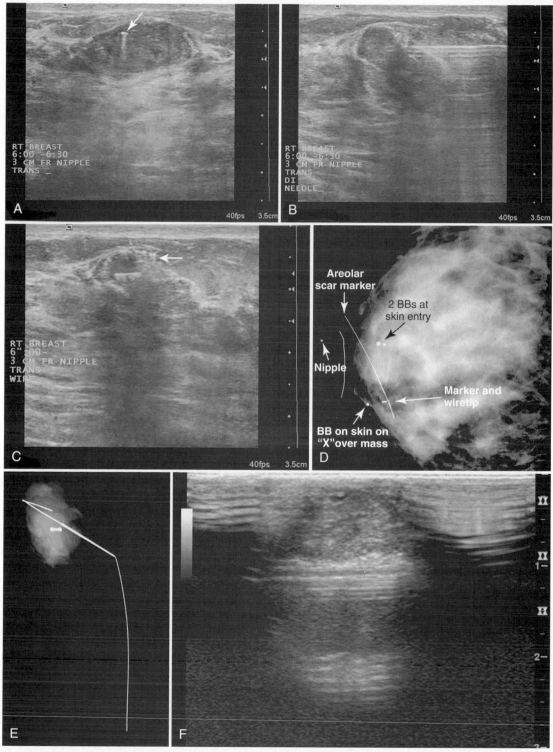

FIGURE 6-5. Ultrasound-guided preoperative needle localization with specimen radiography. In an 18-year-old woman, ultrasound-guided core biopsy of an oval mass in the 6-o'clock position showed pathology suggestive of fibroadenoma versus phyllodes tumor. A marker was placed in the mass. The surgeon requested ultrasound-guided preoperative needle localization. **A,** The ultrasound shows the bright speckle inside the mass (*arrow*), representing the marker placed at the time of the core biopsy. This patient then underwent ultrasound-guided preoperative needle localization for excisional biopsy. **B,** Ultrasound shows the needle within the mass just before wire placement for ultrasound-guided preoperative needle localization. **C,** Ultrasound shows the wire tip (*arrow*) in the mass after wire placement through the needle. **D,** Mammogram after ultrasound-guided needle localization shows the hookwire near the marker in the mass, which is obscured by surrounding dense breast tissue. **E,** After excisional biopsy, the specimen radiograph shows inclusion of the hookwire, dense tissue, and the marker. Just as on the mammogram, the mass is invisible. **F,** Ultrasound of the breast specimen shows inclusion of the mass previously seen within the patient. The surgeon was called in the operating room to confirm that he had removed the mass, marker, hookwire, and hookwire tip. Pathology showed fibroadenoma.

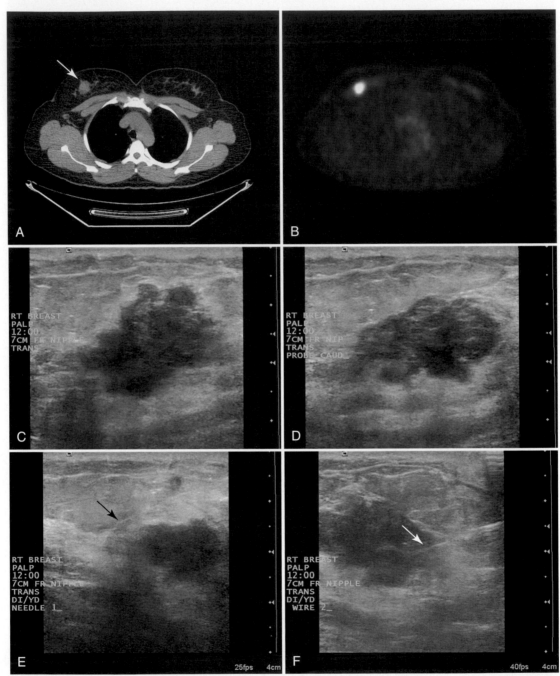

FIGURE 6-6. Ultrasound-guided bracket needle localization. **A,** Positron emission tomography/computed tomography (PET/CT) shows a mass in the right breast on the CT scan (*arrow*). **B,** The mass demontrates increased uptake of fluorodeoxyglucose on the PET scan. **C,** Ultrasound shows a palpable lobulated, hypoechoic, suspicious mass in the 12-o'clock position on the right breast in transverse plane, corresponding to the mass seen on PET/CT. **D,** The mass is slightly wider in its caudal aspect. Core biopsy showed cancer. Because the mass was difficult to see against the dense breast tissue on the mammogram, the surgeon requested ultrasound bracket localization. **E,** Ultrasound bracket localization shows the needle at the medial aspect of the mass (*arrow*). **F,** A second wire can be seen in the lateral aspect of the mass (*arrow*). **G,** Lateral-medial mammogram after localization shows the two wires at either end of the mass (the mass is difficult to see against the dense tissue). Use of the open aperture of the alphanumeric plate avoids pushing the wires further into the breast. Annotations show clusters of three and four BBs marking the skin entry sites. Single and double BBs show the medial and lateral aspects of the mass, marked by an X written on the skin to help the surgeon find the mass in the operating room.

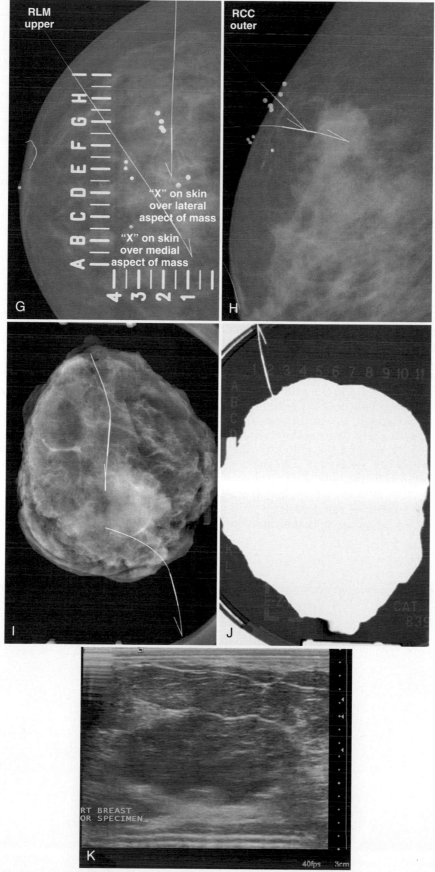

Figure 6-6, cont'd. H, Annotated magnified craniocandal view shows the wires next to the mass. Annotations show clusters of three and four BBs marking the skin entry sites. Single and double BBs show the medial and lateral aspects of the mass, marked by an X written on the skin to help the surgeon find the mass in the operating room. **I,** A specimen radiograph shows inclusion of the mass and the two hookwires. Note that one of the wires no longer inside the specimen was placed within the container to show that it and its tip were removed. **J,** The same specimen photographed at lighter contrast shows the letters and numbers on the container. The mass is located at coordinates F.0/4.0. **K,** An ultrasound of the breast specimen shows inclusion of the entire mass scanned at coordinates F.0/4.0, showing that the entire mass and its margins were removed.

Pathology Correlation

Later, the radiologist reviews the pathology report to see if the pathology reflects what the radiologist expected, based on the lesion's imaging characteristics. Radiologic–pathologic correlation ensures that the targeted lesion analyzed at pathologic evaluation is concordant with the imaging finding and, specifically, that the pathology report describes a histologic finding that is known to correlate with the imaging findings. For example, if the targeted lesion shows fine pleomorphic calcifications, a diagnosis of malignancy, high-risk lesion, or benign lesion would all be concordant if the targeted calcifications were definitely seen in the specimen radiograph and preferably also on the pathology slides (Fig. 6-7). If the pathology report showed an uncalcified fibroadenoma when the targeted radiographic finding was fine pleomorphic calcifications, the pathologic–radiologic correlation would be discordant, and the case would warrant additional investigation.

Pathologic–radiologic correlation of targeted calcifications is a special subset of breast biopsy correlation. Calcifications from targeted calcifications must be seen on the surgical specimen radiograph for the biopsy to be concordant. Calcifications seen just on histologic slides and not on the specimen radiograph do not represent the calcified lesion being targeted and are not concordant. Calcifications seen on the specimen radiograph are usually seen on pathology slides, but the pathologist may not see them for several reasons.

First, the calcifications may be calcium oxalate and are seen on the slides. Unlike calcium phosphate calcifications, which are easily seen on hematoxylin and eosin (H&E) staining, calcium oxalate is not visualized with H&E staining and requires a special polarized light to show the calcifications.

Second, the calcifications may be in the paraffin blocks. During specimen processing, thin breast tissue samples are embedded in paraffin blocks, which are then sliced and placed on slides for staining. Each block is several millimeters thick, but each slide contains only micromillimeters of paraffin and tissue. The calcifications may still be in the block and may never have been placed on a slide for review. A radiograph of the blocks may show the calcifications, and re-sectioning of that particular block will show the calcifications (Fig. 6-8).

Third, other calcifications may be removed from the specimen if the microtome cutting device that slices the tissue/paraffin block for slides pushes large calcifications out of the specimen at the time of sectioning.

If the targeted calcifications seemed to be present in the specimen radiograph but no calcifications are found in the pathology slides or in the paraffin blocks, a repeat mammogram can determine whether the calcifications are still in the breast and were not removed at surgery. Rarely, the calcifications seen in the specimen radiograph can be incidental calcifications and not the ones that were targeted.

PERCUTANEOUS NEEDLE BIOPSY OF CYSTS, SOLID MASSES, OR CALCIFICATIONS

Breast lesions can be classified as cysts, solid masslike lesions (which include true masses, asymmetries, and areas of architectural distortion), and calcifications. Needle types and cyst aspirations are discussed here, followed by needle biopsies guided by palpation, ultrasound, and stereotactic techniques. Needle biopsies guided by MRI are discussed in Chapter 7. This section then discusses core specimen radiography, marker placement, carbon marking,

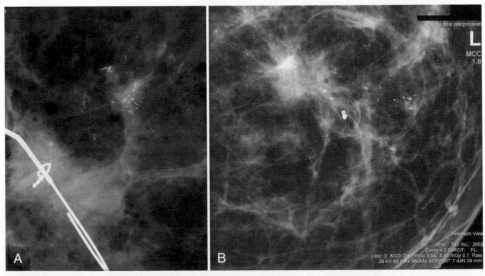

FIGURE 6-7. A, Magnification mammogram shows invasive ductal cancer (IDC) and ductal carcinoma in situ (DCIS) as a mass and calcifications previously sampled by stereotactic biopsy. The magnified craniocaudal mammogram shows a spiculated mass, residual calcifications, air, and a metallic marker. This area was localized for surgical excisional biopsy. **B,** After preoperative localization and excisional biopsy, magnified, cropped specimen radiograph shows the hookwire, hookwire tip, marker, the mass, and calcifications. The uncropped specimen radiograph (not shown) showed that the entire mass and calcifications were removed. Because IDC and DCIS had been shown by stereotactic core biopsy, the radiologist expects IDC, DCIS, and calcifications in the pathology report. Pathology showed IDC, DCIS, calcifications, and postbiopsy change, which was concordant with imaging.

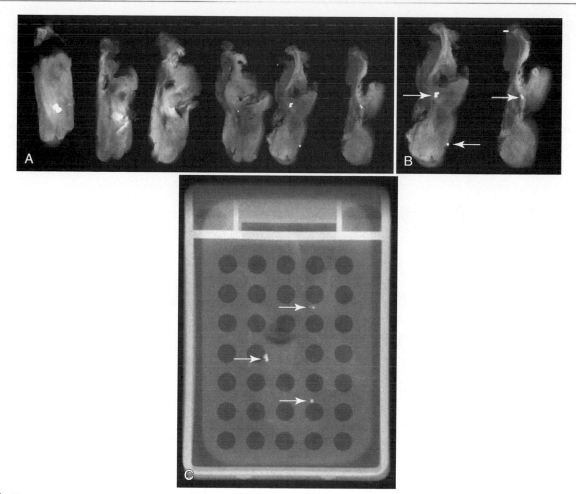

FIGURE 6-8. Tissue specimen radiography in pathology department. **A,** Radiograph of six tissue specimens sectioned from an excisional breast biopsy performed for calcifications. Calcifications are found in all six specimens. **B,** Magnified view of two tissue specimens containing calcifications (*arrows*). **C,** Pathology technologists place the tissue pieces in paraffin in a plastic tissue cassette. This paraffin block radiograph shows the calcifications (*arrows*) from the two tissue specimens shown in part **B**. Pathology showed fibrocystic change and calcifications. If the slides from this cassette did not show calcifications, the pathologists would have taken additional samples from this cassette. (Images courtesy of Dr. Gerald Berry, Stanford University, Palo Alto, CA.)

patient safety and comfort after biopsy, complete lesion removal, calcification and epithelial displacement, pathology correlation, high-risk lesions, follow-up of benign lesions, complications, differences between core and vacuum needle biopsies, and patient follow-up, audits, and noncompliance.

Needle Types

The types of biopsy needles used for specific breast lesions and guidance methods vary around the world. A trend toward progressively larger needles and more tissue samples per biopsy site has been noted, especially in the United States. Three main types of needles are used for percutaneous biopsies (Table 6-1). Fine-needle aspiration (FNA) needles, usually 25- to 20-gauge, are used for cyst aspirations and for solid breast masses. The aspirated material requires interpretation by expert cytopathologists. FNA is usually done with ultrasound or palpation guidance with at least four needle passes. FNA is less commonly done in the United States compared to Europe and Asia.

TABLE 6-1. Needles Used for Percutaneous Breast Biopsies

Needle Type	Usual Gauge	Biopsy Use
Fine-needle aspiration	25- to 20-gauge	Cyst aspiration. Solid mass highly likely to be either benign or malignant
Automated large-core	18- to 14-gauge	Ultrasound-guided biopsy. Uncommon for stereotactic biopsy
Directional vacuum-assisted	14- to 7-gauge	Stereotactic biopsy. Uncommon but growing use for ultrasound-guided biopsy

Automated large-core (core) needles in 18- to 14-gauge (Fig. 6-9A and B) commonly are used to biopsy masses with ultrasound or palpation guidance. In some facilities, especially outside the United States, core needles are used with stereotactic guidance to biopsy masses or calcifications. An automated large-core biopsy needle obtains a single specimen with each pass of the needle, and 2 to 12

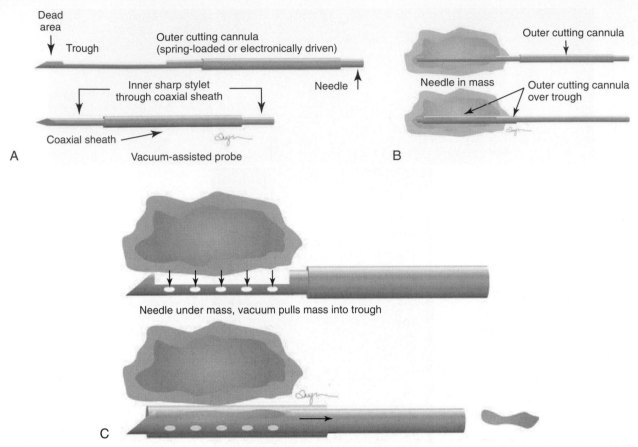

FIGURE 6-9. Needle types and coaxial guide for core needle biopsy. **A,** Schematic of core biopsy needle parts showing the needle, coaxial sheath, and inner stylet. **B,** Schematic of how to use a multifire core biopsy needle for breast biopsies. The outer cutting cannula shoots over the trough and cuts the mass. The entire needle is removed each time. **C,** Schematic of a vacuum-assisted probe for needle core biopsy. The outer cutting cannula shoots over the trough and cuts the mass. The vacuum transports the specimen to the needle end for removal. There may be one or multiple insertions, depending on the vendor.

specimens are obtained by firing the needle multiple times. Pathologists who are comfortable interpreting surgically excised breast biopsy tissue can interpret the histologic material obtained.

Directional vacuum-assisted (vacuum) needles (see Fig. 6-9C) are available in 7- to 14-gauge and are used for stereotactic, ultrasound-guided, and MRI-guided biopsies. Depending on the manufacturer, vacuum biopsy can be done with just one needle pass, and multiple specimens are obtained by rotating the collection aperture of the needle to obtain between 6 and 18 specimens. Other directional vacuum-assisted needles obtain single vacuum specimens with each pass, requiring multiple insertions. In some facilities, vacuum biopsies are used to excise benign lesions such as fibroadenomas to avoid the need for surgical excision or imaging follow-up, once the fibroadenoma has been diagnosed by core needle biopsy and adequate sampling.

Both single-insertion and multi-insertion needles can be used with or without a coaxial guide (Fig. 6-10A). The coaxial guides are usually used with ultrasound or MRI guidance. The purpose of the coaxial guide is to provide a path to the target that the radiologist can use again and again without retraumatizing the breast tissue. The coaxial device consists of an inner sharp stylet and an outer sheath.

The coaxial device is placed through the tissue so that the stylet tip/sheath edge is at or in the lesion. Then the radiologist removes the stylet, leaving a sheath that provides a "tunnel" through the breast tissue directly to the lesion. The radiologist then places the biopsy needle through the sheath into the lesion and takes samples. The radiologist can repeatedly place the biopsy needle through the sheath without having to disturb the surrounding breast tissue. Coaxial biopsies can be done with the sheath near the mass or through the mass (see Fig. 6-10B).

Cyst Aspiration

Masses on mammograms often prompt requests for breast ultrasound and cyst aspiration. To do a cyst aspiration the radiologist advances a fine needle into the cyst by palpation or image guidance. If the cyst is tense, fluid wells up into the needle hub. To aspirate the cyst, the radiologist attaches a syringe to the needle and draws fluid into the syringe until no more fluid can be obtained. Cyst aspiration can be done by ultrasound (Fig. 6-11) or, less commonly, by x-ray guidance using a fenestrated compression plate and mammography. If cyst aspiration is done under ultrasound, the radiologist should be able to watch the cyst disappear in real time.

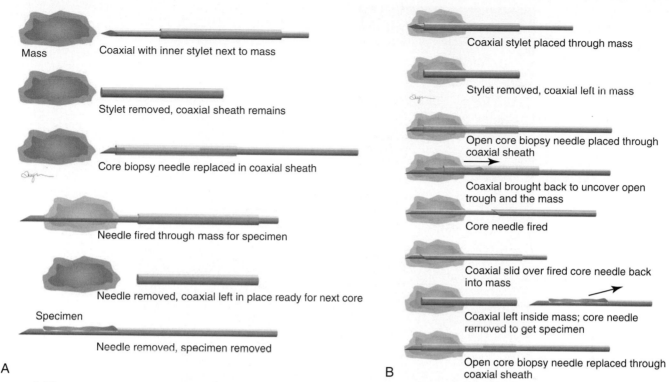

A

Mass
Coaxial with inner stylet next to mass

Stylet removed, coaxial sheath remains

Core biopsy needle replaced in coaxial sheath

Needle fired through mass for specimen

Needle removed, coaxial left in place ready for next core

Specimen
Needle removed, specimen removed

B

Coaxial stylet placed through mass

Stylet removed, coaxial left in mass

Open core biopsy needle placed through coaxial sheath

Coaxial brought back to uncover open trough and the mass

Core needle fired

Coaxial slid over fired core needle back into mass

Coaxial left inside mass; core needle removed to get specimen

Open core biopsy needle replaced through coaxial sheath

FIGURE 6-10. **A,** Schematic of how to use a coaxial sheath next to a mass for ultrasound-guided core biopsies. The radiologist places a coaxial containing a sharp, inner stylet through the breast tissue next to a mass. The radiologist removes the stylet, places a core biopsy needle through the coaxial sheath, fires the needle through the mass, and withdraws the needle. The coaxial sheath is left adjacent to the mass, providing a tunnel through the breast tissue. The radiologist removes the specimen from the needle and can replace the needle through the coaxial sheath for the next core. **B,** Schematic of how to use a coaxial sheath inside a mass for ultrasound-guided core biopsies. The radiologist places a coaxial containing a sharp, inner stylet into a mass. The radiologist removes the stylet, places an open core biopsy needle through the coaxial sheath, withdraws the coaxial to expose the biopsy trough inside the mass, and fires the needle to take the sample. Before withdrawing the biopsy needle, the radiologist threads the coaxial sheath over the fired needle and leaves the sheath inside the mass. The core biopsy needle can now be replaced into the sheath to take the next sample.

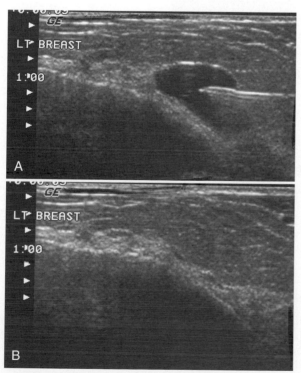

FIGURE 6-11. Cyst aspiration. **A,** Ultrasound shows a needle in a cyst near an implant. **B,** The follow-up ultrasound shows that the cyst is gone.

Aspirated fluid is sent for cytologic evaluation only if an intracystic mass is present or the fluid is bloody. A large series of cyst aspirations by Tabar and colleagues showed that cyst fluid cytology is often falsely negative, even in the presence of an intracystic mass. In these cases, the pneumocystogram was enough to diagnose an intracystic mass and prompt biopsy of the rare intracystic cancer.

Pneumocystograms are mammograms obtained after the radiologist injects air into a cyst cavity. The pneumocystogram shows the air-filled cyst cavity on the mammogram, enabling the radiologist to make sure that a mass prompting biopsy on the mammogram corresponds to the aspirated cyst and to exclude an intracystic mass. Air is thought to be therapeutic in preventing cyst recurrence (Fig. 6-12). To do a pneumocystogram, the radiologist aspirates the cyst first. Once the fluid has been aspirated completely, the radiologist disengages the syringe while carefully holding the needle tip in the decompressed, flattened cyst cavity. The radiologist attaches an air-filled syringe to the needle, injects a small amount of air into the cyst cavity, takes the needle out, and obtains CC and mediolateral mammograms immediately. A normal pneumocystogram should show an air-filled, thin-walled, round or oval cavity without intracystic solid masses or mural nodules.

Although radiologists can usually tell if a cyst on ultrasound corresponds to a specific mammographic mass, this correlation can be tricky. When the correlation is unclear

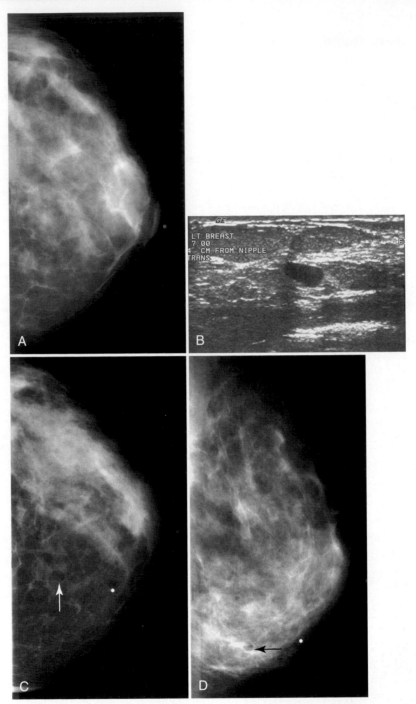

FIGURE 6-12. Pneumocystogram. **A,** A craniocaudal (CC) mammogram shows an oval breast mass in the inner portion of the breast. **B,** Ultrasound shows a complicated cyst versus a solid oval mass. After cyst aspiration under ultrasound guidance, air was placed in the cyst cavity. CC **(C)** and lateral **(D)** pneumocystogram mammograms show air (*arrows*) replacing fluid in the mass, which confirms that the finding on the mammogram represents a cyst that was aspirated.

and the radiologist has chosen not to do a pneumocystogram, the radiologist orders a postaspiration mammogram to see if the "cyst" disappears. The mass should be gone on the postaspiration mammogram if the aspirated cyst is the mammographic mass. If the mass still shows on the postaspiration mammogram, the mammographic finding is separate from the cyst and needs further investigation (Fig. 6-13).

Palpation Guidance

FNA or core biopsy can be performed on palpable masses. With this method, CC and mediolateral mammograms and other imaging studies are reviewed. Palpation-guided procedures are similar to ultrasound-guided procedures, but there is no visualization of the lesion or needle during the procedure. The lesion must be discretely palpable and

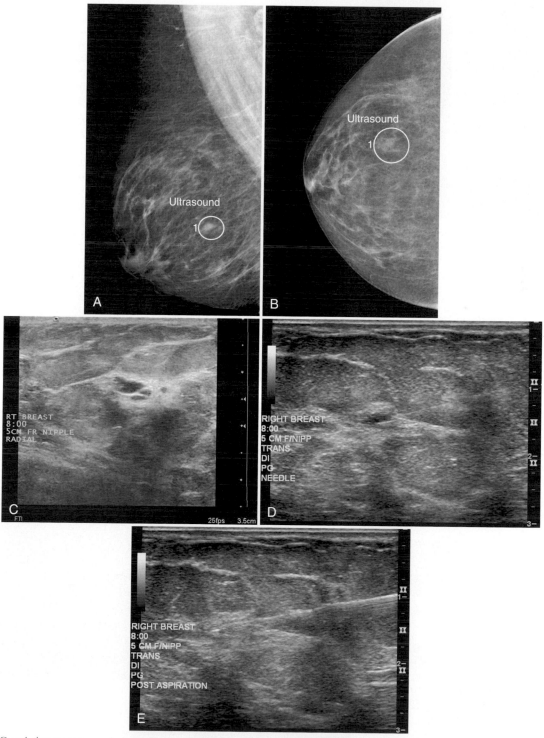

FIGURE 6-13. Correlating mammography and ultrasound after cyst aspiration. Right mediolateral oblique (MLO) (**A**) and craniocaudal (CC) (**B**) views show a possible mass on screening mammography (*circles*). **C,** Ultrasound shows a probable multiseptated, complicated cyst in the expected location of the mammographic mass. **D,** Fine needle aspiration under ultrasound shows the needle in the mass. **E,** Cyst fluid was aspirated and the mass disappeared.

Continued

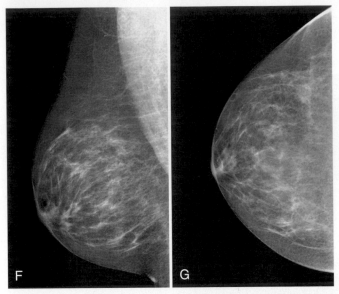

FIGURE 6-13, cont'd. Postaspiration MLO (**F**) and CC (**G**) views show that the mammographic mass disappeared, indicating that the ultrasound and mammographic findings represented the same simple cyst.

well away from the chest wall for the biopsy to be done with accuracy and safety. This procedure is usually reserved for cysts and solid masses that are almost definitely malignant or benign by imaging and palpation criteria.

Ultrasound Guidance

When compared with stereotactic biopsy, ultrasound-guided biopsy has the advantage of using readily available equipment and is fast and cost-effective. The first step in ultrasound-guided biopsy is to find the questioned lesion for biopsy. This commonly occurs when a mass on the mammogram prompts an ultrasound to further characterize the mass and localize it for biopsy. When correlating the mammogram to the ultrasound, the mass can be far away from the chest wall on the mammogram and lie next to the pectoralis muscle on the ultrasound. This occurs because the breast tissue is compressed far away from the chest wall when the patient stands up for the mammogram. On ultrasound, the breast falls dependently onto the chest wall when the patient lies down (Fig. 6-14A).

When planning ultrasound-guided needle biopsies, it is important to keep the needle tip away from the chest wall to prevent pneumothorax. Unlike upright preoperative x-ray–guided needle localization or prone stereotactic

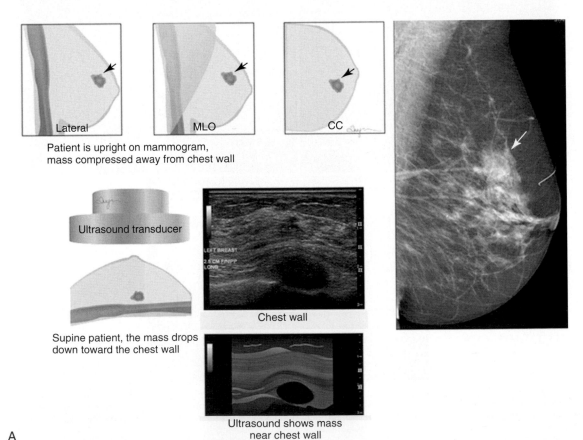

FIGURE 6-14. Schematics of how masses appearing to be far away from the chest wall on mammography may be found near the chest wall on ultrasound and how to keep the needle tip away from the chest wall on ultrasound-guided core biopsy **A,** Schematic mammograms show a mass in the upper inner quadrant that appears to be far from the chest wall. However, mammograms are obtained with compression; when the patient lies supine, the mass falls dependently against the chest wall. On ultrasound, the mass may be closer to the chest wall than expected from the mammogram.

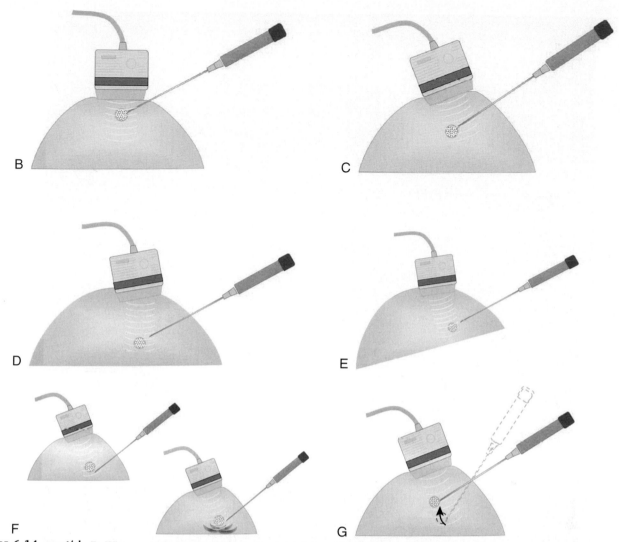

FIGURE 6-14, cont'd. B, With superficial lesions, the needle tip and throw are usually far away from the chest wall. **C,** With deeper lesions, the needle angle is steeper, and the radiologist judges whether the needle "throw" will penetrate the lung. **D,** When the patient is flat and the lesion is even deeper, the needle trajectory can point toward the chest wall. **E,** To change the needle trajectory, the patient can be angled so that her chest wall parallels the needle track/throw. **F,** Injecting anesthetic underneath the lesion can lift it away from the chest wall for biopsy. **G,** Inserting the needle tip into the lesion and redirecting the throw of the needle avoids placing the needle tip into the chest wall. (**B** to **G,** Courtesy of Dr. Sunita Pal, Stanford Radiology, Stanford, CA.)

localization, the ultrasound-guided biopsy is done supine and the needle is not necessarily parallel to the chest wall. Further complicating matters, some core biopsy needles "throw" the cutting trough 2.5 cm further into the tissue beyond the needle tip. Thus, planning a safe ultrasound-guided needle biopsy trajectory must take into account both the needle tip and the needle "throw" trajectory. To plan a safe procedure, the radiologist rolls the patient on the table so that the needle trajectory is as parallel to the chest wall as possible and not at a steep angle aiming toward the lungs. Patient positioning can take some time, but it is worth the few minutes to position the patient accurately to avoid an untoward complication. Another way to keep the needle away from the chest wall is to inject anesthetic underneath the targeted mass to lift it away from the pectoralis muscle. Alternatively, in some cases, the radiologist can stick the biopsy needle tip into the mass

and lift it into a safer trajectory before firing the needle (see Fig. 6-14B to G).

For ultrasound-guided FNA, the radiologist introduces a needle in the plane of the transducer axis to show the entire shaft of the needle, its tip, and the lesion. Once the needle is within the lesion, the radiologist aspirates the mass with a vigorous to-and-fro movement to obtain material for cytologic evaluation and then withdraws the needle. At least four passes should be performed; optimally, the material should be analyzed immediately to ensure that adequate cellular material has been obtained for diagnosis. After aspiration, direct pressure is applied to the site (Fig. 6-15).

To perform a core biopsy under ultrasound guidance, the radiologist localizes the lesion by ultrasound and chooses the course of needle insertion that offers the most accuracy and safety. While anesthetizing the core biopsy

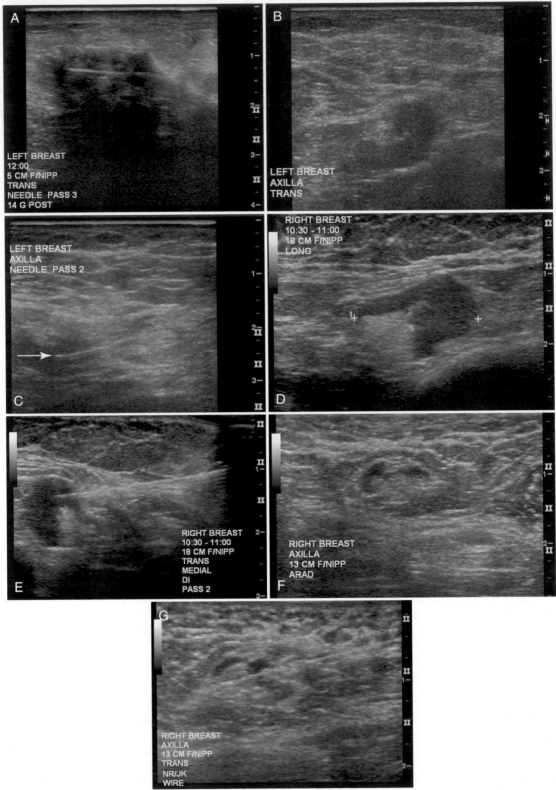

FIGURE 6-15. Fine-needle aspiration of axillary lymphadenopathy in a patient with invasive ductal cancer. **A,** Initial ultrasound shows a large invasive ductal cancer in the upper left breast undergoing ultrasound-guided core biopsy. **B,** Ultrasound of the left axilla in this patient shows a lymph node with an enlarged, thickened cortex, suspicious for metastatic disease. **C,** Fine-needle aspiration under ultrasound guidance shows the needle tip in the lymph node cortex (*arrow*). Cytology showed lymph node metastases. **D,** In another patient, the right axillary lymph node has an irregular, thickened cortex and a compressed fatty hilum. **E,** Ultrasound shows the fine-needle tip in the lymph node. Cytology showed metastatic disease from invasive ductal cancer. **F,** In another patient, a lymph node has an irregular cortex. Fine-needle aspiration showed metastatic disease. **G,** To make sure this irregular lymph node was removed at surgery, the surgeon requested preoperative needle localization. The ultrasound shows a hookwire traversing the lymph node at ultrasound-guided needle localization. Pathology showed metastatic disease.

track under direct ultrasound guidance, the radiologist uses the anesthesia needle to get an idea of how dense the breast feels and to see the needle trajectory. The radiologist also calculates the core needle "throw" to determine where to place the core needle tip "pre-fire" so the core trough will be in the middle of the lesion "postfire."

Then, under direct ultrasound visualization, the radiologist introduces the core biopsy needle into the breast. If the lesion is large enough, the radiologist introduces the needle into the edge of the lesion to hold it in place. Otherwise, the radiologist may choose to fire the needle through the mass with or without a coaxial system. In any case, the radiologist fires the biopsy core needle under direct visualization and harvests the cores. Optimally, at least three to five tissue specimens are obtained from different parts of the mass. After sampling, the radiologist places a metallic marker into the mass, and the technologist holds direct pressure on the breast to establish hemostasis. After hemostasis is established, the technologist bandages the wound and takes orthogonal mammograms to show the marker and any residual mass (Fig. 6-16).

A vacuum biopsy is similar to an automated multifire core biopsy, but the vacuum needle is usually placed under or occasionally inside the lesion. The probe "vacuums" tissue into the trough to be sampled. The vacuum technique carries a special caveat regarding the skin. If the probe is too close to the skin, the skin can be "vacuumed" into the trough and sampled, causing skin injury, requiring a suture or, in extreme cases, a skin graft. During a needle biopsy using vacuum technique, the radiologist obtains several samples, concentrating on aiming the trough at the mass (Fig. 6-17). Afterward, the radiologist can place a marker in the mass either through the probe or (depending on the manufacturer) by using a marker that has its own separate needle.

If a mass previously cored under ultrasound guidance must be removed, the radiologist localizes the mass or marker under ultrasound, places a wire, then takes orthogonal mammograms to show the wire and marker, and waits for the excised tissue specimen (Fig. 6-18).

Stereotactic Guidance

This method uses a compression device with a small aperture and an x-ray tube that has the ability to take two stereotactic views about 15 degrees off perpendicular (Fig. 6-19A to I). The patient is in a prone, upright, or decubitus position with the breast compressed by a fenestrated compression paddle for stereotactic needle biopsy. The radiologist reviews prebiopsy CC and mediolateral mammograms to determine the lesion's location on orthogonal views. The breast is then firmly compressed with the compression paddle aperture placed on the skin surface closest to the breast lesion. After taking a straight-on scout view that visualizes the lesion, the stereotactic technologist takes two stereo views of the lesion. The radiologist locates the lesion on the stereo views and passes a needle into the breast to a calculated depth. Prefire stereotactic images, which should show the tip of the biopsy needle at the edge of the lesion, are obtained. The radiologist then fires the needle deeper into the breast and reviews postfire stereotactic images to ensure that the trough of the needle is within the breast lesion. After the radiologist collects multiple specimens, he or she reviews the core specimen radiograph to make sure that the calcifications or mass has been sampled. The tissue specimens are labeled and sent to the pathology laboratory. At this point the radiologist decides whether to deploy a metallic marker into the biopsy cavity. If the radiologist deploys a marker, the technologist takes additional stereotactic images to confirm marker deployment before releasing the patient from compression. The technologist maintains direct pressure on the biopsy site after release of the compression paddle to achieve hemostasis, places a bandage, and obtains immediate postbiopsy upright CC and mediolateral mammograms. These show the biopsy cavity, confirm removal of all or a portion of the calcifications or mass, and show the location of the marker and its position relative to the targeted findings.

Burbank in 1996 and Jackman and Marzoni in 2003 discussed various techniques used to successfully biopsy lesions in technically challenging situations.

Core Specimen Radiography

Magnification specimen radiography is mandatory after stereotactic biopsy of calcifications and optional after biopsy of a mass to ensure that the lesion that prompted biopsy has been adequately sampled or removed (see Fig. 6-19J and K). If the targeted lesion is not present in the specimen, the radiologist obtains more specimens. Specimen radiography is not usually done after ultrasound-guided core biopsy unless the biopsy is targeting radiographically detectable calcifications (see Fig. 6-19L to R).

At times, specimen radiography may be equivocal in determining if the specimens include the lesion prompting biopsy, especially for masses. In such cases, the radiologist compares the breast specimen pathology report with the specimen radiograph. If there is a discrepancy between the appearance of the mammographic finding and the pathology report, the radiologist reviews the patient's immediate postbiopsy mammograms to see whether the lesion that prompted biopsy has been sampled or removed.

Calcifications from a biopsied calcific cluster must be evident on the core specimen radiograph for the imaging and histologic findings to be concordant. Most, but not all, calcifications seen on a specimen radiograph are also seen on histologic slides. If the radiologist was targeting calcifications and no calcifications are seen on the specimen radiograph, the ensuing pathology report will not be representative of the calcifications prompting biopsy (which are probably still inside the breast). However, the pathology report may still report calcifications even if they are absent on the core specimen radiograph because pathologists can see tiny calcifications on breast specimen slides that cannot be seen by core specimen radiography. These calcifications are usually smaller than 100 microns and are seen on the slides by serendipity. Thus, patients who undergo biopsy of calcifications and have specimen radiographs that show no calcifications need rebiopsy, even if the pathology report describes calcifications.

Text continued on p. 223

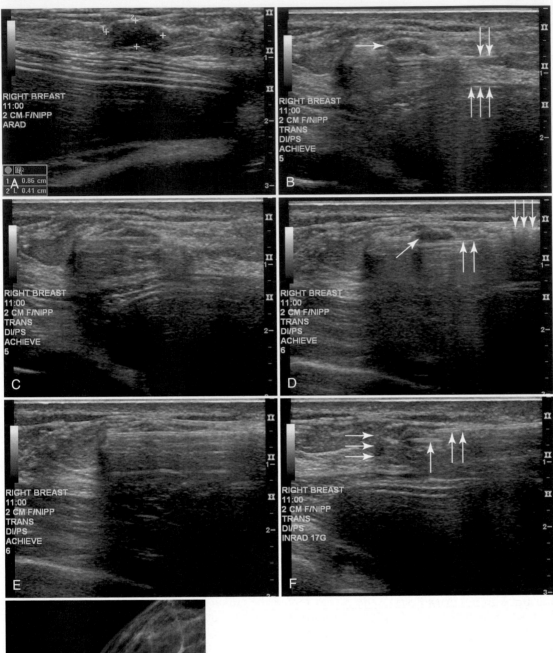

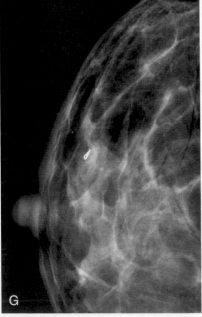

FIGURE 6-16. Use of the coaxial to core a mass adjacent to an implant. **A,** Ultrasound shows an oval mass on top of a breast implant, for which core biopsy was recommended. **B,** Ultrasound-guided core biopsy shows the trough of the needle (*double arrows*) traversing an oval mass (*single arrow*) on top of an implant (*triple arrows*). **C,** Postfire ultrasound shows the needle traversing the mass. At this point, a coaxial was placed over the needle, securing the needle's original position within the mass. **D,** The needle was replaced in the coaxial sheath and the coaxial (*triple arrows*) was withdrawn to expose the trough (*double arrows*) and allow the mass (*single arrow*) to fall within it. **E,** Postfire ultrasound with the coaxial sheath extended over the needle shows both the needle and coaxial traversing the mass. **F,** Ultrasound showing a needle threaded through the coaxial sheath (*double arrows*) placing a marker (*single arrow*) in the mass (*triple arrows*). **G,** Cropped implant-displaced digital lateral mammogram shows dense tissue and the marker. Histology showed fibroadenoma.

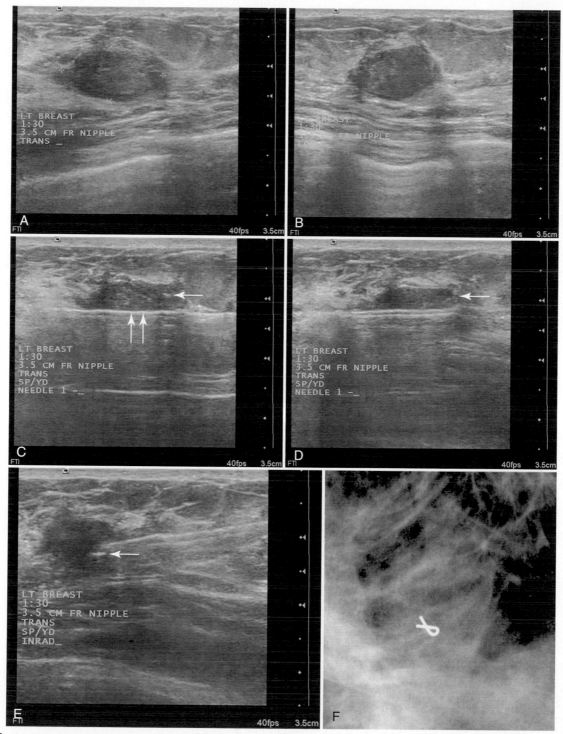

FIGURE 6-17. Vacuum-assisted core biopsy under ultrasound. A young patient has a new palpable mass in the left breast; biopsy was recommended. Transverse (**A**) and longitudinal (**B**) ultrasounds show an oval solid mass near the chest wall. **C,** To perform the ultrasound-guided vacuum-assisted biopsy, the radiologist injected lidocaine between the mass and the chest wall to lift it away from the pectoralis muscle. The radiologist then inserted the vacuum-assisted probe, shown here traversing the mass. Note the amount of mass (*arrow*) above the probe (*double arrow*). **D,** After vacuum-assisted sampling, in which the vacuum draws the mass into the probe and cuts off the tissue in the trough, there is less mass (*arrow*) above the probe after tissue removal. **E,** After biopsy, the ultrasound shows the needle placing a marker (*arrow*) within the mass. **F,** Magnified digital mammogram shows the marker within dense tissue, and the mass is not seen. Histology showed fibroadenoma.

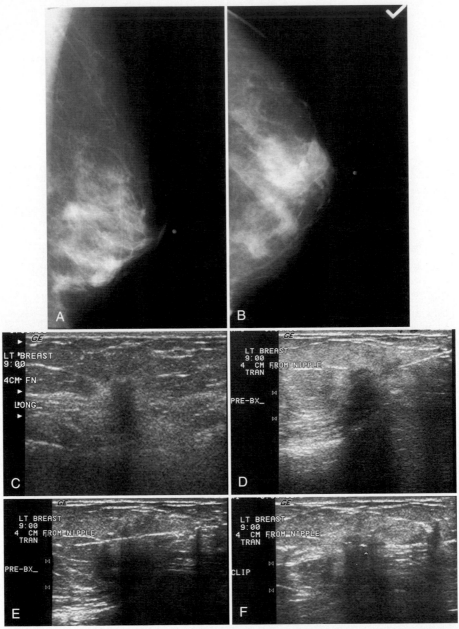

FIGURE 6-18. Ultrasound-guided core biopsy with marker placement and subsequent needle localization. Mediolateral (**A**) and craniocaudal (CC) (**B**) mammograms show a spiculated mass in the midportion of the left breast at the 9-o'clock position. **C**, Ultrasound shows a hypoechoic, spiculated shadowing mass. **D**, Ultrasound-guided needle placement shows the tip of the core biopsy needle before biopsy just proximal to the mass. Note that the trajectory of the needle is well away from the chest wall and will not produce a pneumothorax. **E**, A postfire ultrasound scan shows the needle traversing the mass and the expected location of the sampling trough inside the mass. All postfire films are imaged. **F**, A marker is placed in the mass and is displayed as a bright echo in the middle of the mass.

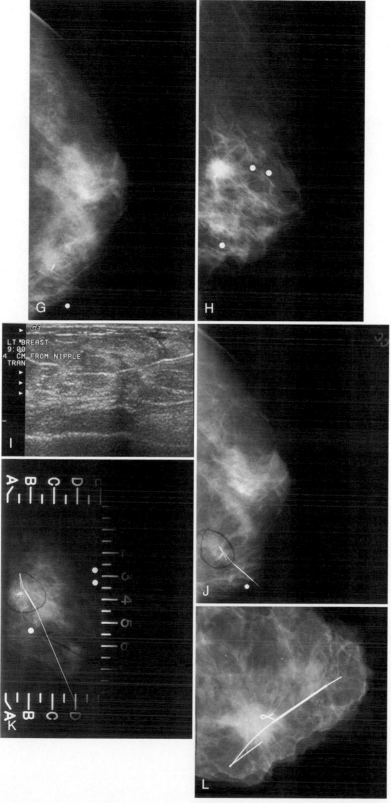

FIGURE 6-18, cont'd. Follow-up CC (**G**) and mediolateral (**H**) views show the marker in the mass. A single marker shows the skin entry site for the core needle, and two BBs show the location of the mass on the skin. **I,** Subsequent ultrasound-guided needle localization shows a wire in the mass. CC (**J**) and lateral (**K**) mammograms taken after ultrasound-guided needle localization show the wire tip in the mass. **L,** The specimen radiograph shows the mass, hookwire tip, and the marker. Pathologic examination revealed invasive ductal cancer and lobular carcinoma in situ; one of three sentinel lymph nodes was positive.

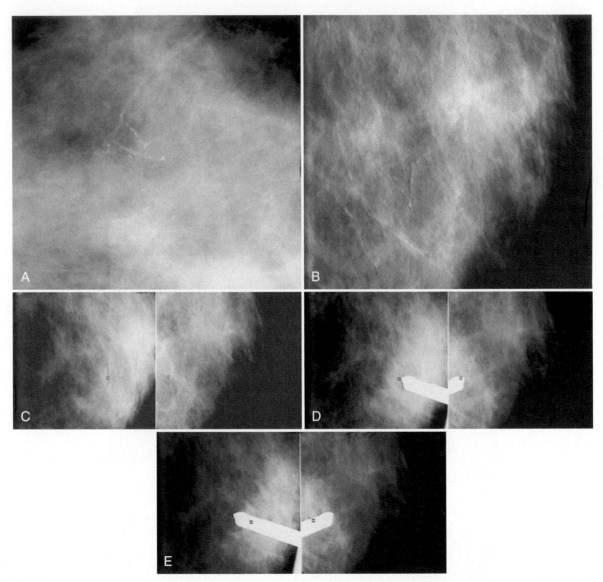

FIGURE 6-19. Eleven-gauge stereotactic vacuum-assisted core biopsy and marker placement. **A,** A mammogram shows suspicious branching micro-calcifications. **B,** A stereotactic straight-on scout view shows the suspicious microcalcifications in digital format. **C,** A 15-degree stereotactic view shows that the calcifications are within the aperture of the compression plate. **D,** Prefire films demonstrate that the stereotactic needle is directed toward the calcifications. **E,** Postfire stereotactic views show that the needle is traversing the suspicious microcalcifications.

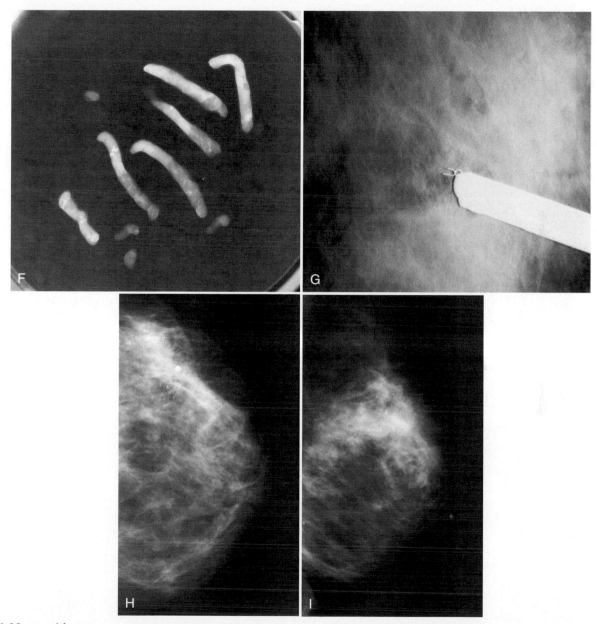

FIGURE 6-19, cont'd. F, A specimen radiograph shows inclusion of the suspicious microcalcifications corresponding to the mammographic finding. **G,** A stereotactic view at marker placement demonstrates that the marker is near the biopsy cavity on the stereotactic view. Immediate postbiopsy craniocaudal (CC) **(H)** and lateral **(I)** mammograms show that the marker is near the biopsy site and that air is present in the biopsy site.

Continued

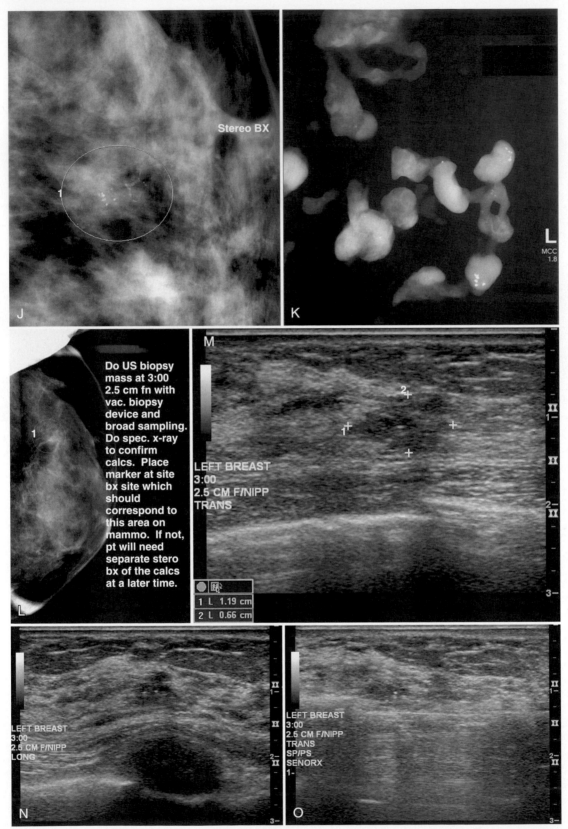

FIGURE 6-19, cont'd. **J,** Cropped digital magnification CC mammogram shows fine pleomorphic calcifications marked for stereotactic needle biopsy. **K,** Cropped magnified digital specimen radiograph shows inclusion of the suspicious calcifications. Pathology showed invasive ductal cancer and DCIS with calcifications. **L to R,** Ultrasound-guided core biopsy of calcifications with core specimen radiography. **L,** CC mammogram shows calcifications in the outer left breast. Note the radiologist has annotated the mammogram with instructions on how to manage this patient. Ultrasound later showed a mass and calcifications in this location. Transverse (**M**) and longitudinal (**N**) ultrasounds show a 1.1-cm hypoechoic mass containing calcifications. **O,** The ultrasound shows the vacuum-assisted core needle trough below the mass and calcifications.

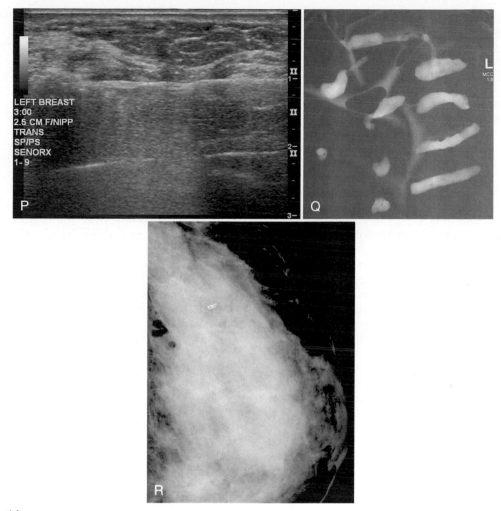

FIGURE 6-19, cont'd. **P,** Nine samples were obtained by vacuum-assisted core biopsy, and the ultrasound shows less of the mass and calcifications above the trough. **Q,** Core specimen radiographs of samples show the calcifications first seen on the mammogram. **R,** Postbiopsy mammogram shows the marker on the outer breast, absence of the calcifications, and air near the chest wall from the biopsy. Biopsy showed DCIS.

Marker Placement, Movement, and Compatibility with Ultrasound and MRI

Immediate postbiopsy insertion of a metallic marker at the biopsy site is usually indicated in core or vacuum needle biopsies guided by stereotactic technique. If a residual mass or calcifications is still left on postbiopsy stereotactic images after adequate sampling, a marker may not be needed. The marker is needed in case a cancer, high-risk lesion, or discordant benign lesion is diagnosed and the patient needs subsequent surgical excision of the needle biopsy site. With ultrasound- and MRI-guided biopsies, a metallic marker is often placed after biopsy even if some of the biopsied lesion is still evident. The marker helps to correlate the ultrasound, MRI, and mammogram findings.

After stereotactic biopsy and marker placement, the radiologist reviews stereotactic images before releasing breast compression to be sure the marker has deployed and is at or near the biopsy site. As a rule of thumb, our facility deploys a second marker if the first is more than 7 mm in depth (either deeper or more superficial) away from the initial biopsy site. For ultrasound-guided biopsies,

ultrasound-visible markers are used to be sure the marker has deployed accurately.

However, there is no practical way after MRI-guided biopsy to be sure the marker has deployed accurately by using MRI only. Even though an MRI scan done immediately after marker placement can show the signal void from the metallic marker, air introduced by the biopsy can also cause a signal void that simulates metallic markers. A post-MRI procedure mammogram will determine if the marker was deployed but not if it is accurately placed.

For stereotactic core biopsies, upright orthogonal CC and lateral mammograms obtained immediately after stereotactic biopsy show the location of the marker in relation to the biopsy site. Usually, the marker is located in or near the biopsy site. If the marker is some distance away from the site (i.e., inaccurate initial deployment), there is no practical way to insert a second marker. If the patient with an inaccurately placed marker needs surgical excision of the biopsy site, it may help to proceed with surgery as quickly as possible, hoping that a postbiopsy hematoma can be visualized by ultrasound or mammography to help guide the needle localization.

For ultrasound- or MRI-guided biopsies, upright orthogonal mammograms are obtained immediately after biopsy to correlate with prebiopsy mammogram images and to see the metallic marker's location in the breast.

If biopsy is performed on two sites in the same breast, markers with two unique shapes can be used to differentiate the two different sites. Rarely, patients request removal of a biopsy marker, which can be performed percutaneously with a vacuum-assisted biopsy device.

Various types of markers are available, including those containing stainless steel or titanium alone and those with metal embedded in plugs of various types. Terms for these markers include both *clips* and *markers*. The initial marking devices, which truly clipped to the edge of the biopsy cavity, are correctly said to be *clips*. Later, marking devices were developed to fall into the cavity without clipping to tissue; these are more correctly called *markers*. In scientific literature, the terms *markers* or *clip/markers* refer to both types of devices but are used inconsistently. The marker plugs are composed of Gelfoam, bovine or porcine collagen, suture-type material, or other materials. If markers containing bovine or porcine collagen are used, the patient should be asked about allergies to either beef or pork before deploying the markers.

A variety of problems are associated with the markers (Box 6-4). The first potential problem, nondeployment, is uncommon. It was anecdotally noted that some plugs may get stuck during deployment, making it impossible to push the plunger in or difficult to withdraw or close the needle. This problem is possibly due to the plugs filling with fluid, expanding in the deployment device, and getting stuck in the trough. For vacuum-assisted needles, the deployment device can get stuck on a retained fragment in the vacuum needle.

The second and most common potential problem is inaccurate initial deployment of the marker. An even rarer problem is delayed migration of the marker (i.e., it moves from the initial site to a different site in the breast). This can occur whether the initial deployment was accurate or inaccurate. Both inaccurate initial deployment and delayed migration are primarily along the axis of needle biopsy insertion (i.e., the z-axis).

Because there is no way to predict delayed migration, we advise upright orthogonal mammogram views immediately before x-ray–guided needle localization. The radiologist compares the marker on those images with the lesion position on prebiopsy mammograms and the marker (and postbiopsy changes) on the immediate poststereotactic biopsy mammograms. This will determine if the marker has moved.

If the marker was inaccurately deployed or has later migrated away from an original biopsy site, the radiologist determines the location of the original targeted lesion by using breast architecture and landmarks. The goal of subsequent localization is to remove the targeted biopsy site, including any residual cancer (Fig. 6-20). Whether it is necessary to also localize and remove the inaccurately positioned marker is controversial, but it should be considered if the needle biopsy revealed cancer. If the needle biopsy revealed a high-risk lesion or a discordant benign lesion, the inaccurately positioned marker presumably does not need to be removed. When the marker is in an inaccurate position, some facilities use presurgical or intraoperative ultrasound to try to identify the needle biopsy site.

Some markers placed by stereotaxis are embedded in plugs visible by ultrasound. Facilities may use ultrasound to localize these plugs for subsequent needle localization after stereotactic biopsy. After an ultrasound-guided biopsy, facilities may use markers visible by ultrasound. This allows the physician placing the marker to see whether the marker has deployed.

MRI is increasingly being used to stage the breast for cancer and to plan surgical management. Because biopsy site markers placed by stereotaxis, ultrasound, or MRI may be imaged by subsequent MRI studies, understanding of marker MRI compatibility and safety, and of marker artifacts, is becoming increasingly important. Accordingly, all facilities should use MRI-compatible metallic markers when markers are placed with any modality because MRI might be performed later. Metallic markers cause a signal void on MRI, and the size of the signal void varies according to the marker type and pulse sequence (Fig. 6-21). There is a difference between MRI marker compatibility and safety. *MRI compatibility* means that the marker can be used in the MRI magnet and will cause little artifact. *Marker safety* means that the marker will produce no harm to the patient in the magnet. Some markers are MRI compatible but still cause large artifacts of up to 2 cm, thus rendering the MRI less readable than when using other markers. MRI testing of markers for artifact by using phantoms on the facility's pulse sequences is a simple way to determine the marker artifact and the size of the signal void. This should be done before inserting metallic markers for marking tumors or biopsy sites. However, correlation between MRI, ultrasound, and mammography can be challenging, when markers or even wires are placed for preoperative localization (Fig. 6-22).

Carbon Marking

This method uses activated charcoal USP (Mallinckrodt, Phillipsburg, NJ) sterilized and suspended as a 4% weight/weight aqueous suspension. It is mixed with 0.3 mL sterile saline or water and injected in a to-and-fro motion after core biopsy along the stereotactic or ultrasound needle track to yield a dark line of carbon particles in the breast. This line of carbon particles can be used as a guide for excisional biopsy days to weeks after the percutaneous biopsy. It is used as an alternative to a postbiopsy metallic marker, mainly in Europe.

BOX 6-4. Possible Post Needle Biopsy Marker Problems

Nondeployment (rare and recognized on stereo views while the breast is still in compression)

Inaccurate initial deployment (common and recognized on views on the biopsy day)

Delayed migration from initial deployment site (rare and recognized on views taken days to months after biopsy)

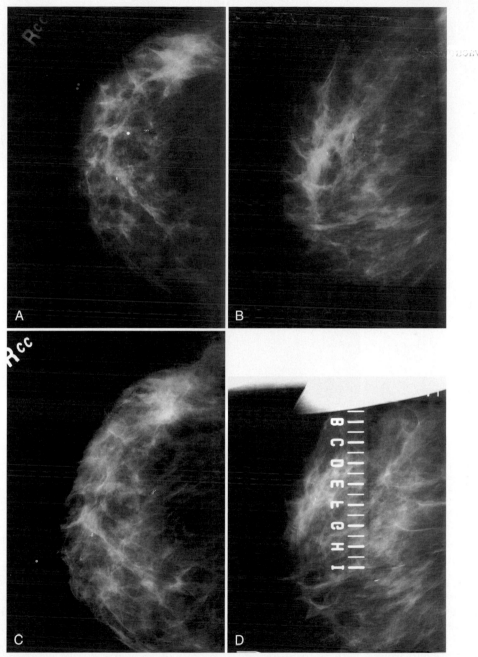

FIGURE 6-20. Value of two different types of markers for two stereotactic biopsy sites and marker migration. Because this patient had two suspicious microcalcification clusters, two different markers were placed at stereotactic biopsy. Craniocaudal (CC) (**A**) and mediolateral (**B**) mammograms show the difference in marker configuration, which clearly identifies the biopsy site. If the same type of marker had been placed in both sites, it would be difficult to determine the location of each biopsy site on subsequent mammograms. Cancer was found in the upper biopsy site, and the lower biopsy site was benign. Two months later, preoperative CC (**C**) and lateral (**D**) views show that the upper marker has migrated to the inferior portion of the breast. Because cancer was taken from the upper biopsy site, breast architecture was used to target the original upper biopsy site for excision because the marker is now in a different quadrant. This case shows the importance of correlation of the prestereotactic biopsy scout mammogram, the immediate postmarker placement mammogram, which documents orientation of the marker to the biopsy site, and scout mammograms before preoperative needle localization.

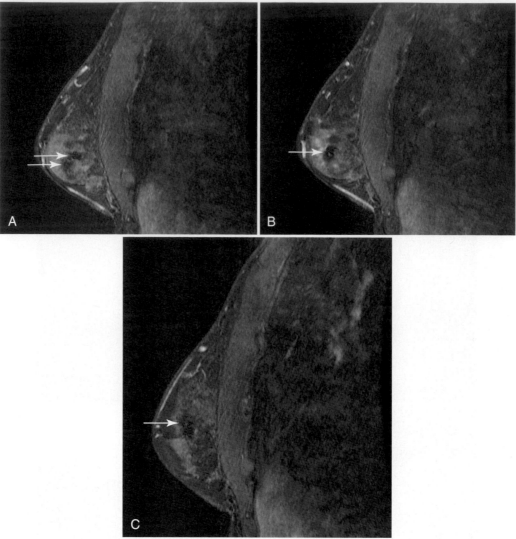

FIGURE 6-21. Signal void on breast magnetic resonance imaging (MRI) due to metallic markers placed from stereotactic core biopsy. **A,** Postcontrast 3-D spectral-spatial excitation magnetization transfer (3DSSMT) breast MRI shows signal voids as dark areas (*arrows*) in a patient who had four stereotactic core biopsies with metallic markers placed. **B** and **C,** Postcontrast 3DSSMT breast MRI slices showing signal voids (*arrows*) in the same patient from the other metallic markers.

Patient Safety and Comfort after Biopsy

After needle biopsy, hemostasis is achieved by direct pressure. In some institutions, after hemostasis is confirmed, the patient is taught how to "hold pressure" on the biopsy site so that she knows what to do if subsequent untoward bleeding occurs. After adequate hemostasis is achieved, some institutions close the wound with Steri-Strips and cover the Steri-Strips with Opsite, a self-adhesive polyurethane film sterile material used to cover operative wounds. Opsite prevents the Steri-Strips from getting wet and keeps the wound clean and dry. The patient can take a shower with the Opsite on but is instructed not to "scrub" the Opsite, take a bath, swim, or engage in other activities that might immerse the wound site. The patient is told to expect a quarter-sized spot of blood on the Steri-Strips and a bruise at the biopsy site that may travel to dependent sites; the patient is told to put direct pressure on the biopsy site if oozing or unexpected bleeding occurs. The patient is instructed to remove the Opsite and Steri-Strips after 4

to 7 days. Some facilities also bind the breast with wrap-around bandages or commercially available binders (commonly used after mastectomy) to hold the breasts tight to the chest wall. These bandages restrict breast motion while the patient is awake and limit breast motion during the night. Patients are also told that the biopsy site may feel bigger because of a blood clot in the biopsy site.

Part of recovery is pain control. If the patient is not allergic to acetaminophen and has no liver problems, she may take acetaminophen initially and then every 6 hours as needed, up to 4 g/day. Rarely, stronger medication such as Tylenol No. 3 (acetaminophen with codeine) or Vicodin (acetaminophen with hydrocodone), may be prescribed for pain. Any pain medications (usually aspirin or nonsteroidal anti-inflammatory drugs [NSAIDs]) withheld for 7 days before biopsy are to be avoided for 3 days after biopsy to decrease the risk of bleeding. After the technologist puts an ice pack on the biopsy site, the patient is told to leave the ice on for 60 minutes initially and then for 10 minutes every hour until bedtime. She is advised *not* to keep it on

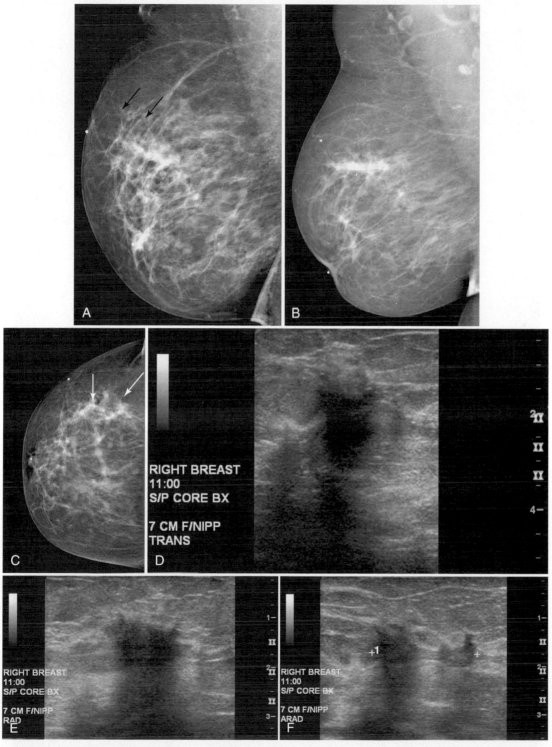

FIGURE 6-22. Correlation of mammogram, ultrasound, and magnetic resonance imaging (MRI) on wire localization. **A,** Right mediolateral oblique (MLO) digital mammogram shows architectural distortion in the upper right breast (*arrows*) and a skin marker on the distortion because there was a palpable mass. **B,** Slightly lighter technique MLO shows the distortion to greater advantage. **C,** Craniocaudal (CC) mammogram shows the architectural distortion after core biopsy with a marker in it (*arrows*). **D,** Ultrasound in the upper outer quadrant shows an irregular, hypoechoic, shadowing mass corresponding to the mammographic finding. Core biopsy showed invasive lobular cancer. **E,** Radial scan of the invasive lobular cancer on ultrasound. **F,** Two other satellite masses representing invasive lobular cancer in the same quadrant on ultrasound. *Continued*

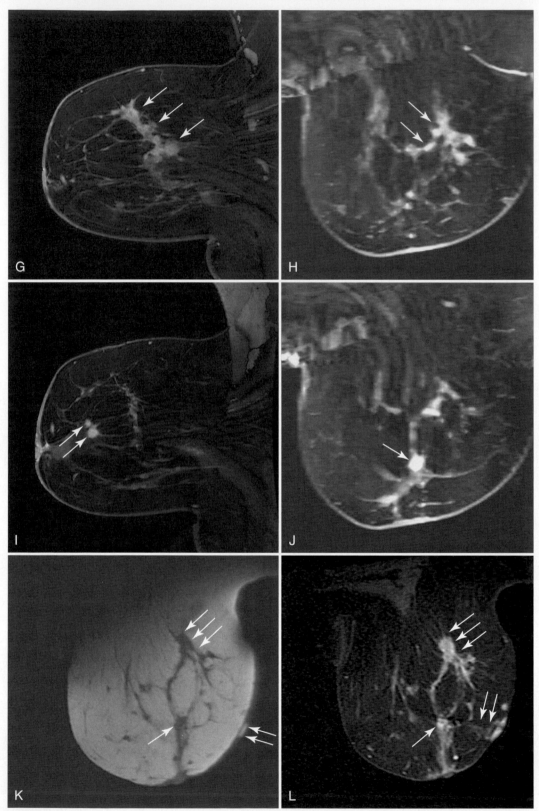

Figure 6-22, cont'd. G, Contrast-enhanced 3-D spectral-spatial excitation magnetization transfer (3DSSMT) MRI shows an irregular spiculated mass (*arrows*) representing the invasive lobular cancer seen on the MLO mammogram. The kinetic curve showed a rapid wash-in and late washout. **H,** Postcontrast 3DSSMT axial reformat shows the irregular enhancing cancer in the outer breast, similar to its appearance on the CC mammogram (*arrows*). **I,** Sagittal 3DSSMT postcontrast MRI shows two unexpected incidental spiculated enhancing lesions (IELs) in the midbreast on another slice, far away from the upper outer quadrant invasive lobular cancer (*arrows*). These were not evident on the mammogram, nor found with certainty by ultrasound. **J,** Postcontrast 3DSSMT axial reformat MRI shows one of the two spiculated IEL masses suspicious for cancer (*arrow*). **K,** Axial non-contrast T1-weighted MRI on the day of the MRI-guided needle localization shows the low signal architectural distortion representing invasive lobular cancer (*triple arrows*), the unenhanced IELs (*single arrow*) and the fiducial on the skin marking the planned needle entry site (*double arrows*). **L,** Post-contrast Dixon technique axial MRI shows the enhancing palpable spiculated invasive lobular cancer (*triple arrows*), the signal void from the needle traversing the satellite lesion (*double arrows*), and the enhancing IEL (*arrow*).

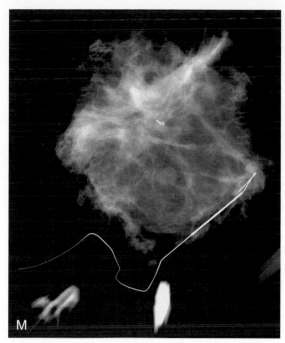

FIGURE 6-22, cont'd. M, Specimen radiograph shows inclusion of the hookwire and hookwire tip in the possible dense mass and architectural distortion in the dense tissue with the marker within it. Pathology showed invasive lobular cancer near the marker and at the hookwire tip.

longer because of the possibility of frostbite. The ice helps decrease postbiopsy discomfort and bleeding. To keep the ice pack in place, the patient may put the ice pack inside her brassiere or use a commercially available breast binder. Afterward, patients are given verbal and written postbiopsy wound care instructions and a phone number to call for problems. Each time the 10-minute ice pack is removed, the patient is told to look at the bandage (which may require using a mirror). If the amount of blood has increased since the last inspection, the patient is told to again firmly compress the biopsy site for 10 more minutes. Patients are instructed on where and how to obtain their biopsy result. Most patients do well with these instructions. Some facilities call the patient later in the afternoon, early evening, or the next day as a courtesy call to see how the patient is doing and to answer any questions.

Complete Lesion Removal

Core biopsy samples showing cancer routinely undergo subsequent excisional biopsy to remove residual cancer at the biopsy location. Even if the entire radiographic finding has been removed by percutaneous biopsy, occult residual cancer has been demonstrated in the needle biopsy site in 73% (15/23) of cases at subsequent surgery.

How is the core biopsy site localized when the entire lesion has been removed and no marker was placed in the biopsy site, or a marker was placed but is not at the biopsy site (either from inaccurate initial placement or delayed migration)? Because air can move along the biopsy track, air alone is not enough to identify the biopsy site. Although a hematoma may sometimes be mammographically seen in the immediate postbiopsy period, it usually persists for

just a few days or weeks. Studies have shown no mammographically detectable findings some months after a stereotactic core or vacuum needle biopsy.

Brenner suggests using landmarks within the breast to localize the approximate stereotactic biopsy site. Others have suggested localizing the fluid collection in the biopsy site by ultrasound. Although this may work in the immediate postbiopsy period, fluid can be reabsorbed if the excisional biopsy is delayed by several weeks, and using the fluid alone may not be reliable.

Calcification and Epithelial Displacement

Percutaneous biopsy needles rarely displace calcifications to locations distant from the original biopsy site. It is controversial whether displaced metallic markers or displaced calcifications far from the biopsy site require surgical excision when the percutaneous biopsy specimen shows cancer.

Epithelial displacement of breast cancer cells into benign tissue along the needle track may occur with any gauge biopsy needle. These displaced tumor cells may simulate breast cancer invasion or a second focus of tumor unless the pathologist knows there was a prior core biopsy. Pathologists should be informed that a needle biopsy has been performed so that they do not mistakenly diagnose displaced epithelium as invasive cancer in a ductal carcinoma in situ (DCIS) lesion or erroneously stage a tumor as multifocal when only one cancerous site is present. Epithelial displacement is more common with FNA or core biopsy (where the needle is removed from the breast with each needle pass) than with vacuum biopsy (where the external part of the needle stays in the breast until the rotational biopsy is finished). To our knowledge, epithelial displacement has not been evaluated with the type of vacuum biopsy needle that is inserted several times, but we would assume that displacement would be similar to that seen with a core biopsy needle that is inserted several times. The displaced epithelial cancer cells are thought to rarely, if ever, acquire a blood supply and grow as metastatic disease along the needle track, in draining lymph nodes, or systemically elsewhere in the body.

Pathology Correlation

Routine correlation between the mammographic appearance of the breast lesion and the pathology report is an essential part of quality assurance to reduce the number of false-negative results and to excise cancers. Biopsies that are initially benign (exclusive of high-risk lesions) and later proven to be carcinoma at that same site are called *false-negative biopsies.* Liberman and colleagues and Jackman and colleagues have separately defined the false-negative rate as all false-negative lesions in a study divided by all breast cancers found at any time in the study. Immediate false-negatives occur if an initial benign biopsy is discordant and immediate repeat biopsy reveals cancer. Delayed false-negatives occur if the benign biopsy is considered concordant and lesion growth at follow-up imaging leads to later rebiopsy and discovery of the missed cancer.

False-negative biopsies occur with any kind of biopsy. They are most thoroughly reported for stereotactic biopsies done in prone position with automated large-core multiple-insertion needles and with single-insertion directional vacuum-assisted needles. False-negatives have also been thoroughly studied for image-guided diagnostic surgical biopsies. In separate literature reviews, Jackman and colleagues found the mean false-negative rates to be 1% for stereotactic 11-gauge vacuum-assisted needle biopsy, 4% for stereotactic 14-gauge automated large-core needle biopsy, and 2% for image-guided needle-localized diagnostic surgical excision.

False-negative rates are less well-defined for other image-guided percutaneous biopsies, but are approximately 2% to 2.5% for ultrasound-guided needle biopsies (with both vacuum-assisted and automated large-core needles).

Liberman and colleagues emphasized in 2000 that benign histologic diagnoses that do not explain the imaging findings must be considered discordant and should lead to repeat biopsy done by surgical excision or a more aggressive needle core biopsy (Box 6-5). American College of Radiology Breast Imaging Reporting and Data System (BI-RADS®) category 5 lesions with a benign histologic diagnosis are discordant. Specific benign diagnoses for mass lesions include fibroadenomas, lymph nodes, and benign cysts. There are no specific diagnoses for nonmass lesions whether the nonmass lesions are calcified or uncalcified. With nonspecific benign diagnoses, one relies on the quality of the needle biopsy to determine if the diagnosis is concordant. As discussed, biopsy of calcifications must include adequate sampling or removal of the calcifications as determined on specimen radiographs of the core or vacuum biopsy samples (looking for calcifications) and postbiopsy stereotactic or upright images (looking for reduction or absence of calcifications seen before biopsy compared to after biopsy).

Discordance is hardest to determine with BI-RADS® category 4 noncalcified mass and nonmass lesions. When needle pathology is benign on stereotactic, ultrasound, or MRI-guided needle biopsy, a subjective combination of confidence with the accuracy of the needle biopsy and decreased size of the lesion after biopsy are used to make that decision.

Surgical excision is advised for all DCIS lesions, the same as for invasive cancer. Women with invasive cancer also undergo axillary node sampling or dissection at initial therapeutic surgery, but women with DCIS usually do not undergo axillary node biopsy. A moderate percentage of patients with DCIS diagnosed at needle biopsy may later need axillary node dissection because invasive cancer is diagnosed at subsequent excisional biopsy. Biopsy specimens showing DCIS at initial biopsy and invasive cancer at subsequent surgical excision (called *DCIS underestimates*) occurred at prone stereotactic biopsy in 20% of DCIS lesions diagnosed with 14-gauge core biopsy and in 11% of DCIS lesions diagnosed with 11-gauge vacuum biopsy.

DCIS underestimates with ultrasound-guided biopsies have been less thoroughly studied, but those underestimates are also decreased with 11-gauge vacuum biopsy compared to 14-gauge core biopsy. DCIS underestimates also occur with diagnostic surgical biopsies, but we do not know the overall rate. When just those with positive or close histologic margins for DCIS have a repeat operation (meaning there is a large selection bias) the surgical DCIS underestimate rate is 11%.

High-Risk Lesions, Including Controversies

There are no universally accepted criteria to decide which lesions diagnosed at core or vacuum needle biopsy are high-risk and should undergo surgical excision to determine the presence of an associated cancer underestimated by the biopsy. Sickles defines a "probably benign" BI-RADS® category 3 mammographic lesion as a finding with a less than 2% chance of malignancy that can be followed with imaging. In 2002, Jackman and colleagues suggested that the less than 2% chance of malignancy could be used to decide if specific histologic lesions diagnosed at needle biopsy could be followed or needed excision. This was initially applied to atypical ductal hyperplasia (ADH) lesions and has subsequently been accepted by many as a practical way to decide what to do with both ADH and non-ADH lesions. Those with a greater than 2% chance of malignancy at follow-up would be considered high-risk and would be sent for surgical excision. Those with a less than 2% chance of malignancy at follow-up would be considered benign and would be carefully followed with imaging.

Lesions that can underestimate the associated presence of cancer are called high-risk lesions, and they occur in roughly 10% of percutaneous biopsies. Half of the high-risk lesions are ADH. Biopsies showing ADH at initial biopsy and cancer at subsequent surgical excision (termed *ADH underestimates*) occurred at prone stereotactic biopsy in 44% of ADH lesions diagnosed with 14-gauge large-core needle biopsy and 19% of ADH lesions diagnosed with 11-gauge vacuum-assisted biopsy. Although pathologists have trouble distinguishing between ADH and low-grade DCIS, the ADH underestimates are a more significant problem. The cancers found with the ADH underestimates were invasive carcinoma in 25% of cases and any grade DCIS in the other 75%. Jackman and colleagues showed that there are no patient, lesion, or biopsy risk factors that might obviate excision after stereotactic core biopsy showing ADH.

More controversy exists about the need for surgical excision of non-ADH lesions. Most authors in the scientific

---

Box 6-5. Discordant Needle Biopsy Results

Malignant and high-risk diagnoses may not completely characterize the lesion, but they are not discordant

Benign diagnoses can be discordant if:

The histologic diagnosis does not explain the imaging findings

A BI-RADS® category 5 lesion is histologically benign

An adequate sample of calcifications is not seen on the specimen radiograph from a calcific cluster

The radiologist is not confident the biopsy was done with accuracy

The lesion is not smaller postbiopsy

literature report that lobular carcinoma in situ (LCIS), atypical lobular hyperplasia (ALH), and any other lesions with atypia (such as flat epithelial atypia, papillary lesions with atypia, and radial scar with atypia) need excision because cancer is often found at surgical excision (Box 6-6).

Large studies by Brenner and colleagues and Becker and colleagues strongly suggest that radial scars without atypia do not need excision if the biopsy was done with a vacuum-assisted device (as opposed to a large-core device) with removal of at least 12 specimens. It is important that the patient comply with imaging follow-up. Imaging follow-up should be done, as it is for benign concordant percutaneous biopsies, 6, 12, 24, and perhaps 36 months after biopsy to be sure a cancer was not missed. Radial scars without atypia that are diagnosed with a core needle instead of vacuum needle or removal of less than 12 specimens should prompt surgical excision.

Papillary lesions without atypia might be safe to follow without excision if the biopsy criteria outlined for radial scars are met, but there are no large studies to prove that. Currently individual decisions are made to either excise or follow papillary lesions, mucocele-like lesions, and pseudoangiomatous stromal hyperplasia (PASH), if they have no atypia (see Box 6-6). However, PASH or hemangiomas that have possible features of angiosarcoma need surgical excision.

Columnar lesions without atypia, including columnar alterations with prominent apical snouts and secretions, are usually considered benign and do not need excision.

Phyllodes tumor, although generally benign, has a small percentage of malignant forms that are diagnosed only by complete histologic examination. Phyllodes tumor also tends to recur in the biopsy site and should be completely excised by surgery. This means all phyllodes tumors should be excised.

BOX 6-6. High-Risk Lesions Diagnosed at Needle Biopsy and Need for Surgical Excision

Almost universal agreement about need to excise:
  Atypical ductal hyperplasia
  Phyllodes tumor
Majority agreement about need to excise:
  Lobular carcinoma in situ
  Atypical lobular hyperplasia
  Papillary lesion with atypia
  Radial scar with atypia
  Flat epithelial atypia
  Other lesions with atypia
Mixed opinion about need to excise:
  Papillary lesion without atypia
  Radial scar without atypia (excision probably not needed if vacuum biopsy and removal of 12 or more specimens)
  PASH without atypia or histologic concern for angiosarcoma

PASH, pseudoangiomatous stromal hyperplasia.

ADH underestimates are less thoroughly studied with ultrasound-guided biopsies, but those underestimates are also decreased with 11-gauge vacuum biopsy compared to 14-gauge core biopsy. ADH underestimates also occur with diagnostic surgical biopsies, but we do not know the overall rate. When just those with positive or close histologic margins for ADH have a repeat operation (meaning there is a large selection bias), Arora and colleagues found a surgical ADH underestimate rate of 27%.

Follow-Up of Benign Lesions

Long-term studies of benign concordant lesions diagnosed at core or vacuum biopsy can occasionally be falsely negative and emphasize the importance of a good follow-up program to minimize the potential for missing cancer. Postbiopsy follow-up imaging, using the same imaging modality that guided the needle biopsy, should be done at 6, 12, 24, and perhaps 36 months postbiopsy for all benign concordant lesions. Specific concordant lesions diagnosed as fibroadenoma or lymph node can have the initial follow-up at 12 months rather than 6 months. If the lesion increases in size at follow-up imaging, the lesion should undergo repeat biopsy by needle or surgical excision.

Complications

Complications are discussed in the "Informed Consent" section of this chapter and are also listed in Box 6-2.

Vasovagal reactions occur more frequently with presurgical needle localization because most are done upright with the patient fasting and often dehydrated. Thus, all personnel in the procedure room must be able to recognize and treat a vasovagal reaction and be able to release the breast from compression for mammographic procedures. A stretcher and resuscitation cart should be in close vicinity to the procedure room, and the patient should never be unaccompanied in the room during the procedure. The patient must be able to respond, be alert, be able to remain motionless during the procedure, and be able to cooperate with the radiologist during the procedure.

Methods to decrease untoward bleeding include familiarity with the patient's current prescribed medications and over-the-counter self-prescribed drugs, herbs, and vitamins, as well as when the patient should stop taking them. The radiologist works with the referring physician to determine whether administration of Coumadin (warfarin), heparin, or Plavix (clopidogrel) can be safely curtailed. At many facilities patients are instructed to stop taking all pain medications except for acetaminophen for 1 week before the biopsy because aspirin, NSAIDs, and other medications can inactivate platelets. Some institutions instruct patients to also stop taking all herbal medications (particularly Ginkgo biloba, which potentiates anticoagulants), vitamin E, and fish oils for 1 week before the biopsy.

At the other extreme of not stopping medications before needle biopsy, Melotti and Berg reported needle biopsies in 18 patients undergoing anticoagulation therapy. The patients were taking warfarin ($n = 11$), heparin ($n = 1$), or aspirin ($n = 6$). Hematomas measuring 13 to 40 mm occurred in 3 of 8 anticoagulated patients undergoing ste-reotactic 11-gauge vacuum biopsy. A 10-mm hematoma occurred in 1 of 10 anticoagulated patients undergoing ultrasound-guided 14-gauge core biopsy. Their study suggests that needle biopsy can be performed in anticoagulated patients if the need for biopsy is urgent, but that hematomas may occur after the biopsy.

For ultrasound-guided biopsies, pneumothorax is an unusual but reported complication. The risk of pneumothorax increases if the patient is unable to hold still or is coughing, if the angle needed to biopsy the lesion is very steep, if the lesion is on the chest wall, and particularly if the lesion lies between ribs. Pneumothorax has been reported as a complication of both fine-needle breast aspiration and large-core biopsy. It is imperative that the radiologist identifies the chest wall and pleura before the biopsy to evaluate the trajectory of the needle throw. Taking the extra time to roll the patient into the perfect position so that the needle trajectory is parallel to the chest wall is especially important. When there is a possibility of pneumothorax during the biopsy, the radiologist should obtain informed consent from the patient specifically for the possibility that the "needle could puncture the lung and result in the need for an emergency room visit and possible stay in the hospital, which is very unusual." Knowledge of pneumothorax and its consequences, as well as strict instructions to the patient to remain immobile during the biopsy, are important for informed consent. If there are serious concerns about pneumothorax during a procedure, one should consider using a needle that has the needle tip inserted to the deepest point without firing. The external cutting part of the needle then fires from the "pre-fire" position to shear off the tissue specimen. The cutting part of the needle stops at the needle tip and has no "throw" beyond the tip. Another alternative is to not do a core needle biopsy and to proceed with needle localization and surgical excision.

Differences between Core and Vacuum Needle Biopsies

In two seminal articles, Parker and colleagues introduced 14-gauge automated large-core needle biopsies guided by prone stereotactic technique in 1991 and by ultrasound in 1993 as practical alternatives to image-guided needle localization and diagnostic surgical excision of nonpalpable lesions. Parker and colleagues then reported successful use of those biopsy methods in multiple institutions in 1994. Burbank introduced directional vacuum-assisted needle biopsies in 1996 as a way to remove more biopsy tissue more rapidly, more accurately, and with less bleeding. Vacuum needles were initially 14-gauge and are now available in 7- to 14-gauge sizes.

The weight of the individual specimens is about 17 mg with 14-gauge core, 37 mg with 14-gauge vacuum, 95 mg with 11-gauge vacuum, and 120 mg with 9-gauge vacuum biopsy devices. The core biopsy needles and some vacuum needles are removed from the breast after acquisition of each tissue sample and re-fired into the breast to obtain each new sample. The most frequently used vacuum biopsy needles are inserted once into the breast, unless a very large lesion requires multiple skin entry sites for accurate sampling.

For stereotactic biopsy, the collection trough of the vacuum needle is rotated "around the clock" to acquire tissue from different parts of the lesion and surrounding tissue, with the external part of the needle staying in the breast and the internal cutting part of the needle extracting tissue out of the breast. For ultrasound-guided biopsy, the collection trough is aimed at the lesion and rotated though just a few clock positions to acquire tissue from different parts of the lesion. The vacuum portion of the biopsy device both pulls in breast tissue to be biopsied (which is a major factor in a vacuum biopsy specimen weighing about twice as much as a core biopsy specimen from the same gauge needle) and vacuums blood out of the breast away from the biopsy site (allowing one to extract more tissue and less blood). In addition, the vacuum biopsy specimens are extracted contiguously. All of these factors make the vacuum biopsy faster and more accurate if initial targeting is correct.

The increased accuracy of vacuum needle biopsy is most dramatic in reducing the calcification miss rate, as judged on specimen radiographs from stereotactic biopsy of calcification lesions. The negative radiograph specimen rate for calcifications using prone stereotactic guidance is 14% with 14-gauge core needle biopsy and 1% with 11-gauge vacuum needle biopsy. These compare with a miss rate of 4% for x-ray–guided needle localization and surgical excision calcification.

As discussed, prone stereotactic biopsies performed with 11-gauge vacuum needles rather than 14-gauge core needles have decreased false-negative rates and decreased underestimation rates for both DCIS and ADH. Ultrasound-guided needle biopsies performed with 11-gauge vacuum needles rather than 14-gauge core needles also have decreased underestimation rate for both DCIS and ADH. There is, however, no proven decrease in the false-negative rate with vacuum biopsies compared to core biopsies done with ultrasound guidance. There is so much selection bias in the literature, however, that valid comparison of the false-negative rate with ultrasound guidance is impossible. Also, wide variation exists in how often different institutions use vacuum needles for ultrasound-guided needle biopsies.

Ultrasound-guided biopsies are usually done with core needles, but biopsy with vacuum needles is being done with increased frequency in the United States. This is most common for lesions that can be difficult to see after extraction of one or two samples (e.g., small lesions, obscure masses, and complex cystic masses [i.e., those with cystic and solid components that may be difficult to see if the fluid is drained from the mass during the course of the biopsy]). They are also used in some institutions for lesions perceived to be in a dangerous location (e.g., close to the chest wall or a prominent vessel) because of a desire to insert the biopsy needle only once into the breast and aim the collection aperture away from the anatomic structure of concern while acquiring tissue.

MRI-guided needle biopsies are done almost exclusively with vacuum needles, but can be done with core biopsy needles. MRI-guided biopsies are covered in Chapter 7.

Patient Audits, Follow-Up, and Noncompliance

Lesions diagnosed as high-risk (most commonly ADH but also the non-ADH lesions discussed above) at core or vacuum needle biopsy and cancer at excision are considered to be high-risk underestimates. They are neither true positives nor false negatives and thus preclude measuring true sensitivity and specificity. Burbank and Parker published an auditing solution to this dilemma in 1998.

It is important to audit the results from one's own needle biopsy practice to compare with the literature. Most importantly one should determine the false-negative rate with each imaging modality, which requires long-term follow-up. One can more quickly and easily determine the calcification lesion miss rate (from specimen radiographs), the DCIS underestimation rate, and the ADH underestimation rate.

In addition, standard imaging surveillance after the needle biopsy is essential to diagnose missed cancers. Follow-up details are defined in the section "Follow-up of Benign Lesions" in this chapter. The initial informed consent should indicate that imaging follow-up is expected and that the patient is to return for all three or four visits after the procedure.

The problem of follow-up and compliance with follow-up is a difficult one even in the best of hands. Pal and colleagues showed that as many as 40% of women do not return for all their follow-up mammograms after benign results and 15% do not complete the recommended surgery after an abnormal needle biopsy. Jackman and colleagues, however, managed to have the patient return for at least one postbiopsy mammogram in 99% (295/298) of benign concordant lesions having stereotactic core needle biopsy that did not undergo surgical excision. This was achieved with a vigorous, time-consuming follow-up protocol that is not practical for routine use.

As a result of the Mammography Quality Standards Act of 1992, U.S. federal law mandates follow-up on all abnormal mammograms. However, tracking in clinical practice is complicated, time-consuming, and expensive, with multiple costs for personnel, computer updates, and mailing. This requirement is a cause of frustration for many radiologists despite computerized follow-up programs. Goodman and colleagues showed that women's outcomes may be difficult to track as a result of relocation, changing of insurance, decisions by their referring physicians contrary to recommended follow-up, or other reasons. Those same tracking problems occur after benign concordant needle biopsies. Accordingly, informed consent before biopsy assumes even more importance so that proper patient management can be implemented.

KEY ELEMENTS

Know the location of the target lesion in three dimensions.
 Do not attempt biopsy of a lesion not known to be genuine or one whose location in the breast is not known.
Most nonpalpable lesions are now diagnosed by image-guided percutaneous needle biopsy and not by diagnostic surgical excision.

Specimen radiography of x-ray– or ultrasound-localized surgical specimens should show the lesion, hookwire, hookwire tip, and any associated metallic markers. The findings are called to the surgeon in the operating room.

For ultrasound-localized surgical specimens, specimen ultrasound can be done if the lesion is not seen on the specimen radiograph.

Reasons that calcifications may not be visualized on the histologic slides include nonremoval, calcium oxalate, location in the paraffin block, or displacement out of the specimen by the microtome.

Risks of core biopsy include hematoma (fairly common but rarely significant), and rarely untoward bleeding, infection, pneumothorax, pseudoaneurysm formation, implant rupture, milk fistula (if the patient is pregnant or nursing), and vasovagal reactions.

Correlation between the pathology results and imaging studies establishes concordance.

If the lesion targeted was calcifications, the specimen radiograph shows no calcifications, and the pathology report describes calcifications, the pathology report has described tiny, serendipitously found 100-micron calcifications that have nothing to do with the target, and the patient needs to undergo rebiopsy.

Markers are fairly often inaccurately deployed in the breast after needle biopsy but rarely migrate significantly after placement.

Surgical excisional biopsy is recommended for core or vacuum biopsy specimens showing invasive cancer, DCIS, ADH, LCIS, ALH, any atypical lesions (including flat epithelial atypia, atypical radial scar lesions, and atypical papillary lesions), phyllodes tumors, and discordant benign lesions.

It is controversial whether surgical excisional biopsy should always be performed after obtaining core or vacuum biopsy samples showing radial scar, papillary lesions, and PASH without atypia.

SUGGESTED READINGS

Adler DD, Ligut RJ, Granstrom P, et al: Follow-up of benign results of stereotactic core breast biopsy, *Acad Radiol* 7:248–253, 2000.

Agoff SN, Lawton TJ: Papillary lesions of the breast with and without atypical ductal hyperplasia: can we accurately predict benign behavior from core needle biopsy? *Am J Clin Pathol* 122:440–443, 2004.

Arora S, Menes TS, Moung C, et al: Atypical ductal hyperplasia at margin of breast biopsy—is re-excision indicated? *Ann Surg Oncol* 15:843–847, 2008. Epub 7 Nov 2007.

Arpino G, Allred DC, Mohsin SK, et al: Lobular neoplasia on core-needle biopsy—clinical significance, *Cancer* 101:242–250, 2004.

Arpino G, Laucirica R, Elledge RM: Premalignant and in situ breast disease: biology and clinical implications, *Ann Intern Med* 143:446–457, 2005.

Bates T, Davidson T, Mansel RE: Litigation for pneumothorax as a complication of fine-needle aspiration of the breast, *Br J Surg* 89:134–137, 2002.

Bazzocchi M, Francescutti GE, Zuiani C, et al: Breast pseudoaneurysm in a woman after core biopsy: percutaneous treatment with alcohol, *AJR Am J Roentgenol* 179:696, 2002.

Becker L, Trop I, David J, et al: Management of radial scars found at percutaneous breast biopsy, *Can Assoc Radiol J* 57:72–78, 2006.

Berg WA: Image-guided breast biopsy and management of high-risk lesions, *Radiol Clin North Am* 42:935–946, 2004.

Berg WA, Krebs TL, Campassi C, et al: Evaluation of 14- and 11-gauge directional, vacuum-assisted biopsy probes and 14-gauge biopsy guns in a breast parenchymal model, *Radiology* 205:203–208, 1997.

Berkowitz JE, Gatewood OM, Donovan GB, et al: Dermal breast calcifications: localization with template-guided placement of skin marker, *Radiology* 163:282, 1987.

Birdwell RL, Ikeda DM, Brenner RJ: Methods of compliance with Mammography Quality Standards Act regulations for tracking positive mammograms: survey results, *AJR Am J Roentgenol* 172:691–696, 1999.

Birdwell RL, Jackman RJ: Clip or marker migration 5–10 weeks after stereotactic 11-gauge vacuum-assisted breast biopsy: report of two cases, *Radiology* 229:541–544, 2003.

Bober SE, Russell DG: Increasing breast tissue depth during stereotactic needle biopsy, *AJR Am J Roentgenol* 174:1085–1086, 2000.

Bolivar AV, Alonso-Bartolome P, Garcia EO, et al: Ultrasound-guided core needle biopsy of nonpalpable breast lesions: a prospective analysis in 204 cases, *Acta Radiol* 46:690–695, 2005.

Bonnett M, Wallis T, Rossmann M, et al: Histopathologic analysis of atypical lesions in image-guided core breast biopsies, *Mod Pathol* 16:154–160, 2003.

Brem RF, Lechner MC, Jackman RJ, et al: Lobular neoplasia at percutaneous breast biopsy: variables associated with carcinoma at surgical excision, *AJR Am J Roentgenol* 190:637–641, 2008.

Brem RF, Schoonjans JM: Local anesthesia in stereotactic, vacuum-assisted breast biopsy, *Breast J* 7:72–73, 2001.

Brenner RJ: Lesions entirely removed during stereotactic biopsy: preoperative localization on the basis of mammographic landmarks and feasibility of freehand technique—initial experience, *Radiology* 214:585–590, 2000.

Brenner RJ: Percutaneous removal of postbiopsy marking clip in the breast using stereotactic technique, *AJR Am J Roentgenol* 176:417–419, 2001.

Brenner RJ, Bassett LW, Fajardo LL, et al: Stereotactic core-needle breast biopsy: a multi-institutional prospective trial, *Radiology* 218:866–872, 2001.

Brenner RJ, Jackman RJ, Parker SH, et al: Percutaneous core needle biopsy of radial scars of the breast: when is excision necessary? *AJR Am J Roentgenol* 179:1179–1184, 2002.

Burbank F: Stereotactic breast biopsy: its history, its present, and its future, *Am Surg* 62:128–150, 1996.

Burbank F: Mammographic findings after 14-gauge automated needle and 14-gauge directional, vacuum-assisted stereotactic breast biopsies, *Radiology* 204:153–156, 1997.

Burbank F: Stereotactic breast biopsy: comparison of 14- and 11-gauge Mammotome probe performance and complication rates, *Am Surg* 63:988-995, 1997.

Burbank F, Forcier N: Tissue marking clip for stereotactic breast biopsy: initial placement accuracy, long-term stability, and usefulness as a guide for wire localization, *Radiology* 205:407–415, 1997.

Burbank F, Parker SH: Methods for evaluating the quality of an image-guided breast biopsy program, *Sem Breast Dis* 1:71–83, 1998.

Burbank F, Parker SH, Fogarty TJ: Stereotactic breast biopsy: improved tissue harvesting with the Mammotome, *Am Surg* 62:738–744, 1996.

Burnside ES, Sohlich RE, Sickles EA: Movement of a biopsy-site marker clip after completion of stereotactic directional vacuum-assisted breast biopsy: case report, *Radiology* 221:504–507, 2001.

Carder PJ, Garvican J, Haigh I, et al: Needle core biopsy can reliably distinguish between benign and malignant papillary lesions of the breast, *Histopathology* 46:320–327, 2005.

Carr JJ, Hemler PF, Halford PW, et al: Stereotactic localization of breast lesions: how it works and methods to improve accuracy, *Radiographics* 21:463–473, 2001.

Cassano E, Urban LA, Pizzamiglio M, et al: Ultrasound-guided vacuum-assisted core breast biopsy: experience with 406 cases, *Breast Cancer Res Treat* 102:103–110, 2007. Epub 13 Jul 2006.

Charles M, Edge SB, Winston JS, et al: Effect of stereotactic core needle biopsy on pathologic measurement of tumor size of T1 invasive breast carcinomas presenting as mammographic masses, *Cancer* 97:2137, 2003.

Cho N, Moon WK, Cha JH, et al: Sonographically guided core biopsy of the breast: comparison of 14-gauge automated gun and 11-gauge directional vacuum-assisted biopsy methods, *Korean J Radiol* 6:102–109, 2005.

Cohen MA: Cancer upgrades at excisional biopsy after diagnosis of atypical lobular hyperplasia or lobular carcinoma in situ at core-needle biopsy: some reasons why, *Radiology* 231:617–621, 2004.

Collins LC, Connolly JL, Page DL, et al: Diagnostic agreement in the evaluation of image-guided breast core needle biopsies: results from a randomized clinical trial, *Am J Surg Pathol* 28:126–131, 2004.

Crowe JP Jr, Patrick RJ, Rybicki LA, et al: Does ultrasound core breast biopsy predict histologic finding on excisional biopsy? *Am J Surg* 186:397–399, 2003.

Crystal P, Koretz M, Shcharynsky S, et al: Accuracy of sonographically guided 14-gauge core-needle biopsy: results of 715 consecutive breast biopsies with at least two-year follow-up of benign lesions, *J Clin Ultrasound* 33:47–52, 2005.

Dahlstrom JE, Sutton S, Jain S: Histologic–radiologic correlation of mammographically detected microcalcification in stereotactic core biopsies, *Am J Surg Pathol* 22:256–259, 1998.

de Lucena CE, Dos Santos Junior JL, de Lima Resende CA, et al: Ultrasound-guided core needle biopsy of breast masses: how many cores are necessary to diagnose cancer? *J Clin Ultrasound* 35:363–366, 2007.

Dershaw DD: Does LCIS or ALH without other high-risk lesions diagnosed on core biopsy require surgical excision? *Breast J* 9:1–3, 2003.

Dershaw DD, Morris EA, Liberman L, et al: Nondiagnostic stereotaxic core breast biopsy: results of rebiopsy, *Radiology* 198:323–325, 1996.

Deutch BM, Schwartz MR, Fodera T, et al: Stereotactic core breast biopsy of a minimal carcinoma complicated by a large hematoma: a management dilemma, *Radiology* 202:431–433, 1997.

Diaz LK, Wiley EL, Venta LA: Are malignant cells displaced by large-gauge needle core biopsy of the breast? *AJR Am J Roentgenol* 173:1303–1313, 1999.

Dillon MF, Hill AD, Quinn CM, et al: The accuracy of ultrasound, stereotactic, and clinical core biopsies in the diagnosis of breast cancer, with an analysis of false-negative cases, *Ann Surg* 242:701–707, 2005.

Dondalski M, Bernstein JR: Disappearing breast calcifications: mammographic–pathologic discrepancy due to calcium oxalate, *South Med J* 85:1252–1254, 1992.

Duchesne N, Parker SH, Lechner MC, et al: Multicenter evaluation of a new ultrasound-guided biopsy device: improved ergonomics, sampling and rebiopsy rates, *Breast J* 13:36–43, 2007.

Elsheikh TM, Silverman JF: Follow-up surgical excision is indicated when breast core needle biopsies show atypical lobular hyperplasia or lobular carcinoma in situ: a correlative study of 33 patients with review of the literature, *Am J Surg Pathol* 29:534–543, 2005.

Fahrbach K, Sledge I, Cella C, et al: A comparison of the accuracy of two minimally invasive breast biopsy methods: a systematic literature review and meta-analysis, *Arch Gynecol Obstet* 274:63–73, 2006. Epub 6 Apr 2006.

Fine RE, Boyd BA, Whitworth PW, et al: Percutaneous removal of benign breast masses using a vacuum-assisted hand-held device with ultrasound guidance, *Am J Surg* 184:332–336, 2002.

Frenna TH, Meyer JE, Sonnenfeld MR: US of breast biopsy specimens, *Radiology* 190:573, 1994.

Friedman PD, Sanders LM, Menendez C, et al: Retrieval of lost microcalcifications during stereotactic vacuum-assisted core biopsy, *AJR Am J Roentgenol* 180:275–280, 2003.

Golub RM, Bennett CL, Stinson T, et al: Cost minimization study of image-guided core biopsy versus surgical excisional biopsy for women with abnormal mammograms, *J Clin Oncol* 22:2430–2437, 2004.

Goodman KA, Birdwell RL, Ikeda DM: Compliance with recommended follow-up after percutaneous breast core biopsy, *AJR Am J Roentgenol* 170:89–92, 1998.

Grady I, Gorsuch H, Wilburn-Bailey S: Ultrasound-guided, vacuum-assisted, percutaneous excision of breast lesions: an accurate technique in the diagnosis of atypical ductal hyperplasia, *J Am Coll Surg* 201:14–17, 2005.

Grin A, Horne G, Ennis M, et al: Measuring extent of ductal carcinoma in situ in breast excision specimens: a comparison of 4 methods, *Arch Pathol Lab Med* 133:31, 2009.

Guerra-Wallace MM, Christensen WN, White RL Jr: A retrospective study of columnar alteration with prominent apical snouts and secretions and the association with cancer, *Am J Surg* 188:395–398, 2004.

Harris AT: Clip migration within 8 days of 11-gauge vacuum-assisted stereotactic breast biopsy: case report, *Radiology* 228:552–554, 2003.

Harvey JA, Moran RE, DeAngelis GA: Technique and pitfalls of ultrasound-guided core-needle biopsy of the breast, *Semin Ultrasound CT MR* 21:362–374, 2000.

Helvie MA, Ikeda DM, Adler DD: Localization and needle aspiration of breast lesions: complications in 370 cases, *AJR Am J Roentgenol* 157:711–714, 1991.

Hoda SA, Rosen PP: Practical considerations in the pathologic diagnosis of needle core biopsies of breast, *Am J Clin Pathol* 118:101–108, 2002.

Huber S, Wagner M, Medl M, et al: Benign breast lesions: minimally invasive vacuum-assisted biopsy with 11-gauge needles—patient acceptance and effect on follow-up imaging findings, *Radiology* 226:783–790, 2003.

Husien AM: Stereotactic localization mammography: interpreting the check film, *Clin Radiol* 45:387–389, 1992.

Ikeda DM, Helvie MA, Adler DD, et al: The role of fine-needle aspiration and pneumocystography in the treatment of impalpable breast cysts, *AJR Am J Roentgenol* 158:1239–1241, 1992.

Irfan K, Brem RF: Surgical and mammographic follow-up of papillary lesions and atypical lobular hyperplasia diagnosed with stereotactic vacuum-assisted biopsy, *Breast J* 8:230–233, 2002.

Ivan D, Selinko V, Sahin AA, et al: Accuracy of core needle biopsy diagnosis in assessing papillary breast lesions: histologic predictors of malignancy, *Mod Pathol* 17:165–171, 2004.

Jackman RJ, Birdwell RL, Ikeda DM: Atypical ductal hyperplasia: can some lesions be defined as probably benign after stereotactic 11-gauge vacuum-assisted biopsy, eliminating the recommendation for surgical excision? *Radiology* 224:548–554, 2002.

Jackman RJ, Burbank F, Parker SH, et al: Stereotactic breast biopsy of nonpalpable lesions: determinants of ductal carcinoma in situ underestimation rates, *Radiology* 218:497–502, 2001.

Jackman RJ, Lamm RL: Stereotactic histologic biopsy in breasts with implants, *Radiology* 222:157–614, 2002.

Jackman RJ, Marzoni FA Jr: Needle-localized breast biopsy: why do we fail? *Radiology* 204:677–684, 1997.

Jackman RJ, Marzoni FA Jr: Stereotactic histologic biopsy with patients prone: technical feasibility in 98% of mammographically detected lesions, *AJR Am J Roentgenol* 180:785–794, 2003.

Jackman RJ, Marzoni FA Jr, Rosenberg J: False-negative diagnoses at stereotactic vacuum-assisted needle breast biopsy: long-term follow-up of 1,280 lesions and review of the literature, *AJR Am J Roentgenol* 192:341–351, 2009.

Jackman RJ, Nowels KW, Rodriguez-Soto J, et al: Stereotactic, automated, large-core needle biopsy of nonpalpable breast lesions: false-negative and histologic underestimation rates after long-term follow-up, *Radiology* 210:799–805, 1999.

Jackman RJ, Rodriguez-Soto J: Breast microcalcifications: retrieval failure at prone stereotactic core and vacuum breast biopsy—frequency, causes, and outcome, *Radiology* 239:61–70, 2006.

Jacobs TW, Connolly JL, Schnitt SJ: Nonmalignant lesions in breast core needle biopsies: to excise or not to excise? *Am J Surg Pathol* 26:1095–1110, 2002.

Jang M, Cho N, Moon WK, et al: Underestimation of atypical ductal hyperplasia at sonographically guided core biopsy of the breast, *AJR Am J Roentgenol* 191:1347–1351, 2008.

Kass R, Kumar G, Klimberg S, et al: Clip migration in stereotactic biopsy, *Am J Surg* 184:325–331, 2002.

Kettritz U, Rotter K, Schreer I, et al: Stereotactic vacuum-assisted breast biopsy in 2,874 patients: a multicenter study, *Cancer* 100:245–251, 2004.

Kim HS, Kim MJ, Kim EK, et al: US-guided vacuum-assisted biopsy of microcalcifications in breast lesions and long-term follow-up results, *Korean J Radiol* 9:503–509, 2008.

Kim JY, Han BK, Choe YH, et al: Benign and malignant mucocele-like tumors of the breast: mammographic and sonographic appearances, *AJR Am J Roentgenol* 185:1310–1316, 2005.

Kim MJ, Kim EK, Kwak JY, et al: Nonmalignant papillary lesions of the breast at US-guided directional vacuum-assisted removal: a preliminary report, *Eur Radiol* 18:1774–1783, 2008.

Ko ES, Cho N, Cha JH, et al: Sonographically guided 14-gauge core needle biopsy for papillary lesions of the breast, *Korean J Radiol* 8:206–211, 2007.

Lagios MD: Prognostic features of breast carcinoma from stereotactic biopsy material, *Sem Breast Disease* 1:101, 1998.

Lai JT, Burrowes P, MacGregor JH: Diagnostic accuracy of a stereotaxically guided vacuum-assisted large-core breast biopsy program in Canada, *Can Assoc Radiol J* 52:223–227, 2001.

Lamm RL, Jackman RJ: Mammographic abnormalities caused by percutaneous stereotactic biopsy of histologically benign lesions evident on follow-up mammograms, *AJR Am J Roentgenol* 174:753–756, 2000.

Lannin DR, Ponn T, Andrejeva L, et al: Should all breast cancers be diagnosed by needle biopsy? *Am J Surg* 192:450–454, 2006.

Lee CH, Carter D, Philpotts LE, et al: Ductal carcinoma in situ diagnosed with stereotactic core needle biopsy: can invasion be predicted? *Radiology* 217:466–470, 2000.

Lee CH, Egglin TK, Philpotts L, et al: Cost-effectiveness of stereotactic core needle biopsy: analysis by means of mammographic findings, *Radiology* 202:849–854, 1997.

Lee CH, Philpotts LE, Horvath LG, et al: Follow-up of breast lesions diagnosed as benign with stereotactic core-needle biopsy: frequency of mammographic change and false-negative rate, *Radiology* 212:189–194, 1999.

Lee SG, Piccoli CW, Hughes JS: Displacement of microcalcifications during stereotactic 11-gauge directional vacuum-assisted biopsy with marking clip placement: case report, *Radiology* 219:495–497, 2001.

Lehman CD, Shook JE: Position of clip placement after vacuum-assisted breast biopsy: is a unilateral two-view postbiopsy mammogram necessary? *Breast J* 9:272–276, 2003.

Liberman L: Percutaneous image-guided core breast biopsy, *Radiol Clin North Am* 40:483–500, 2002.

Liberman L, Benton CL, Dershaw DD, et al: Learning curve for stereotactic breast biopsy: how many cases are enough? *AJR Am J Roentgenol* 176:721–727, 2001.

Liberman L, Bracero N, Vuolo MA, et al: Percutaneous large-core biopsy of papillary breast lesions, *AJR Am J Roentgenol* 172:331–337, 1999.

Liberman L, Dershaw DD, Glassman JR: Analysis of cancers not diagnosed at stereotactic core breast biopsy, *Radiology* 203:151–157, 1997.

Liberman L, Dershaw DD, Rosen PP, et al: Percutaneous removal of malignant mammographic lesions at stereotactic vacuum-assisted biopsy, *Radiology* 206:711–715, 1998.

Liberman L, Drotman M, Morris EA, et al: Imaging–histologic discordance at percutaneous breast biopsy, *Cancer* 89:2538–2546, 2000.

Liberman L, Ernberg LA, Heerdt A, et al: Palpable breast masses: is there a role for percutaneous imaging-guided core biopsy? *AJR Am J Roentgenol* 175:779–787, 2000.

Liberman L, Feng TL, Dershaw DD, et al: US-guided core breast biopsy: use and cost-effectiveness, *Radiology* 208:717–723, 1998.

Liberman L, Kaplan J, Van Zee KJ, et al: Bracketing wires for preoperative breast needle localization, *AJR Am J Roentgenol* 177:565–572, 2001.

Liberman L, Kaplan JB, Morris EA, et al: To excise or to sample the mammographic target: what is the goal of stereotactic 11-gauge vacuum-assisted breast biopsy? *AJR Am J Roentgenol* 179:679–683, 2002.

Liberman L, Sama M, Susnik B, et al: Lobular carcinoma in situ at percutaneous breast biopsy: surgical biopsy findings, *AJR Am J Roentgenol* 173:291–299, 1999.

Liberman L, Smolkin JH, Dershaw DD, et al: Calcification retrieval at stereotactic, 11-gauge, directional, vacuum-assisted breast biopsy, *Radiology* 208:251–260, 1998.

Liberman L, Tornos C, Huzjan R, et al: Is surgical excision warranted after benign, concordant diagnosis of papilloma at percutaneous breast biopsy? *AJR Am J Roentgenol* 186:1328–1334, 2006.

Liberman L, Vuolo M, Dershaw DD, et al: Epithelial displacement after stereotactic 11-gauge directional vacuum-assisted breast biopsy, *AJR Am J Roentgenol* 172:677–681, 1999.

Liberman L, Zakowski MF, Avery S, et al: Complete percutaneous excision of infiltrating carcinoma at stereotactic breast biopsy: how can tumor size be assessed? *AJR Am J Roentgenol* 173:1315–1322, 1999.

Lomoschitz FM, Helbich TH, Rudas M, et al: Stereotactic 11-gauge vacuum-assisted breast biopsy: influence of number of specimens on diagnostic accuracy, *Radiology* 232:897–903, 2004. Epub 23 Jul 2004.

Londero V, Zuiani C, Linda A, et al: Lobular neoplasia: core needle breast biopsy underestimation of malignancy in relation to radiologic and pathologic features, *Breast* 17:623–630, 2008.

Lourenco AP, Mainiero MB, Lazarus E, et al: Stereotactic breast biopsy: comparison of histologic underestimation rates with 11- and 9-gauge vacuum-assisted breast biopsy. *AJR Am J Roentgenol* 189:W275–W279, 2007.

Mahoney MC, Robinson-Smith TM, Shaughnessy EA: Lobular neoplasia at 11-gauge vacuum-assisted stereotactic biopsy: correlation with surgical excisional biopsy and mammographic follow-up, *AJR Am J Roentgenol* 187:949–954, 2006.

Mainiero MB, Koelliker SL, Lazarus E, et al: Ultrasound-guided large core needle biopsy of the breast: frequency and results of repeat biopsy, *J Women's Imaging* 4:52–57, 2002.

March DE, Coughlin BF, Barham RB, et al: Breast masses: removal of all US evidence during biopsy by using a handheld vacuum-assisted device—initial experience, *Radiology* 227:549–555, 2003.

McNamara MP Jr, Boden T: Pseudoaneurysm of the breast related to 18-gauge core biopsy: successful repair using sonographically guided thrombin injection, *AJR Am J Roentgenol* 179:924–926, 2002.

Meloni GB, Dessole S, Becchere MP, et al: Ultrasound-guided mammotome vacuum biopsy for the diagnosis of impalpable breast lesions, *Ultrasound Obstet Gynecol* 18:520–524, 2001.

Melotti MK, Berg WA: Core needle breast biopsy in patients undergoing anticoagulation therapy: preliminary results, *AJR Am J Roentgenol* 174:245–249, 2000.

Mercado CL, Hamele-Bena D, Oken SM, et al: Papillary lesions of the breast at percutaneous core-needle biopsy, *Radiology* 238:801–808, 2006.

Mercado CL, Hamele-Bena D, Singer C, et al: Papillary lesions of the breast: evaluation with stereotactic directional vacuum-assisted biopsy, *Radiology* 221:650–655, 2001.

Michalopoulos NV, Zagouri F, Sergentanis TN, et al: Needle tract seeding after vacuum-assisted breast biopsy, *Acta Radiol* 49:267–270, 2008.

Morris EA, Liberman L, Trevisan SG, et al: Histologic heterogeneity of masses at percutaneous breast biopsy, *Breast J* 8:187–191, 2002.

Mullen DJ, Eisen RN, Newman RD, et al: The use of carbon marking after stereotactic large-core-needle breast biopsy, *Radiology* 218:255–260, 2001.

Nagi CS, O'Donnell JE, Tismenetsky M, et al: Lobular neoplasia on core needle biopsy does not require excision, *Cancer* 112:2152–2158, 2008.

Pal S, Ikeda DM, Birdwell RL: Compliance with recommended follow-up after fine-needle aspiration biopsy of nonpalpable breast lesions: a retrospective study, *Radiology* 201:71–74, 1996.

Parker SH, Burbank F, Jackman RJ, et al: Percutaneous large-core breast biopsy: a multi-institutional study, *Radiology* 193:359–364, 1994.

Parker SH, Jobe WE, Dennis MA, et al: US-guided automated large-core breast biopsy, *Radiology* 187:507–511, 1993.

Parker SH, Klaus AJ, McWey PJ, et al: Sonographically guided directional vacuum-assisted breast biopsy using a handheld device, *AJR Am J Roentgenol* 177:405–408, 2001.

Parker SH, Lovin JD, Jobe WE, et al: Nonpalpable breast lesions: stereotactic automated large-core biopsies, *Radiology* 180:403–407, 1991.

Perez-Fuentes JA, Longobardi IR, Acosta VF, et al: Sonographically guided directional vacuum-assisted breast biopsy: preliminary experience in Venezuela, *AJR Am J Roentgenol* 177:1459–1463, 2001.

Pfarl G, Helbich TH, Riedl CC, et al: Stereotactic 11-gauge vacuum-assisted breast biopsy: a validation study, *AJR Am J Roentgenol* 179:1503–1507, 2002.

Philpotts LE, Hooley RJ, Lee CH: Comparison of automated versus vacuum-assisted biopsy methods for sonographically guided core biopsy of the breast, *AJR Am J Roentgenol* 180:347–351, 2003.

Philpotts LE, Lee CH, Horvath LJ, et al: Canceled stereotactic core-needle biopsy of the breast: analysis of 89 cases, *Radiology* 205:423–428, 1997.

Philpotts LE, Shaheen NA, Jain KS, et al: Uncommon high-risk lesions of the breast diagnosed at stereotactic core-needle biopsy: clinical importance, *Radiology* 216:831–837, 2000.

Pijnappel RM, Peeters PH, van den Donk M, et al: Diagnostic strategies in nonpalpable breast lesions, *Eur J Cancer* 38:550–555, 2002.

Pijnappel RM, van den Donk M, Holland R, et al: Diagnostic accuracy for different strategies of image-guided breast intervention in cases of nonpalpable breast lesions, *Br J Cancer* 90:595–600, 2004.

Pisano ED, Fajardo LL, Caudry DJ, et al: Fine-needle aspiration biopsy of nonpalpable breast lesions in a multicenter clinical trial: results from the Radiologic Diagnostic Oncology Group V, *Radiology* 219:785–792, 2001.

Pisano ED, Fajardo LL, Tsimikas J, et al: Rate of insufficient samples for fine-needle aspiration for nonpalpable breast lesions in a multicenter clinical trial: the Radiologic Diagnostic Oncology Group 5 Study. The RDOG5 investigators, *Cancer* 82:679–688, 1998.

Poellinger A, Bick U, Freund T, et al: Evaluation of 11-gauge and 9-gauge vacuum-assisted breast biopsy systems in a breast parenchymal model, *Acad Radiol* 14:677–684, 2007.

Rebner M, Helvie MA, Pennes DR, et al: Paraffin tissue block radiography: adjunct to breast specimen radiography, *Radiology* 173:695–696, 1989.

Renshaw AA: Can mucinous lesions of the breast be reliably diagnosed by core needle biopsy? *Am J Clin Pathol* 118:82–84, 2002.

Renshaw AA, Cartagena N, Derhagopian RP, et al: Lobular neoplasia in breast core needle biopsy specimens is not associated with an increased risk of ductal carcinoma in situ or invasive carcinoma, *Am J Clin Pathol* 117:797–799, 2002.

Renshaw AA, Derhagopian RP, Martinez P, et al: Lobular neoplasia in breast core needle biopsy specimens is associated with a low risk of ductal carcinoma in situ or invasive carcinoma on subsequent excision, *Am J Clin Pathol* 126:310–313, 2006.

Renshaw AA, Derhagopian RP, Tizol-Blanco DM, et al: Papillomas and atypical papillomas in breast core needle biopsy specimens: risk of carcinoma in subsequent excision, *Am J Clin Pathol* 122:217–221, 2004.

Rizzo M, Lund MJ, Oprea G, et al: Surgical follow-up and clinical presentation of 142 breast papillary lesions diagnosed by ultrasound-guided core-needle biopsy, *Ann Surg Oncol* 15:1040–1047, 2008.

Rosen EL, Bentley RC, Baker JA, et al: Imaging-guided core needle biopsy of papillary lesions of the breast, *AJR Am J Roentgenol* 179:1185–1192, 2002.

Rosen EL, Vo TT: Metallic clip deployment during stereotactic breast biopsy: retrospective analysis, *Radiology* 218:510–516, 2001.

Ross BA, Ikeda DM, Jackman RJ, et al: Milk of calcium in the breast: appearance on prone stereotactic imaging, *Breast J* 7:53–55, 2001.

Sauer G, Deissler H, Strunz K, et al: Ultrasound-guided large-core needle biopsies of breast lesions: analysis of 962 cases to determine the number of samples for reliable tumor classification, *Br J Cancer* 92:231–235, 2005.

Schnitt SJ, Connolly JL, Tavassoli FA, et al: Interobserver reproducibility in the diagnosis of ductal proliferative breast lesions using standardized criteria, *Am J Surg Pathol* 16:1133–1143, 1992.

Schnitt SJ, Vincent-Salomon A: Columnar cell lesions of the breast, *Adv Anat Pathol* 10:113–124, 2003.

Schoonjans JM, Brem RF: Fourteen-gauge ultrasonographically guided large-core needle biopsy of breast masses, *J Ultrasound Med* 20:967–972, 2001.

Schueller G, Jaromi S, Ponhold L, et al: US-guided 14-gauge core-needle breast biopsy: results of a validation study in 1352 cases, *Radiology* 248:406–413, 2008.

Shin HJ, Kim HH, Kim SM, et al: Papillary lesions of the breast diagnosed at percutaneous sonographically guided biopsy: comparison of sonographic features and biopsy methods, *AJR Am J Roentgenol* 190:630–636, 2008.

Shin SJ, Rosen PP: Excisional biopsy should be performed if lobular carcinoma in situ is seen on needle core biopsy, *Arch Pathol Lab Med* 126:697–701, 2002.

Sickles EA: Periodic mammographic follow-up of probably benign lesions: results in 3,184 consecutive cases, *Radiology* 179:463–468, 1991.

Sickles EA: Management of probably benign breast lesions, *Radiol Clin North Am* 33:1123–1130, 1995.

Simon JR, Kalbhen CL, Cooper RA, et al: Accuracy and complication rates of US-guided vacuum-assisted core breast biopsy: initial results, *Radiology* 215:694–697, 2000.

Smathers RL: Marking the cavity site after stereotactic core needle breast biopsy, *AJR Am J Roentgenol* 180:355–356, 2003.

Smith DN, Rosenfield Darling ML, et al: The utility of ultrasonographically guided large-core needle biopsy: results from 500 consecutive breast biopsies, *J Ultrasound Med* 20:43–49, 2001.

Smith LF, Henry-Tilman R, Rubio T, et al: Intraoperative localization after stereotactic breast biopsy without a needle, *Am J Surg* 182:584–589, 2001.

Sneige N, Lim SC, Whitman GJ, et al: Atypical ductal hyperplasia diagnosis by directional vacuum-assisted stereotactic biopsy of breast microcalcifications. Considerations for surgical excision, *Am J Clin Pathol* 119:248–523, 2003.

Soo MS, Baker JA, Rosen EL, et al: Sonographically guided biopsy of suspicious microcalcifications of the breast: a pilot study, *AJR Am J Roentgenol* 178:1007–1015, 2002.

Soo MS, Baker JA, Rosen EL: Sonographic detection and sonographically guided biopsy of breast microcalcifications, *AJR Am J Roentgenol* 180:941–948, 2003.

Stomper PC, Davis SP, Weidner N, et al: Clinically occult, noncalcified breast cancer: serial radiologic–pathologic correlation in 27 cases, *Radiology* 169:621–626, 1988.

Sydnor MK, Wilson JD, Hijaz TA, et al: Underestimation of the presence of breast carcinoma in papillary lesions initially diagnosed at core-needle biopsy, *Radiology* 242:58–62, 2007.

Tabar L, Pentek Z, Dean PB: The diagnostic and therapeutic value of breast cyst puncture and pneumocystography, *Radiology* 141:659–663, 1981.

Tartter PI, Bleiweiss IJ, Levchenko S: Factors associated with clear biopsy margins and clear reexcision margins in breast cancer specimens from candidates for breast conservation, *J Am Coll Surg* 185:268–273, 1997.

Teh WL, Wilson AR, Evans AJ, et al: Ultrasound guided core biopsy of suspicious mammographic calcifications using high frequency and power Doppler ultrasound, *Clin Radiol* 55:390–394, 2000.

Thompson WR, Bowen JR, Dorman BA, et al: Mammographic localization and biopsy of nonpalpable breast lesions. A 5-year study, *Arch Surg* 126:730–734, 1991.

Tornos C, Silva E, el-Naggar A, Pritzker KP: Calcium oxalate crystals in breast biopsies. The missing microcalcifications, *Am J Surg Pathol* 14:961–968, 1990.

Verkooijen HM: Core Biopsy after Radiological Localisation (COBRA) Study Group. Diagnostic accuracy of stereotactic large-core needle biopsy for nonpalpable breast disease: results of a multicenter prospective study with 95% surgical confirmation, *Int J Cancer* 99:853–859, 2002.

Verkooijen HM, Peterse JL, Schipper ME, et al: Interobserver variability between general and expert pathologists during the histopathological assessment of large-core needle and open biopsies of nonpalpable breast lesions, *Eur J Cancer* 39:2187–2191, 2003.

Whaley DH, Adamczyk DL, Jensen EA: Sonographically guided needle localization after stereotactic breast biopsy, *AJR Am J Roentgenol* 180:352–354, 2003.

Yang JH, Lee WS, Kim SW, et al: Effect of core-needle biopsy vs. fine-needle aspiration on pathologic measurement of tumor size in breast cancer, *Arch Surg* 140:125, 2005.

Yeh IT, Dimitrov D, Otto P, et al: Pathologic review of atypical hyperplasia identified by image-guided breast needle core biopsy. Correlation with excision specimen, *Arch Pathol Lab Med* 127:49–54, 2003.

Youk JH, Kim EK, Kim MJ, et al: Sonographically guided 14-gauge core needle biopsy of breast masses: a review of 2,420 cases with long-term follow-up, *AJR Am J Roentgenol* 190:202–207, 2008.

Youk JH, Kim EK, Kim MJ: Atypical ductal hyperplasia diagnosed at sonographically guided 14-gauge core needle biopsy of breast mass, *AJR Am J Roentgenol* 192:1135–1141, 2009.

Zografos GC, Zagouri F, Sergentanis TN, et al: Diagnosing papillary lesions using vacuum-assisted breast biopsy: should conservative or surgical management follow? *Onkologie* 31:653–656, 2008.

Quizzes

6-1. Fill in the requirements for nonpalpable percutaneous breast lesion biopsy.

_____

_____

_____

_____

_____

_____

For answers, see Box 6-1.

6-2. Fill in the possible complications from breast biopsy.

_____

_____

_____

_____

_____

_____

For answers, see Box 6-2.

6-3. Fill in the types of benign discordant needle biopsies.

_____

_____

_____

_____

_____

For answers, see Box 6-5.

6-4. Fill in the high-risk lesions with almost total or majority agreement about the need for excision.

_____

_____

_____

_____

_____

_____

_____

For answers, see Box 6-6.

CHAPTER 7

Magnetic Resonance Imaging of Breast Cancer and MRI-Guided Breast Biopsy

Bruce L. Daniel and Debra M. Ikeda

▬ BASIC PRINCIPLES

Magnetic resonance imaging (MRI) uses repeated radio-frequency pulses in concert with precise spatial modulation of a strong magnetic field to image the distribution and nuclear magnetic resonance characteristics of hydrogen atoms within human tissue. MRI provides either two-dimensional thin slices or three-dimensional (3-D) volumetric tomographic images without ionizing radiation. Like mammography, MRI is comprehensive, reproducible, and operator independent. Like sonography, MRI is not limited by dense breast tissue.

Different MRI pulse sequences can be used to create images that reflect different tissue properties, such as T1, T2, or T2* relaxation times, proton density, apparent diffusion coefficient (ADC), and others. Pulse sequences can also be made specific for particular tissues, such as fat, water, or silicone, by a variety of techniques. MRI is exquisitely sensitive to paramagnetic substances, such as intravenously injected gadolinium chelate contrast agents. Even minimal concentrations of these agents in tissues substantially shorten the T1 relaxation time and thereby result in high signal on T1-weighted images and improved tissue differentiation.

Breast Cancer

Invasive breast tumors are characterized by an ingrowth of neovascularity at their periphery. Tumor angiogenesis is associated with increased perfusion and abnormal leaky endothelium, leading to preferential enhancement of tumors versus normal breast tissue (Box 7-1). With bolus administration of an intravenous (IV) contrast agent, increased vascular flow and the rapid exchange rate of contrast between blood and the extracellular compartment cause invasive breast tumors to enhance more rapidly and more avidly than normal fibroglandular tissue, even in patients with dense breasts. Thus, invasive breast cancers have high signal intensity and are brighter than the surrounding normal tissue on the first postcontrast scan, which ideally should be obtained about 90 seconds after injection. As a result, MRI exquisitely reveals invasive tumors that are occult on mammography (Fig. 7-1). The sensitivity of MRI for invasive breast cancer is extremely high—over 90%. However, as discussed in detail in this chapter,

contrast enhancement on MRI is seen in many benign conditions as well; the specificity of MRI varies between 39% and 95%. As detailed in this chapter, morphology, T1 and T2 characteristics, and the time course of contrast enhancement help differentiate benign from malignant lesions (Table 7-1).

▬ TECHNIQUE

Patient Preparation

Benign hormone-related enhancement of normal breast tissue, called *background enhancement*, occurs before the onset of menses and can lead to false-positive studies. When possible, patients should be imaged 7 to 10 days after the onset of their menstrual cycle, when spurious contrast enhancement of normal breast tissue is at its nadir (Box 7-2).

Before MRI scanning, the patient fills out an MRI safety form to exclude contraindications of entering the strong magnetic field, such as ferromagnetic vascular clips, metallic ocular fragments, pacemakers, and implanted electromechanical devices. A qualified person reviews the standardized MRI safety form before scanning (Fig. 7-2).

As with mammography, an MRI-specific breast history form is helpful to detail patient breast risk factors, family history, breast lumps, scars, or other areas of complaint. The technologist places MRI-compatible markers on the patient's breast to indicate lumps or areas of concern and annotates them on the history form. The patient details the location, date, and results of previous breast biopsies because recent healing breast biopsies may normally show enhancement and are a cause of false-positive results. The patient also documents any use of exogenous hormone therapy and the phase of the menstrual cycle or menopause, because those factors may cause spurious background enhancement of normal tissue, which can produce false-positive results.

Equipment

An IV catheter is placed before scanning and is continuously flushed by using the keep vein open (KVO) setting of an MRI-compatible remote power injector. Placement of the catheter in the antecubital fossa contralateral to any known, previous, or suspected malignancy is preferred. The patient is placed prone on a dedicated breast coil (Fig. 7-3A). Prone positioning minimizes respiratory motion in the breast. Phased-array breast coils maximize the signal-to-noise ratio of the image. Patient discomfort is the primary cause of motion; the majority of patients remain most comfortable for the duration of the entire scan with both arms at their sides and wearing hearing protection (see Fig. 7-3B). The technologist spends considerable time discussing the importance of "holding still" with the patient to obtain the best scan. The patient then works

with the technologist to obtain a comfortable position within the breast coil. Optional mild breast stabilization, or "compression," may be used to reduce breast motion and decrease the volume of tissue to be scanned so that the whole breast is included. However, firm compression (as used routinely for mammography) should be avoided because it may negatively affect contrast enhancement. Scanners with a magnetic field strength of 1.5 Tesla (T) or 3.0 T provide the best signal-to-noise ratio. Magnets with high-performance gradients enable the fastest, highest-resolution scans (Box 7-3).

MRI Protocols

Conventional breast MRI begins with T1-weighted images to define the position and anatomy of the breast. T1-weighted images using the signal from the "body coil" rather than the breast coil enable basic evaluation of the axillae, anterior mediastinum, chest wall, and supraclavicular fossa for enlarged regional lymph nodes. Thereafter, a dedicated breast coil signal should be used to perform all subsequent sequences. T2-weighted fast spin-echo (FSE)

BOX 7-1. Principles of Breast Cancer MRI

Contrast-enhanced MRI is extremely sensitive for tumor angiogenesis, regardless of radiographic breast density.

Tumor angiogenesis leads to preferential enhancement of cancers with intravenous contrast.

Lesion morphology helps distinguish cancer from benign conditions.

The time-course of contrast enhancement helps distinguish invasive cancer from other conditions:

"Most" cancers initially enhance rapidly (*rapid washin*).

Cancers subsequently have a stable signal intensity (*plateau*) or gradually declining signal intensity (*washout*).

Benign conditions enhance usually gradually and continuously.

BOX 7-2. Patient Selection and Preparation

MRI should be performed on day 7-14 after onset of menses minimizes false-positive enhancement.

Patients should be screened for safety of MRI, including pacemakers or other implanted devices.

Patients should document previous and current breast problems on a breast history form.

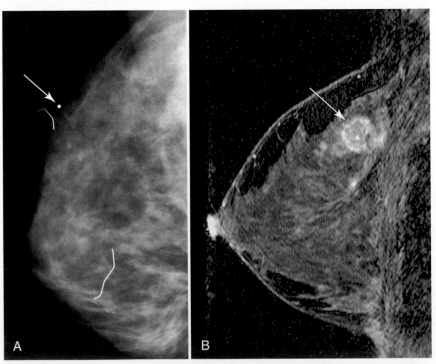

FIGURE 7-1. Mammographically occult breast cancer. **A,** Mediolateral oblique mammogram in a woman with a palpable mass in the upper portion of the breast indicated by a metallic skin marker (*arrow*) revealed only dense tissue. **B,** Contrast-enhanced water-specific 3-D magnetic resonance image demonstrated a 1-cm rim-enhancing lesion (*arrow*). Lumpectomy revealed a 1-cm invasive ductal carcinoma.

TABLE 7-1. Typical T1, T2, and Kinetic Curves for Cancer and Benign Masses on Breast MRI

	Axial T1-Weighted Localizer, Noncontrast, No Fat Suppression	T2-Weighted Noncontrast, Fat-Suppressed	Initial Kinetic Contrast Enhancement Curve	Late Kinetic Contrast Enhancement Curve
Cancer	Dark	Dark*	Rapid	Plateau or washout
Lymph node[†]	Dark cortex Bright fat in hilum	Bright cortex Dark fat in hilum	Rapid	Washout
FA: myxoid[‡]	Dark	Bright	Slow or rapid	Persistent
FA: old, sclerotic	Dark	Dark	Slow	Persistent
Papilloma	Dark	Dark/bright	Rapid	Washout
Mucinous cancer	Dark	Bright	Rapid	Plateau or washout
Ductal carcinoma in situ	Dark	Dark	Variable Kinetic morphology important Focal area, linear, ductal segmental regional, asymmetric, clumped	Variable
Old scar	Dark	Dark	None/slow	None/persistent
Cyst[§]	Dark	Bright	None	None
Fat necrosis[§]	Dark (may have bright fat in center)	Dark (may have dark fat in center)	Rim Rapid for the first 18 mo Slow or none after 18 mo	Persistent or none

*Rarely invasive ductal carcinoma can be T2 bright; these are usually dark or isointense compared to glandular tissue.
[†]Lymph nodes usually upper outer quadrant near blood vessel.
[‡]20% of fibroadenoma (FA) have dark septations.
[§]Inflamed cysts and fat necrosis may have rim enhancement.

BOX 7-3. Equipment for Breast MRI

Remote-controlled power injector connected to the antecubital IV line on KVO (keep vein open) setting
Dedicated breast coil
 Prone position minimizes respiratory motion
 Small volume maximizes signal-to-noise ratio
 Multiple receiver channels enable parallel imaging acceleration
 Mild stabilization or no compression used; firm compression may alter contrast enhancement.
1.5 T magnet with high-performance gradient system
 3.0 T magnets may increase signal to noise ratio but are limited by tissue heating and radiofrequency transmit field inhomogeneity

images are then obtained to characterize the breast and any lesions. T2-weighted scans using an FSE, turbo spin-echo (TSE), or rapid acquisition with relaxation inhibition (RARE) technique, produce high-quality images within reasonable scan times of 5 to 6 minutes. High fat signal on T2-weighted FSE images can be prevented with fat suppression and is most successful if unilateral scanning is performed (Table 7-2).

Considerable variation exists worldwide in methods used for the contrast-enhanced portion of the examination. Most investigators agree that both the time course of enhancement provided by dynamic scanning and the morphology of lesions revealed by high-spatial resolution scanning provide distinct and useful information about the risk of malignancy in enhancing lesions. However, commercially available MRI pulse sequences necessitate a compromise between the dynamic and high-spatial resolution approaches. Currently, most scans are done with repeated T1-weighted, fat-saturated, 3-D spoiled gradient-echo (SPGR) scans. Slice thickness and resolution are selected to give maximum resolution and bilateral whole-breast coverage within a 60- to 90-second scan duration. Parallel imaging and intermittent/partial fat saturation substantially speed up imaging, allowing much higher resolution within the same scan time.

Volumetric T1-weighted 3-D SPGR imaging is repeated as rapidly as possible before, during, and for approximately 5 to 7 minutes after administration of a rapid IV bolus of 0.1 mmol/kg gadolinium contrast agent. Most investigators use axial or coronal images with a rectangular field of view to maximize efficiency. Images may be processed by subtracting the precontrast baseline images from subsequent dynamic images to reveal areas of enhancement. Region-of-interest analysis is used to assess the time course of contrast enhancement. Subtraction processing suppresses signal from bright fat because adipose tissue does not enhance significantly. Spatial resolution is limited by the need for rapid scan times and the large field of view required for bilateral scanning.

Proper shimming of the magnet and choice of center frequency are essential to ensure adequate fat suppression. Bilateral high-spatial resolution imaging is now possible on most scanners because of the development of hardware and software required for bilateral shimming and because coverage is possible with reasonable scan times.

In bilateral combined dynamic and high-spatial resolution imaging, sophisticated protocols and scanning

MAGNETIC RESONANCE (MR) PROCEDURE SCREENING FORM FOR PATIENTS

Date _____/_____/_____   Patient Number _____

Name _____ Age _____ Height _____ Weight _____
      Last name   First name   Middle Initial

Date of Birth _____/_____/_____   Male ❑ Female ❑   Body Part to be Examined _____
         month day   year

Address _____   Telephone (home) (_____) _____-_____

City   _____   Telephone (work) (_____) _____-_____

State   _____ Zip Code _____

Reason for MRI and/or Symptoms _____

Referring Physician _____   Telephone (_____) _____-_____

---

1. Have you had prior surgery or an operation (e.g., arthroscopy, endoscopy, etc.) of any kind? ❑ No ❑ Yes
   If yes, please indicate the date and type of surgery:
   Date _____/_____/_____   Type of surgery _____
   Date _____/_____/_____   Type of surgery _____
2. Have you had a prior diagnostic imaging study or examination (MRI, CT, Ultrasound, X-ray, etc.)? ❑No ❑ Yes
   If yes, please list: Body part   Date   Facility
   MRI   _____ ____/____/____ _____
   CT/CAT Scan _____ ____/____/____ _____
   X-Ray   _____ ____/____/____ _____
   Ultrasound   _____ ____/____/____ _____
   Nuclear Medicine _____ ____/____/____ _____
   Other_____ _____ ____/____/____ _____

3. Have you experienced any problem related to a previous MRI examination or MR procedure? ❑ No ❑ Yes
   If yes, please describe: _____
4. Have you had an injury to the eye involving a metallic object or fragment (e.g., metallic slivers, shavings, foreign body, etc.)? ❑ No ❑ Yes
   If yes, please describe: _____
5. Have you ever been injured by a metallic object or foreign body (e.g., BB, bullet, shrapnel, etc.)? ❑ No ❑ Yes
   If yes, please describe: _____
6. Are you currently taking or have you recently taken any medication or drug? ❑ No ❑ Yes
   If yes, please list:_____
7. Are you allergic to any medication? ❑ No ❑ Yes
   If yes, please list:_____
8. Do you have a history of asthma, allergic reaction, respiratory disease, or reaction to a contrast medium or dye used for an MRI, CT, or X-ray examination? ❑ No ❑ Yes
9. Do you have anemia or any disease(s) that affects your blood, a history of renal (kidney) disease, or seizures? ❑ No ❑ Yes
   If yes, please describe: _____

For female patients:
10. Date of last menstrual period:_____/_____/_____   Post menopausal? ❑ No ❑ Yes
11. Are you pregnant or experiencing a late menstrual period? ❑ No ❑ Yes
12. Are you taking oral contraceptives or receiving hormonal treatment? ❑ No ❑ Yes
13. Are you taking any type of fertility medication or having fertility treatments? ❑ No ❑ Yes
    If yes, please describe: _____
14. Are you currently breastfeeding? ❑ No ❑ Yes

A

© F.G. Shellock, 2002   www.IMRSER.org

FIGURE 7-2. A and B, Magnetic resonance imaging (MRI) safety form. As part of routine safety interview procedures before MRI, patients fill out a history form to screen for implanted devices or other conditions that might affect the safety of MRI. (Courtesy of Dr. Frank Shellock, MRI-Safety.com. Reprinted by permission.)

WARNING: Certain implants, devices, or objects may be hazardous to you and/or may interfere with the MR procedure (i.e., MRI, MR angiography, functional MRI, MR spectroscopy). **Do not enter** the MR system room or MR environment if you have any question or concern regarding an implant, device, or object. Consult the MRI Technologist or Radiologist BEFORE entering the MR system room. **The MR system magnet is ALWAYS on.**

Please indicate if you have any of the following:

☐ Yes ☐ No	Aneurysm clip(s)	
☐ Yes ☐ No	Cardiac pacemaker	
☐ Yes ☐ No	Implanted cardioverter defibrillator (ICD)	
☐ Yes ☐ No	Electronic implant or device	
☐ Yes ☐ No	Magnetically-activated implant or device	
☐ Yes ☐ No	Neurostimulation system	
☐ Yes ☐ No	Spinal cord stimulator	
☐ Yes ☐ No	Internal electrodes or wires	
☐ Yes ☐ No	Bone growth/bone fusion stimulator	
☐ Yes ☐ No	Cochlear, otologic, or other ear implant	
☐ Yes ☐ No	Insulin or other infusion pump	
☐ Yes ☐ No	Implanted drug infusion device	
☐ Yes ☐ No	Any type of prosthesis (eye, penile, etc.)	
☐ Yes ☐ No	Heart valve prosthesis	
☐ Yes ☐ No	Eyelid spring or wire	
☐ Yes ☐ No	Artificial or prosthetic limb	
☐ Yes ☐ No	Metallic stent, filter, or coil	
☐ Yes ☐ No	Shunt (spinal or intraventricular)	
☐ Yes ☐ No	Vascular access port and/or catheter	
☐ Yes ☐ No	Radiation seeds or implants	
☐ Yes ☐ No	Swan-Ganz or thermodilution catheter	
☐ Yes ☐ No	Medication patch (Nicotine, Nitroglycerine)	
☐ Yes ☐ No	Any metallic fragment or foreign body	
☐ Yes ☐ No	Wire mesh implant	
☐ Yes ☐ No	Tissue expander (e.g., breast)	
☐ Yes ☐ No	Surgical staples, clips, or metallic sutures	
☐ Yes ☐ No	Joint replacement (hip, knee, etc.)	
☐ Yes ☐ No	Bone/joint pin, screw, nail, wire, plate, etc.	
☐ Yes ☐ No	IUD, diaphragm, or pessary	
☐ Yes ☐ No	Dentures or partial plates	
☐ Yes ☐ No	Tattoo or permanent makeup	
☐ Yes ☐ No	Body piercing jewelry	
☐ Yes ☐ No	Hearing aid	
	(Remove before entering MR system room)	
☐ Yes ☐ No	Other implant _____	
☐ Yes ☐ No	Breathing problem or motion disorder	
☐ Yes ☐ No	Claustrophobia	

Please mark on the figure(s) below the location of any implant or metal inside of or on your body.

RIGHT   LEFT   LEFT   RIGHT

⚠ **IMPORTANT INSTRUCTIONS**

Before entering the MR environment or MR system room, you must remove all metallic objects including hearing aids, dentures, partial plates, keys, beeper, cell phone, eyeglasses, hair pins, barrettes, jewelry, body piercing jewelry, watch, safety pins, paperclips, money clip, credit cards, bank cards, magnetic strip cards, coins, pens, pocket knife, nail clipper, tools, clothing with metal fasteners, & clothing with metallic threads.

Please consult the MRI Technologist or Radiologist if you have any question or concern BEFORE you enter the MR system room.

NOTE: You may be advised or required to wear earplugs or other hearing protection during the MR procedure to prevent possible problems or hazards related to acoustic noise.

I attest that the above information is correct to the best of my knowledge. I read and understand the contents of this form and had the opportunity to ask questions regarding the information on this form and regarding the MR procedure that I am about to undergo.

Signature of Person Completing Form: _____   Date ____/____/____
                                              Signature

Form Completed By: ☐ Patient ☐ Relative ☐ Nurse _____   _____
                                                        Print name   Relationship to patient

Form Information Reviewed By: _____   _____
                                        Print name   Signature

☐ MRI Technologist   ☐ Nurse   ☐ Radiologist   ☐ Other_____

© F.G. Shellock, 2002   www.IMRSER.org

B

FIGURE 7-2, cont'd.

techniques capture both rapid dynamic and high-spatial resolution images of both breasts during and after IV contrast injection. Approaches include time-resolved imaging of contrast kinetics (TRICKS) and interleaved protocols, in which dynamic scanning is interrupted for high-spatial resolution imaging. These protocols provide very high-quality images but they require rapid switching between different pulse sequences.

The American College of Radiology (ACR) now has guidelines for the performance of breast MRI and in 2010 launched a breast MRI accreditation program. The ACR MRI program recommends that facilities be able to obtain bilateral studies and be able to perform MRI-guided biopsies.

THE NORMAL BREAST MRI

Normal Breast MRI Findings

Typical images from a normal patient who underwent both bilateral dynamic and high-spatial resolution imaging are provided in Figure 7-4. On T1-weighted noncontrast-enhanced images, aqueous tissues (including skin, fibroglandular tissue, muscle, and lymph nodes) have moderately low signal intensity when compared with the higher signal intensity of fat, which has a short T1 relaxation time. In the absence of previous surgery or pathology, a layer of subcutaneous and retromammary fat completely surrounds the mammary gland tissue except where it enters the

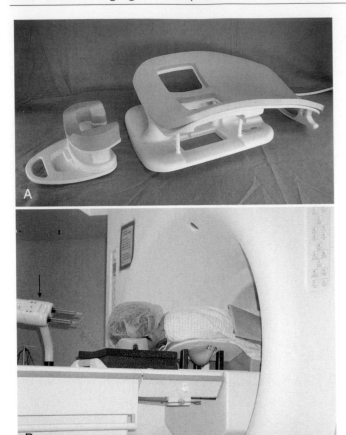

FIGURE 7-3. Dedicated breast coil and 1.5-Tesla (T) scanner. Prone positioning with the breasts in the apertures of a dedicated, phased-array breast coil (**A**) improves image quality by maximizing the signal-to-noise ratio of the image and minimizing respiratory motion. Imaging at 1.5 T enables more robust fat suppression and produces a higher signal-to-noise ratio than imaging at lower field strengths does. **B,** Conventional closed-bore scanners have stronger, faster gradient systems than open magnetic resonance imaging systems do; these systems enable faster scans with more slices and higher spatial resolution. Use of a remote power injector (*arrow*) enables administration of contrast during the dynamic scan protocol while the patient is within the magnet. (**A,** Courtesy of Tom Tynes, MRI-Devices Inc, Waukesha, WI. Used by permission.)

nipple–areola complex. The mammary gland itself is composed of a mix of low-signal fibroglandular tissue and high-signal fat lobules. The mix and distribution of fat and fibroglandular tissue vary greatly between patients—from dense, uniformly glandular tissue with almost no visible fat, to heterogeneous, to predominantly fatty tissue separated by thin strands or septa of fibroglandular tissue. In the ACR Breast Imaging Reporting and Data System (BI-RADS®) MRI lexicon the amount of dense glandular tissue by volume is described in the same terms as used in the mammography lexicon. These include *almost all fat* (0% to 25% dense), *scattered fibroglandular tissue* (25% to 50% dense), *heterogeneously dense* (50% to 75% dense), or *dense* (>75% dense) (Box 7-4 and Fig. 7-5).

T2-weighted noncontrast-enhanced images reveal heterogeneous fibroglandular tissue that is usually higher in signal intensity than adjacent muscle but still not as bright as the small subcutaneous blood vessels commonly seen at the periphery of the breast or as pure fluid (i.e., cysts, ducts).

TABLE 7-2. Basic Bilateral Protocol for Breast Cancer MRI

Series	Description	Purpose
1	Axial T1 or STIR	Show lymph nodes and overall anatomy; localization
2	Fast T2*	Map cysts, ducts; assess lesion T2
[3]	Diffusion-weighted EPI[†]	Assess lesion ADC
4	3-D T1 fat-saturated spoiled gradient echo; 90 seconds or less[‡]	Baseline prior to contrast injection
5	Repeat series 4 over 7–12 min with contrast[§]	Assess contrast enhancement morphology and kinetics
[6]	¹H spectroscopy[¶]	Measure choline
N/A	Postprocessing	Enhancement curves, subtraction, 3-D, measurements, parametric maps

Sagittal imaging for all scans except series 1 allows smallest field of view (~20 cm for most patients) and thus highest resolution.
Frequency encoding in the anteroposterior direction minimizes artifacts from cardiac and respiratory motion in the breast.
Series in brackets are optional, and not yet standard of care.
*T2: Fast spin-echo (FSE, RARE, TSE, etc.) with effective TE 80–100 ms and TR at least 3000 ms provides good T2 weighting. Use 3- to 4-mm-thick slices and 256×192 matrix or higher for small FOV sagittal images. Fat saturation improves conspicuity of bright lesions on T2, although nonfat-suppressed T2 imaging allows fat signal intensity to be used as a reference signal intensity. Volume shimming improves fat suppression.
†B-values have not been standardized yet, but most investigators use 500–1000 with good results. Parallel imaging may reduce distortions in echo planar imaging.
‡Both fat suppression and high spatial resolution (<2 mm in all directions) are essential to assess lesion morphology. Rapid imaging (60–90 sec per scan or less) is necessary to assess contrast uptake kinetics. Use "fast" spoiled 3-D gradient echo (TR ≤ 6 ms; FA ~ 15° for T1 weighting). Intermittent "special" fat saturation pulses speed imaging substantially over conventional fat saturation. Fractional k-space ("1/2 NEX," etc.), and parallel imaging (SENSE/IPAT, etc.) maximize resolution obtained during the limited scan time.
§Repeat rapidly for dynamic scans totaling approximately 7 minutes or more. Inject 0.1 mmol/kg standard low molecular weight gadolinium contrast agent (e.g., Gd-DTPA, gadoteridol, etc.) at 2 mL/sec followed by 20 mL flush (normal saline) at the start of the acquisition. Avoid negatively charged gadolinium agents if protocol includes spectroscopy, because they may reduce choline signal. (Lenkinski B, Wang X, Elian M, Goldberg SN: Interaction of gadolinium-based MR contrast agents with choline: implications for MR spectroscopy (MRS) of the breast, *Magn Reson Med* 61(6):1286–1292, 2009.
¶Single-voxel choline spectroscopy. A minimum voxel size of 1 cm × 1 cm × 1 cm is recommended for adequate signal-to-noise. Localized shimming and high-quality spatial saturation pulses, fat suppression, and partial water suppression improve quality of spectra.
1H, proton (hydrogen nucleus); ADC, apparent diffusion coefficient; EPI, echo-planar imaging; FOV, field of view; FSE, fast spin echo; Gd-DTPA, gadolinium diethylenetriamine pentaacetic acid; IPAT, integrated parallel acquisition techniques; NEX, number of excitations or signal averages; RARE, rapid acquisition with refocused echoes; SENSE, sensitivity encoding; STIR, short tau inversion recovery; TE, echo time; TR, repetition time; TSE, turbo spin echo.

BOX 7-4. Breast Density by Volume

Fatty: 0% to 25%
Scattered fibroglandular: 25% to 50%
Heterogeneously dense: 50% to 75%
Dense: >75%

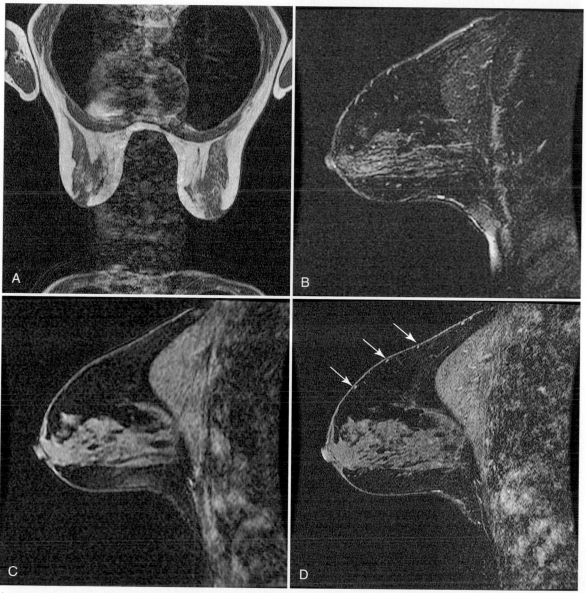

FIGURE 7-4. Normal breast magnetic resonance imaging (MRI). **A,** Axial T1-weighted spin-echo images reveal high-signal fat within the breast and axilla. Soft tissues, including skin, fibroglandular tissue, lymph nodes, and muscles, are dark. **B,** Sagittal, fat-saturated, T2-weighted fast spin-echo images reveal dark signal within fat and moderately low signal within the pectoralis muscle. Glandular tissue has mixed T2-weighted signal intensity. **C,** Precontrast water-specific 3-D spectral-spatial excitation magnetization transfer (3DSSMT) reveals dark fat and moderately low fibroglandular and muscle tissue signal. **D,** High-spatial resolution 3DSSMT after the intravenous administration of a 0.1-mmol/kg bolus of contrast reveals enhancing peripheral vessels (*arrows*) and mild nipple enhancement.

Continued

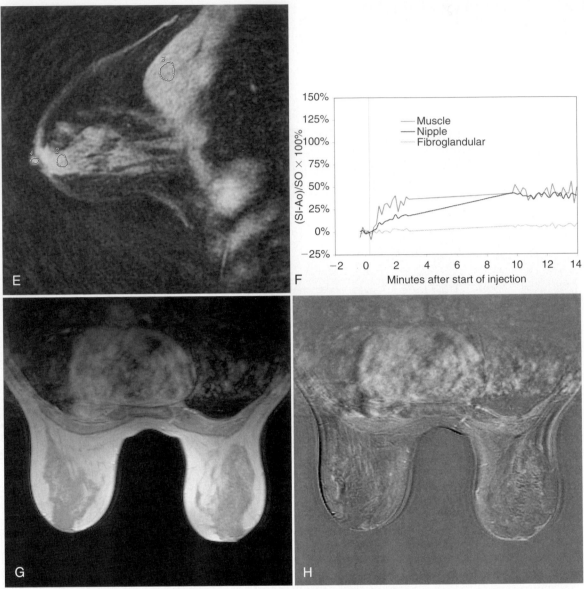

FIGURE 7-4, cont'd. E, Rapid dynamic 3-D spiral imaging reveals mild (<50%) gradual enhancement in the nipple and fibroglandular tissue and mild (<50%) rapid enhancement in the pectoralis muscle (**F**). Subtraction processing of early postcontrast multiplanar two-dimensional spoiled gradient echo images (**G**) minus precontrast baseline images (**H**) reveals diffuse low-level fibroglandular and muscle enhancement.

After contrast injection, normal glandular tissue enhances to variable degrees. Normal fibroglandular breast tissue enhancement is called *background enhancement* in the BI-RADS® lexicon. An understanding of normal background enhancement is important because normal background enhancement can obscure cancers and make the MRI harder to read. *Background enhancement* describes slowly enhancing breast tissue within the breast. Specifically, normal fibroglandular tissue enhances with nonmass-like patterns, including stippled enhancement (tiny <5 mm foci of enhancement separated by normal tissue); scattered, regional, or multiple regions; or diffused stippled enhancement throughout both breasts. The areas of enhancement are usually separated by nonenhancing normal breast tissue between the normal background enhancing foci. In the BI-RADS® lexicon, the amount of background enhancement is described as a percentage of enhancing breast tissue with respect to the volume of the entire breast. Background enhancement is categorized in

> **BOX 7-5. Background Enhancement**
>
> None: 0
> Minimal: 1% to 25%
> Mild: 25% to 50%
> Moderate: 50% to 75%
> Marked: >75%
>
> Note: Background enhancement details how much of the breast is enhancing, which may obscure a breast cancer.

quartiles. The descriptors include *none* (0%), *minimal* (1% to 25%), *mild* (25% to 50%), *moderate* (50% to 75%), and *marked* (>75%) (Box 7-5 and Fig. 7-6).

The amount of background enhancement depends on the patient's hormonal status, stage of the menstrual cycle, and whether the patient is premenopausal or postmenopausal. For example, in premenopausal women, normal breast tissue enhances the most right before the

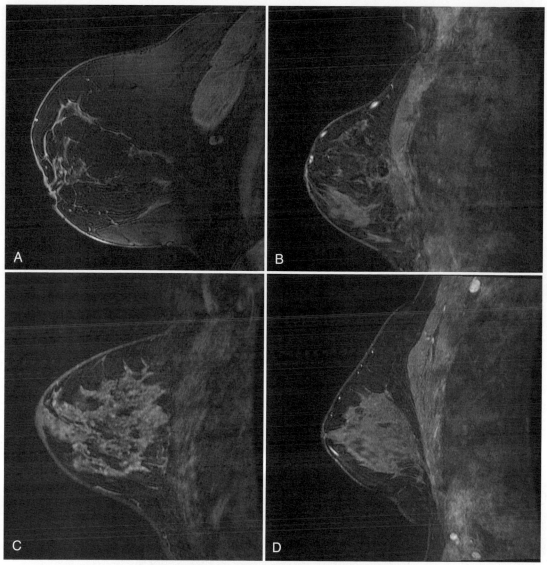

FIGURE 7-5. Examples of normal breast magnetic resonance imaging (MRI) density by volume on noncontrast sagittal 3-D spectral-spatial excitation magnetization transfer (3DSSMT) scans. **A,** Fatty sagittal postcontrast MRI shows mostly fatty tissue (0% to 25% density). **B,** Scattered fibroglandular tissue (25% to 50%). **C,** Heterogeneously dense breast tissue (50% to 75%). **D,** Dense glandular tissue (>75%).

onset of menses. The normal breast tissue enhances the least 7 to 10 days after the onset of menses. Postmenopausal women on exogenous hormone therapy may enhance greatly. However, the amount of background enhancement depends *not only* on how much the tissue enhances, but also on the actual volume of dense breast tissue present. For example, a woman with extremely dense breast tissue, in which most of the breast is composed of fibroglandular tissue, may enhance from 0% to 100%. This woman might have minimal to marked background enhancement, because more than 75% of her breast is capable of enhancing. However, if the breast has only scattered fibroglandular tissue (25% to 50% dense), the greatest amount of background enhancement possible is *mild background enhancement,* or 25% to 50% enhancement, because only 25% to 50% of the breast is dense enough to enhance within and the remaining 50% is fat. Of note, cancers can occur in both dense and fatty parts of any breast.

Reporting normal background enhancement gives a clinician and other radiologists an idea of how likely it would be for the normal enhancing structures to hide a breast cancer and how confident the radiologist is in detecting breast cancer on the MRI.

After contrast injection, peripheral small subcutaneous vessels, the nipple, and adjacent retroareolar tissue enhances to variable degrees. The normal nipple enhances along its edge in a thin line; the rest of the nipple is dark, with an occasional dot of enhancement centrally within the nipple itself. The areolar complex is dark on the normal MRI. The normal skin is 2 to 3 mm in thickness and enhances slightly.

The rate and degree to which findings enhance gives a clue to whether the finding is normal or malignant. Dynamic imaging shows that fibroglandular tissue enhances mildly and slowly. Nipple enhancement curves are more avid, but still gradual. Muscle enhances rapidly at first, but never enhances very avidly. Subtraction imaging of a normal breast should show mild glandular and muscle enhancement. Usually cancer is much brighter than the background enhancement and will look much brighter on

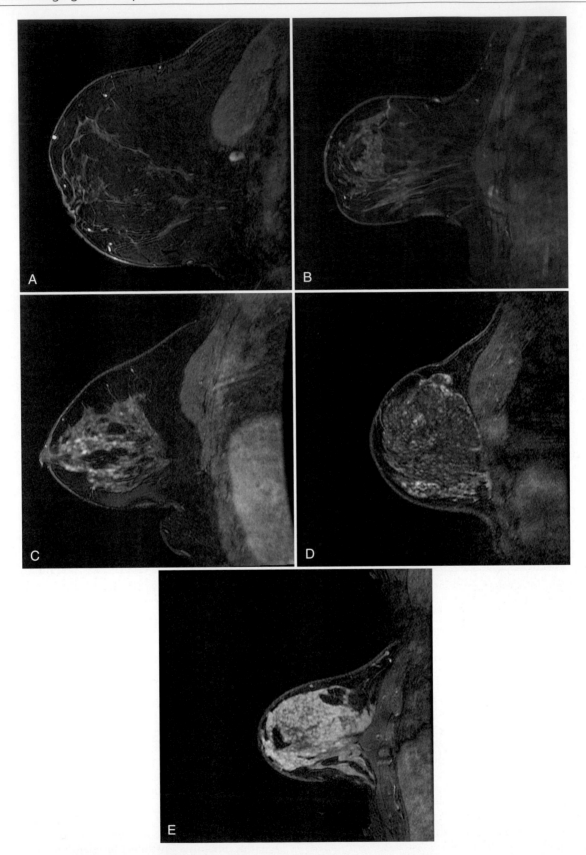

FIGURE 7-6. Background enhancement on contrast-enhanced breast magnetic resonance imaging (MRI). **A,** No abnormal background enhancement. Contrast-enhanced breast MRI shows that the scant glandular tissue does not enhance. There is enhancement of an axillary lymph node. **B,** Minimal enhancement. Scattered fibroglandular tissue with minimal background enhancement. **C,** Mild enhancement. Scattered fibroglandular breast tissue with mild background enhancement. **D,** Heterogeneously dense tissue with moderate background enhancement. **E,** Marked enhancement. Dense glandular tissue with marked background enhancement.

the first postcontrast scan compared to normal tissue. Normal breast tissue kinetic curves show a slow initial rise and a late persistent plateau. This normal slow initial and late persistent curve helps to distinguish normal breast tissue from cancers. Cancers will usually enhance rapidly initially, with a washout or a plateau of signal intensity in the delayed phase.

Common Breast MRI Artifacts

Ghosting from cardiac or respiratory motion occurs in the phase-encoding direction (Table 7-3). It can be prevented from obscuring breast tissue by careful selection of phase- and frequency-encoding directions. Poor fat suppression is usually due to poor shimming or incorrect choice of the excitation center frequency, especially in patients with silicone implants (Fig. 7-7) or non–MRI-compatible

TABLE 7-3. Common Artifacts

Artifact	Cause
Line(s) of noise	Electronic noise/poor room shielding/scan room door open
Ghosting from heart across the breast	Wrong frequency-encoding direction
Blurring	Patient motion
Bright and dark edges on subtraction	Patient motion
Poor enhancement	Slow or failed contrast injection
Poor fat suppression	Poor shimming or center frequency, non-MRI compatible skin marker left on breast

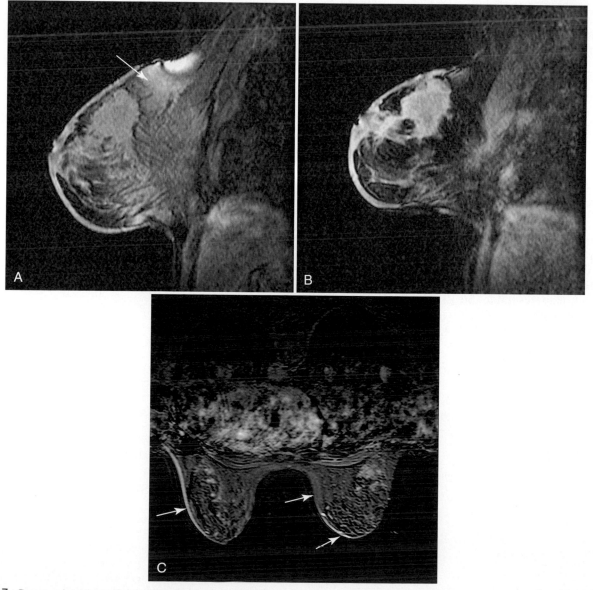

FIGURE 7-7. Common imaging artifacts. **A,** Inconsistent fat suppression on water-selective images is due to poor shimming or incorrect selection of the center frequency (*arrow*), or both. **B,** Repeat shimming and tuning improve fat suppression. **C,** Poor fat suppression on subtraction images is due to patient motion, causing misregistration artifacts at fat–skin or fat–glandular interfaces (*arrows*).

objects, such as BB markers, magnetic tissue expanders, scar markers, and metal infusion ports, in or near the breast. Patient motion may cause blurring of the image, so it is especially important that the patient hold still and breathe quietly during scanning. On subtraction imaging, patient motion causes alternating bright and dark bands at fat–glandular tissue interfaces (see Fig. 7-7).

Poor breast tissue enhancement may be due to failed contrast injection, which can be confirmed by abnormal dynamic enhancement curves from the heart. The heart usually shows normal rapid, avid initial enhancement and rapid washout. In fact, one of the most common errors in contrast-enhanced breast MRI is the result of a poor bolus of IV contrast. Sometimes, the IV line is injected slowly or may even become detached from the vein; as a result, the contrast never enters the patient. To ensure rapid uptake of contrast and washout of signal intensity within the heart, one checks a region of interest over the heart or a large artery for a rapid intake bolus and late washout on the kinetic curve. This is important because only a good bolus of contrast will translate into breast cancer enhancing rapidly on the MRI scans. An abnormal or poor cardiac kinetic curve tells the radiologist that something is wrong with the contrast injection; further investigation is needed to determine why contrast in the heart did not rise in signal intensity rapidly and washout as expected. Scans that show poor contrast enhancement in the heart indicate a problem with the contrast injection and cannot be trusted to show cancer in the breast (Fig. 7-8).

Breast Lesions: Approach and Lexicon

Initial studies of contrast-enhanced MRI reported a sensitivity of more than 90% for invasive breast cancer. The sensitivity of contrast enhancement has remained high for invasive breast cancer. However, achieving high specificity remains difficult because some benign breast conditions enhance more avidly than normal breast tissue and may resemble breast cancer. Specifically, benign fibroadenoma, papilloma, and proliferative fibrocystic change also enhance to a greater degree than normal surrounding breast tissue.

To interpret studies of lesions on MRI, radiologists use a combination of high-spatial resolution scanning (which produces sharp images for analysis of abnormally enhancing findings or produces analysis by lesion morphology) and dynamic imaging (which produces the kinetic curves of an abnormally enhancing finding). In addition, T2-weighted imaging plays a secondary role in distinguishing some benign and malignant lesions (Table 7-4).

Morphology

In the high-spatial resolution approach, lesion morphology is evaluated on fat-nulled, 3-D images to look for characteristic shapes, borders, or internal enhancement patterns characteristic of cancer. With this approach, Nunes and colleagues reported a sensitivity of 96% and a specificity of 80% for cancer. Leong and colleagues reported similar results. The morphologic characteristics of benign and malignant lesions are summarized in Table 7-1 and Box 7-6, and are shown in Figure 7-9. As discussed elsewhere in this chapter, the radiologist first decides if the finding is a mass or a nonmasslike enhancement. Consistent with mammography, masses with spiculated or very irregular borders are suspicious. Bright enhancement, particularly rim enhancement and enhancing septations, is usually suspicious for tumor angiogenesis. A ductal, linear, or segmental pattern of clumped enhancement is suspicious for ductal carcinoma in situ (DCIS), but it can also be seen in benign duct ectasia or fibrocystic change. As with mammography, entirely smooth, oval, or lobulated masses oriented parallel to Cooper ligaments suggest benign lesions, whereas lesions traversing Cooper ligaments are abnormal and suggest invasive ductal cancer. Nonenhancing internal septations in smooth, oval, or lobulated masses are highly specific for a benign fibroadenoma. Nonenhancing lesions are also benign. However, it is important to evaluate the dynamic curves of benign-appearing enhancing masses because round or oval homogeneous cancers mimic benign fibroadenomas. Sometimes the suspicious kinetic curves

TABLE 7-4. T2-Weighted Imaging of Breast Lesions

	T2 > Glandular Tissue or Muscle	T2 ≤ Glandular Tissue
Enhances with contrast	Benign (e.g., lymph node)* Papilloma or hyalinized fibroadenoma	Possible cancer
Nonenhancing	Benign (e.g., cyst or duct)	Benign (e.g., sclerotic fibroadenoma or normal glandular tissue)

*The exceptions are rare mucinous carcinomas and some invasive ductal cancers, which may enhance and have high T2 signal; irregular, rim-enhancing morphology and dynamic enhancement curves may help with diagnosis.

BOX 7-6. Morphologic Features of Enhancing Breast Lesions

FEATURES SUGGESTING BENIGNANCY
Minimal enhancement
Smooth or gently lobulated margin
Most intense enhancement at center
Homogeneous enhancement
Nonenhancing internal septations
Oriented along Cooper ligaments

FEATURES SUGGESTING MALIGNANCY
Bright enhancement
Spiculated, very irregular margin
Rim enhancement
Heterogeneous enhancement
Enhancing septations
Ductal/linear-branching/segmental enhancement
Associated enhancement of adjacent tissue region
Enlarged feeding blood vessel

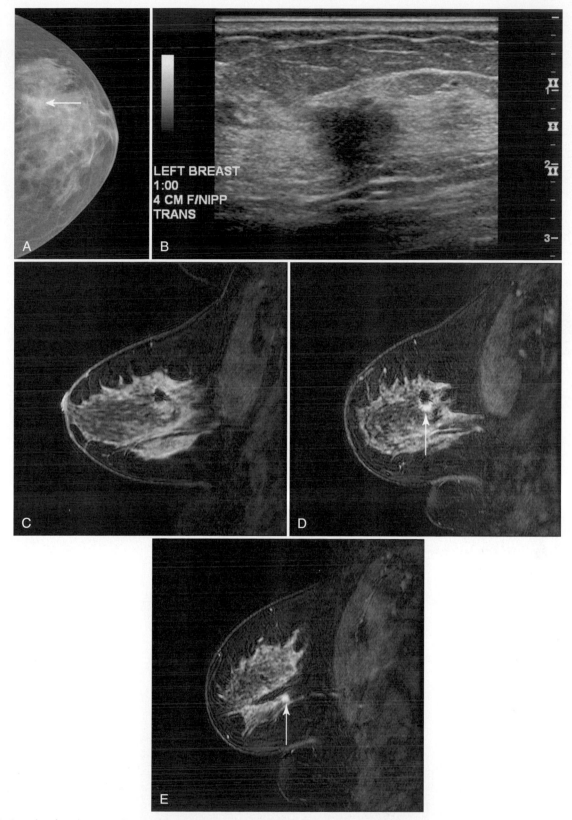

FIGURE 7-8. Invasive ductal cancer (IDC) on ultrasound and signal void on postcontrast sagittal 3-D spectral-spatial excitation magnetization transfer (3DSSMT) magnetic resonance imaging (MRI) scans, missed because of late imaging. **A,** In the outer left breast, a focal asymmetry with possible spiculations (*arrow*) within dense fibroglandular tissue is seen only on the craniocaudal view. **B,** Left breast ultrasound shows a very hypoechoic irregular suspicious breast mass corresponding to the density seen in part **A. C,** Postcontrast sagittal 3DSSMT shows heterogeneously dense breast tissue and marked background enhancement in the left breast. There is signal void from the marker placed in the IDC in the upper breast, but the cancer itself is not seen, possibly obscured by the marker or the surrounding background enhancement. However, it was noted that the scan was delayed and the imaging was done in a later phase approximately 10 minutes after injection. A repeat MRI was done. **D,** Postcontrast sagittal repeat 3DSSMT shows marked background enhancement in the left breast, but because this scan was done at 2½ minutes, it shows an enhancing tumor at the signal void (*arrow*). **E,** In addition, a 6-mm mass is noted inferior to the main cancer; this was not seen previously and was undetectable in the background enhancement (*arrow*).

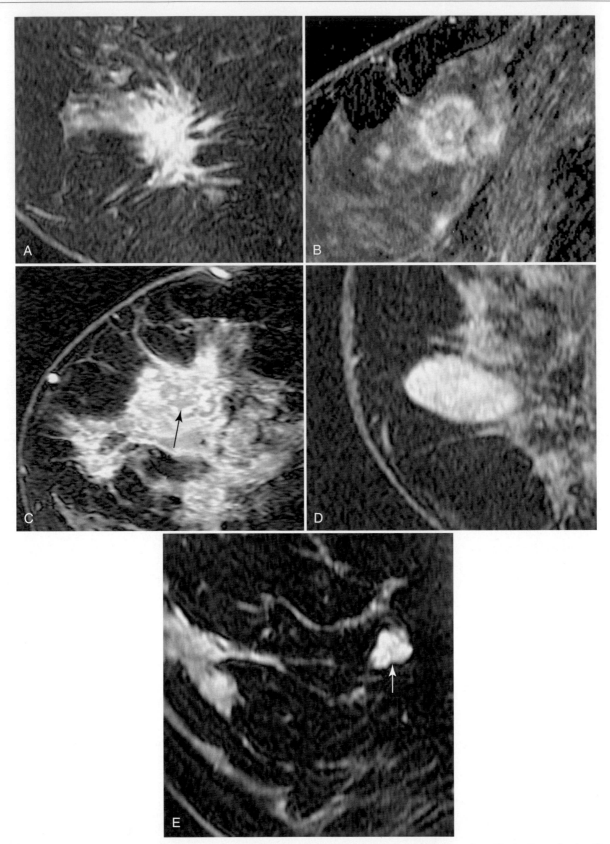

FIGURE 7-9. Morphologic features suggesting malignancy include spiculation (**A**), rim enhancement (**B**, detail from Fig. 7-1B), and enhancing internal septations (**C**, *arrow*). Morphologic features suggesting benignancy include smooth borders (**D**) and nonenhancing internal septations (**E**, *arrow*).

may be the only clue that the morphologically benign mass is a cancer.

Dynamic Contrast Enhancement

In the dynamic MRI approach, one evaluates a lesion's signal intensity as a function of time during the bolus IV administration of contrast material (Box 7-7). The dynamic curves are evaluated according to initial and late enhancement. *Initial enhancement* describes the curve in the first 2 minutes during the bolus or when the curve begins to change. The *late phase of enhancement* occurs after the first 2 minutes or after the curve starts to change. The late-phase curve is described as *persistent, plateau,* or *washout,* in keeping with the ACR BI-RADS® MRI lexicon. The entire spectrum of the time course of enhancement may be categorized from most benign to most suspicious, according to the following scheme of Daniel and colleagues (Fig. 7-10): nonenhancing (type I), gradually enhancing (type II), or rapidly enhancing with a sustained gradual enhancement, plateau, or early washout (types III, IV, and V, respectively). In reference to the curve shapes depicted in Figure 7-7, types I and II typically indicate benignancy and types IV and V indicate a high likelihood of malignancy. Type III curves are indeterminate. Using a similar approach, Kuhl and colleagues reported a sensitivity of 91% and a specificity of 83%. Kuhl type I curves are gradually enhancing with a late persistent plateau. Kuhl type II curves are rapidly enhancing with a late plateau. Kuhl type III curves are rapidly enhancing with a

late rapid washout. There are a few exceptions to these general principles. DCIS may exhibit any of the curve types, including nonenhancing or gradually enhancing curves, shown as types I and II in Figure 7-7. Benign papillomas may exhibit type I, II, III, or even type IV curves shown in Figure 7-7. The geographic distribution of dynamic enhancement also appears to be predictive, with tumors usually enhancing most rapidly at their periphery and benign lesions enhancing most rapidly at the center.

A variety of image-processing techniques have been developed to automate analysis of dynamic images throughout the breast on a pixel-by-pixel basis, including the saturation model, the two-compartment pharmacokinetic model, the "three time point method," and simpler enhancement ratios, wash-in slopes, and washout rates. Stand-alone workstations are available to perform these calculations and produce "functional images" that display abnormal areas of dynamic enhancement on corresponding anatomic images. Most current software determines whether to colorize a lesion based on whether it exceeds a percentage enhancement threshold at approximately 1 minute. The color of the lesion is set to reflect the late enhancement dynamics (i.e., persistent, plateau, and washout).

Not surprisingly, the highest sensitivity and specificity arise when both morphologic information and dynamic enhancement curves are taken into account, with a sensitivity of 95% and a specificity of 86% reported by Daniel and colleagues and a sensitivity of 91% and a specificity of 83% reported by Kinkel and colleagues. Pharmacokinetic scans or physiologic scans are scans that superimpose physiologic information, such as enhancement information, on morphologic images, thereby combining both types of information into one format. This type of scan usually shows the morphologic appearance of a lesion with the physiologic image superimposed in color.

T2-Weighted Imaging

T2-weighted imaging also plays an important role in discriminating which enhancing lesions are likely to be benign or malignant (Fig. 7-11; see also Tables 7-1 and 7-4). Lesions with very high signal, in which the lesion is much brighter than glandular tissue and even higher than fat on nonfat-suppressed T2-weighted FSE images, suggest benign lesions such as cysts, fluid-filled ducts, lymph nodes, or fibroadenomas. Invasive tumor, on the other

---

Box 7-7. Dynamic Contrast Enhancement of Breast Lesions

PATTERNS SUGGESTING BENIGNANCY
No enhancement
Early and late enhancement (persistent, gradual, sustained)
Center enhances first

PATTERNS SUGGESTING MALIGNANCY
Rapid initial enhancement
Late plateau (stable enhancement)
Washout (decreasing late signal intensity)
Periphery enhances first

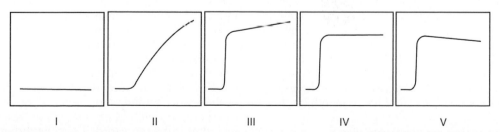

| I | II | III | IV | V |

FIGURE 7-10. Classification of the time course of dynamic contrast enhancement from the most likely benign (type I) through the most likely malignant (type V). No enhancement (type I) or gradual enhancement (type II) suggests a benign lesion. Rapid initial enhancement followed by gradual late enhancement (type III) is indeterminate. Rapid initial enhancement followed by a plateau signal intensity (type IV) or early washout of signal intensity (type V) is suspicious for invasive malignancy. (From Daniel BL, Yen YF, Glover GH, et al: Breast disease: dynamic spiral MR imaging, *Radiology* 209:499–509, 1998.)

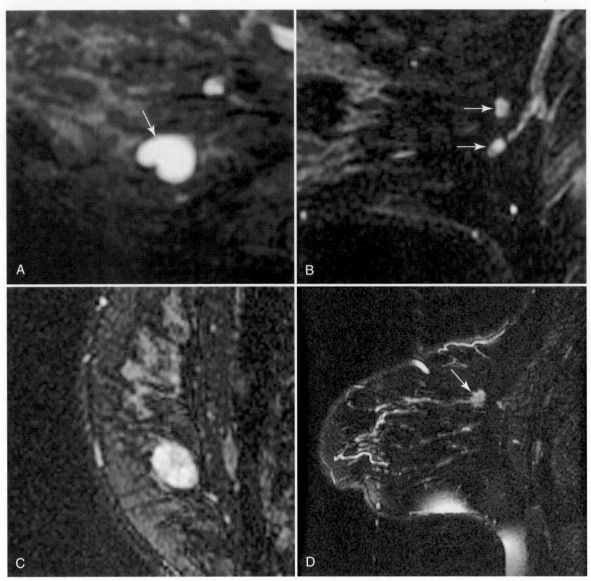

FIGURE 7-11. T2-weighted imaging features of benign and malignant disease. Very high signal on T2-weighted fast spin-echo images that is brighter than fat (on nonfat-suppressed sequences) and substantially brighter than glandular tissue suggests a benign lesion such as a cyst (**A**, *arrow*), intramammary lymph node (**B**, *arrows*), or fibroadenoma (**C**). Low-signal septa are particularly specific for fibroadenoma (see Fig. 7-18A). **D**, Most malignancies, unless frankly necrotic, have a signal intensity that is similar to that of fibroglandular tissue (*arrow*).

hand, usually has a T2 signal similar to that of glandular tissue, that is, higher than muscle but not as high as fluid. Low-signal septations within very high-signal smooth oval or lobulated lesions on T2-weighted imaging also suggest benign fibroadenomas. Exceptions to this "rule" include mucinous cancer, which can be very bright on a T2-weighted image. Some invasive ductal cancers also may be bright on T2-weighted images. These T2-bright cancers may show irregular margins and inhomogeneity; however, it is important to check kinetic curves on all masses because occasionally cancer may be round or oval and have smooth borders.

▬ APPROACH TO INTERPRETATION AND REPORTING OF BREAST MRI

The ACR BI-RADS® provides a valuable standard for the terminology used to analyze breast lesions on MRI (Table

7-5) and is recommended for all breast MRI reporting. First, reporting should include a brief summary of the scan technique, including the scanner, field strength, and pulse sequences used; the specifics of contrast injection; and imaging findings and management recommendations.

To read the MRI, the radiologist reviews the breast history, clinical symptoms, and results of other imaging tests, such as mammogram, ultrasound, and positron emission tomography/computed tomography (Box 7-8). The radiologist then reviews the T1-weighted axial localizer to evaluate any findings outside the breast. These findings can be seen on either coronal or axial scout images, including fat-suppressed T1-weighted noncontrast axial images. Prior studies looking at findings in the thorax or abdomen outside the breast show lymph nodes within the mediastinum, supraclavicular regions, and other areas that the radiologist may not commonly search. Abnormal

TABLE 7-5. American College of Radiology BI-RADS®–MRI Lexicon Terms and Classification Scheme

Lesion type (select one) Focus/foci Mass	Internal Enhancement (Mass and Non-masslike) (select one) Homogeneous (mass) Heterogeneous (mass) Stippled, punctate (non-masslike) Clumped (non-masslike) Reticular, dendritic (non-masslike)
Non-masslike Enhancement Morphology Assessment for Masses (select one in each) *Shape* Round Oval Lobular Irregular	
	Symmetry (use for bilateral scans only) Symmetric Asymmetric
Margin Smooth Irregular Spiculated	Other Findings (report all that apply) Nipple retraction Nipple invasion Precontrast high ductal signal Hematoma/blood Cysts
Enhancement Homogeneous Heterogeneous Rim enhancement Dark internal septation Enhancing internal septation Central enhancement	Skin thickening (focal) Skin thickening (diffuse) Skin invasion Abnormal signal void Edema Lymphadenopathy Pectoralis muscle invasion Chest wall invasion
Non-masslike Enhancement *Distribution Modifiers (select one)* Focal area Linear Ductal Segmental Regional Multiple regions Diffuse	Kinetic Curve Assessment (select one in each) *Initial Rise* Slow Medium Rapid *Delayed Phase* Persistent Plateau Washout

Note: Stippled = nonconfluent < 2 mm dots of enhancement, sand-like. Heterogeneous = confluent and non-confluent, mixed enhancement. Clumped = confluent regions of enhancement, like cobblestones. Homogeneous = confluent, diffuse enhancement.
Reporting of kinetic data should also include the size of the region of interest used to generate the kinetic data and the location (i.e., edge, center, entire lesion), as well as the overall degree of enhancement (i.e., mild, moderate, strong).
Adapted from American College of Radiology: ACR BI-RADS®—MRI, In *ACR Breast Imaging and Reporting and Data System, breast imaging atlas,* Reston, VA, 2003, American College of Radiology.

findings found elsewhere in the body on the breast MRI include lung cancer, bone metastases, liver lesions (most commonly liver cysts or hemangiomas), thyroid masses, and adrenal or renal masses (Fig. 7-12). A systematic search of the T1-weighted axial images and of the thorax (similar to evaluation of computed tomography scans) helps detect unexpected lesions in the thyroid, mediastinum, lungs, liver, spleen, adrenals, kidneys, and the bony thorax.

Most facilities then obtain a T1-weighted precontrast scan, which may be used for subtraction imaging. The T1-weighted precontrast scan provides a source image to let the radiologist know what findings had high signal intensity (sometimes seen in ducts filled with fluid or in blood-filled ducts). In addition, evaluation of the T1-weighted scan allows the radiologist to evaluate shimming of the magnetic field and determine if any abnormally bright areas caused by field inhomogeneity are present.

The radiologist then examines the T2-weighted noncontrast fat-suppressed images to evaluate the bright or high signal intensity findings. This allows the radiologist to see findings that are filled with fluid or have fluid-packed cells, such as cellular fibroadenomas. In addition,

the radiologist can see if fat is present within bright lymph nodes, which helps distinguish them from cancer.

Next, the radiologist looks at imaging findings on the first postcontrast scan. Specifically, the first postcontrast scan should have marked enhancement in the heart, blood vessels, and any rapidly enhancing finding, such as cancer or lymph nodes. The scans are usually obtained with the middle of k-space at approximately 90 seconds after the injection of contrast. The radiologist looks for the whitest part of the image and the background enhancement, which represents enhancement greater than normal background enhancement. Multiple foci in background enhancement represent normal findings; the radiologist judges whether it is normal or abnormal based on morphology, symmetry, kinetics, and change over time (Fig. 7-13). Abnormal enhancement findings would then be classified into either normal findings, for which nothing needs to be done, or abnormal findings, which need to be investigated further.

If the finding needs further investigation, the radiologist then classifies the finding as either a mass or a nonmass. Masses are 3-D objects that have a shape and margin and internal enhancing characteristics. The radiologist

---

BOX 7-8. Organized Approach to Breast MRI Interpretation

Breast history and old imaging reports

Patient breast questionnaire

Scout noncontrast localizer

Review breast and nonbreast anatomy (thyroid, lungs, mediastinum, chest wall, liver, spleen, adrenals, kidneys, bones)

Review axillary lymph nodes (supraclavicular, level I–III, Rotter nodes)

T1-weighted scout noncontrast

T2-weighted scout noncontrast fat-nulled source

First postcontrast scan with fat nulled, suppressed, subtracted

Estimate background enhancement

High signal findings (higher than background)

Region of interest in heart: Check for good IV contrast bolus

If good bolus: check kinetics on important findings

Compare to history, previous MRIs, and other imaging

Report

BOX 7-9. Common False-Positives: Conditions That Simulate Malignancy

Fibrocystic change, hormone-related enhancement, or focal fibrosis, especially if unilateral and regional or if in a ductal/segmental distribution mimicking ductal carcinoma in situ

Radial scar, especially if spiculated and rapidly enhancing

Surgical scar, especially if speculated

Fat necrosis, especially if rim enhancing or lacking macroscopic central fat

Intraductal papilloma, especially if irregular, rapidly enhancing, and not associated with symptoms or a dilated duct

Fibroadenoma, especially if rapidly enhancing (hyalinized) and lacking a high T2 signal

Intramammary lymph node, especially if in an unusual location, lacking a visible fatty hilum, and not associated with a feeding vessel

---

evaluates the mass borders, margins, and enhancing characteristics on the first postcontrast scan, and then evaluates the T2-weighted noncontrast fat-suppressed characteristics of the mass. Last, the radiologist evaluates the kinetic curve and makes a final assessment of the mass's suspicion for breast cancer.

If the finding is a nonmass, it should be further classified using the terms *focus*, *focal area*, *linear*, *ductal*, *segmental*, *regional*, *multiple regions*, or *diffuse enhancement*, as described by the ACR BI-RADS® lexicon (see Table 7-5). The radiologist further evaluates whether the finding is bilaterally symmetric or if it is asymmetric. Asymmetric findings are more likely to be cancer than symmetric findings are. The radiologist then evaluates the pattern of more masslike enhancements because clumped or cobblestonelike enhancement is worrisome for DCIS. In general, DCIS can grow within the ducts and expand them but may not show abnormal kinetic enhancement characteristics. Thus, the radiologist evaluates the nonmasslike enhancement for its kinetic curves. But if the morphology is suspicious, biopsy should be done because DCIS may not show abnormal enhancement kinetics.

Once the radiologist has characterized the finding by its morphology and evaluated its T1 and T2 characteristics, he or she evaluates the kinetic curve characteristics. The radiologist determines the initial signal intensity curve characteristics and classifies it as slow, medium, or fast initial enhancement. They then determine the late signal intensity curve characteristics and classifies them as either continually enhancing (*persistent*), flat (*plateau*), or washout (*washout*).

Table 7-1 shows noncontrast T1 and T2 characteristics of benign and malignant conditions. It also details the

kinetic enhancement features of these conditions. These morphologic, characteristic, and kinetic conditions help distinguish cancer from benign lesions. Cancers are usually dark on both T1 and T2 with an early, rapid enhancement rise and a late plateau or washout. Lymph nodes are typically dark on T1, bright on T2, and also have a rapid initial enhancement and late washout. However, the lymph nodes are usually found in the upper outer quadrant of the breast and have a fatty hilum seen on the T1- and T2-weighted images. A papilloma is indistinguishable from breast cancer and is a common cause for false-positive biopsies. Mucinous cancer is dark on T1 and bright on T2 but can be distinguished from a cellular fibroadenoma by kinetic curves. The mucinous cancer has a rapid initial enhancement and washout in a late phase, whereas the fibroadenoma has a late-phase persistent enhancement curve. Notice that cellular fibroadenomas, mucinous cancer, and cysts are bright on noncontrast T2-weighted scans. However, it is also known that some invasive ductal cancer may be bright on T2-weighted scans, so it is especially important to look at the kinetic curves of any mass. DCIS is mostly detected and diagnosed by its morphology because the kinetic curves in DCIS can be variable.

Last, the radiologist provides a combined report, including an overall assessment of suspicion for cancer (BI-RADS® 036). The report also discusses correlation with any other imaging studies and recommendations for patient management.

Unfortunately, not all benign findings or cancer follow "the rules." Exceptions to the usual enhancement paths are shown in Boxes 7-9 and 7-10.

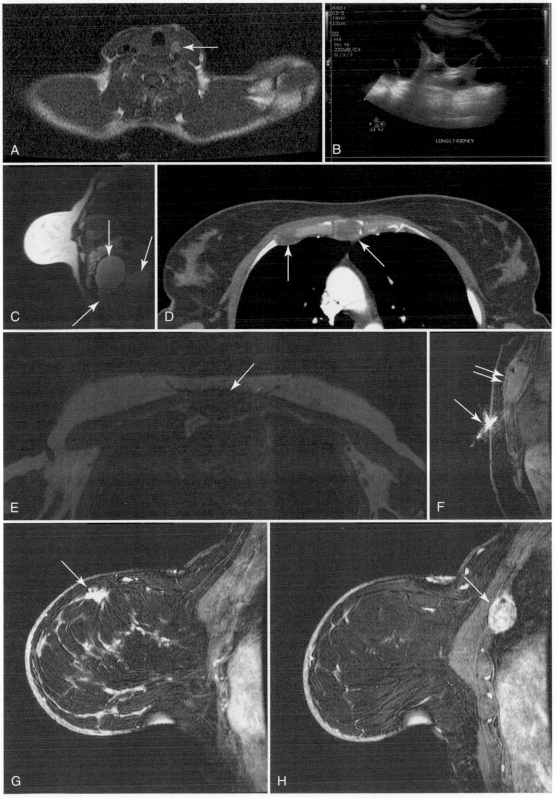

FIGURE 7-12. Incidental findings on breast magnetic resonance imaging (MRI) scans. **A,** Noncontrast T1-weighted MRI to the neck shows a high signal intensity mass in the left thyroid gland (*arrow*). Ultrasound showed colloid cysts in the thyroid. **B,** In another patient with polycystic kidney disease, renal ultrasound showed multiple left kidney cysts. **C,** The sagittal scout image in the patient with polycystic kidney disease shows multiple cysts in the left kidney below the diaphragm (*arrows*). **D,** In a patient with bone metastases, axial computed tomography (CT) scan shows expansive metastases of the sternum and the right rib (*arrows*). **E,** Axial scout localizer for the breast MRI shows the metastasis in the sternum (*arrow*). **F,** Sagittal contrast-enhanced bilateral breast MRI shows enhancement in the metastasis in the sternum with a signal void from a prior biopsy (*double arrows*) and an artifact inferiorly on slides obtained in the midline (*arrow*). **G,** Contrast-enhanced sagittal breast MRI in the same patient shows the spiculated cancer (*arrow*) in the upper right breast. **H,** Sagittal contrast-enhanced breast MRI shows the enhancing right rib metastasis demonstrated on the axial CT scan in part **D.**

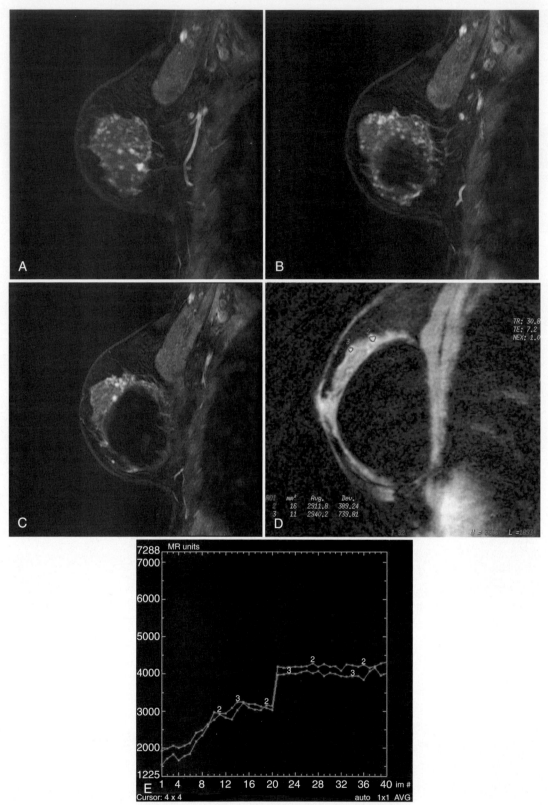

FIGURE 7-13. Normal breast magnetic resonance imaging (MRI) with benign foci and an implant on postcontrast sagittal 3-D spectral-spatial excitation magnetization transfer MRI scans. **A,** Sagittal postcontrast MRI shows multiple round nonspecific foci within dense fibroglandular tissue. **B** and **C,** Other foci are present around the implant on additional slices. **D,** Regions of interest (ROI) on other similar foci on spiral dynamics scans. **E,** Kinetic curves show slow initial enhancement and late plateau of the ROI shown in part **D,** suggestive of benign disease.

BOX 7-10. Common False-Negative Tumors on Breast MRI

Nonenhancing ductal carcinoma in situ (DCIS)
Nonenhancing invasive lobular carcinoma
Smoothly marginated mucinous tumor with bright T2 signal mimicking a fibroadenoma
Residual poorly enhancing tumor, especially DCIS during or after chemotherapy
Gradually enhancing tumor surrounded by simultaneous vigorous background enhancement (e.g., from scanning at the wrong time in the menstrual cycle)

Breast MRI Atlas

Table 7-6 shows a simplified guide to breast MRI interpretation.

Benign Breast Conditions

Fluid-filled cysts and milk ducts are normal and occur frequently (Fig. 7-14). Simple cysts are round or oval with sharp margins. Adjacent cysts may be separated by thin, low-signal septations. Simple cysts have very high T2 signal and display no internal enhancement with contrast, although a faint thin rim of gradual enhancement may be seen on high-resolution images. Occasionally, benign cysts may demonstrate high signal on unenhanced T1-weighted images, with corresponding lower signal on T2-weighted images, presumably because of their protein content. Dilated fluid-filled ducts are linear, radiate from the nipple, and may branch. Their signal and enhancement characteristics are the same as for cysts.

TABLE 7-6. Simplified Breast MRI Interpretation*

	Signal Intensity			Contrast-Enhanced Imaging				
	T1	T2	ADC	Cho	Overall Intensity	Dynamic Pattern: Early/Late	Margin	Internal	Distribution
Invasive ductal carcinoma†	−	−−		+	+++	Rapid/washout or plateau	Rim spiculated or irregular	Heterogeneous; enhancing septae	Mass May have associated segmental enhancement or large vessels
Invasive lobular carcinoma				+	Variable	Variable			Nonmasslike or mass
Mucinous carcinoma		+++	++	+	+	Variable	Rim or irregular		
Ductal carcinoma in situ			−	+	+			Clumped and/or periductal enhancement	Segmental, linear, branching, ductal
Fibroadenoma, hyalinized		+++	+		+++	Rapid/persistent	Smooth	Nonenhancing septae‡	Along Cooper ligaments
Fibroadenoma, sclerotic		−			−	Gradual/persistent	Smooth	Nonenhancing septae‡	Along Cooper ligaments
Cyst	−− or +	+++	++	−	−	None	Smooth		
Duct ectasia	−− or +	+++	+	−	−	−	−		Ductal
Fibrocystic change					Variable	Gradual/persistent	Variable		
Lymph node		++			++	Rapid/washout	Smooth	Central fatty hilum	Along vessels in the upper outer quadrant
Surgical scar					Variable	Gradual/persistent	Irregular		
Postoperative seroma		++	++	−	−		Rim	None	
Fat necrosis					++	Variable	Rim	Central fat	
Intraductal papilloma					++	Variable	Variable	[small]	Associated fluid-filled duct

*The prototype features of common breast conditions (not all features are always present in all lesions).
†Rare bright T2 signal in invasive ductal cancer.
‡Rare; in 20% of cases.
+, increased; ++, moderately increased; +++, markedly increased; −, decreased; −−, moderately decreased; −−−, markedly decreased; ADC, apparent diffusion coefficient; Cho, choline.

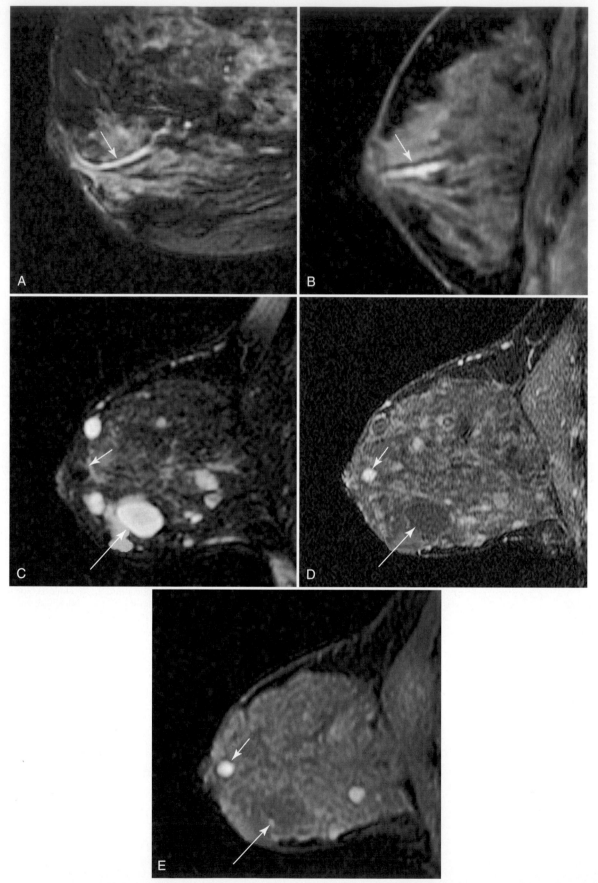

FIGURE 7-14. Normal variants. **A,** Dilated milk ducts cause linear high signal extending from the nipple (*arrow*) on fat-suppressed T2-weighted fast spin-echo images. **B,** Ducts may also demonstrate high signal (*arrow*) on unenhanced T1-weighted images and variable signal on T2-weighted images, presumably because of the high protein content. Unlike ductal carcinoma in situ (see Fig. 7-25), they do not enhance with contrast. **C,** Benign cysts cause focal, well-circumscribed high signal (*large arrow*) on T2-weighted images. **D,** Normal benign cysts do not enhance, but they may be surrounded by a faint rim of gradual enhancement (*large arrow*). **E,** Like ducts, some benign cysts may appear bright (*small arrow*) on unenhanced T1-weighted images.

Hormone-related enhancement occurs in premenopausal women and women taking oral contraceptives (Fig. 7-15), and is a cause for normal background enhancement, which on occasion may be moderate or marked. Usually, diffuse gradual glandular enhancement is seen, and it is commonly bilateral and symmetric. Dynamic enhancement is generally gradual and progressive (Daniel type II, III; Kuhl type I); thus, the appearance is rarely confused with invasive carcinoma on dynamic imaging. Less commonly, hormone-related enhancement may be focal (see Fig. 7-15) and may resemble lobular carcinoma or DCIS. Hormone-related enhancement is minimized by scanning during the second week of a woman's menstrual cycle.

Fibrocystic change is commonly associated with focal (geographic) or regional nonspecific enhancement, especially in premenopausal women (Fig. 7-16), with gradual early enhancement, and with sustained gradual late enhancement. Occasionally, a specific diagnosis can be made by the presence of tiny associated microcysts (see Fig. 7-16). Adjacent cysts do not necessarily exclude carcinoma, however, so careful scrutiny of all enhancing foci remains essential to exclude concurrent malignancy.

Intramammary lymph nodes are common, especially in the upper outer quadrant and along blood vessels (Fig. 7-17). Typically, intramammary nodes are small (≤5 mm) and have uniform high T2 signal. They are sharply circumscribed oval or kidney bean-shaped masses that have a central fatty hilum. On dynamic imaging, they enhance avidly and rapidly, with a rapid initial enhancement and a late-phase plateau or early washout, and hence cannot be distinguished from malignancy based on dynamic criteria alone. However, a definitive diagnosis is usually possible when lesion morphology shows their fatty hilum and close proximity to blood vessels with a "grapes on a vine" appearance. Correlation with sonography may avoid biopsy in cases in which location or morphologic criteria remain inconclusive. MRI is not as reliable as sentinel node sampling in determining the presence or absence of intranodal metastases. Abnormal lymph nodes become rounder, enlarge from prior studies, and lose their fatty hilum. Lymphadenopathy can also be diagnosed when the node becomes completely replaced by metastases and becomes dark (instead of light) on T2.

Fibroadenoma is usually an oval or macrolobulated, sharply marginated, avidly and uniformly enhancing mass (Figs. 7-18 and 7-19). Young cellular fibroadenomas are very bright on noncontrast fat-suppressed T2-weighted scans. Later sclerotic fibroadenomas may be dark on T2-weighted scans. Nonenhancing internal septations are seen occasionally in about 20% of benign cellular fibroadenomas. Of note, nonenhancing internal septations may very rarely be seen in mucinous cancer, so kinetic curves on benign appearing masses should be evaluated to distinguish fibroadenomas from T2-bright mucinous or ductal cancer. On dynamic imaging, most fibroadenomas show early gradual enhancement with sustained late gradual enhancement. Young fibroadenomas may have a more rapidly enhancing curve with sustained late-phase gradual enhancement, and they may occasionally demonstrate a late plateau of signal intensity that overlaps with the appearance of some invasive carcinomas. However, unlike

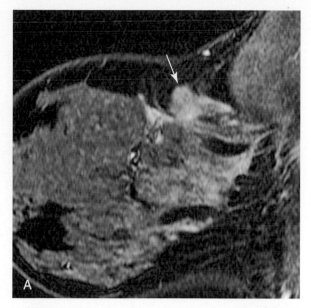

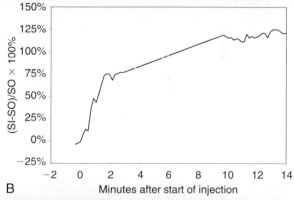

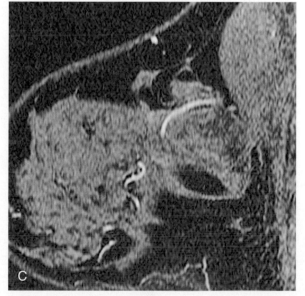

FIGURE 7-15. Hormone-related enhancement. Normal menstrual cycle variations may cause fibroglandular enhancement. **A,** Although hormone-related enhancement is usually mild and diffuse, it may occasionally cause focal intense enhancement that can simulate disease (*arrow*). Even though the persistent late enhancement suggested a benign etiology (**B**), repeat breast magnetic resonance imaging was performed during the second week of the menstrual cycle (**C**) and showed that all previous findings had resolved and were hence presumably related to menstrual cycle variations.

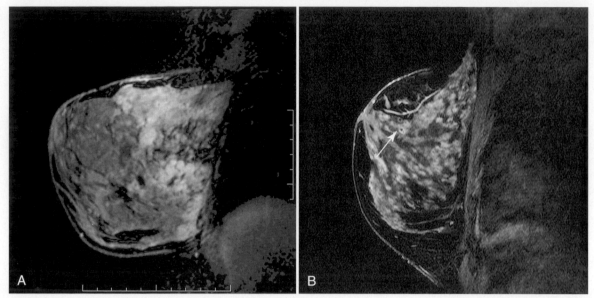

FIGURE 7-16. Fibrocystic change. **A,** Geographic, regional, or diffuse glandular enhancement can be seen in patients with fibrocystic change. **B,** Although variable in appearance, the diagnosis is most readily established when small nonenhancing cysts are scattered throughout the lesion (*arrow*). (**A,** From American College of Radiology: ACR BI-RADS®—MRI, ed 4, In *ACR Breast Imaging and Reporting and Data System, breast imaging atlas,* Reston, VA, 2003, American College of Radiology.)

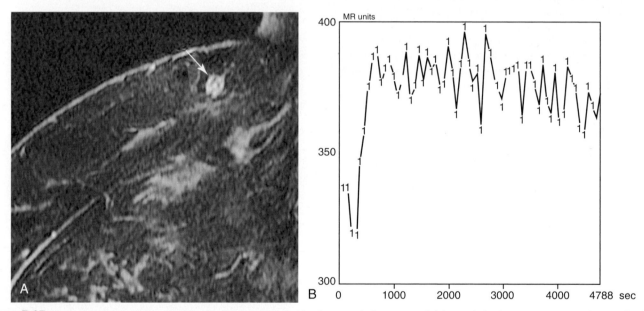

FIGURE 7-17. Intramammary lymph node. Usually small and located in close proximity to superficial vessels in the upper outer quadrant and axillary tail of the breast, lymph nodes demonstrate high signal on T2-weighted images (see Fig. 7-11B). **A,** All lymph nodes enhance rapidly and brightly with contrast (*arrow*), usually with a Daniel type IV or type V time course of enhancement (**B**). A normal fatty hilum can cause central low signal on fat-suppressed or subtracted images that mimics rim enhancement.

many invasive carcinomas, the earliest, most avid enhancement is frequently central rather than peripheral. Among rapidly enhancing well-circumscribed masses, very high T2 signal is suggestive of benign fibroadenoma; the lack of very high T2 signal implies that malignancy cannot be excluded. The rare, well-differentiated phyllodes tumor has an appearance similar to that of fibroadenomas. Degenerating fibroadenomas, seen in older patients, do not enhance significantly and may have irregular internal signal voids that correspond to the large, coarse "popcorn" calcifications seen mammographically.

Intraductal papilloma has a wide variety of appearances. On MRI, a papilloma may have a round masslike structure that has a rapid enhancement initial rise and washout in a late phase that is indistinguishable from breast cancer. Before MRI, most papillomas were identified by the presence of abnormal nipple discharge, an intraductal filling defect on galactography, or an intraductal mass on ultrasound. The analogous "classic" findings on MRI are an avidly enhancing mass at the posterior end of a fluid-filled duct (Fig. 7-20). However, a fluid-filled duct is not necessarily present in all cases, and dynamic enhancement spans

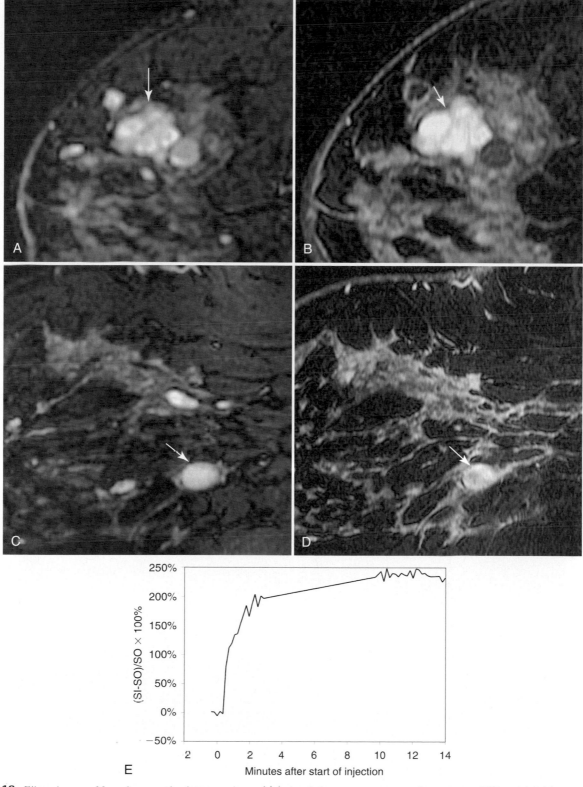

FIGURE 7-18. Fibroadenoma. Note the smooth, sharp margins and lobulated shape on precontrast, fat-suppressed T2-weighted images (**A**, *arrow*) and on contrast-enhanced, water-specific 3-D spectral-spatial excitation magnetization transfer gradient echo images (**B**, *arrow*). The low-signal septations (**A**) that do not enhance (**B**) are particularly specific for fibroadenoma. Frequently, magnetic resonance imaging (MRI) findings are less specific, as in this different case (**C** and **D**), which reveals an ovoid, well-circumscribed high-signal mass on T2-weighted imaging (**C**, *arrow*) that enhances very strongly (**D**, *arrow*) but without specific low-signal septations. **E**, The time course of enhancement is typically rapid initial enhancement followed by sustained late enhancement. MRI-guided core biopsy revealed fibroadenoma.

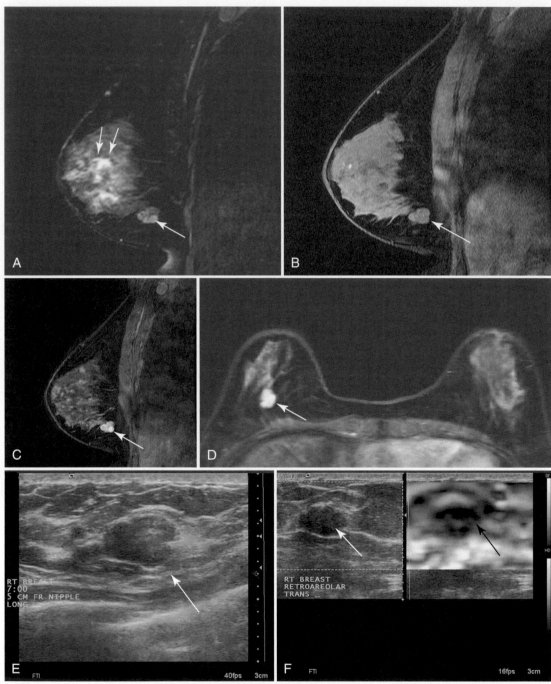

FIGURE 7-19. A, T2-weighted sagittal noncontrast magnetic resonance imaging (MRI) shows a lobulated mass with high signal intensity (*arrow*) in the lower breast and fluid in benign breast ducts (*double arrows*). Noncontrast (**B**) and postcontrast (**C**) sagittal 3-D spectral-spatial excitation magnetization transfer (3DSSMT) MRIs show a lobulated enhancing mass in the lower left breast that is slightly inhomogeneous but has smooth borders (*arrow*). **D,** Axial reconstruction of the 3DSSMT contrast-enhanced breast MRI shows the mass in the lower breast near the chest wall (*arrow*). Enhancement kinetics showed a slow uptake and late persistent curve, suggesting a benign finding. Because the patient had a history of breast cancer, she desired a biopsy of the mass. **E,** Second-look ultrasound of the breast shows an oval lobulated homogeneous mass (*arrow*) in the area of the MRI-detected mass. **F,** B-mode (*left image*) and elastography (*right image*) ultrasound images show that the mass (*arrow*) is about the same size on the strain view, suggesting a benign finding. Biopsy showed fibroadenoma.

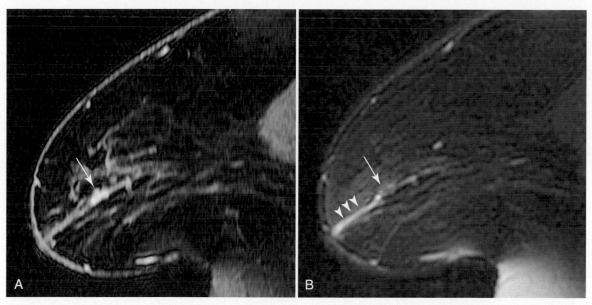

FIGURE 7-20. Intraductal papilloma. **A,** Contrast-enhanced, fat-suppressed, T1-weighted, 3-D gradient echo MRI revealed a small, avidly enhancing retroareolar mass (*arrow*). **B,** A fluid-filled duct (*arrowheads*) extended to the mass (*arrow*) on precontrast, fat-suppressed T2-weighted images. Papillomas may enhance with any time course, including a rapid initial rise with a plateau mimicking invasive carcinoma. This is the classic appearance of intraductal papilloma, although not all papillomas demonstrate all these features. (From Daniel BL, Gardner RW, Birdwell RL, et al: Magnetic resonance imaging of intraductal papilloma of the breast, *Magn Reson Imaging* 21:887–892, 2003.)

the entire range from nonenhancing to washout curves that mimic invasive carcinoma.

Postoperative changes include seroma, hematoma, scar, and fat necrosis. A careful breast history analysis usually enables distinction of these postbiopsy findings from primary breast lesions. Seroma and hematoma resemble cysts with variable intrinsic signal intensity, but they may have more irregular margins. Uniform rimlike enhancement occurs normally; peripheral nodular enhancement suggests residual tumor in the setting of pathologically transected margins. Scars and fat necrosis do not usually enhance beyond 2 years. Fat necrosis is typically manifested as irregular rimlike enhancement surrounding nonenhancing tissue that is identical to fat on all sequences.

Breast Cancers

Invasive ductal carcinoma (IDC) is virtually always manifested as a focal, avidly enhancing mass, which is often irregular but may have any shape. Margins are usually irregular or spiculated (Fig. 7-21), but IDC may be more sharply defined or smooth in some cases. Rim enhancement and enhancing internal septations are particularly suspicious. Dynamic imaging reveals rapid initial enhancement followed by a plateau or early washout of signal intensity and is frequently most worrisome at the periphery of the lesion. T2 signal is similar to that of breast tissue; the lack of high signal distinguishes IDC from benign intramammary lymph nodes and fibroadenomas. However, there are some T2-bright cancers (mucinous cancers and some invasive ductal cancers), so kinetic evaluation is important. True central nonenhancing necrosis is rare. Direct skin or muscle invasion, growth of the tumor through Cooper ligaments, and architectural distortion are secondary signs of carcinoma; axillary lymph nodes that

have become rounder and lost their fatty hila are worrisome for lymphadenopathy (Fig. 7-22).

Infiltrating lobular carcinoma (ILC) has a much more variable appearance than IDC does. A particularly unique appearance is enhancement that follows the course of normal fibroglandular elements without a substantial mass effect (Fig. 7-23), which may lead to a missed diagnosis. ILC can also appear as a solitary mass or a combination of multiple masses with or without enhancing intervening fibroglandular tissue. Rarely, ILC may not enhance enough to be distinguished from surrounding breast tissue. On dynamic imaging, lobular carcinoma may have any pattern; benign patterns of dynamic curves, such as either slow or rapid initial enhancement with sustained late-phase gradual enhancement, do not exclude lobular carcinoma.

Mucinous carcinoma, a rare breast cancer, is a round mass that may have a unique appearance on MRI (Fig. 7-24). The large central pool of mucin does not enhance and has very high T2 signal. Thus, mucinous carcinoma resembles a cyst, but with an irregular, thickened, avidly enhancing rim. Breast abscess may have a similar appearance. Alternatively, it may have irregular internal enhancement.

DCIS has a very wide range of appearances on MRI. The "classic" description is clumped enhancement in a ductal system distribution, including segmental enhancement, or linear/branching enhancement emanating from the nipple (Fig. 7-25). Ductal enhancement per se is present in only a minority of cases. An especially worrisome sign for DCIS includes *clumped enhancement*, which represents enhancement tumor following the duct, simulating a string of pearls or cobblestone appearance. This is due to the cancer growing and expanding the ductal system, without penetrating the duct basement membrane.

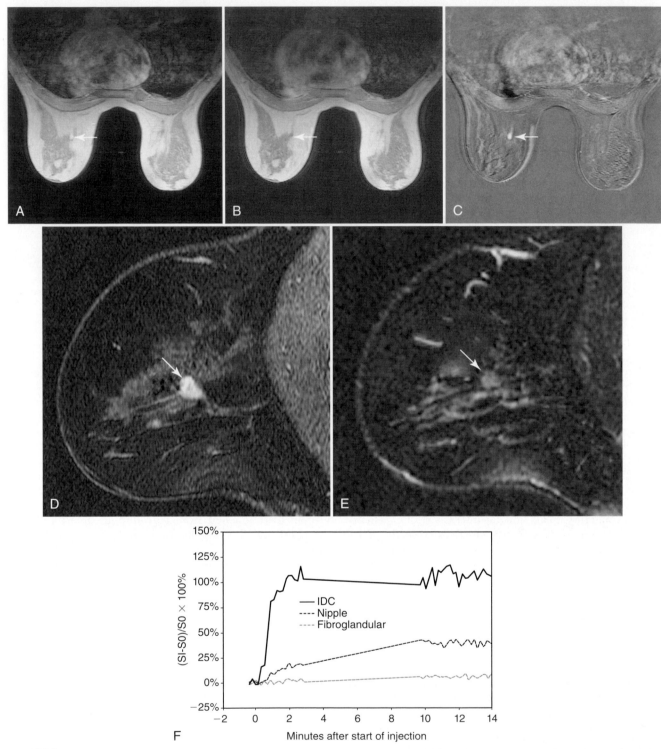

FIGURE 7-21. Invasive ductal carcinoma (IDC). Screening breast magnetic resonance imaging (MRI) using bilateral, dynamic, two-dimensional spoiled gradient echo images revealed focal enhancement (*arrow*) on the initial postcontrast scan (**A**) not seen on the precontrast scan (**B**). **C,** Subtraction processing confirms the suspicious enhancement (*arrow*). **D,** Repeat unilateral, water-specific, high-spatial resolution, contrast-enhanced 3-D gradient echo MRI confirmed the enhancement and revealed suspicious rim enhancement and irregular margins (*arrow*). **E,** The lesion did not have high signal on T2-weighted MRI (*arrow*). **F,** On dynamic imaging, the lesion enhanced intensely and rapidly, with a subsequent plateau of signal intensity.

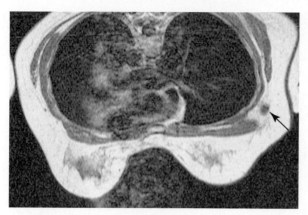

FIGURE 7-22. Enlarged axillary lymph node. T1-weighted, precontrast spin-echo images reveal a 15-mm right axillary soft-tissue mass corresponding to an abnormally enlarged lymph node (*arrow*). Note the absence of a normal fatty hilum. Although magnetic resonance imaging (MRI) may reveal grossly metastatic nodes, as in this case, a normal appearance on MRI does not exclude micrometastases; the sensitivity of MRI is inferior to that of sentinel node sampling.

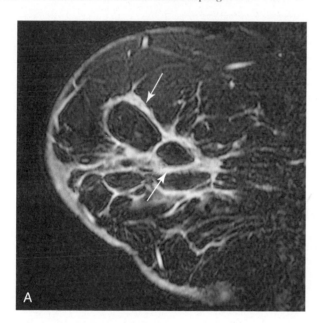

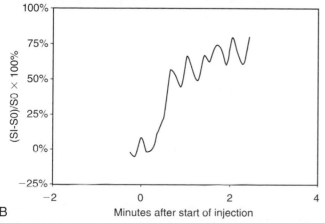

FIGURE 7-23. Infiltrating lobular carcinoma. **A,** Contrast-enhanced, water-selective, 3-D gradient echo images reveal enhancement along the normal fibroglandular elements (*arrows*), without a significant mass effect, findings corresponding to the infiltrating pattern of spread. **B,** Initial enhancement is rapid but is followed by sustained late enhancement.

DCIS also can be manifested as a focal area of clumped enhancement, as a focal mass, as geographic nonspecific enhancement, or even as enhancement indistinguishable from other breast tissue. Dynamic enhancement is also unreliable. DCIS usually enhances with a nonspecific rapid initial enhancement and a sustained gradual enhancement curve. However, any curve type can be seen, including no enhancement or suspicious rapid initial enhancement with a late-phase plateau or early washout. Thus, DCIS may resemble focal fibrocystic change, hormone-related enhancement, intraductal papilloma, or even invasive carcinoma. When associated with an invasive tumor, DCIS commonly appears as a surrounding wedge of enhancing tissue that has a less worrisome dynamic enhancement curve than do invasive tumors. Calcifications cannot be reliably assessed with MRI, and thus mammographic correlation remains essential when attempting to determine the extent or presence of disease. Of note, between 25% and 40% of DCIS may be diagnosed only by pleomorphic calcifications seen on mammography in DCIS that is invisible on the contrast-enhanced MRI. Thus, it is important to biopsy pleomorphic calcifications if they are of concern for cancer because they may be the only sign of malignancy.

Diagnostic Limitations

Although the sensitivity of MRI is very high for invasive carcinoma, significantly higher than mammography or sonography in some settings, substantial diagnostic challenges remain (see Boxes 7-9 and 7-10). Common false positives mimicking DCIS include focal fibrocystic change, hormone-related enhancement, focal fibrosis, and fibroadenomatous change. False positives occasionally mimicking invasive carcinomas include rapidly enhancing intraductal papillomas, avidly enhancing fibroadenomas lacking high T2 signal, intramammary lymph nodes without a fatty hilum, rim-enhancing fat necrosis, radial scar, and enhancing spiculated surgical scars. False negatives remain rare; they are usually due to nonenhancing DCIS or ILC. Recent or ongoing chemotherapy may also reduce the sensitivity of contrast-enhanced MRI.

Small incidental enhancing lesions (IELs) are foci that are smaller than 5 mm, difficult to characterize, and common. Investigators vary in the level of concern they attribute to these lesions. Regardless of size, an initial attempt should be made to characterize each lesion's morphology, dynamic enhancement, and T2 signal because invasive carcinomas, fibroadenoma, and papilloma can also be very small. However, biopsy of an IEL frequently reveals no identifiable explanation. A practical approach to management is to use both the character of individual lesions along with their number and distribution, as well as the patient's clinical setting to determine whether biopsy or follow-up MRI should be performed. In patients at very high risk for occult breast malignancy, such as those with known axillary nodal metastases and normal mammograms and physical examination, even a single relatively nonspecific IEL that is the dominant abnormality in the breast may be the index tumor and should prompt biopsy. In patients with lower risk, multiple bilateral,

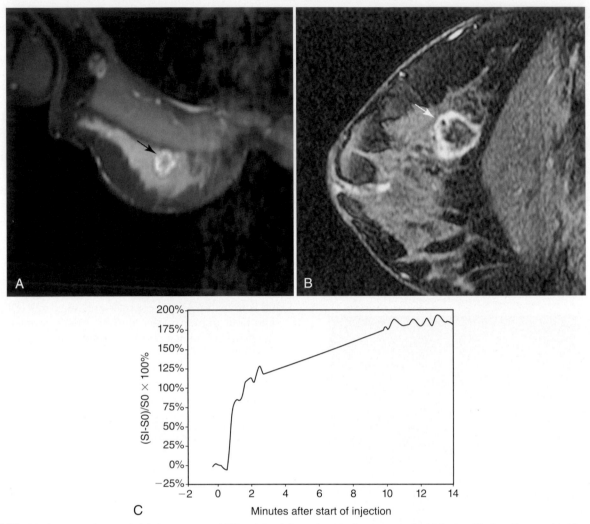

FIGURE 7-24. Mucinous carcinoma. Axial, fat-suppressed T2-weighted fast spin-echo images reveal a high-signal lesion (**A**, *arrow*) with surrounding rim enhancement (*arrow*) on sagittal water-specific 3-D gradient echo images (**B**). **C**, Although the dynamic enhancement of the rim is indeterminate, the nodularity and irregular thickness of the rim are incompatible with a simple cyst. Biopsy revealed invasive carcinoma with mucinous features.

diffusely scattered, nonspecific small IELs have been successfully managed with serial MRI to document stability.

▬ INDICATIONS

Large-scale randomized, controlled trials, similar to the early mammography studies, have not been reported to support the widespread general use of contrast-enhanced breast MRI at this time. However, utility has been demonstrated by smaller studies in many specific situations (Box 7-11).

Screening

Improvements in genetic testing and counseling are identifying an increasing population of women who are at increased risk for the development of breast cancer. Current options include routine clinical and imaging screening with mammography or ultrasound and prophylactic mastectomy. MRI has recently been investigated as an adjunct to conventional imaging for screening. In one of the largest U.S. studies, Morris and colleagues detected 14 tumors in 367 *BRCA1* and *BRCA2* mutation carriers, individuals with a similar risk profile and negative initial mammograms (Fig. 7-26). This led to the 2007 recommendation by the American Cancer Society for cancer screening with MRI in the United States in women with a greater than 20% lifetime risk of breast cancer and in patients who have a history of treated Hodgkin disease (Table 7-7). Optimal MRI screening intervals and the age at which MRI screening should be initiated have yet to be determined.

Women without a documented increased risk for breast cancer benefit less from MRI because the rate of false-positive abnormalities may substantially exceed the rate at which cancers are found; further investigation of these false-positive results may subject these women to significant morbidity. Patients with a history of direct free silicone injections of the breast for augmentation, however, cannot undergo any other type of screening (i.e., clinical breast examination, mammography, or sonography) with

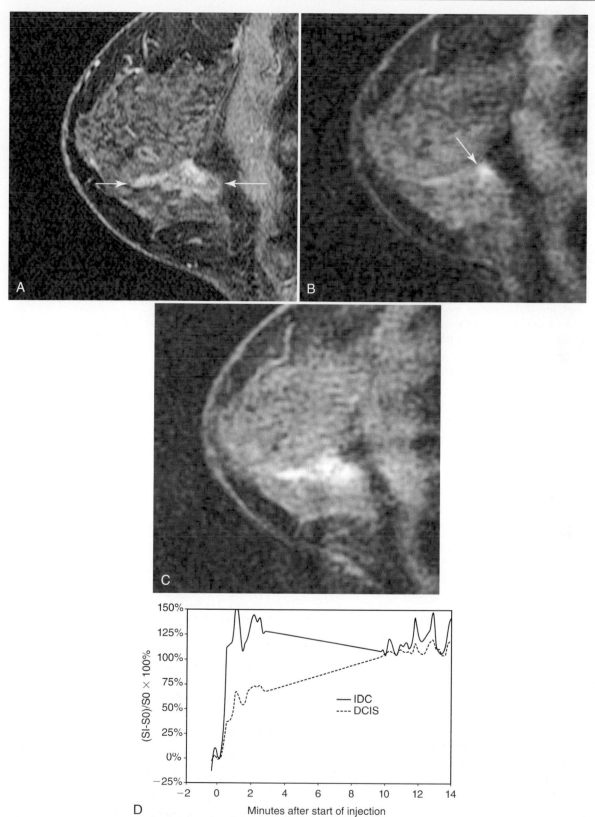

FIGURE 7-25. Ductal carcinoma in situ (DCIS). **A,** Sagittal high-spatial resolution water-selective 3-D magnetic resonance imaging (MRI) reveals enhancement in a segmental distribution corresponding to one ductal system (*arrows*). **B,** Dynamic 3-D spiral MRI reveals a small focus that enhanced on the initial images (*arrow*) sooner than the rest of the lesion, which enhanced on later images (C). **D,** This small focus, which had a washout curve, proved to be a 4-mm focus invasive ductal carcinoma within the DCIS. IDC, invasive ductal carcinoma.

Box 7-11. Accepted Indications for Contrast-Enhanced Breast MRI

SCREENING

ACS recommendations*

BRCA mutation (*BRCA1* or *BRCA2*)

First-degree relative of *BRCA* carrier, but untested

Lifetime risk of approximately 20% to 25% or greater, as defined by BRCAPRO or other models that are largely dependent on family history

Obscured breast tissue (e.g., previous free silicone injection)

Radiation to chest between age 10 and 30 (e.g., for Hodgkin disease)

Li-Fraumeni syndrome (*p53* mutation) and first-degree relatives

Cowden and Bannayan-Riley-Ruvalcaba syndromes and first-degree relatives

DIAGNOSIS

Suspicious lesions seen on only one x-ray mammographic view, not found by sonography

Bloody nipple discharge with negative or failed galactogram

Indeterminate palpable findings with negative mammogram and ultrasound[†]

STAGING

Locate the breast primary in patients with axillary metastases

Detect chest wall invasion

Evaluate opposite breast in patients with new, unilateral breast cancer

Evaluate the extent of cancer in patients with poorly evaluated breast tissue on mammography:

    Dense breasts

    Implants, free silicone injection

Evaluate the extent of cancer in tumors poorly seen on mammography:[†]

    Infiltrating lobular carcinoma

Ductal carcinoma in situ without corresponding microcalcifications

Goals of breast cancer staging MRI:

Plan lumpectomy to reduce the rate of transected tumor at specimen margins

    Detect occult multifocal or multicentric tumor

    Detect occult contralateral tumor

    Detect residual disease when initial lumpectomy is incomplete

MANAGEMENT (ESPECIALLY PATIENTS UNDERGOING NEOADJUVANT CHEMOTHERAPY)

Measure disease before initiating neoadjuvant chemotherapy.

Assess response to treatment after the initial cycle.

Localize potential residual tumor after a complete clinical response.

*Data from Saslow D, Boetes C, Burke W, et al: American Cancer Society guidelines for breast screening with MRI as an adjunct to mammography, *CA Cancer J Clin* 57:75–89, 2007, Table 1.

[†]Some indications are more controversial.

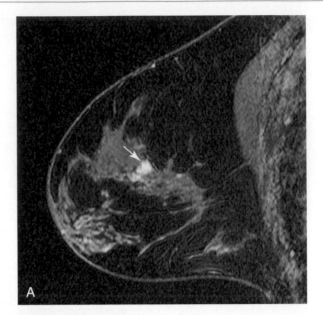

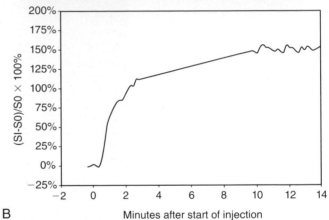

FIGURE 7-26. Ductal carcinoma in situ (DCIS) detected on screening magnetic resonance imaging (MRI). MRI was performed after genetic testing revealed a suspicious *BRCA1* mutation. **A,** An 8-mm focal area of enhancement was noted with irregular margins on high-spatial resolution MRI (*arrow*). **B,** Dynamic imaging demonstrated a nonspecific enhancement curve. Pathologic examination revealed a 6.9-cm region of high-grade comedo DCIS.

confidence and hence may be appropriate screening subjects when counseled accordingly about the risks associated with false-positive lesions.

Diagnosis

MRI is infrequently used to diagnose equivocal findings on mammography, sonography, or physical examination because the cost of MRI, including follow-up MRI, approaches the cost of the more traditional minimally invasive core biopsy. However, in rare instances, lesions are found that are not amenable to conventional biopsy, such as suspicious findings seen on only one mammographic view (Fig. 7-27). MRI is also used to evaluate patients with persistent bloody or cytologically abnormal nipple discharge in whom conventional galactography and ductoscopy were either unrevealing or unsuccessful. In addition, MRI is used to evaluate patients with equivocal findings

TABLE 7-7. Evidence for Breast MRI Screening Among High-Risk Women: Large Trials

Study	n	Sensitivity		Positive Predictive Value for MRI	Stage of MRI-Positive, X-Ray–Negative Tumors					
					Size			Nodes		
		X-Ray	MRI		TIS	T1	≥T2	N0	N1	N2/N3
Netherlands[1]	1909	40%	71%	7%	1	11*	8*	19	1†	
Canada[2]	236	36%	77%	46%	3	9	2	7		1
United Kingdom[3]	649	40%	77%	10%	0	15	4	13	1	1
Germany[4]	529	33%	91%	50%	5	14	0	19		
United States[5]	390	25%	100%	13%	1	2		3		

Results aggregated from Saslow D, Boetes C, Burke W, et al: American Cancer Society guidelines for breast screening with MRI as an adjunct to mammography, *CA Cancer J Clin* 57:75–89, 2007 and the individually cited references.
[1]Kriege M, Brekelmans CT, Boetes C, et al: Efficacy of MRI and mammography for breast-cancer screening in women with a familial or genetic predisposition, *N Engl J Med* 351:427–437, 2004.
[2]Warner E, Plewes DB, Shumak RS, et al: Comparison of breast magnetic resonance imaging, mammography, and ultrasound for surveillance of women at high risk for hereditary breast cancer, *J Clin Oncol* 19:3524–3531, 2001.
[3]Leach MO, Boggis CR, Dixon AK, et al: Screening with magnetic resonance imaging and mammography of a UK population at high familial risk of breast cancer: a prospective multicentre cohort study (MARIBS), Lancet 365:1769–1778, 2005.
[4]Kuhl CK, Schrading S, Leutner CC, et al: Mammography, breast ultrasound, and magnetic resonance imaging for surveillance of women at high familial risk for breast cancer, *J Clin Oncol* 23:8469–8476, 2005.
[5]Lehman CD, Blume JD, Thickman D, et al: Added cancer yield of MRI in screening the contralateral breast of women recently diagnosed with breast cancer: results from the International Breast Magnetic Resonance Consortium (IBMC) trial, *J Surg Oncol* 92:9–16, 2005.
*Netherlands trial[1] did not use the AJCC size threshold of "≤2 cm" to define T1 invasive tumors. Instead they reported that "11 of 19 invasive tumors [detected by MRI but missed by x-ray mammography] were smaller than 10 mm."
†This study reported that "only 1 [of the 20 tumors found only by MRI] was associated with a positive node." The number of positive nodes in this one case was not reported.

on physical examination that are mammographically and sonographically occult. However, the potential for false-positive and equivocal findings that generate biopsy or follow-up MRI must be balanced against the accuracy of simple palpation-based biopsy in this setting.

Staging

MRI is frequently used preoperatively to image the extent of biopsy-proven breast cancer, especially in patients contemplating breast-conserving therapy. Controversy exists over whether all patients who have breast cancer should undergo breast MRI as part of the staging process. In fact, several articles indicate that the MRI may cause false-positive biopsies as well as fail to improve the resection rate at the first surgery. However, although not routinely indicated as part of the local staging process in all newly diagnosed carcinomas, MRI is commonly used in selected subgroups, including the following:

- Patients with biopsy-proven axillary lymph node metastases of breast cancer origin and normal mammograms and ultrasound (Fig. 7-28). Although the primary treatment of these patients remains systemic therapy, MRI may identify an occult primary breast tumor that can be treated with breast-conserving therapy.
- Patients with equivocal chest wall invasion on imaging or physical examination (Fig. 7-29).
- Patients with breast tissue that is suboptimally imaged by mammography, especially those with dense breast tissue, silicone implants, or silicone injections obscuring the breast.
- Patients with tumors that are poorly seen on conventional mammography, including ILC or DCIS without corresponding microcalcifications.
- Patients who are going to undergo accelerated partial breast irradiation, in which only the breast cancer biopsy cavity and the margins around the cavity are treated with radiation therapy rather than whole-breast radiation.

In these patients, MRI may be used to plan the shape of the lumpectomy in an attempt to minimize the chance of transecting tumor margins. MRI may also reveal mammographically occult multifocal carcinoma (Fig. 7-30) and thereby prompt wider local excision. In addition, MRI may reveal occult multicentric or bilateral carcinoma (Fig. 7-31). Recent papers indicate that mammographically occult contralateral carcinoma is detected in 3.8% to 5.4% of patients with unilateral carcinoma. In these circumstances, preoperative biopsy is critical to pathologically confirm multicentric carcinoma or bilateral carcinoma because MRI findings can be nonspecific and may even lead to more extensive surgery than necessary in occasional patients.

Although MRI is most easily interpreted when performed in the absence of recent surgery because of the potential overlap of postsurgical healing scars and imaging findings of tumor, it has been successfully used to map the extent of residual disease in patients with transected tumor detected at the margins of an initial excisional biopsy specimen. Asymmetric and nodular enhancement or enhancement that is noncontiguous with the biopsy site is suspicious.

Formal outcome studies demonstrating the benefit of staging MRI as an adjunct to conventional breast-conserving therapy are still in progress; however, controversy persists regarding the exact role and benefit of staging breast cancer by MRI given the high success rate of traditional breast-conserving therapy without MRI.

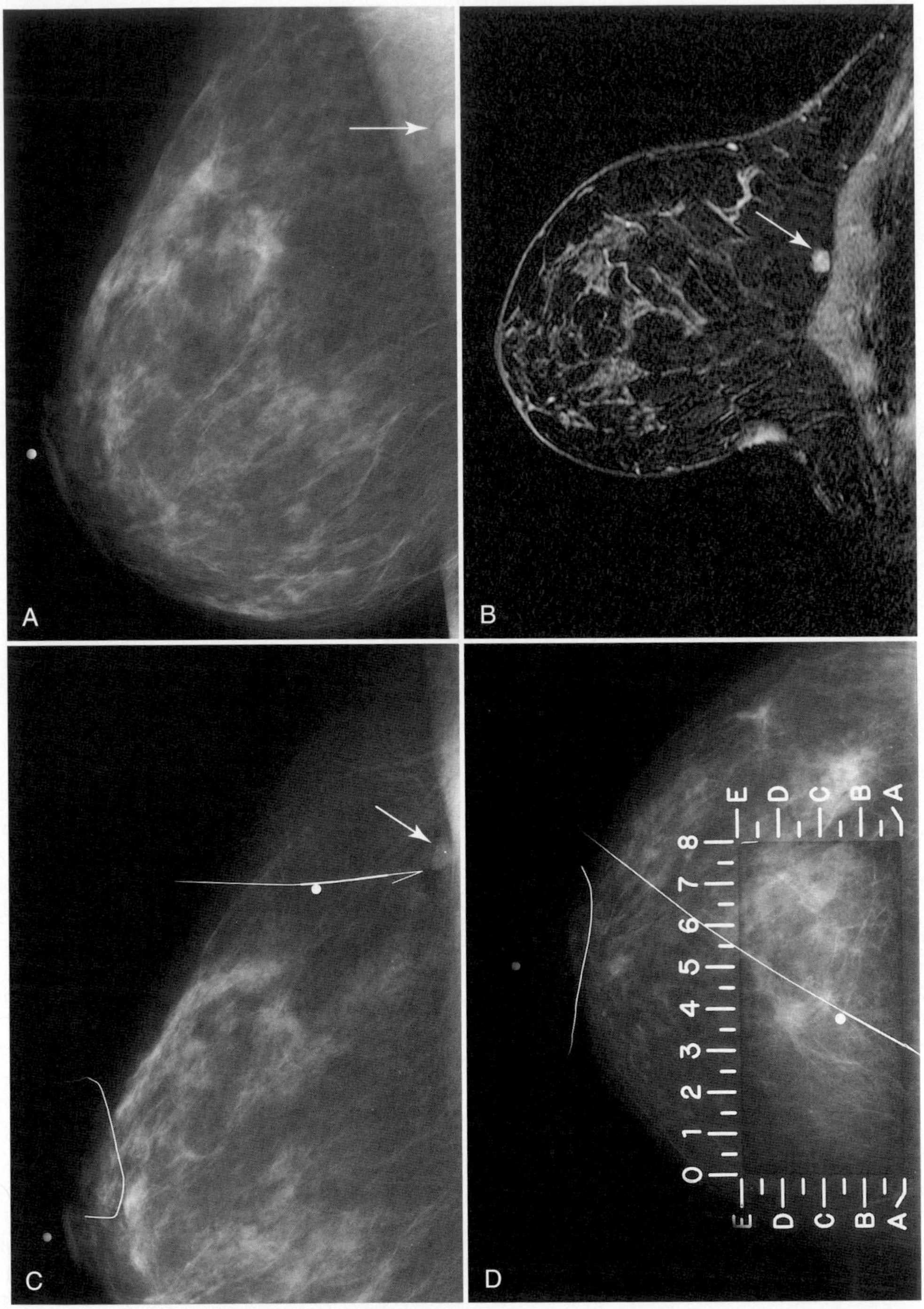

FIGURE 7-27. Magnetic resonance imaging (MRI) of a suspicious mass seen on one x-ray mammographic view. **A,** A suspicious mass was noted in the superior aspect of the breast, near the chest wall on the mediolateral oblique (MLO) mammogram only (*arrow*). **B,** Water-selective 3-D gradient echo MRI revealed a focal enhancing mass (*arrow*). Preoperative MRI-guided wire localization was performed (not shown). **C,** After localization, an MLO mammogram confirmed that localization was successful and the lesion (*arrow*) was too close to the chest wall to be seen on craniocaudal views (**D**). Pathologic evaluation revealed a small fibroadenoma. (From Offodile RS, Daniel BL, Jeffrey SS, et al: Magnetic resonance imaging of suspicious breast masses seen on one mammographic view, *Breast J* 10(5):416–422, 2004.)

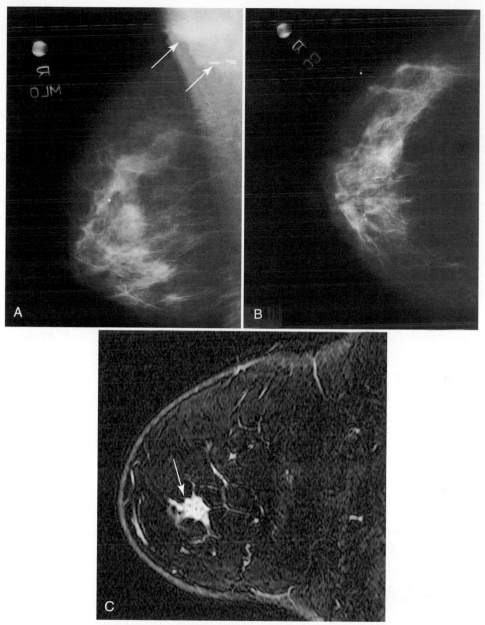

FIGURE 7-28. Mammographically occult breast cancer in a patient with axillary node metastases. Mediolateral oblique (**A**) and craniocaudal (**B**) mammograms revealed only postoperative changes in the right axilla (**A**, *arrows*) in this patient with a history of metastatic breast cancer discovered on recent excision of a palpable axillary node. **C,** Sagittal water-selective contrast-enhanced magnetic resonance imaging (MRI) revealed an 11-mm focal mass in the lateral portion of the breast (*arrow*). MRI-guided, wire-localized excision revealed a 9-mm invasive ductal carcinoma that was excised with tumor-free margins.

Management

Patients undergoing neoadjuvant chemotherapy are frequently imaged with breast MRI. Pretreatment scans provide the most accurate nonsurgical 3-D measurements of the extent of tumor. Scans performed after the first one or two cycles can detect a treatment response that may predict whether completion of chemotherapy will be successful. In patients who do respond, MRI after completion of chemotherapy can be used to identify and localize residual tumor, even in patients who have had a complete clinical response (Fig. 7-32). It is important to note that in these circumstances, the dynamic enhancement of tumors may be less specific and may even resem-

ble benign disease. Indeed, any residual enhancement at the site of a previously known tumor is suspicious. Because of the poor specificity of MRI findings after chemotherapy, pretreatment MRI is essential as a baseline for comparison.

MRI has also been investigated for its ability to detect local breast cancer recurrence. Debate persists regarding the duration of enhancement in benign postsurgical scars, although enhancement clearly decreases substantially over the first 2 years. Nevertheless, interpretation is best performed on serial MRI scans to assess whether enhancement is normally decreasing over time or suspiciously increasing over time.

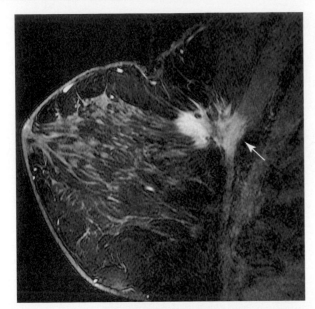

FIGURE 7-29. Chest wall invasion. Contrast-enhanced, 3-D water-specific breast magnetic resonance imaging reveals a large spiculated mass in the posterior of the breast. The enhancing tissue traverses the normal retromammary fat plane to abut the chest wall. The focal enhancement of the pectoralis muscle (*arrow*) is consistent with invasion and indicates locally advanced disease. (From American College of Radiology: ACR BI-RADS®—MRI, ed 4, In *ACR Breast Imaging and Reporting and Data System, breast imaging atlas*, Reston, VA, 2003, American College of Radiology.)

toward the specific area of abnormality noted on MRI. If a corresponding lesion is seen, ultrasound-guided core needle biopsy is easily performed. Careful attention to technique is essential to ensure that the MRI abnormality corresponds to the sonographic lesion, given the difference in patient position and breast configuration between the two methods.

Studies evaluating MRI-detected findings with sonography show that ultrasound demonstrates a finding in between 23% and 90%. A 2010 study by Abe and colleagues showed that 57% (115/202) of MRI-detected findings were seen by ultrasound. Of the remaining 87 lesions undetected by ultrasound, II were cancer. Other studies by Ko and colleagues (2007), Linda and colleagues (2008), and Destounis and colleagues (2009) showed that 90%, 82%, and 70% of 10, 173, and 182 MRI-detected findings, respectively, were seen on second-look ultrasound.

The largest study designed to evaluate which MRI lesion should undergo targeted ultrasound for purposes of biopsy, Meissnitzer and colleagues showed in 2009 that 290 of 519 MRI-detected lesions (56%) were seen with second-look ultrasound, with masses more likely to be seen compared to nonmass lesions (62% of masses versus 31% of nonmass lesions). This study showed that MRI-detected lesions were most likely to be seen with

▬ MRI-GUIDED BIOPSY

Second-Look Ultrasound

Lesions that are detected by MRI must frequently be biopsied (Box 7-12). The easiest method of biopsy is to perform a "second-look" ultrasound examination directed

---

BOX 7-12. Options for Biopsy of MRI Abnormalities

Second-look ultrasound-guided biopsy
MRI-guided needle localization
MRI-guided core needle biopsy

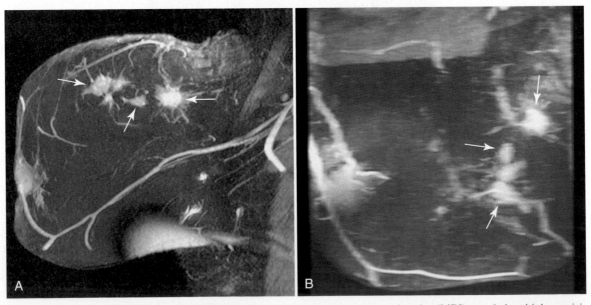

FIGURE 7-30. Multifocal carcinoma. Water-specific, contrast-enhanced 3-D magnetic resonance imaging (MRI) revealed multiple suspicious enhancing masses in the upper outer quadrant (*arrows*), as shown on these 2-cm–thick slab, maximum intensity projections in the sagittal (**A**) and axial (**B**) planes. MRI-guided lumpectomy confirmed multifocal invasive carcinoma.

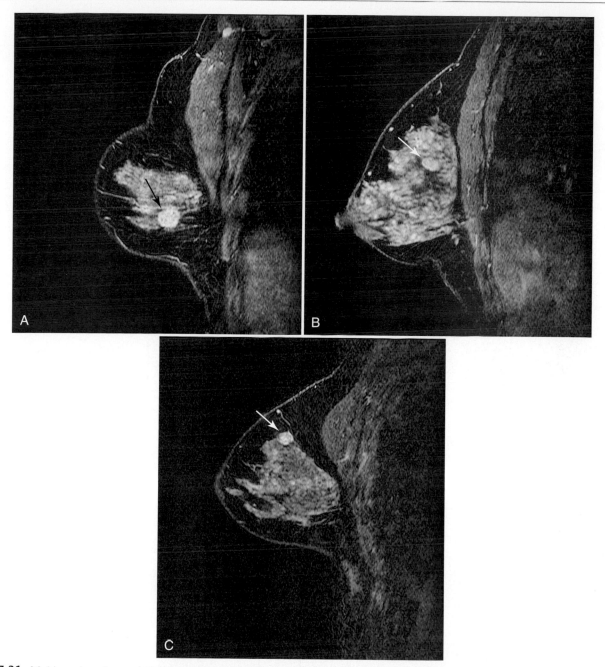

FIGURE 7-31. Multicentric and contralateral breast lesions. **A,** Water-selective magnetic resonance imaging (MRI) confirmed a 1.5-cm palpable invasive ductal carcinoma in the lower outer portion of the right breast (*arrow*) of a patient with normal bilateral mammograms. **B,** In addition, a suspicious upper inner quadrant enhancing focus (*arrow*) was shown to be stromal fibrosis and fibrocystic changes by MRI-guided, wire-localized biopsy. **C,** MRI of the asymptomatic left breast also demonstrated a brightly enhancing focus (*arrow*) that proved to be an 8-mm invasive ductal carcinoma at MRI-guided biopsy.

ultrasound if the MRI finding was a mass (rather than a nonmass), if it was large, if it was BI-RADS® category 5, if the mass had rim enhancement, or if it was a nonmass with clumped enhancement. Furthermore, Meissnitzer's study showed that 10 of 80 findings were discordant on a follow-up MRI after ultrasound-guided biopsy for second-look sonographic findings thought to represent the MRI target. This means that the "concordant" second-look ultrasound biopsy did not sample the MRI-detected

abnormality. Of the 9 out of 10 patients who underwent subsequent MRI-guided core biopsy, 5 had cancers. For these patients, biopsy must be performed under direct MRI guidance.

Preoperative Needle Localization

The simplest method of MRI-guided biopsy is preoperative MRI-guided needle localization and hookwire marking

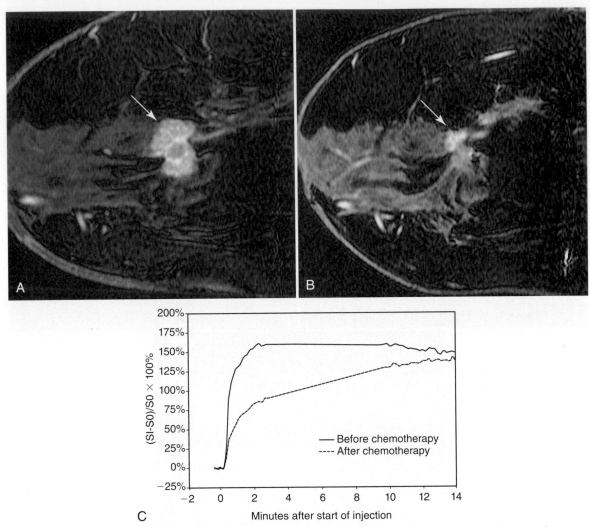

FIGURE 7-32. Response to neoadjuvant chemotherapy. **A,** Initial contrast-enhanced, water-selective 3-D gradient echo magnetic resonance imaging (MRI) confirmed a discrete, central avidly enhancing mass approximately 2.5 cm in diameter consistent with biopsy-proven invasive ductal carcinoma (*arrow*). **B,** Follow-up MRI after a complete clinical response to neoadjuvant chemotherapy revealed a small residual mass (*arrow*). **C,** Note that after chemotherapy, the time course of contrast enhancement of the residual tumor had a benign shape, a marked change in comparison to the suspicious pretreatment curve.

(Fig. 7-33). With the use of an open breast coil and sterile technique, an 18- or 20-gauge MRI-compatible needle is inserted in the breast and directed toward the abnormality. A variety of methods have been proposed to determine the correct needle trajectory, including grid-coordinate positioning devices and freehand methods. Contrast-enhanced scans are critical to confirm correct needle placement and target localization. Procedure speed is important because lesions commonly do not enhance preferentially over breast tissue more than 5 to 10 minutes after injection.

A postprocedure, presurgery mammogram is recommended for three reasons. First, most breast surgeons are more familiar with the use of mammograms in planning the surgical approach. Second, mammography may reveal a mass or calcifications at the MRI-guided, wire-localized lesion that was not previously appreciated as suspicious and can therefore be looked for on intraopera-

tive specimen radiographs, thus maximizing the chance for accurate surgical excision. Third, mammograms document the location of the MRI-guided biopsy and hence provide a critical baseline for future postoperative mammograms.

Correlating the MRI, mammographic, and ultrasound finding can be challenging. Use of markers or clips after core biopsy can be extremely helpful to identify findings cored under ultrasound, MRI, or stereotactic core biopsy, especially if the patient is to undergo excision of cancer seen on more than one modality (Fig. 7-34).

On occasion, the target may not be seen during the preoperative needle localization procedure. This may be due to a variety of reasons, including vigorous breast compression, which does not allow inflow of contrast material to enhance the lesion; spurious enhancement of a lesion due to hormonal influences; or nonvisualization for unknown reasons. In most cases, definite localization can

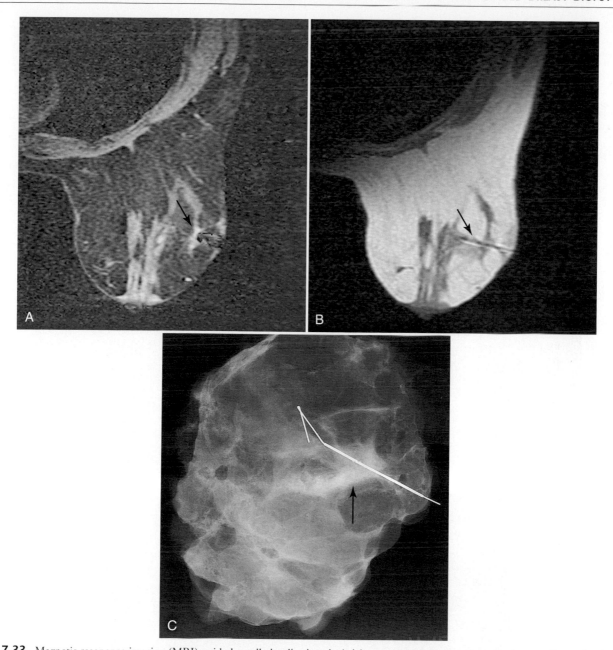

FIGURE 7-33. Magnetic resonance imaging (MRI)-guided needle localization. **A,** Axial, contrast-enhanced, water-selective two-dimensional gradient echo MRI reveals an MRI-compatible localizing needle abutting the suspicious focus of contrast enhancement (*arrow*) described in Figure 7-28. **B,** An axial T1-weighted fast spin-echo image after hookwire deployment reveals the mass centered on the stiffener of the hookwire (*arrow*). **C,** Radiography of the excised specimen demonstrated nonspecific glandular tissue adjacent to the hookwire (*arrow*). Pathologic examination revealed invasive ductal carcinoma.

proceed based on surrounding breast architecture rather than targeting the enhanced lesion if such architecture exists. Otherwise, a 1-month follow-up contrast-enhanced MRI study will confirm or exclude whether the enhancing lesion still exists. On occasion, breast cancers may not enhance on the day of preoperative needle localization. In these cases, the short-term MRI follow-up may be helpful to confirm the lesion, and that the need for biopsy still exists.

Based on published data, contrast-enhanced breast MRI preoperative needle localization true-positive results range between 20% and 40%, similar to mammographically detected breast lesion needle localization data.

Percutaneous Core Biopsy

Percutaneous core needle biopsy (Fig. 7-35) can be performed under direct MRI guidance by both grid-coordinate and freehand methods. Devices include MRI-compatible 14-gauge titanium needles and vacuum-assisted biopsy devices. The imaging artifacts associated with core biopsy needles and the potential for breast motion remain limitations to reliable biopsy of sub-centimeter lesions given the current technology.

MRI-guided core biopsy can be especially helpful after a breast cancer diagnosis if MRI detects a possible second

Text continued on p 283

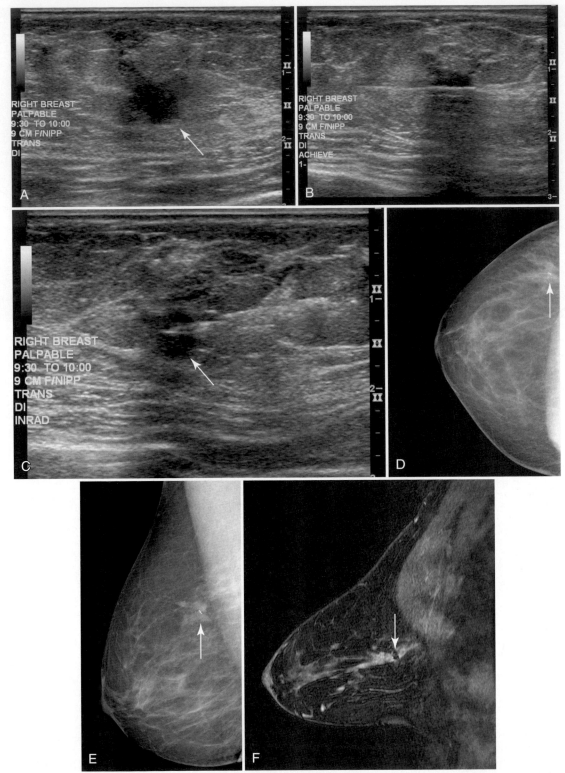

FIGURE 7-34. Core biopsy and needle localization of invasive ductal cancer (IDC) and ductal carcinoma in situ (DCIS) on postcontrast sagittal 3-D spectral-spatial excitation magnetization transfer (3DSSMT) magnetic resonance imaging (MRI) scans and ultrasound. **A,** Ultrasound shows a palpable spiculated mass (*arrow*) in the upper outer quadrant of the right breast, worrisome for cancer. **B,** Ultrasound-guided core biopsy showed IDC. **C,** Ultrasound showing marker (*arrow*) placement during the core biopsy. Craniocaudal (CC) (**D**) and mediolateral oblique (**E**) digital mammograms after the core biopsy show the marker in the upper outer right breast in a suspicious spiculated mass (*arrows*). Biopsy showed IDC. **F,** Postcontrast sagittal 3DSSMT MRI scan shows linear enhancement extending from the midbreast to the chest wall. There is a signal void (*arrow*) in the thickened portion of enhancement, representing the biopsied cancer and the marker placed by ultrasound.

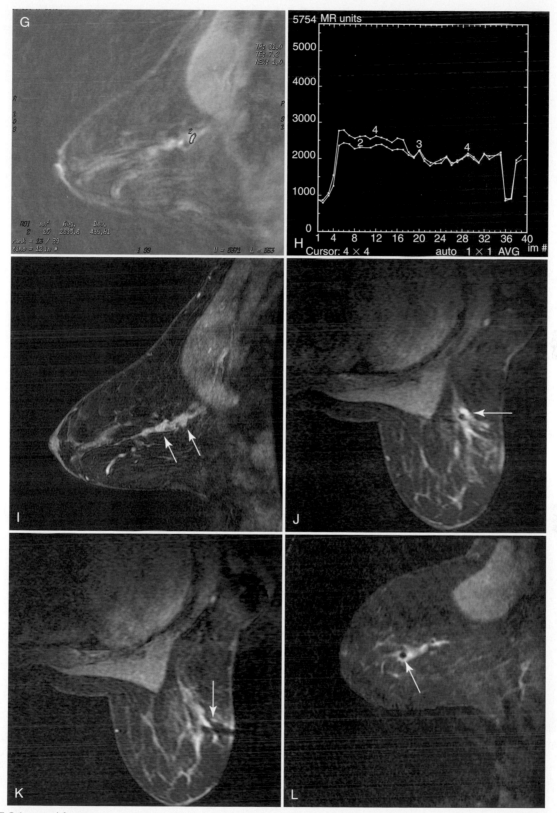

FIGURE 7-34, cont'd. The corresponding region of interest (**G**) and kinetic curve (**H**) show rapid initial enhancement and washout compatible with the known invasive cancer. **I,** In an adjacent sagittal MRI slice, the linear enhancement extends anterior and posterior to the known cancer (*arrows*), worrisome for DCIS, even though kinetic enhancement curves were unremarkable. To determine if the linear enhancement represented DCIS, an MRI-guided core biopsy was done. **J,** Three-point Dixon axial postcontrast MRI during a vacuum-assisted, MRI-guided core biopsy shows the invasive cancer and signal void in the posterior breast (*arrow*). Three-point Dixon axial (**K**) and sagittal (**L**) postcontrast MRI slices shows the 10-gauge obturator and sheath (dark linear signal void; *arrow*) traversing the linear enhancement about 3 cm anterior to the IDC during an MRI-guided core biopsy. After the core biopsy a ring-shaped marker was placed in the biopsy site under MRI guidance. Core biopsy showed DCIS. *Continued*

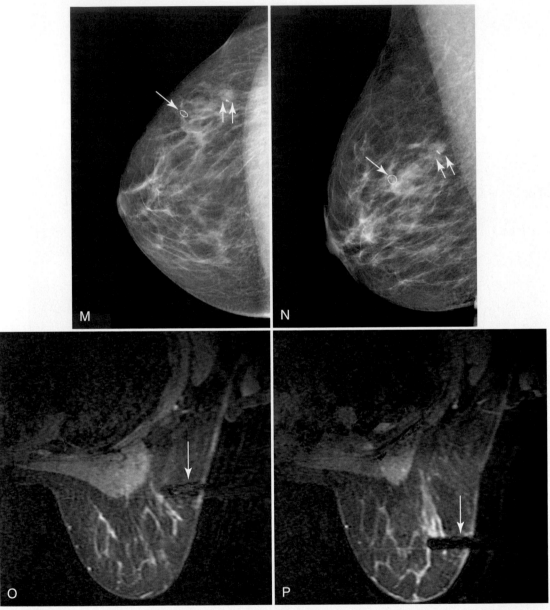

FIGURE 7-34, cont'd. CC (**M**) and mediolateral (**N**) mammograms after MRI-guided biopsy show the ring-shaped metal marker (*arrow*) within the biopsy site (DCIS). Note the known cancer and marker posteriorly, near the chest wall (*arrows*). MRI-guided bracket needle localization of the linear enhancement was recommended to include both the IDC and the linear enhancement. **O,** The postcontrast three-point Dixon preoperative needle localization axial MRI scan shows a wire signal void traversing the posterior invasive cancer (*arrow*) and a wire traversing the anterior aspect of the linear enhancement (**P**), bracketing the area to be excised.

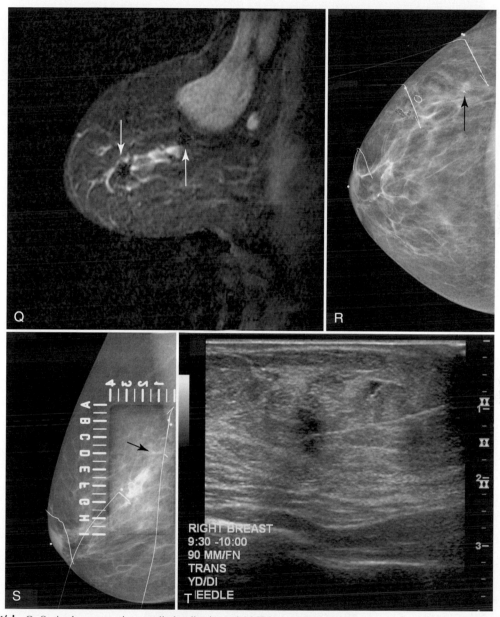

FIGURE 7-34, cont'd. Q, Sagittal preoperative needle localization axial MRI scan shows the signal void from the bracketing wires of the posterior mass and the anterior edge of the ductal enhancement (*arrows*). CC (**R**) and mediolateral (**S**) mammograms after MRI-guided needle localization show the posterior wire is superior to the spiculated mass by at least 2 cm; the surgeon could possibly miss the IDC (*arrows*). It was decided to place a third wire into the IDC by ultrasound. **T,** Ultrasound-guided needle localization of the spiculated mass shows a wire passing to the mass. *Continued*

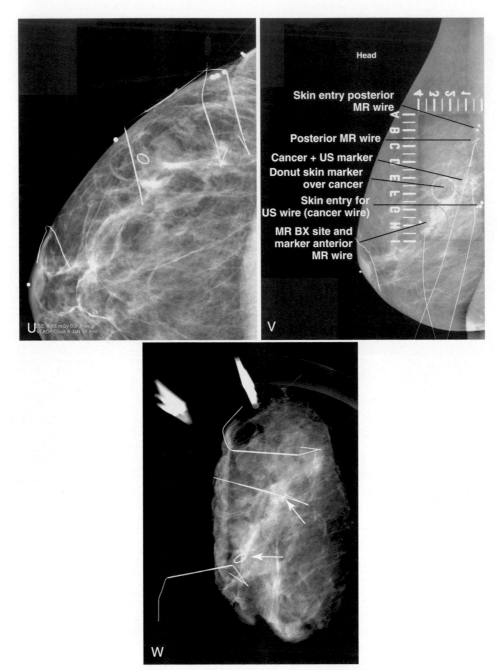

FIGURE 7-34, cont'd. CC (**U**) and mediolateral (**V**) mammograms after ultrasound-guided needle localization show a third wire in the spiculated mass on films marked for the surgeon. **W,** Specimen radiograph shows inclusion of three hookwires, three hookwire tips, and the two markers (*arrows*). Pathology showed IDC and DCIS.

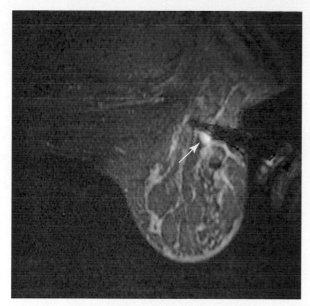

FIGURE 7-35. Magnetic resonance imaging (MRI)-guided vacuum-assisted core needle biopsy. Axial, water-selective, two-dimensional gradient echo MRI revealed the inner trocar of a 14-gauge titanium biopsy needle extended through the focally enhancing mass (*arrow*) noted in Figure 7-19C to E. Pathologic evaluation revealed benign fibroadenoma.

cancer not seen on any other modality. This is particularly true in the postbiopsy surgical patient who has already undergone one operation and now seeks definitive surgical therapy (Fig. 7-36).

MRI-compatible clips may be deployed after MRI-guided core needle biopsy to mark the site of biopsy. When benign results are obtained that do not specifically correspond to the expected appearance of the MRI lesion, repeat MRI-guided needle-localized surgical biopsy or follow-up MRI must be performed. The use of the MRI-guided markers or markers placed under ultrasound that are later imaged by MRI or mammography can help guide the surgeon to excise the entire tumor and any associated DCIS (Fig. 7-37).

Diffusion-Weighted MRI

Diffusion-weighted imaging (DWI) measures water molecule mobility in vivo on unenhanced breast MRI sequences (Fig. 7-38). DWI evaluates tissue biophysical characteristics, such as the microstructure of breast tissue, cell density, membrane integrity, and extracellular matrix composition. Preliminary studies show a lower apparent diffusion coefficient (ADC) on DWI studies of breast cancers (Table 7-8). A higher ADC was observed in benign breast lesions and normal tissue. It was thought that a higher cell density in breast cancer causes an increased restriction of the extracellular matrix, with the resultant increased signal fraction coming from intracellular water. A preliminary study by Partridge and colleagues showed that increased positive predictive value might be achieved by combining ADC and conventional contrast-enhanced MRI criteria. The studies will need to be validated with larger populations.

■ KEY ELEMENTS

Contrast enhancement in breast cancers is due to angiogenesis.

Indications for breast MRI are breast cancer screening in high-risk patients (*BRCA1*, *BRCA2*, or equivalent); breast cancer staging to detect mammographically occult bilateral, multicentric, multifocal, or locally extensive disease; poorly visualized tumors on mammography; diagnosis of suspicious findings that cannot be fully evaluated with conventional imaging; and before and after neoadjuvant chemotherapy.

Chemotherapy produces a potential pitfall in interpretation because it can decrease tumor conspicuity and change suspicious enhancement curves to benign persistent curves despite the persistence of viable, residual cancer.

Proper technique includes a dedicated breast coil, a contrast bolus followed by a saline flush, fat suppression, or subtraction.

Both morphology and enhancement curves are important in interpretation of MRI.

Abnormal enhancement is defined as enhancement brighter than normal surrounding glandular tissue on the first postcontrast scan or early in the initial enhancement phase.

ACR BI-RADS® terms for morphologic features of abnormal enhancement include *focus*, *focal area*, *mass*, *linear*, *ductal*, *segmental*, *regional*, *multiple regions*, and *diffuse enhancement*.

Suspicious morphologic findings on MRI include an irregular shape, irregular or spiculated margins, rim enhancement, and enhancing internal septations.

Associated findings of focal skin thickening, satellite lesions, lymphadenopathy, and skin or chest wall invasion are suspicious for cancer in the appropriate clinical setting.

Suspicious enhancement curves include a rapid initial rise and abrupt transition to a late-phase plateau or washout; the curve shape is also called a "square root sign" or a "cancer corner."

Benign enhancement curves include a slow initial rise and a late persistent enhancement phase.

Fibroadenomas are usually bright on T2-weighted images if myxoid and dark on T2-weighted images if sclerotic and may have dark internal septations and a persistent late enhancement phase.

DCIS may be difficult to distinguish from fibrocystic changes.

Classic patterns for DCIS include clumped enhancement in a ductal, linear, or segmental distribution, particularly if it is asymmetric.

DCIS does not always display rapid initial enhancement with a plateau or washout.

Pitfalls in interpreting rim enhancement include fat necrosis and inflamed cysts; precontrast T2-weighted images can reduce false positives.

Pitfalls in interpreting benign-appearing masses include cancers with a benign morphology and a suspicious enhancement curve.

Mastitis and inflammatory cancer both produce breast edema and abnormal enhancement.

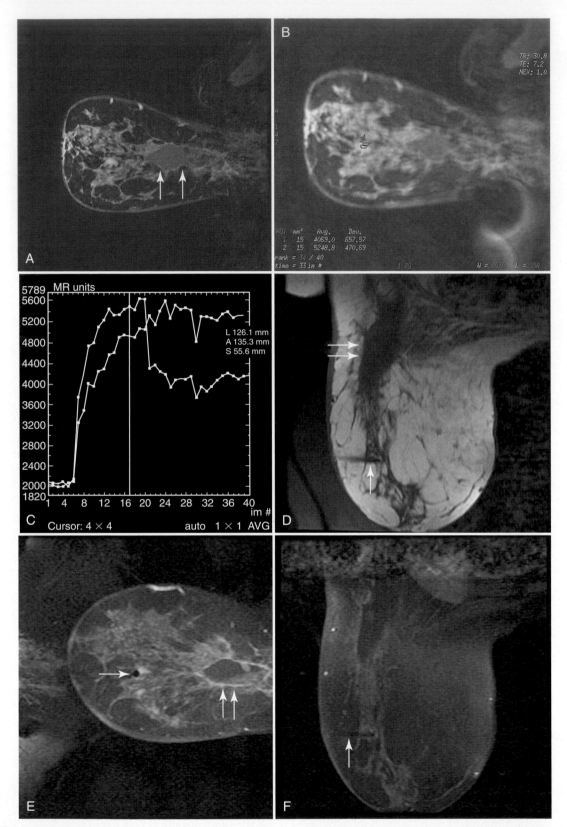

FIGURE 7-36. Magnetic resonance imaging (MRI)-guided core biopsy for incidental enhancing lesion (IEL) after lumpectomy for invasive ductal cancer (IDC). This patient had a lumpectomy for IDC, resulting in a seroma in the posterior breast. The MRI was done to look for additional foci of cancer. **A,** Postcontrast sagittal 3-D spectral-spatial excitation magnetization transfer (3DSSMT) MRI scan shows the seroma (*arrows*) and a nonspecific mass 3.5 cm anterior to the seroma. The region of interest (ROI) (**B**) and corresponding kinetic curve (**C**) show rapid initial enhancement and plateau, worrisome for cancer. Note, two ROI were placed on the slice because the patient moved between the two scans: one line represents the initial kinetic curve for the lesion; the other line represents the kinetic curve for the late, "wash-out" phase. This shows that motion artifact can have spurious results if motion correction is not employed. To determine if the IEL was cancer, MRI-guided core biopsy was done. **D,** Axial T1-weighted nonfat-suppressed noncontrast MRI shows the needle (*arrow*) adjacent to the expected location of the IEL based on reconstructed axial images from the diagnostic 3DSSMT MRI. Incidentally, note the seroma in the posterior aspect of the breast (*double arrows*). **E,** Sagittal three-point Dixon postcontrast MRI-guided vacuum-assisted core biopsy scan shows signal void (*arrow*) adjacent to the IEL in the anterior breast. In this case, the needle biopsy trough is aimed toward the patient's chest wall to sample the IEL. Note the seroma from excisional biopsy for IDC (*double arrows*), rim enhancement around the biopsy site, the fluid/fluid level, and the fibrin ball in the superior aspect of the cavity. **F,** Axial three-point Dixon postcontrast MRI shows the needle (*arrow*) adjacent to the IEL. Core needle biopsy showed a second focus of IDC.

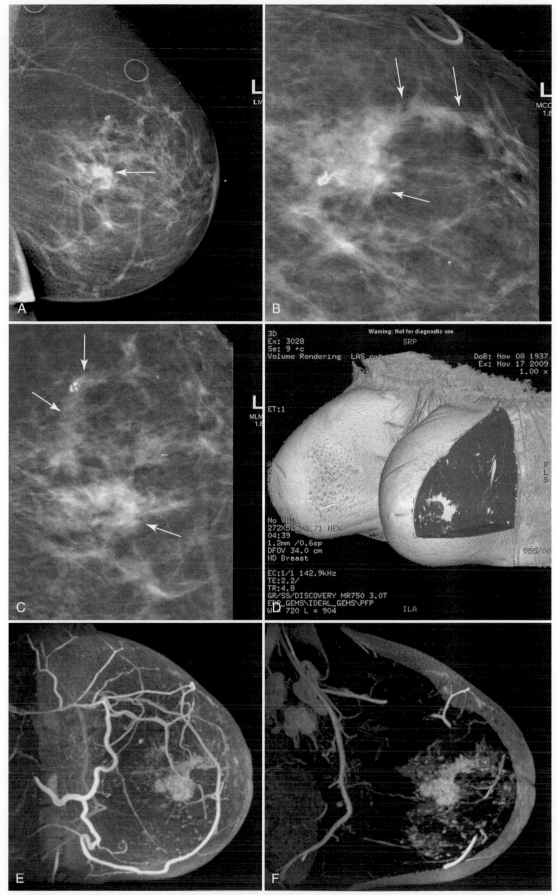

Figure 7-37. Correlation of mammography, ultrasound, and 3 Tesla (T) magnetic resonance imaging (MRI) for needle localization. **A,** Lateral mammogram in a 72-year-old woman with a palpable mass in the outer left breast shows a dense mass (*arrow*) in the midbreast at the 3-o'clock position. **B,** Magnified cropped left craniocaudal mammogram shows the spiculated mass (*arrow*) and curvilinear area of dense tissue lateral and anterior to the spiculated mass (*arrows*). This curvilinear density was later shown to represent noncalcified ductal carcinoma in situ (DCIS). *Continued*

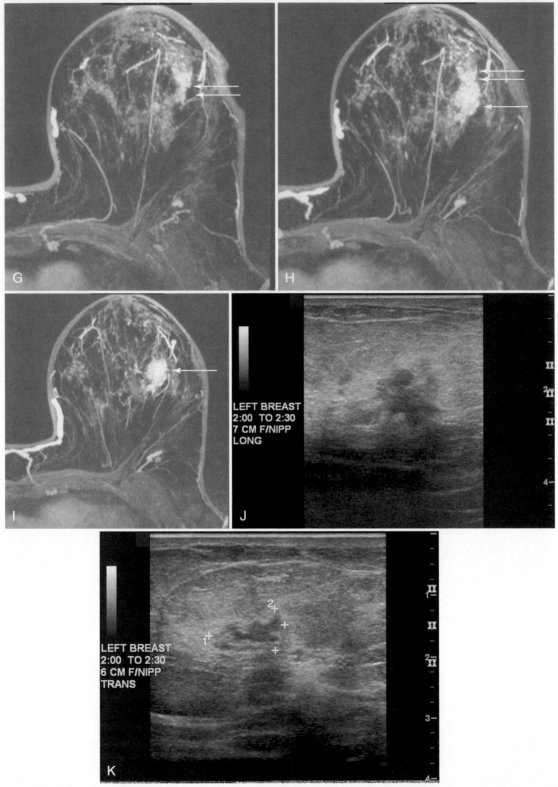

FIGURE 7-37, cont'd. **C,** Lateral cropped magnification mammogram shows the spiculated mass (*arrow*) and curvilinear density extending superior to the mass (*arrows*). **D,** Shaded cut surface display postcontrast 3T 3-D spectral-spatial excitation magnetization transfer (3DSSMT) MRI shows a spiculated mass with clumped enhancement extending superiorly in a curvilinear distribution, corresponding to the findings shown on the mammograms in parts **B** and **C. E,** Maximal intensity projection (MIP) 3DSSMT MRI shows the mass and clumped enhancement representing invasive ductal cancer and DCIS on biopsy. Note scattered foci of nonspecific enhancement elsewhere in the breast. **F,** Thick slab MIP cut surface display shows the invasive ductal cancer, associated DCIS, and axillary adenopathy in greater detail. **G to I,** Thick slab axial reconstructions of breast cancer and DCIS. Three slices from axial reconstruction 3T MRI show the irregular invasive ductal cancer mass (*arrow*) and clumped ductal enhancement DCIS extending from the mass (*double arrows*), corresponding to the mammographic findings on the craniocaudal mammogram in part **B. J,** Second-look ultrasound directed to the left breast shows the invasive ductal cancer seen on the MRI and on the mammogram. **K,** Second-look ultrasound superior to the cancer shows nodular hypoechoic ductal findings corresponding to the clumped DCIS enhancement seen on MRI. Ultrasound-guided core biopsy of the nodular hypoechoic ductal findings showed DCIS. A marker was placed in the DCIS under ultrasound.

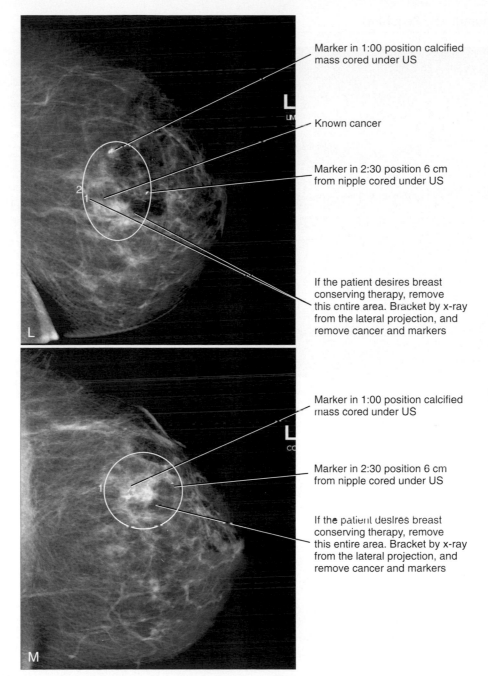

FIGURE 7-37, cont'd. Scout annotated lateral mammogram for preoperative needle localization (**L**) and scout craniocaudal mammogram (**M**). Of note, a calcified benign-appearing mass was also cored under ultrasound superior to the cancer and found to be benign. The invasive cancer and the DCIS were localized under x-ray guidance using mammographic landmarks, and invasive ductal cancer and DCIS with clear margins were found at surgery.

TABLE 7-8. Diffusion-Weighted Echo Planar Imaging of Breast Lesions

Study	n	B-Values	ADC Threshold × 10^{-3} (mm²/sec)	Sensitivity	Specificity
Guo et al.[1]	52	0, 250, 500, 750, 1000	1.3	93%	88%
Woodhams et al.[2]	191	0, 750, 1000	1.6	93%	46%
Rubesova et al.[3]	87	0, 200, 400, 600, 1000	1.13	86%	86%
Marini et al.[4]	81	0, 1000	1.1 (mean diffusivity)	80%	81%
Hatenaka et al.[5]	140	0, 500, 1000	1.48	84%	81%
Yabuchi et al.[6]	192	0, 500, 1000	1.1	~83%	~86%

[1]Guo Y, Cai YQ, Cai ZL, et al: Differentiation of clinically benign and malignant breast lesions using diffusion-weighted imaging, *J Magn Reson Imaging* 16:172–178, 2002.
[2]Woodhams R, Matsunaga K, Kan S, et al: ADC mapping of benign and malignant breast tumors, *Magn Reson Med Sci* 4:35–42, 2005.
[3]Rubesova E, Grell AS, De Maertelaer V, et al. Quantitative diffusion imaging in breast cancer: a clinical prospective study, *J Magn Reson Imaging* 24:319–324, 2006.
[4]Marini C, Iacconi C, Giannelli M, et al: Quantitative diffusion-weighted MR imaging in the differential diagnosis of breast lesion, *Eur Radiol* 17:2646–2655, 2007.
[5]Hatenaka M, Soeda H, Yabuuchi H, et al: Apparent diffusion coefficients of breast tumors: clinical application. *Magn Med Sci* 7(1):23–29, 2008.
[6]Yabuuchi H, Matsuo Y, Okafuji T, et al: Enhanced mass on contrast-enhanced breast MR imaging: lesion characterization using combination of dynamic contrast-enhanced and diffusion-weighted MR images, *J Magn Reson Imaging* 28:1157–1165, 2008.
ADC, apparent diffusion coefficient.

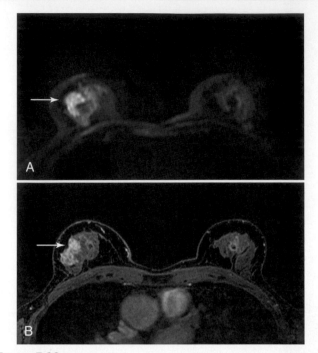

FIGURE 7-38. A 65-year-old woman with invasive ductal cancer of the right breast seen on diffusion-weighted imaging (DWI). **A,** Noncontrast DWI spin-echo echoplanar image obtained with a *b*-value of 600 at 3.0 Tesla (TR/TE 2000/76 ms, matrix 128 × 256, with 8 signal averages, 5-mm slice thickness). An invasive ductal cancer is present in the right breast and is high signal on the DWI (*arrow*). The restricted diffusion in the tumor leads to intrinsically high signal intensity even before contrast administration. **B,** For comparison, subsequent high spatial resolution water-selective T1-weighted contrast-enhanced 3-D spoiled gradient echo image of the same breast cancer (*arrow*).

Papillomas and lymph nodes may have rapid initial rise and plateau or washout patterns and can thus be a cause of false-positive findings that generate biopsy.

MRI-guided preoperative needle localization and MRI-guided core biopsy must be performed rapidly because the signal intensity of the tumor may be indistinguishable from surrounding enhancing breast tissue within 10 minutes.

■ SUGGESTED READINGS

Abe H, Schmidt RA, Shah RN, et al: MRI-directed ("second-look") ultrasound examination for breast lesions detected initially on MRI: MR and sonographic findings, *AJR Am J Roentgenol* 194(2):370–377, 2010.

Agoston AT, Daniel BL, Herfkens RJ, et al: Intensity-modulated parametric mapping for simultaneous display of rapid dynamic and high-spatial resolution breast MR imaging data, *Radiographics* 21:217–226, 2001.

American College of Radiology: *ACR Breast Imaging Reporting and Data System*, Breast Imaging Atlas. Reston, VA, 2003, American College of Radiology.

Balu-Maestro C, Chapellier C, Bleuse A, et al: Imaging in evaluation of response to neoadjuvant breast cancer treatment benefits of MRI, *Breast Cancer Res Treat* 72:145–152, 2002.

Bedrosian I, Mick R, Orel SG, et al: Changes in the surgical management of patients with breast carcinoma based on preoperative magnetic resonance imaging, *Cancer* 98:468–473, 2003.

Bedrosian I, Schlencker J, Spitz FR, et al: Magnetic resonance imaging-guided biopsy of mammographically and clinically occult breast lesions, *Ann Surg Oncol* 9:457–461, 2002.

Beran L, Liang W, Nims T, et al: Correlation of targeted ultrasound with magnetic resonance imaging abnormalities of the breast, *Am J Surg* 190:592–594, 2005.

Berg WA, Blume JD, Cormack JB, Mendelson EB: Operator dependence of physician-performed whole-breast US: lesion detection and characterization, *Radiology* 241:355–365, 2006.

Boetes C, Mus RD, Holland R, et al: Breast tumors: comparative accuracy of MR imaging relative to mammography and US for demonstrating extent, *Radiology* 197:743–747, 1995.

Brenner RJ: Needle localization of breast lesions: localizing data, *AJR Am J Roentgenol* 179:1643-1644, 2002.

Brinck U, Fischer U, Korabiowska M, et al: The variability of fibroadenoma in contrast-enhanced dynamic MR mammography, *AJR Am J Roentgenol* 168:1331–1334, 1997.

Brown J, Buckley D, Coulthard A, et al: Magnetic resonance imaging screening in women at genetic risk of breast cancer: imaging and analysis protocol for the UK Multicentre Study. UK MRI Breast Screening Study Advisory Group, *Magn Reson Imaging* 18:765–776, 2000.

Brown J, Smith RC, Lee CH: Incidental enhancing lesions found on MR imaging of the breast, *AJR Am J Roentgenol* 176:1249–1254, 2001.

Buadu LD, Murakami J, Murayama S, et al: Breast lesions: correlation of contrast medium enhancement patterns on MR images with histopathologic findings and tumor angiogenesis, *Radiology* 200:639–649, 1996.

Chenevert TL, Helvie MA, Aisen AM, et al: Dynamic three-dimensional imaging with partial k-space sampling: initial application for gadolinium-enhanced rate characterization of breast lesions, *Radiology* 196:135–142, 1995.

Cohen EK, Leonhardt CM, Shumak RS, et al: Magnetic resonance imaging in potential postsurgical recurrence of breast cancer: pitfalls and limitations, *Can Assoc Radiol J* 47:171–176, 1996.

Daniel BL, Birdwell RL, Black JW, et al: Interactive MR-guided, 14-gauge core-needle biopsy of enhancing lesions in a breast phantom mode, *Acad Radiol* 4:508–512, 1997.

Daniel BL, Birdwell RL, Butts K, et al: Freehand iMRI-guided large-gauge core needle biopsy: a new minimally invasive technique for diagnosis of enhancing breast lesions, *J Magn Reson Imaging* 13:896–902, 2001.

Daniel BL, Birdwell RL, Ikeda DM, et al: Breast lesion localization: a freehand, interactive MR imaging-guided technique, *Radiology* 207:455–463, 1998.

Daniel B, Herfkens R: Intraoperative MR imaging: can image guidance improve therapy? *Acad Radiol* 9:875–877, 2002.

Daniel BL, Yen YF, Glover GH, et al: Breast disease: dynamic spiral MR imaging, *Radiology* 209:499–509, 1998.

Degani H, Chetrit-Dadiani M, Bogin L, Furman-Haran E: Magnetic resonance imaging of tumor vasculature, *Thromb Haemost* 89:25–33, 2003.

Degani H, Gusis V, Weinstein D, et al: Mapping pathophysiological features of breast tumors by MRI at high spatial resolution, *Nat Med* 3:780–782, 1997.

Demartini WB, Eby PR, Peacock S, Lehman CD: Utility of targeted sonography for breast lesions that were suspicious on MRI, *AJR Am J Roentgenol* 192:1128–1134, 2009.

Destounis S, Arieno A, Somerville PA, et al: Community-based practice experience of unsuspected breast magnetic resonance imaging abnormalities evaluated with second-look sonography, *J Ultrasound Med* 28:1337–1346, 2009.

El Khouli RH, Macura KJ, Jacobs MA, et al: Dynamic contrast-enhanced MRI of the breast: quantitative method for kinetic curve type assessment, *AJR Am J Roentgenol* 193:W295–W300, 2009.

Elmore JG, Armstrong K, Lehman CD, Fletcher SW: Screening for breast cancer, *JAMA* 293:1245–1256, 2005.

Esserman L, Hylton N, Yassa L, et al: Utility of magnetic resonance imaging in the management of breast cancer: evidence for improved preoperative staging, *J Clin Oncol* 17:110–119, 1999.

Guo Y, Cai YQ, Cai ZL, et al: Differentiation of clinically benign and malignant breast lesions using diffusion-weighted imaging, *J Magn Reson Imaging* 16:172–178, 2002.

Gutierrez RL, DeMartini WB, Eby PR, et al: BI-RADS lesion characteristics predict likelihood of malignancy in breast MRI for masses but not for nonmasslike enhancement, *AJR Am J Roentgenol* 193:994–1000, 2009.

Harms SE, Flamig DP, Hesley KL, et al: MR imaging of the breast with rotating delivery of excitation off resonance: clinical experience with pathologic correlation, *Radiology* 187:493–501, 1993.

Hashimoto BE: Sonographic assessment of breast calcifications, *Curr Probl Diagn Radiol* 35:213–218, 2006.

Hashimoto BE, Morgan GN, Kramer DJ, Lee M: Systematic approach to difficult problems in breast sonography, *Ultrasound Q* 24:31–38, 2008.

Heywang SH, Wolf A, Pruss E, et al: MR imaging of the breast with Gd-DTPA: use and limitations, *Radiology* 171:95–103, 1989.

Hochman MG, Orel SG, Powell CM, et al: Fibroadenomas: MR imaging appearances with radiologic–histopathologic correlation, *Radiology* 204:123–129, 1997.

Houssami N, Ciatto S, Macaskill P, et al: Accuracy and surgical impact of magnetic resonance imaging in breast cancer staging: systematic review and meta-analysis in detection of multifocal and multicentric cancer, *J Clin Oncol* 26:3248–3258, 2008.

Hrung JM, Langlotz CP, Orel SG, et al: Cost-effectiveness of MR imaging and core-needle biopsy in the preoperative work-up of suspicious breast lesions, *Radiology* 213:39–49, 1999.

Hrung JM, Sonnad SS, Schwartz JS, Langlotz CP: Accuracy of MR imaging in the work-up of suspicious breast lesions: a diagnostic meta-analysis, *Acad Radiol* 6:387–397, 1999.

Hwang ES, Kinkel K, Esserman LJ, et al: Magnetic resonance imaging in patients diagnosed with ductal carcinoma in situ: value in the diagnosis of residual disease, occult invasion, and multicentricity, *Ann Surg Oncol* 10:381–388, 2003.

Ikeda DM, Baker DR, Daniel BL: Magnetic resonance imaging of breast cancer: clinical indications and breast MRI reporting system, *J Magn Reson Imaging* 12:975–983, 2000.

Ikeda DM, Hylton NM, Kinkel K, et al: Development, standardization, and testing of a lexicon for reporting contrast-enhanced breast magnetic resonance imaging studies, *J Magn Reson Imaging* 13:889–895, 2001.

Kelcz F, Santyr GE, Cron GO, Mongin SJ: Application of a quantitative model to differentiate benign from malignant breast lesions detected by dynamic, gadolinium-enhanced MRI, *J Magn Reson Imaging* 6:743–752, 1996.

Kinkel K, Helbich TH, Esserman LJ, et al: Dynamic high-spatial resolution MR imaging of suspicious breast lesions: diagnostic criteria and interobserver variability, *AJR Am J Roentgenol* 175:35–43, 2000.

Kinoshita T, Odagiri K, Andoh K, et al: Evaluation of small internal mammary lymph node metastases in breast cancer by MRI, *Radiat Med* 17:189–193, 1999.

Kinoshita T, Yashiro N, Yoshigi J, et al: Inflammatory intramammary lymph node mimicking the malignant lesion in dynamic MRI: a case report, *Clin Imaging* 26:258–262, 2002.

Kinoshita T, Yashiro N, Ihara N, et al: Diffusion-weighted half-Fourier single-shot turbo spin echo imaging in breast tumors: differentiation of invasive ductal carcinoma from fibroadenoma, *J Comput Assist Tomogr* 26:1042–1046, 2002.

Ko EY, Han BK, Shin JH, Kang SS: Breast MRI for evaluating patients with metastatic axillary lymph node and initially negative mammography and sonography, *Korean J Radiol* 8:382–389, 2007.

Kriege M, Brekelmans CT, Boetes C, et al: Efficacy of MRI and mammography for breast-cancer screening in women with a familial or genetic predisposition, *N Engl J Med* 351:427–437, 2004.

Kuhl CK: High-risk screening: multi-modality surveillance of women at high risk for breast cancer (proven or suspected carriers of a breast cancer susceptibility gene), *J Exp Clin Cancer Res* 21(3 Suppl):103–106, 2002.

Kuhl CK: Interventional breast MRI: needle localisation and core biopsies, *J Exp Clin Cancer Res* 21(3 Suppl):65–68, 2002.

Kuhl CK, Bieling HB, Gieseke J, et al: Healthy premenopausal breast parenchyma in dynamic contrast enhanced MR imaging of the breast: normal contrast medium enhancement and cyclical-phase dependency, *Radiology* 203:137–144, 1997.

Kuhl CK, Elevelt A, Leutner CC, et al: Interventional breast MR imaging: clinical use of a stereotactic localization and biopsy device, *Radiology* 204:667–675, 1997.

Kuhl CK, Klaschik S, Mielcarek P, et al: Do T2-weighted pulse sequences help with the differential diagnosis of enhancing lesions in dynamic breast MRI? *J Magn Reson Imaging* 9:187–196, 1999.

Kuhl CK, Mielcareck P, Klaschik S, et al: Dynamic breast MR imaging: are signal intensity time course data useful for differential diagnosis of enhancing lesions? *Radiology* 211:101–110, 1999.

Kuhl CK, Schild HH: Dynamic image interpretation of MRI of the breast, *J Magn Reson Imaging* 12:965–974, 2000.

Kuhl CK, Schmutzler RK, Leutner CC, et al: Breast MR imaging screening in 192 women proved or suspected to be carriers of a breast cancer susceptibility gene: preliminary results, *Radiology* 215:267–279, 2000.

Kuhl CK, Schrading S, Leutner CC, et al: Mammography, breast ultrasound, and magnetic resonance imaging for surveillance of women at high familial risk for breast cancer, *J Clin Oncol* 23:8469–8476, 2005.

Leach MO, Boggis CR, Dixon AK, et al: Screening with magnetic resonance imaging and mammography of a UK population at high familial risk of breast cancer: a prospective multicentre cohort study (MARIBS), *Lancet* 365:1769–1778, 2005.

Le Bihan D, Turner R, Douek P, Patronas N: Diffusion MR imaging: clinical applications, *AJR Am J Roentgenol* 159:591–599, 1992.

Lehman CD, Blume JD, Thickman D, et al: Added cancer yield of MRI in screening the contralateral breast of women recently diagnosed with breast cancer: results from the International Breast Magnetic Resonance Consortium (IBMC) trial, *J Surg Oncol* 92:9–16, 2005.

Lehman CD, Blume JD, Weatherall P, et al: Screening women at high risk for breast cancer with mammography and magnetic resonance imaging, *Cancer* 103:1898–1905, 2005.

Lehman CD, DeMartini W, Anderson BO, Edge SB: Indications for breast MRI in the patient with newly diagnosed breast cancer, *J Natl Compr Canc Netw* 7:193–201, 2009.

Leong CS, Daniel BL, Herfkens RJ, et al: Characterization of breast lesion morphology with delayed 3DSSMT: An adjunct to dynamic breast MRI, *J Magn Reson Imaging* 11:87–96, 2000.

Li J, Dershaw DD, Lee CH, et al: MRI follow-up after concordant, histologically benign diagnosis of breast lesions sampled by MRI-guided biopsy, *AJR Am J Roentgenol* 193:850–855, 2009.

Liberman L, Morris EA, Benton CL, et al: Probably benign lesions at breast magnetic resonance imaging: preliminary experience in high-risk women, *Cancer* 98:377–388, 2003.

Liberman L, Morris EA, Dershaw DD, et al: MR imaging of the ipsilateral breast in women with percutaneously proven breast cancer, *AJR Am J Roentgenol* 180:901–910, 2003.

Liberman L, Morris EA, Dershaw DD, et al: Ductal enhancement on MR imaging of the breast, *AJR Am J Roentgenol* 181:519–525, 2003.

Liberman L, Morris EA, Dershaw DD, et al: Fast MRI-guided vacuum-assisted breast biopsy: initial experience, *AJR Am J Roentgenol* 181:1283–1293, 2003.

Liberman L, Morris EA, Kim CM, et al: MR imaging findings in the contralateral breast of women with recently diagnosed breast cancer, *AJR Am J Roentgenol* 180:333–341, 2003.

Liberman L, Morris EA, Lee MJ, et al: Breast lesions detected on MR imaging: Features and positive predictive value. *AJR Am J Roentgenol* 179:171–178, 2002.

Linda A, Zuiani C, Londero V, Bazzocchi M: Outcome of initially only magnetic resonance mammography-detected findings with and without correlate at second-look sonography: distribution according to patient history of breast cancer and lesion size, *Breast* 17:51–57, 2008.

Lyng H, Haraldseth O, Rofstad EK: Measurement of cell density and necrotic fraction in human melanoma xenografts by diffusion weighted magnetic resonance imaging, *Magn Reson Med* 43:828–836, 2000.

Marini C, Iacconi C, Giannelli M, et al: Quantitative diffusion-weighted MR imaging in the differential diagnosis of breast lesion, *Eur Radiol* 17:2646–2655, 2007.

Meissnitzer M, Dershaw DD, Lee CH, Morris EA: Targeted ultrasound of the breast in women with abnormal MRI findings for whom biopsy has been recommended, *AJR Am J Roentgenol* 193:1025–1029, 2009.

Monzawa S, Yokokawa M, Sakuma T, et al: Mucinous carcinoma of the breast: MRI features of pure and mixed forms with histopathologic correlation, *AJR Am J Roentgenol* 192:W125–W131, 2009.

Morris EA: Illustrated breast MR lexicon, *Semin Roentgenol* 36:238–249, 2001.

Morris EA, Liberman L, Ballon DJ, et al: MRI of occult breast carcinoma in a high-risk population, *AJR Am J Roentgenol* 181:619–626, 2003.

Morris EA, Liberman L, Dershaw DD, et al: Preoperative MR imaging-guided needle localization of breast lesions, *AJR Am J Roentgenol* 178:1211–1220, 2002.

Morris EA, Schwartz LH, Drotman MB, et al: Evaluation of pectoralis major muscle in patients with posterior breast tumors on breast MR images: early experience, *Radiology* 214:67–72, 2000.

Moy L, Elias K, Patel V, et al: Is breast MRI helpful in the evaluation of inconclusive mammographic findings? *AJR Am J Roentgenol* 193:986–993, 2009.

Muller-Schimpfle M, Ohmenhauser K, Sand J, et al: Dynamic 3D-MR mammography: is there a benefit of sophisticated evaluation of enhancement curves for clinical routine? *J Magn Reson Imaging* 7:236–240, 1997.

Nicholson BT, Harvey JA, Cohen MA: Nipple–areolar complex: normal anatomy and benign and malignant processes, *Radiographics* 29:509–523, 2009.

Nunes LW, Englander SA, Charafeddine R, Schnall MD: Optimal post-contrast timing of breast MR image acquisition for architectural feature analysis, *J Magn Reson Imaging* 16:42–50, 2002.

Nunes LW, Schnall MD, Orel SG: Update of breast MR imaging architectural interpretation model, *Radiology* 219:484–494, 2001.

Obdeijn IM, Brouwers-Kuyper EM, Tilanus-Linthorst MM, et al: MR imaging-guided sonography followed by *Breast J* fine-needle aspiration cytology in occult carcinoma of the breast, *AJR Am J Roentgenol* 174:1079–1084, 2000.

Offodile RS, Daniel BL, Jeffrey SS, et al: Magnetic resonance imaging of suspicious breast masses seen on one mammographic view, *Breast J* 10(5):416–422, 2004.

Orel SG, Dougherty CS, Reynolds C, et al: MR imaging in patients with nipple discharge: initial experience, *Radiology* 216:248–254, 2000.

Partridge SC, DeMartini WB, Kurland BF, et al: Quantitative diffusion-weighted imaging as an adjunct to conventional breast MRI for improved positive predictive value, *AJR Am J Roentgenol* 193:1716–1722, 2009.

Partridge SC, Gibbs JE, Lu Y, et al: Accuracy of MR imaging for revealing residual breast cancer in patients who have undergone neoadjuvant chemotherapy, *AJR Am J Roentgenol* 179:1193–1199, 2002.

Partridge SC, McKinnon GC, Henry RG, Hylton NM: Menstrual cycle variation of apparent diffusion coefficients measured in the normal breast using MRI, *J Magn Reson Imaging* 14:433–438, 2001.

Pereira FP, Martins G, Figueiredo E, et al: Assessment of breast lesions with diffusion-weighted MRI: comparing the use of different *b* values, *AJR Am J Roentgenol* 193:1030–1035, 2009.

Perlet C, Schneider P, Amaya B, et al: MR-guided vacuum biopsy of 206 contrast-enhancing breast lesions, *Rofo Fortschr Geb Rontgenstr Neuen Bildgeb Verfahr* 174:88–95, 2002.

Qayyum A, Birdwell RL, Daniel BL, et al: MR imaging features of infiltrating lobular carcinoma of the breast: histopathologic correlation, *AJR Am J Roentgenol* 178:1227–1232, 2002.

Ralleigh G, Walker AE, Hall-Craggs MA, et al: MR imaging of the skin and nipple of the breast: differentiation between tumour recurrence and post-treatment change, *Eur Radiol* 11:1651–1658, 2001.

Rieber A, Zeitler H, Rosenthal H, et al: MRI of breast cancer: influence of chemotherapy on sensitivity, *Br J Radiol* 70:452–458, 1997.

Rodenko GN, Harms SE, Pruneda JM, et al: MR imaging in the management before surgery of lobular carcinoma of the breast: correlation with pathology, *AJR Am J Roentgenol* 167:1415–1419, 1996.

Rubesova E, Grell AS, De Maertelaer V, et al: Quantitative diffusion imaging in breast cancer: a clinical prospective study, *J Magn Reson Imaging* 24:319–324, 2006.

Saslow D, Boetes C, Burke W, et al: American Cancer Society guidelines for breast screening with MRI as an adjunct to mammography, *CA Cancer J Clin* 57:75–89, 2007.

Schnall MD, Blume J, Bluemke DA, et al: MRI detection of distinct incidental cancer in women with primary breast cancer studied in IBMC 6883, *J Surg Oncol* 92:32–38, 2005.

Schnall MD, Rosten S, Englander S, et al: A combined architectural and kinetic interpretation model for breast MR images, *Acad Radiol* 8:591–597, 2001.

Sinha S, Lucas-Quesada FA, Sinha U, et al: In vivo diffusion-weighted MRI of the breast: potential for lesion characterization, *J Magn Reson Imaging* 15:693–704, 2002.

Slanetz PJ, Edmister WB, Yeh ED, et al: Occult contralateral breast carcinoma incidentally detected by breast magnetic resonance imaging, *Breast J* 8:145–148, 2002.

Soderstrom CE, Harms SE, Farrell RS Jr, et al: Detection with MR imaging of residual tumor in the breast soon after surgery, *AJR Am J Roentgenol* 168:485–488, 1997.

Stoutjesdijk MJ, Boetes C, Jager GJ, et al: Magnetic resonance imaging and mammography in women with a hereditary risk of breast cancer, *J Natl Cancer Inst* 93:1095–1102, 2001.

Sugahara T, Korogi Y, Kochi M, et al: Usefulness of diffusion-weighted MRI with echo-planar technique in the evaluation of cellularity in gliomas, *J Magn Reson Imaging* 9:53–60, 1999.

Talele AC, Slanetz PJ, Edmister WB, et al: The lactating breast: MRI findings and literature review, *Breast J* 9:237–240, 2003.

Tan JE, Orel SG, Schnall MD, et al: Role of magnetic resonance imaging and magnetic resonance imaging-guided surgery in the evaluation of patients with early-stage breast cancer for breast conservation treatment, *Am J Clin Oncol* 22:414–418, 1999.

Teifke A, Lehr HA, Vomweg TW, et al: Outcome analysis and rational management of enhancing lesions incidentally detected on contrast-enhanced MRI of the breast, *AJR Am J Roentgenol* 181:655–662, 2003.

Tendulkar RD, Chellman-Jeffers M, Rybicki LA, et al: Preoperative breast magnetic resonance imaging in early breast cancer: implications for partial breast irradiation, *Cancer* 115:1621–1630, 2009.

Tilanus-Linthorst MM, Bartels CC, Obdeijn AI, Oudkerk M: Earlier detection of breast cancer by surveillance of women at familial risk, *Eur J Cancer* 36:514–519, 2000.

Tilanus-Linthorst MM, Obdeijn AI, Bontenbal M, Oudkerk M: MRI in patients with axillary metastases of occult breast carcinoma, *Breast Cancer Res Treat* 44:179–182, 1997.

Trecate G, Tess JD, Vergnaghi D, et al: Lobular breast cancer: how useful is breast magnetic resonance imaging? *Tumori* 87:232–238, 2001.

Tsuboi N, Ogawa Y, Inomata T, et al: Changes in the findings of dynamic MRI by preoperative CAF chemotherapy for patients with breast cancer of stage II and III: pathologic correlation, *Oncol Rep* 6:727–732, 1999.

Viehweg P, Heinig A, Lampe D, et al: Retrospective analysis for evaluation of the value of contrast-enhanced MRI in patients treated with breast conservative therapy, *MAGMA* 7:141–152, 1998.

Viehweg P, Lampe D, Buchmann J, Heywang-Kobrunner SH: In situ and minimally invasive breast cancer: morphologic and kinetic features on contrast-enhanced MR imaging, *MAGMA* 11:129–137, 2000.

Viehweg P, Paprosch I, Strassinopoulou M, Heywang-Kobrunner SH: Contrast-enhanced magnetic resonance imaging of the breast: interpretation guidelines, *Top Magn Reson Imaging* 9:17–43, 1998.

Warner E, Plewes DB, Shumak RS, et al: Comparison of breast magnetic resonance imaging, mammography, and ultrasound for surveillance of women at high risk for hereditary breast cancer, *J Clin Oncol* 19:3524–3531, 2001.

Wenkel E, Geppert C, Schulz-Wendtland R, et al: Diffusion weighted imaging in breast MRI: comparison of two different pulse sequences, *Acad Radiol* 14:1077–1083, 2007.

Wiratkapun C, Duke D, Nordmann AS, et al: Indeterminate or suspicious breast lesions detected initially with MR imaging: value of MRI-directed breast ultrasound, *Acad Radiol* 15:618–625, 2008.

Woodhams R, Matsunaga K, Kan S, et al: ADC mapping of benign and malignant breast tumors, *Magn Reson Med Sci* 4:35–42, 2005.

Yabuuchi H, Matsuo Y, Okafuji T, et al: Enhanced mass on contrast-enhanced breast MR imaging: lesion characterization using combination of dynamic contrast-enhanced and diffusion-weighted MR images, *J Magn Reson Imaging* 28:1157–1165, 2008.

Quizzes

7-1. Fill in the principles of breast cancer MRI.

_____

_____

_____

_____

_____

_____

For answers, see Box 7-1.

7-2. Fill in the requirements for patient selection and preparation.

_____

_____

_____

For answers, see Box 7-2.

7-3. Fill in the equipment for breast MRI.

_____

_____

_____

_____

_____

_____

For answers, see Box 7-3.

7-4. Fill in the breast density by volume.

_____ _____

_____ _____

_____ _____

_____ _____

For answers, see Box 7-4.

7-5. Fill in the background enhancement.

_____ _____

_____ _____

_____ _____

_____ _____

_____ _____

For answers, see Box 7-5.

7-6. Fill in the morphologic features of enhancing breast lesions.

FEATURES SUGGESTING BENIGNANCY

_____

_____

_____

_____

_____

_____

FEATURES SUGGESTING MALIGNANCY

_____

_____

_____

_____

_____

_____

_____

_____

For answers, see Box 7-6.

7-7. Fill in the dynamic contrast enhancement of breast lesions.

PATTERNS SUGGESTING A BENIGN LESION

_____

_____

_____

PATTERNS SUGGESTING MALIGNANCY

_____

_____

_____

_____

For answers, see Box 7-7.

7-8. Fill in the organized approach to breast MRI interpretation.

_____

_____

_____

_____

_____

_____

_____

_____

_____

_____

_____

_____

For answers, see Box 7-8.

7-9. Fill in the common false-positive conditions that simulate malignancy.

_____

_____

_____

_____

_____

_____

For answers, see Box 7-9.

7-10. Fill in the common false-negative tumors on breast MRI.

_____

_____

_____

_____

_____

For answers, see Box 7-10.

7-11. Fill in the accepted indications for contrast-enhanced breast MRI.

SCREENING

_____

_____

_____

_____

_____

_____

_____

DIAGNOSIS

_____

_____

_____

STAGING

_____

_____

_____

_____

_____

_____

_____

_____

_____

_____

_____

_____

_____

MANAGEMENT

_____

_____

_____

For answers, see Box 7-11.

7-12. Fill in the options for biopsy of MRI abnormalities.

_____

_____

_____

For answers, see Box 7-12.

7-13. Fill in the T1, T2, and kinetic curves for cancer and benign masses on breast MRI.

	Axial T1-Weighted Localizer Noncontrast No Fat Suppression	T2-Weighted Noncontrast Fat-Suppressed	Initial Kinetic Contrast Enhancement Curve	Late Kinetic Contrast Enhancement Curve
Cancer				
Lymph node				
Fibroadenoma: myxoid				
Fibroadenoma: old, sclerotic				
Papilloma				
Mucinous cancer				
Ductal carcinoma in situ				
Old scar				
Cyst				
Fat necrosis				

For answers, see Table 7-1.

7-14. Fill in the basic bilateral protocol for breast cancer MR imaging.

SERIES DESCRIPTION   **PURPOSE**

1 _____   _____

2 _____   _____

[3] _____   _____

4 _____   _____

5 _____   _____

[6] _____   _____

N/A _____   _____

For answers, see Table 7-2.

7-15. Fill in the common artifacts.

ARTIFACT	CAUSE
_____	_____
_____	_____
_____	_____
_____	_____
_____	_____
_____	_____

For answers, see Table 7-3.

7-16. Fill in the T2-weighted imaging of breast lesions.

	T2 > GLANDULAR TISSUE OR MUSCLE	**T2 ≤ GLANDULAR TISSUE**
Enhances with contrast	_____	_____
	_____	
Nonenhancing	_____	_____

For answers, see Table 7-4.

7-17. Fill in the ACR BI-RADS®–MRI lexicon terms and classification scheme.

Lesion Type (Select One)
Mass

NON-MASSLIKE ENHANCEMENT
MORPHOLOGY ASSESSMENT
FOR MASSES
(SELECT ONE IN EACH)

Shape	**Enhancement**
_____	_____
_____	_____
_____	_____
_____	_____
Margin	_____
_____	_____
_____	
_____	

NON-MASSLIKE ENHANCEMENT

Distribution Modifiers (select one)

_____

_____

_____

_____

_____

_____

_____

Internal Enhancement (Mass and Non-masslike) (select one)

_____

_____

_____

_____

SYMMETRY (USE FOR BILATERAL SCANS ONLY)

_____

_____

For answers, see Table 7-5.

OTHER FINDINGS (REPORT ALL THAT APPLY)

_____

_____

_____

_____

_____

_____

_____

_____

_____

KINETIC CURVE ASSESSMENT (SELECT ONE IN EACH)

Initial Rise

_____

_____

_____

Delayed Phase

_____

_____

_____

CHAPTER 8

Breast Cancer Treatment-Related Imaging and the Postoperative Breast

Debra M. Ikeda, Kathleen C. Horst, and Frederick M. Dirbas

This chapter provides an overview of clinically driven breast cancer evaluation; the sequence of events after a breast cancer diagnosis; locoregional breast cancer treatment options, including sentinel lymph node (SLN) biopsy; the normal postoperative breast; postradiation therapy change; ipsilateral breast tumor recurrence (IBTR) after lumpectomy; and the appearance of the breast after mastectomy with or without reconstruction.

Palpable or image-detected breast abnormalities constitute the majority of consultations for breast specialists. After assessment, the specialist usually orders a complete imaging workup of suspicious findings and may ask for a fine-needle aspiration (FNA) or percutaneous core biopsy if the findings are worrisome enough. If results of percutaneous biopsy are indeterminate or discordant, or if the patient prefers, a diagnosis may be established by open surgical breast biopsy.

No matter how breast cancer is diagnosed, follow-up treatment depends on the tumor size and stage. If the tumor is large, women may undergo neoadjuvant chemotherapy (i.e., chemotherapy given before excision of the primary tumor). Neoadjuvant chemotherapy shrinks the tumor and allows the medical oncologist to determine the chemotherapy's effectiveness in vivo. If the tumor shrinks to a small enough size, the woman may undergo breast-conserving therapy and radiation therapy, rather than mastectomy.

If the breast cancer is small, surgical management is almost always recommended initially to remove the cancer. Lumpectomy (almost always followed by breast radiotherapy) and mastectomy are the two principal options for local therapy. Survival is the same with either approach. Of the two, lumpectomy (also referred to as *breast-conserving surgery, partial mastectomy,* or *quadrantectomy*) is more commonly preferred. Mastectomy may be performed in a variety of fashions, such as using skin-sparing techniques, and can be performed with or without breast reconstruction.

At the time of surgery, SLN biopsy commonly accompanies removal of the primary tumor to determine if axillary lymph nodes harbor metastases. A full axillary node dissection (levels I and II are commonly performed today) follows if the sentinel node harbors anything more than isolated tumor cells (*AJCC Staging Manual*).

Whole-breast radiotherapy usually is performed after lumpectomy to eliminate microscopic residual disease remaining in the breast. The purpose of radiotherapy is to suppress tumor recurrence in the remaining breast parenchyma in general and in the tissue around the lumpectomy cavity in particular. This typically involves 6 weeks of whole-breast radiotherapy with an electron beam boost dose to further eradicate any residual cells near the surgical margins. Clinical studies evaluating radiotherapy doses delivered over shorter time periods are now under way and include hypofractionated schedules (e.g., treatment delivered over approximately 3 weeks) and accelerated partial-breast irradiation (APBI), in which the radiotherapy period ranges from 5 days to a single dose given at the time of lumpectomy. If successful, these new radiotherapy approaches will allow much shorter radiotherapy treatment periods for most women.

It is important to understand how patients progress from workup to cancer diagnosis and through treatment and how surgery, radiation, and systemic therapy, affect imaging of the treated breast. This chapter details each of these steps.

■ COMBINED CLINICAL AND IMAGING WORKUP OF BREAST ABNORMALITIES

Once the referring physician finds a suspicious breast mass or receives a suspicious mammographic report, the patient undergoes a thorough history and a focused breast examination. Usually a breast cancer specialist (commonly a general surgeon with an interest in breast cancer, a dedicated breast surgeon, or a surgical oncologist) then estimates the patient's risk of having breast cancer, seeks patterns of familial breast cancer, and helps the patient to make an informed decision about imaging versus immediate intervention.

Most patients are then referred for a thorough diagnostic imaging workup. Patients with suspicious palpable abnormalities undergo ultrasound, with or without mammography, depending on age, family history, and level of concern over the finding. For example, ultrasound would likely be the sole imaging modality in an 18-year-old woman with a new breast lump and no family history of breast cancer. On the other hand, ultrasound and mammography would likely be used for a 25-year-old woman with a new palpable lesion and an extensive family history of breast cancer in young relatives. The final decision as to whether or not to incorporate mammography into a very young patient's workup is a shared responsibility of the clinician directing the breast workup, the radiologist performing the initial imaging (ultrasound in this case), and the patient. Breast magnetic resonance imaging (MRI) is used sparingly during the initial evaluation of a palpable finding, unless there is an extensive family history, in which case it serves a dual role as both a diagnostic tool on the affected breast and a screening tool on the contralateral breast.

For patients with nonpalpable findings on screening mammography, workup always includes diagnostic mammography. For suspicious calcifications alone, the radiologist usually obtains magnification mammograms, often not needing ultrasound. An exception might be extensive pleomorphic microcalcifications, in which ultrasound might be used to search for masses within the area that could be indicative of invasive cancer, prompting biopsy. However, if there is an image-detected mass, area of architectural distortion, or palpable mass, the radiologist usually uses both mammography and ultrasound to evaluate the abnormality, estimate its size, and direct later biopsy. Breast MRI may be valuable in selected cases, as discussed in Chapter 7. Ideally, the radiologist correlates all physical and imaging findings in the report to form a composite picture of all potential abnormalities and their level of suspicion on mammography, ultrasound, and MRI.

Using the combined report, the directing clinician and radiologist plan percutaneous or open biopsy to sample all areas of concern. This sequence varies from patient to patient. This may be as simple as FNA in a young woman with a single area of fibrocystic nodularity and a normal ultrasound or as complex as numerous core biopsies or surgical biopsies in one or both breasts using palpation or image guidance for localization.

Although there are no hard and fast rules about what defines a "suspicious" palpable abnormality, in general cancers are firm or hard, asymmetric compared with the opposite breast, irregular in shape, and feel as if they are rising up out of the breast tissue, rather than spreading out in the substance of the breast. Physical examination, ultrasound/mammography, and FNA are generally considered the "minimum" intervention for a suspicious palpable finding and in combination are referred to as the *triple test*. For suspicious palpable findings in which all components of the triple test are negative, the risk of malignancy is considered approximately 3% or less. Even if all components of the triple test are normal, it is extremely important to inform the patient that there is a low, but measurable, false-negative rate for the triple test and that surgical excision can be performed to completely exclude the possibility of malignancy. This discussion is ideally documented in the medical record. Patients with likely benign palpable findings, unremarkable imaging, and normal percutaneous sampling with FNA (i.e., a negative triple test) usually undergo a single follow-up visit 3 to 6 months later with the referring physician. Patients who undergo image-guided core biopsy usually undergo repeat imaging 6, 12, and 24 months later to assess stability of any residual findings. Progressive findings on repeat palpation or breast imaging at follow-up prompt surgical excision.

For suspicious *image-detected* nonpalpable lesions, image-guided FNA, percutaneous core biopsy, or wire-localized excisional biopsy is generally considered the "minimum" intervention. Percutaneous needle core biopsy has become the more common choice. Here, too, it is important to inform the patient of the limitations of percutaneous core biopsy—specifically, that there is a small false-negative rate with needle biopsy. Wire-localized surgical biopsy is usually recommended to exclude malignancy if percutaneous biopsy is indeterminate or discordant with imaging findings. For an anxious patient, wire-localized surgical excision may be a better option initially; the surgeon will usually document this discussion in the medical record, too. For some patients with lesions close to the chest wall or nipple, wire-localized excisional biopsy may also be the safer initial approach.

■ BREAST CANCER DIAGNOSIS AND TREATMENT

When a combined clinical and imaging workup leads to a breast cancer diagnosis, treatment planning usually involves a consideration of surgery, chemotherapy, and radiation therapy, with the goal to remove all the cancer from the breast, optimize chances for locoregional control, and eradicate occult foci of metastatic disease via systemic treatment (e.g., hormone therapy, chemotherapy), if indicated. The team of breast imagers, surgeons, medical oncologists, pathologists, radiation oncologists, and breast reconstruction surgeons plan the sequence in which surgery, chemotherapy, and radiation occurs. The pathology report is a key component on which treatment is based. The report states tumor histology; size; estrogen, progesterone, and *her2neu* receptor status; and lymph node involvement. Traditionally, breast tumors are staged using the TNM (*t*umor, lymph *n*ode, *m*etastasis) Classification on Breast Cancer from the American Joint Committee on Cancer (currently in the 7th edition) (Table 8-1). The treatment plan is based on this classification. A clinical decision algorithm is also available from the National Comprehensive Cancer Network regarding the full spectrum of care; Adjuvant! Online is an Internet-based tool that provides guidance regarding prognosis and the potential benefit of different chemotherapy protocols. Additional tests based on tumor gene signatures are emerging (OncoType DX and MammaPrint) and are the subject of two large randomized trials, one in the United States and the other in Europe. Gene expression profiling may play an increasingly important role in the future; preliminary data suggest improvement in separating high- and low-risk patients.

Locoregional control of the cancer means that the patient undergoes surgical removal of the cancer with a margin of normal breast tissue. (Although the definition of an acceptable margin varies from institution to institution, the more commonly followed models range from simple nontransection [tumor not on inked margin] to 2 mm of normal tissue at the margin.) The patient achieves this locoregional control by either breast-conserving surgery, usually followed by whole-breast irradiation, or mastectomy. As shown by Protocol B-06 conducted by the National Surgical Adjuvant Breast and Bowel Project (NSABP), both approaches yield equivalent local control

TABLE 8-1. TNM Staging Classification for Breast Cancer

Primary Tumor (T)*	
TX	Primary tumor cannot be assessed
T0	No evidence of primary tumor
Tis	Carcinoma in situ
Tis (DCIS)	Ductal carcinoma in situ
Tis (LCIS)	Lobular carcinoma in situ
Tis (Paget)	Paget disease of the nipple *not* associated with invasive carcinoma and/or carcinoma in situ (DCIS and/or LCIS) in the underlying breast parenchyma. Carcinomas in the breast parenchyma associated with Paget disease are categorized based on the size and characteristics of the parenchymal disease, although the presence of Paget disease should still be noted
T1	Tumor ≤ 2 cm in greatest dimension
T1mic	Microinvasion ≤ 0.1 cm in greatest dimension
T1a	Tumor > 0.1 cm but ≤0.5 cm in greatest dimension
T1b	Tumor > 0.5 cm but ≤1 cm in greatest dimension
T1c	Tumor > 1 cm but ≤2 cm in greatest dimension
T2	Tumor > 2 cm but ≤5 cm in greatest dimension
T3	Tumor > 5 cm in greatest dimension
T4	Tumor of any size with direct extension to the chest wall and/or skin (ulceration or skin nodules)[†]
T4a	Extension to the chest wall not including only pectoralis muscle adherence/invasion
T4b	Ulceration and/or ipsilateral satellite nodules and/or edema (including *peau d'orange*) of the skin, which do not meet the criteria for inflammatory carcinoma
T4c	Both T4a and T4b
T4d	Inflammatory carcinoma

Regional Lymph Nodes (N)*	
NX	Regional lymph nodes cannot be assessed (e.g., previously removed)
N0	No regional lymph node metastases
N1	Metastasis to movable ipsilateral level I, II axillary lymph node(s)
N2	Metastases in ipsilateral level I, II axillary lymph nodes that are clinically fixed or matted; or in clinically detected[‡] ipsilateral internal mammary nodes in the *absence* of clinically evident axillary lymph node metastases
N2a	Metastases in ipsilateral level I, II axillary lymph nodes fixed to one another (matted) or to other structures
N2b	Metastases only in clinically detected[‡] ipsilateral internal mammary nodes and in the *absence* of clinically evident level I, II axillary lymph node metastases
N3	Metastases in ipsilateral infraclavicular (level III axillary) lymph node(s) with or without level I, II axillary lymph node involvement; or in clinically detected[‡] ipsilateral internal mammary lymph node(s) with clinically evident level I, II axillary lymph node metastases; or metastases in ipsilateral supraclavicular lymph node(s) with or without axillary or internal mammary lymph node involvement
N3a	Metastases in ipsilateral infraclavicular lymph node(s)

Regional Lymph Nodes—cont'd	
N3b	Metastases in ipsilateral internal mammary lymph node(s) and axillary lymph node(s)
N3c	Metastases in ipsilateral supraclavicular lymph node(s)

Pathologic (pN)[§]	
pNX	Regional lymph nodes cannot be assessed (e.g., previously removed, or not removed for pathologic study)
pN0	No regional lymph node metastasis identified histologically

Note: Isolated tumor cell clusters (ITC) are defined as small clusters of cells not greater than 0.2 mm, or single tumor cells, or a cluster of fewer than 200 cells in a single histologic cross-section. ITCs may be detected by routine histology or by immunohistochemical (IHC) methods. Nodes containing only ITCs are excluded from the total positive node count for purposes of N classification but should be included in the total number of nodes evaluated.

pN0(i−)	No regional lymph node metastases histologically, negative IHC
pN0(i+)	Malignant cells in regional lymph node(s) no greater than 0.2 mm (detected by H&E or IHC including ITC)
pN0(mol−)	No regional lymph node metastases histologically, negative molecular findings (RT-PCR)
pN0(mol+)	Positive molecular findings (RT-PCR), but no regional lymph node metastases detected by histology or IHC
pN1	Micrometastases; or metastases in 1–3 axillary lymph nodes; and/or in internal mammary nodes with metastases detected by sentinel lymph node biopsy but not clinically detected[‖]
pN1mi	Micrometastases (greater than 0.2 mm and/or more than 200 cells, but none greater than 2 mm)
pN1a	Metastases in 1–3 axillary lymph nodes, at least one metastasis greater than 2 mm
pN1b	Metastases in internal mammary nodes with micrometastases or macrometastases detected by sentinel lymph node biopsy but not clinically detected[‖]
pN1c	Metastases in 1–3 axillary lymph nodes and in internal mammary lymph nodes with micrometastases or macrometastases detected by sentinel lymph node biopsy but not clinically detected
pN2	Metastases in 4–9 axillary lymph nodes; or in clinically detected[¶] internal mammary lymph nodes in the *absence* of axillary lymph node metastases
pN2a	Metastases in 4–9 axillary lymph nodes (at least one tumor deposit greater than 2 mm)
pN2b	Metastases in clinically detected[¶] internal mammary lymph nodes in the *absence* of axillary lymph node metastases
pN3	Metastases in 10 or more axillary lymph nodes; or in infraclavicular (level III axillary) lymph nodes; or in clinically detected[¶] ipsilateral internal mammary lymph nodes in the *presence* of 1 or more positive level I, II axillary lymph nodes; or in more than 3 axillary lymph nodes and in internal mammary lymph nodes with micrometastases or macrometastases detected by sentinel lymph node biopsy but not clinically detected[‖]; or in ipsilateral supraclavicular lymph nodes

TABLE 8-1. TNM Staging Classification for Breast Cancer—cont'd

Pathologic—cont'd		Distant Metastases—cont'd			
pN3a	Metastases in 10 or more axillary lymph nodes (at least 1 tumor deposit greater than 2 mm); or metastases to the infraclavicular (level III axillary lymph) nodes	M1	Distant detectable metastases as determined by classic clinical and radiographic means and/or histologically proven larger than 0.2 mm		
pN3b	Metastases in clinically detected[¶] ipsilateral internal mammary lymph nodes in the *presence* of 1 or more positive axillary lymph nodes; or in more than 3 axillary lymph nodes and in internal mammary lymph nodes with micrometastases or macrometastases detected by sentinel lymph node biopsy but not clinically detected[‖]	**Anatomic Stage/Prognostic Group**			
		0	Tis	N0	M0
		IA	T1**	N0	M0
		IB	I0	N1mi	M0
			I1**	N1mi	M0
pN3c	Metastases in ipsilateral supraclavicular lymph nodes	IIA	T0	N1[††]	M0
			T1**	N1[††]	M0
Post-treatment ypN			T2	N0	M0
Post-treatment yp "N" should be evaluated as for clinical (pretreatment) "N" methods above. The modifier "sn" is used only if a sentinel node evaluation was performed after treatment. If no subscript is attached, it is assumed that the axillary nodal evaluation was by axillary node dissection (AND)		IIB	T2	N1	M0
			T3	N0	M0
The X classification will be used (ypNX) if no yp post-treatment SN or AND was performed		IIIA	T0	N2	M0
			T1**	N2	M0
N categories are the same as those used for pN			T2	N2	M0
			T3	N1, N2	M0
Distant Metastases (M)		IIIB	T4	N0, N1, N2	M0
M0	No clinical or radiographic evidence of distant metastases	IIIC	Any T	N3	M0
cM0(i+)	No clinical or radiographic evidence of distant metastases, but deposits of molecularly or microscopically detected tumor cells in circulating blood, bone marrow, or other nonregional nodal tissue that are no larger than 0.2 mm in a patient without symptoms or signs of metastases	IV	Any T	Any N	M1

*The T classification of the primary tumor is the same regardless of whether it is based on clinical or pathologic criteria, or both. Size should be measured to the nearest millimeter. If the tumor size is slightly less than or greater than a cutoff for a given T classification, it is recommended that the size be rounded to the millimeter reading that is closest to the cutoff. For example, a reported size of 1.1 mm is reported as 1 mm, or a size of 2.01 cm is reported as 2 cm. Designation should be made with the subscript "c" or "p" modifier to indicate whether the T classification was determined by clinical (physical examination or radiologic) or pathologic measurements, respectively. In general, pathologic determination should take precedence over clinical determination of T size.

[†]Invasion of the dermis alone does not qualify as T4.

[‡]*Clinically detected* is defined as detected by imaging studies (excluding lymphoscintigraphy) or by clinical examination and having characteristics highly suspicious for malignancy or a presumed pathologic macrometastasis based on fine needle aspiration biopsy with cytologic examination. Confirmation of clinically detected metastatic disease by fine needle aspiration without excision biopsy is designated with an (f) suffix, for example, cN3a(f). Excisional biopsy of a lymph node or biopsy of a sentinel node, in the absence of assignment of a pT, is classified as a clinical N, for example, cN1. Information regarding the confirmation of the nodal status will be designated in site-specific factors as clinical, fine needle aspiration, core biopsy, or sentinel lymph node biopsy. Pathologic classification (pN) is used for excision or sentinel lymph node biopsy only in conjunction with a pathologic T assignment.

[§]Classification is based on axillary lymph node dissection with or without sentinel lymph node biopsy. Classification based solely on sentinel lymph node biopsy without subsequent axillary lymph node dissection is designated (sn) for "sentinel node," for example, pN0(sn).

[‖]"Not clinically detected" is defined as not detected by imaging studies (excluding lymphoscintigraphy) or not detected by clinical examination.

[¶]"Clinically detected" is defined as detected by imaging studies (excluding lymphoscintigraphy) or by clinical examination and having characteristics highly suspicious for malignancy or a presumed pathologic macrometastasis based on fine needle aspiration biopsy with cytologic examination.

**T1 includes T1mi.

[††]T0 and T1 tumors with nodal micrometastases only are excluded from stage IIA and are classified stage IB.

M0 includes M0(i+).

The designation pM0 is not valid; any M0 should be clinical.

If a patient presents with M1 prior to neoadjuvant systemic therapy, the stage is considered stage IV and remains stage IV regardless of response to neoadjuvant therapy.

Stage designation may be changed if postsurgical imaging studies reveal the presence of distant metastases, provided that the studies are carried out within 4 months of diagnosis in the absence of disease progression and provided that the patient has not received neoadjuvant therapy.

Postneoadjuvant therapy is designated with "yc" or "yp" prefix. Of note, no stage group is assigned if there is a complete pathologic response (CR) to neoadjuvant therapy, for example, ypT0ypN0cM0.

H&E, hematoxylin and eosin stain; RT-PCR: reverse transcriptase/polymerase chain reaction.

From American Joint Committee on Cancer (AJCC): Breast. In Edge SB, Byrd Dr, Compton CC, et al, editors: AJCC *cancer staging manual*, ed 3, New York, 2010, Springer, 2010, pp 358–361.

and identical survival rates in women with tumors 4 cm or smaller in diameter whether the axillary lymph nodes are positive or negative for metastatic disease.

The radiologist helps the team select candidates for breast-conserving surgery or mastectomy by estimating the location and extent of disease. The critical information the surgeon requests relates to lesion location and size. This allows the surgeon to form a three-dimensional (3-D) representation of normal versus malignant tissue, develop a mental image of the tumor within the breast, estimate the amount of additional tissue needed to obtain tumor-free margins, and plan the incision (surgical approach) with the goal of maximizing probability of tumor removal while preserving cosmesis as best as possible. For example, it is difficult to remove an extensive ductal carcinoma in situ (DCIS) completely with microscopically clear margins, and these patients are usually treated with mastectomy. Increasingly, there is interest (though no good randomized data to support) in removing multiple lesions from the same breast while preserving the breast. *Multifocal disease* refers to lesions in the same quadrant; *multicentric disease* refers to lesions in separate quadrants. As a straightforward example, a 3-mm satellite lesion is almost always amenable to resection with a primary lesion using breast-conserving techniques with an acceptable cosmetic outcome. In contradistinction, a pair of 3- to 4-cm lesions on opposite sides of the breast are usually treated with mastectomy. There are no hard and fast rules for excising multiple lesions with breast conservation, and excellent clinical judgment must be used. For this reason, in the setting of multiple lesions, the surgeon requests information regarding the number and size of the lesions, as well as their geographic relationship to each other. If too many foci of invasive cancer or extensive DCIS are present, the patient is not a candidate for breast-conserving surgery because the surgeon would have a hard time excising all the cancer and because of concern over an elevated risk of IBTR.

In general, surgeons perform mastectomy when the entire cancer cannot be excised with a good cosmetic result (as just discussed), if the woman has a contraindication to radiotherapy, or if it is the patient's desire. Usually, patients are offered ipsilateral breast reconstruction with an autologous tissue flap or a tissue expander after mastectomy, unless there is a medical contraindication to reconstruction (e.g., multiple co-morbidities). Because the contralateral breast is often larger than the reconstructed breast, patients may also need reduction mammoplasty on the contralateral side. Characteristic appearances of reduction mammoplasty and breast reconstruction are discussed in Chapter 9.

If the patient has breast-conserving surgery, she usually undergoes postsurgical whole-breast irradiation to achieve control of residual microscopic disease. Relative contraindications to radiation therapy include pregnancy, previous radiation therapy, and collagen vascular disease (Box 8-1). Axillary nodal involvement is not a contraindication. Six randomized trials of lumpectomy and radiation therapy showed that the frequency of local recurrence and overall survival rates are generally comparable to mastectomy. However, IBTRs are reported in 5% of patients at 5 years and in 10% to 15% at 10 years after completion of therapy. Treatment failures (i.e., IBTR) usually undergo salvage mastectomy.

Invasive IBTR usually occurs in the lumpectomy site or quadrant within the first 7 years, but rarely earlier than 18 months after treatment. IBTR after 7 years will more likely occur in any quadrant, not necessarily at the original site, and is usually considered a new cancer. IBTR near the original lumpectomy site is associated more frequently with systemic relapse than IBTR in other quadrants, which more often reflect a new primary tumor. IBTR is considered more likely in women who have invasive ductal cancer with an extensive intraductal component, residual disease in the breast, extensive DCIS, lymphatic or vascular invasion, or multicentricity, and is more common in younger women (Box 8-2).

▬ EVALUATION OF AXILLARY LYMPH NODES

The treatment of invasive breast cancer has historically involved removal of ipsilateral axillary lymph nodes. This was natural, because most women receiving treatment for breast cancer 100 years ago had nodal involvement. With earlier detection of breast cancer, nodal involvement is no longer the norm. In fact, approximately 65% to 70% of women with newly diagnosed invasive breast cancer have normal lymph nodes and therefore will not derive any benefit from axillary lymph node dissection (ALND).

ALND is also problematic from the standpoint of side effects. It exposes patients to the risk of major complications such as lymphedema, shoulder dysfunction, and sensory changes in and around the axilla. To address this problem, routine level I/level II ALND (Table 8-2) has evolved to use the SLN biopsy as an initial screen for nodal involvement in patients who are clinically node-negative.

SLN biopsy was initially described for patients with penile cancer, but did not attract much attention until it was broadly adopted for use in melanoma patients. SLN biopsy is performed by injecting a tracer material, either a radionuclide, blue dye, or both into the breast either preoperatively or perioperatively and by looking for evidence of the tracer in one or more sentinel nodes (Box 8-3).

SLN biopsy alone does not eliminate, but does significantly decrease, the risk of developing the common complications of lymphedema. A level I/level II ALND is now most commonly performed contingent on identification of tumor in one of the sentinel lymph nodes.

The role of the radiologist is to understand the rationale for SLN biopsy and to facilitate its performance. First, the radiologist should *not* inject tracer *into* the biopsy cavity or

---

BOX 8-2. Factors Affecting the Frequency of In-Breast Tumor Recurrence after Radiation Therapy

Invasive ductal cancer with an extensive intraductal component
Residual tumor in the breast
Younger women
Large ductal carcinoma in situ tumors
Lymphatic or vascular invasion
Multicentricity

BOX 8-1. Contraindications to Whole-Breast Radiation Therapy

Pregnancy
Previous breast radiation therapy
Multicentric or diffuse disease
Collagen vascular disease
Poor cosmetic result (relative contraindication)

TABLE 8-2. Location of Lymph Nodes Draining the Breast

Level	Location
I	Infralateral to lateral edge of the pectoralis minor muscle
II	Behind the pectoralis minor muscle
III	Between the pectoralis minor and subclavius muscles (Halsted ligament)

the tumor; tracer injected into a biopsy site cavity is likely to remain in the cavity rather than be transported into the lymphatics. The most common tracers are technetium-99 sulfur colloid and lymphazurin blue; some also use methylene blue dye.

Preoperative lymphoscintigraphy is used in some facilities to assist preoperative localization of sentinel lymph nodes in the axilla or in extra-axillary sites (Fig. 8-1A to C). Most commonly these extra-axillary sites will be in the supraclavicular, infraclavicular, or internal mammary groups. If tracer does not identify an axillary SLN, the surgeon may choose to harvest an SLN from one of these other sites. Some facilities do not remove an internal mammary SLN or other nonaxillary SLN due to the very low frequency of isolated positive biopsies (usually <3%) and the relatively few cases that would result in meaningful changes in prognosis or therapy. Perhaps not surprisingly, institutions that harvest both axillary and internal mammary sentinel lymph nodes have demonstrated a poorer prognosis when lymph nodes at both sites are involved.

Although there are differences of opinion as to the "optimal" location of tracer injection, as well as "optimal" tracer modality, there is general agreement from randomized studies that the technique is sensitive and specific enough to obviate the need for a full ALND in patients whose sentinel nodes test negative for tumor. In general, the SLN is harvested at the time of surgery and tested with touch preparation or frozen section intraoperatively. If there are tumor cells in the SLN, the surgeon proceeds to a completion level I/level II ALND. Nonvisualization of the SLN on lymphoscintigraphy does not preclude SLN identification by the surgeon in the operating room. The SLN may be within thick adipose tissue that can only be identified by the gamma probe in the operating room. The yield for SLN identification in the operating room when it cannot be visualized on lymphoscintigraphy can be increased if blue dye is also used.

Intraoperative evaluation of sentinel lymph nodes occasionally yields false-positive findings. More commonly, false-negative findings occur. This can precipitate return of the patient to the operating room weeks after the original SLN biopsy for completion ALND.

Based on current American Joint Committee on Cancer (AJCC) guidelines, nodal staging is based on the maximal size of the single largest tumor deposit in an SLN (if the SLN is the only involved node) as well as the number of involved lymph nodes. The descriptive category for the smallest extent of disease, isolated tumor cells, means that no single tumor deposit in an axillary node is larger than 0.2 mm. Patients with isolated tumor cells are considered to have normal nodes and are usually not treated with a completion ALND. Proceeding from SLN biopsy alone to the wider axillary node clearance typically requires micrometastatic (>0.2- to 2-mm tumor cell cluster in an SLN) or macrometastatic (>2-mm focus) disease within one SLN. Management of the axilla is performed independent of the decision to pursue lumpectomy or mastectomy.

Not all patients are candidates for SLN biopsy. For example, patients who present with clinically involved axillary nodes usually proceed directly to ALND. However, it is important to exercise caution in declaring an axillary lymph node as clinically positive. With the increased frequency of percutaneous core biopsy, more and more patients are presenting to breast cancer specialists with enlarged "reactive" nodes. A recent study by experienced breast surgeons demonstrated that clinical examination in this setting often overestimates the probability that lymph nodes are involved, which in turn could overestimate the number of patients who proceed directly to ALND. Although SLN biopsy has been widely adopted as a precursor to a full ALND for most patients, many have sought to use imaging studies to obviate the need for SLN biopsy or ALND. Toward this end, investigators have assessed the preoperative appearance of nodes on mammography, ultrasound, MRI, and even positron emission tomography. Among these, only positron emission tomography with a high standardized uptake value may provide near-definitive proof of nodal involvement preoperatively in the absence of percutaneous sampling. Here, too, one must be careful to distinguish between a reactive node versus an uninvolved node.

One preoperative axillary imaging method that has gained a following is axillary lymph node ultrasound with percutaneous FNA of suspicious nodes (see Fig. 8-1D to G). Although this test is not a routine part of the initial breast imaging evaluation, there is a new appreciation for preoperative evaluation of ipsilateral axillary lymph nodes in the setting of breast cancer. Axillary ultrasound is particularly helpful when the results of clinical examination of the axilla are suspicious for cancer. Several studies have recently been published using ultrasound-guided FNA or core biopsy to document nodal involvement preoperatively, thus allowing the surgeon to bypass SLN biopsy. This can obviate several known issues with intraoperative assessment of sentinel lymph nodes, such as the time needed to harvest one or more nodes, the intraoperative time needed for pathology to evaluate the node and, most important, the potential for false-negative touch preparation or frozen section at the time of surgery, which can lead to reoperation at a later date.

CLINICAL AND BREAST IMAGING FACTORS IN DETERMINING APPROPRIATE LOCAL THERAPY: LUMPECTOMY OR MASTECTOMY

The therapeutic options for local control of a breast malignancy are lumpectomy (almost always followed by radiotherapy) and mastectomy. Lumpectomy (followed by whole-breast radiotherapy) was introduced approximately 40 years ago and offers equivalent survival to mastectomy. Mastectomy has a slightly lower risk of local recurrence than lumpectomy and obviates the need for radiotherapy

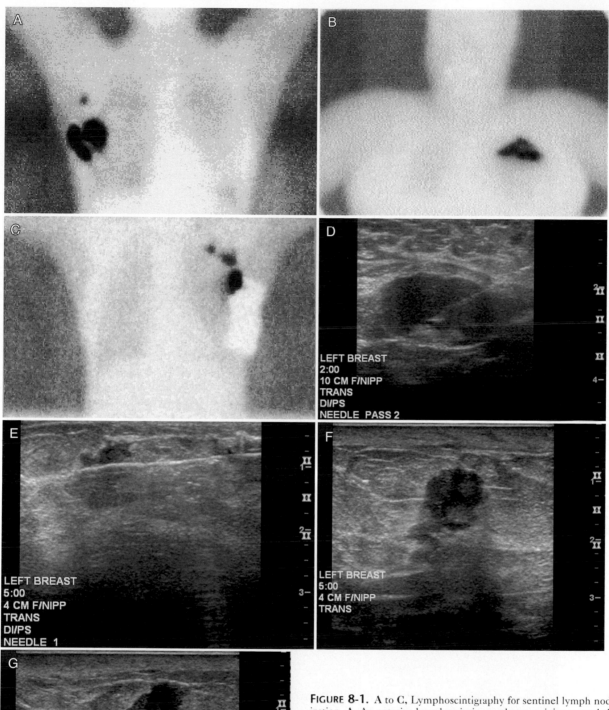

FIGURE 8-1. A to **C,** Lymphoscintigraphy for sentinel lymph node (SLN) visualization. **A,** An anterior lymphoscintigram shows activity around the tumor and in the axillary SLN. **B,** The lymphoscintigram shows radionuclide injected into the biopsy cavity rather than around it; the radiotracer stayed in the biopsy cavity because it could not be transported to the breast lymphatics. **C,** A lymphoscintigram shows activity in the infraclavicular nodes medial to the tumor site. Note the shielding around the injection site and tumor to improve SLN detection. **D** to **G,** Ultrasound to evaluate for lymphadenopathy. **D,** Ultrasound shows a fine needle aspirating an abnormal lymph node with a very thick cortex that flattened the normal fatty hilum. Aspiration showed breast cancer metastases. **E,** Ultrasound shows a core biopsy of a low axillary lymph node that has irregular superficial margins. Biopsy showed cancer metastases. Breast cancer that metastasized to the lymph nodes (**D** and **E**) on transverse (**F**) and longitudinal (**G**) ultrasound. The mass is taller than wide, with microlobulated superficial margins, suspicious for cancer. Invasive ductal cancer was found at biopsy.

in most patients. The use of postmastectomy radiotherapy is controversial in premenopausal women with one to three involved nodes (see the meta-analysis of randomized studies with and without radiotherapy by the Early Breast Cancer Trialists' Collaborative Group, *Lancet* 2005), but it is a common recommendation for women with tumors larger than 5 cm or with four or more involved nodes. The equivalence in overall survival between lumpectomy with radiotherapy and mastectomy was shown in Protocol B-06 conducted by the NSABP and the Milan I trial conducted in Italy.

The breast imager plays a critical role in aiding the surgeon to make the right therapeutic choice by showing how much cancer is in the breast. There is virtually no disagreement that patients with a unifocal DCIS or invasive cancer may be treated with breast conservation therapy if the entire tumor can be removed with a good cosmetic result and if there are no relative contraindications to radiation therapy (i.e., pregnancy, collagen vascular disease, poorly defined or multicentric disease) or prior radiotherapy involving the breast (Fig. 8-2).

The controversy regarding the best surgical approach concerns patients with multifocal disease. Some physicians believe that mastectomy is the proper choice for such patients. This preference may be due to results from the original clinical trials comparing lumpectomy with mastec-

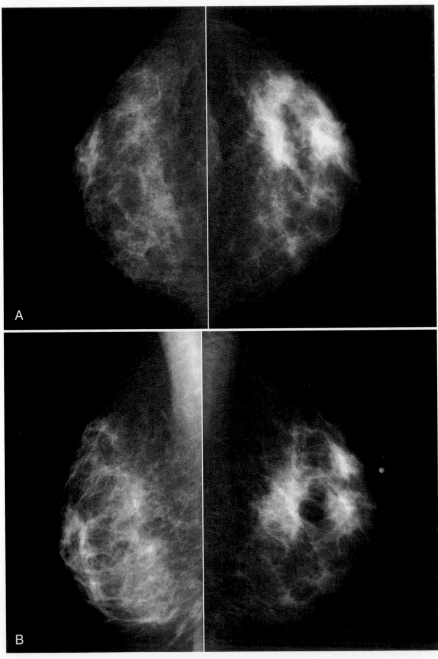

FIGURE 8-2. Mammography showing a poor candidate for breast conservation. Although this patient felt only one mass in her left breast, craniocaudal (**A**) and mediolateral oblique (**B**) mammograms show three spiculated masses over a large region, thus rendering this patient a poor candidate for breast conservation.

tomy, which involved almost exclusively women with unifocal breast cancers. Hence, the safety of breast conservation with respect to local recurrence, distant metastasis, and survival is not as well documented in women with multifocal disease. Still, surgeons are increasingly offering breast conservation to patients with multifocal disease. Thus, there is no hard and fast rule regarding how many satellite lesions, or what distance between lesions, constitutes an absolute indication for mastectomy. It is the physician's clinical judgment to avoid predisposing the patient to IBTR; recent data suggest that an IBTR may increase the risk of distant metastasis and death from breast cancer.

Whether the surgeon offers lumpectomy to patients with unifocal disease alone or to patients with multifocal disease, tumor-free margins are a must. For example, offering a woman breast conservation may be reasonable if she has multifocal invasive carcinoma with sub-centimeter lesions 3 mm apart and margins that are tumor-free by several millimeters. On the other hand, breast conservation may not be offered if a patient has multifocal high-grade DCIS scattered over an area of 5 to 6 cm with only a 1-mm margin; in this example, one would be concerned about additional multifocal disease just beyond the surgical margin.

The definition of *tumor-free margin* varies among institutions, with some accepting the NSABP model of nontransection, and others requiring a 2-mm or greater tumor-free margin. In general, the margin status must be carefully considered in patients with multifocal disease. Ideally, these patients should have the multiple lesions resected in continuity to gain the best histologic understanding of size, extent, and relationship of lesions to one another, and of the true margins.

Proof of multicentric disease has been handled by some surgeons with breast conservation, but the more accepted, and proven, route is with mastectomy as initial treatment. As stated previously, no prospective, randomized study to date has evaluated the safety and effectiveness of breast conservation therapy in the setting of multifocal or multicentric disease. Retrospective studies have been published suggesting that this approach may be safe by demonstrating comparable local recurrence rates in multifocal as well as unifocal disease, whereas others suggest higher IBTR rates. These studies are not powered to draw definitive conclusions but do suggest that such a randomized study in the future may be worthwhile.

PREOPERATIVE IMAGING

Mammography, ultrasound, and MRI for tumor extent are important tools for selecting appropriate breast conservation therapy candidates and planning surgery (Table 8-3). Mammography is the mainstay for determining extent of disease. Mammography identifies diffuse or multicentric disease by finding suspicious breast masses and pleomorphic calcifications. Mammography also can identify benign, extensive, innumerable bilateral calcifications that could hide early tumor recurrence. Such calcifications are a relative contraindication to breast conservation therapy. Furthermore, mammography finds DCIS that is invisible to MRI. Specifically, approximately 25% of DCIS cases are

TABLE 8-3. Breast Imaging Relating to Breast-Conserving Therapy

Timing	Reason	Technique(s)
Preoperative	Ipsilateral tumor extent and contralateral tumor	Bilateral mammography US or MRI as warranted
	Establish diagnosis	Percutaneous biopsy
Perioperative	Tumor excision	Preoperative needle localization (as needed) Specimen radiography
	SLN identification	Radionuclide injection Lymphoscintigraphy (as needed)
Preradiation	Check for residual tumor	Ipsilateral unilateral mammogram US or MRI as needed
Postradiation	Baseline/tumor recurrence	Ipsilateral unilateral mammogram (initial one at 6 mo, then every 6–12 mo)
	Evaluate ipsilateral and contralateral breast	Bilateral mammogram (12 mo)
	Clinical problem	Ipsilateral unilateral mammogram US or MRI as needed

MRI, magnetic resonance imaging; SLN, sentinel lymph node; US, ultrasound. Modified from Dershaw DD: The conservatively treated breast. In Bassett LW, Jackson VP, Fu KL, Fu YS, editors: *Diagnosis of diseases of the breast*. Philadelphia, 1997, WB Saunders, p. 553.

false-negative on MRI and are discovered only by visualizing pleomorphic calcifications on the mammogram.

On the other hand, MRI has been especially useful in predicting tumor extent before the first surgical procedure (Fig. 8-3). Some investigators have claimed particular effectiveness of MRI in women with invasive lobular carcinoma or showing tumor invasion into the pectoralis muscle or chest wall (Fig. 8-4). With respect to invasive lobular carcinoma, several studies have suggested that MRI may be more effective in detecting the extent of disease than physical examination, mammography, and ultrasound. However, false-negative studies in these series have led to mixed opinions regarding the routine use of MRI in staging invasive lobular carcinoma.

Chest wall tumor invasion on MRI was shown by obliteration of the fat plane between the tumor and the pectoralis muscle, with muscle enhancement, and was proven in 5 of 5 cases at surgery (Morris et al, 2000). No muscle involvement was seen at surgery when muscle enhancement was absent in 14 of 14 cases.

MRI also helps exclude candidates for APBI when it finds more than one focus of cancer. Bedrosian and colleagues (2003) reported a 95% tumor detection rate with MRI and a change in surgical management in 26% (69/267) of patients requiring wider/separate excision or mastectomy, with pathologic verification in 71% (49/69).

Overall, these studies show that MRI may be helpful in surgical planning, but they also indicate that MRI prompts a number of unnecessary biopsies because of a relative lack of specificity. MRI also has false-negative results in invasive lobular carcinoma and DCIS. Other data show that MRI

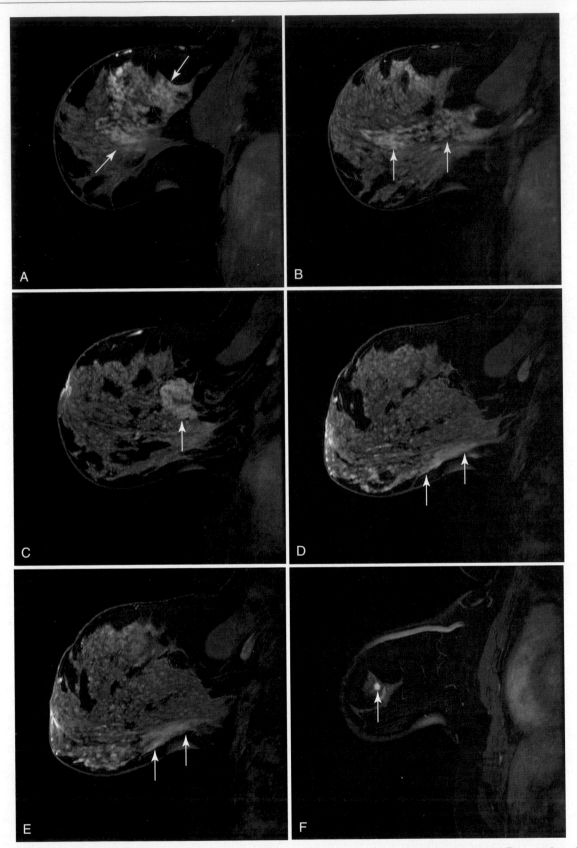

FIGURE 8-3. Magnetic resonance imaging (MRI) showing a poor candidate for breast conservation. **A to C,** Postcontrast 3-D spectral-spatial excitation magnetization transfer (3DSSMT) MRI slices of the right breast show a mass near the chest wall (*arrow;* invasive ductal cancer) in part **C** and adjacent segmental clumped enhancement (*arrows*) over more than two thirds of the upper left breast in parts **A** and **B,** worrisome for ductal carcinoma in situ (DCIS). **D** and **E,** In the opposite breast there is linear enhancement (*arrows*) in the lower breast, also worrisome for DCIS. **F,** In the extreme medial left breast there is a round, suspicious mass (*arrows*) that had rapid initial enhancement and late washout on kinetic curves, worrisome for invasive ductal cancer. Biopsies of the outer right breast showed invasive ductal cancer and DCIS (**A** to **C**); core biopsy of the left segmental enhancement showed DCIS (**D** and **E**) and invasive ductal cancer in the inner left breast mass (**F**). Because of the widespread cancer in both breasts, the patient is not a candidate for breast conservation.

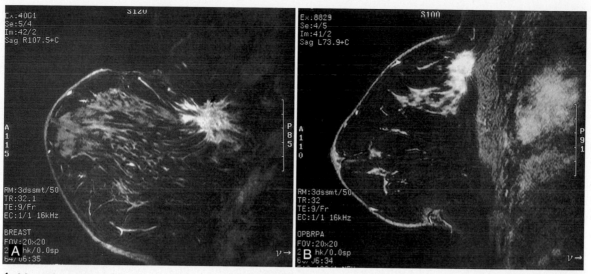

FIGURE 8-4. Magnetic resonance imaging (MRI) showing extension into the pectoralis muscle. **A,** Sagittal, contrast-enhanced, 3-D spectral-spatial excitation magnetization transfer (3DSSMT) MRI shows a spiculated posterior enhancing mass extending into and enhancing the pectoralis muscle. **B,** MRI showing tumor on top of the pectoralis muscle. In contrast to part **A,** sagittal, contrast-enhanced, 3DSSMT MRI shows an irregular enhancing mass abutting the pectoralis muscle but without enhancing it, thus suggesting no tumor invasion. Although the surgeon may take some of the pectoralis muscle at surgery to achieve clear margins, the tumor does not extend into the muscle or chest wall.

may be associated with treatment delay and an increased mastectomy rate and does not decrease the number of fewer positive margins at surgery. The use of pretreatment MRI before definitive breast cancer surgery remains controversial, particularly if one anticipates whole-breast radiotherapy. The literature on this subject is extensive.

When imaging is complete, additional dialogue with the breast imaging team or additional review of imaging studies may be necessary to help the surgeon, medical oncologist, or radiation oncologist properly counsel the patient regarding appropriate treatment options. This involves a review of the original workup to ensure that all potential abnormalities on physical examination have been evaluated and that the breast imaging workup has been completed (such as up-to-date contralateral mammography as well as additional ultrasound or mammographic imaging for lesions previously considered of secondary concern). The thorough combination of abnormalities identified by palpation or on breast imaging helps ensure that any suspicious foci of tumor are evaluated and incorporated into the treatment plan.

■ NORMAL POSTOPERATIVE IMAGING CHANGES AFTER BREAST BIOPSY OR LUMPECTOMY

To perform a local excision for diagnostic or therapeutic purposes, the surgeon makes a skin incision, removes the mass or wire-localized abnormality, and then closes the subcutaneous tissues and skin. More tissue is excised when removing a cancer to obtain a margin of normal tissue. Usually, the surgeon allows the surgical cavity to fill in with fluid and granulation tissue.

As a rule, mammograms are not often obtained immediately after diagnostic surgical excisional biopsy. However, in the rare cases when a mammogram is obtained within a few days of surgery, mammography shows a round or oval mass in the postoperative site representing a seroma or

hematoma, with or without air. This mass represents the biopsy cavity, filled with fluid that should resolve over time (Fig. 8-5A and B). The adjacent breast tissue shows thickening of trabeculae in subcutaneous fat and increased density caused by local edema or hemorrhage. Skin thickening at the incision is usually present. On MRI the biopsy site is filled with blood or seroma. The fluid in the biopsy cavity is high signal intensity on T2-weighted noncontrast fat-suppressed images (see Fig 8-5C to E).

Over the subsequent weeks, the postoperative site resorbs the air and fluid collection; the collection is replaced by fibrosis and scarring, with residual focal skin thickening and breast edema. On MRI the immediate postbiopsy cavity is a fluid-filled structure with surrounding normal healing tissue enhancement for up to 18 months after the biopsy. The biopsy cavity shows high signal intensity, architectural distortion, and a scar that can simulate cancer (Fig. 8-6 and Box 8-4). The biopsy site usually contains fluid from the seroma, which will be bright on T2-weighted images on MRI. Rim enhancement around the biopsy site is normal even if there is no residual tumor and is due to healing. In the ipsilateral axilla, reactive lymph nodes may develop that cannot be distinguished from metastatic disease (Fig. 8-7). MRI after surgery may reveal cancer at

---

Box 8-4. Enhancement on MRI after Biopsy

Up to 9 months after biopsy and radiation therapy, there is strong enhancement in the biopsy site. From 10 to 18 months after therapy, the enhancement slowly subsides, with no significant enhancement in 94% of cases.

From Heywang-Kobrunner SH, Schlegel A, Beck R, et al: Contrast-enhanced MRI of the breast after limited surgery and radiation therapy, *J Comput Assist Tomogr* 17:891–900, 1993.

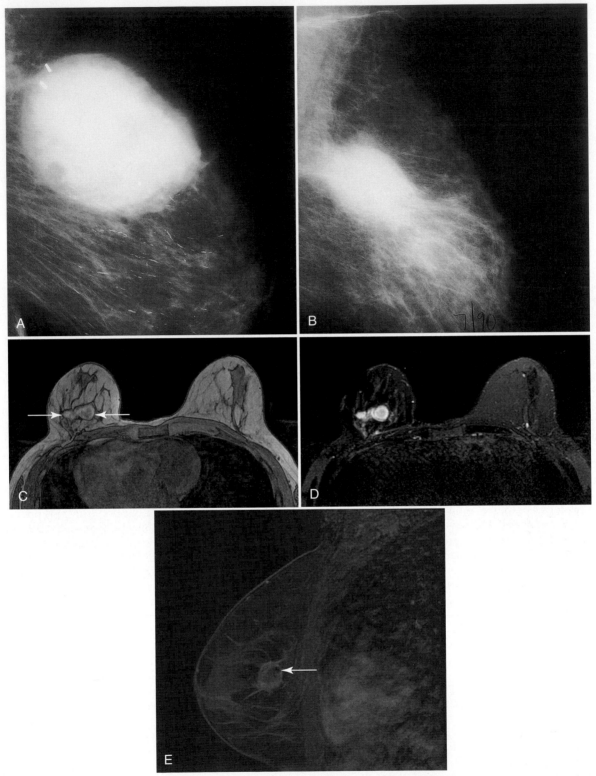

FIGURE 8-5. Normal postbiopsy changes. **A,** A postbiopsy mediolateral oblique (MLO) view shows a large oval mass representing a huge seroma/hematoma after biopsy for cancer, with two adjacent surgical clips. **B,** Four years later, the MLO views shows the seroma/hematoma is smaller; the two surgical clips are obscured. **C to E,** Normal hematoma on magnetic resonance imaging (MRI). **C,** Precontrast axial nonfat-suppressed T1-weighted MRI shows high signal intensity in the biopsy cavity in the left breast soon after surgery (*arrows*). **D,** Precontrast axial fat-suppressed T2-weighted MRI shows high signal intensity in the postbiopsy cavity representing blood and fluid. **E,** Postcontrast sagittal vibrant MRI shows rim enhancement around the hematoma that contains a small round signal void (air, *arrow*).

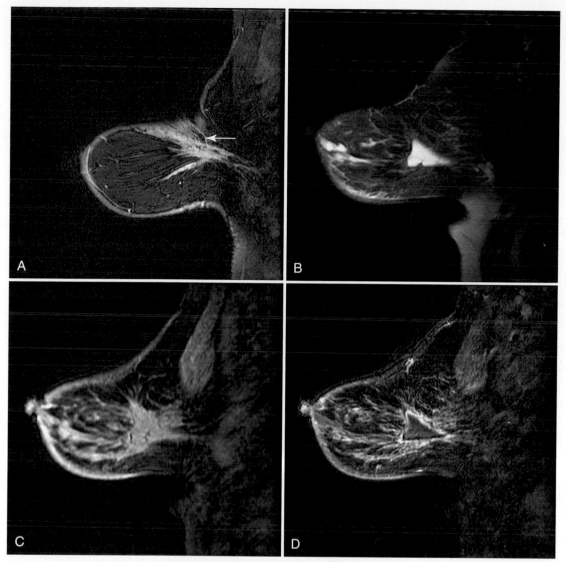

FIGURE 8-6. Normal postbiopsy changes on magnetic resonance imaging (MRI). **A,** Postcontrast sagittal 3-D spectral-spatial excitation magnetization transfer (3DSSMT) MRI shows enhancing architectural distortion extending from the skin into the upper breast, representing a normal postbiopsy scar. Note the signal void in the biopsy scar due to methemoglobin (*arrow*) and skin thickening. **B,** In another recently postoperative patient treated for cancer, precontrast sagittal fat-suppressed T2-weighted MRI shows high signal intensity fluid in the biopsy cavity, bright fluid in the retroareolar ducts, and thickened skin with subcutaneous thick fluid-filled trabeculae, compatible with breast edema. **C,** Precontrast sagittal 3DSSMT MRI shows the gray fluid-filled postbiopsy scar. **D,** Postcontrast sagittal 3DSSMT MRI shows rim enhancement around the dark fluid-filled seroma and associated breast edema. Note that there are no additional masses in this breast to suggest multifocal cancer.

the margin edge by showing clumped enhancement or an eccentric residual mass. Although immediate postbiopsy MRI for cancer staging may depict cancer at the biopsy margin, it is more often used to look for cancer elsewhere in the breast away from the biopsy site.

Normal postoperative findings on mammography include architectural distortion, increased density, and parenchymal scarring in at least 50% of patients (Box 8-5). These findings diminish in severity over time (Fig. 8-8A to I). After 3 to 5 years, the findings should be stable on subsequent mammograms. On the mammogram, in 50% to 55% of cases, the biopsy cavity resolves so completely that it leaves no scar or distortion in the underlying breast parenchyma, and only comparison with prebiopsy mammograms indicates that breast tissue is missing. In other cases, the scar appears as a chronic architectural distortion or a spiculated mass more evident on one projection than the other.

The remaining 45% to 50% of patients continue to have variable mammographic findings ranging from spiculated masslike scars to slight architectural distortion (see Fig. 8-8J and K). In still other, more rare cases, seroma cavities persist, appearing as a round or oval mass.

Postbiopsy scars often have a spiculated masslike appearance that can simulate cancer. Spiculated masses should be viewed with suspicion unless one knows that a biopsy was performed in that location. For this reason, it is important to document the date and location in the breast of previous biopsies on the breast history sheet. Some facilities also place a linear metallic scar marker directly on the skin's biopsy scar before taking the mammogram to show the previous biopsy site. On the mammogram, the linear metallic scar marker on the skin will be near the underlying scar. The skin scar may not be immediately adjacent to the scar inside the breast because

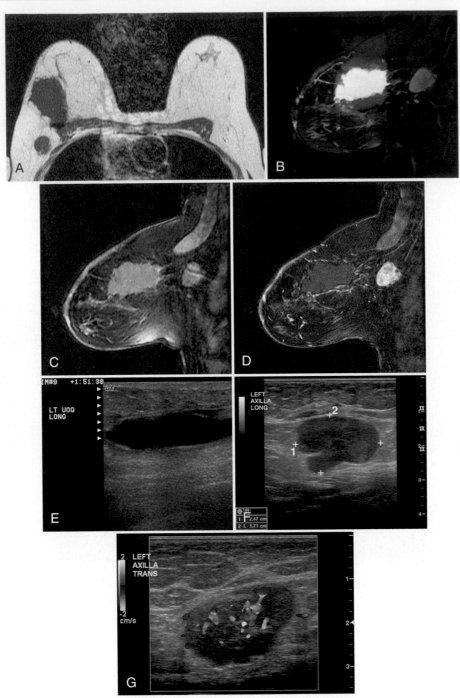

FIGURE 8-7. Postbiopsy changes on magnetic resonance imaging (MRI) with abnormal lymphadenopathy. **A,** Precontrast axial nonfat-suppressed T1-weighted MRI shows low signal intensity representing fluid in the biopsy cavity soon after surgery. A large lymph node in the left axilla has lost its fatty hilum and is worrisome for metastatic disease. **B,** Precontrast fat-suppressed sagittal T2-weighted MRI shows the high signal seroma and the lymph node in the left axilla near the chest wall. Note that the lymph node has abnormal low signal intensity, indicating lymphadenopathy. Normal lymph nodes will usually show a thin high signal intensity cortex with a fatty hilum. **C,** Precontrast sagittal 3-D spectral-spatial excitation magnetization transfer (3DSSMT) MRI shows the seroma and the lymph node in the left axilla. **D,** Postcontrast sagittal 3DSSMT MRI shows the nonenhancing seroma and the enhancing abnormal lymph node in the left axilla. **E,** Postbiopsy ultrasound shows the fluid-filled biopsy cavity in the left breast corresponding to the fluid cavity seen on MRI. **F,** Ultrasound of the abnormal lymph node seen on the MRI shows a thick cortical heterogeneous rim and flattening of the fatty hilum by the abnormal metastatic disease in the lymph node. **G,** Doppler ultrasound shows marked vascular flow within the lymph node. The usually thick rim, heterogeneity of the cortex, flattening of the fatty hilum, and increased vascular flow are all abnormal findings worrisome for metastatic disease. Biopsy of the lymph node showed metastatic disease.

Box 8-5. Normal Postoperative Findings for Benign Disease

Focal skin change (early)

Increased focal density (edema) near the biopsy site (early)

Oval fluid or fluid/air collection (early)

Complete resolution of biopsy findings (late; 50% to 55% of all cases)

Time when findings resolve: 3 to 5 years after biopsy

Postoperative findings seen after 3 to 5 years (45% to 50% of all cases)

Architectural distortion (48%)

Skin thickening/deformity (17%)

Parenchymal scarring (15%)

Scars: poorly defined masses with spiculation

Data from Brenner RJ, Pfaff JM: Mammographic changes after excisional breast biopsy for benign disease, *AJR Am J Roentgenol* 167:1047–1052, 1996; and Sickles EA, Herzog KA: Mammography of the postsurgical breast, *AJR Am J Roentgenol* 136:585–588, 1981.

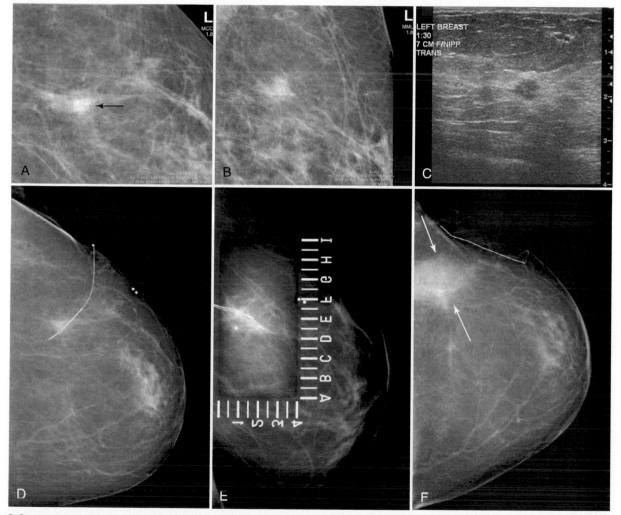

FIGURE 8-8. **A to E,** Prebiopsy mammogram and normal postbiopsy changes. Magnified craniocaudal (CC) (**A**) and mediolateral (**B**) mammograms show an ill-defined mass with a few calcifications in the outer left breast. **C,** Ultrasound shows an ill-defined hypoechoic mass in the left breast. Core biopsy showed invasive ductal cancer. Left CC (**D**) and mediolateral (**E**) mammograms show a wire through the mass before excisional biopsy. Pathology showed invasive ductal cancer with negative margins. Two years later, postbiopsy CC (**F**) and mediolateral (**G**) views show mild architectural distortion, skin deformity, and an ill-defined scar (*arrows*) below a linear metallic scar marker over the skin where the cancer was removed. Notice skin thickening and architectural distortion in the left axilla from sentinel lymph node dissection. *Continued*

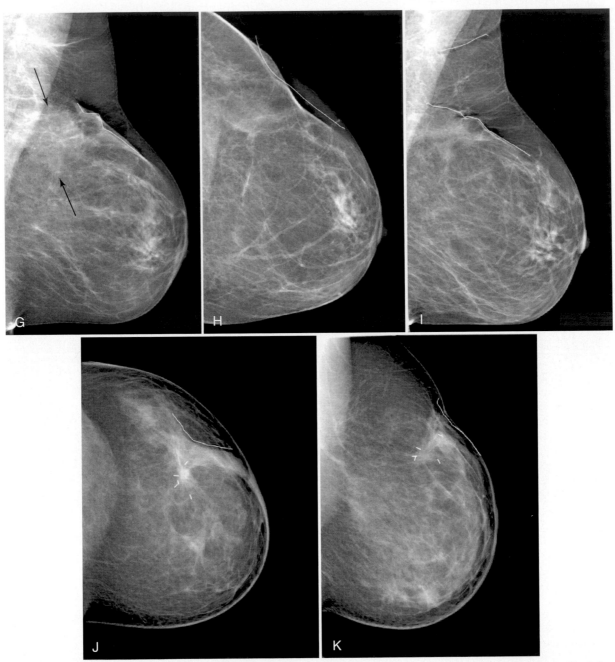

FIGURE 8-8, cont'd. Five years later, postbiopsy CC (**H**) and mediolateral (**I**) views show only mild architectural distortion and skin deformity, with resolution of most of the skin thickening and scarring shown in parts **F** and **G**. In another patient, normal postbiopsy scarring with metallic clips in the biopsy site for radiation therapy are shown on CC (**J**) and mediolateral (**K**) mammograms. Note the scar looks like a spiculated mass on the CC view and less like a mass on the mediolateral view, which is typical for scars and distinguishes them from true masses, which appear masslike (same size, density, and shape) on *both* views. A linear metallic scar marker is seen on the skin above the scar, showing that the scar correlates with the incision site.

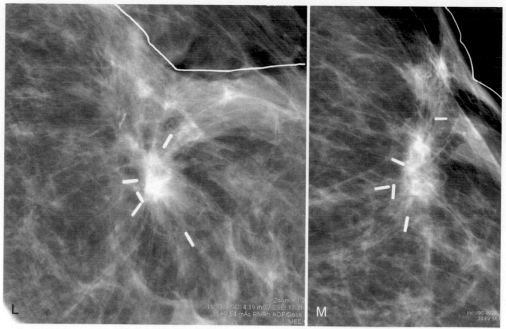

FIGURE 8-8, cont'd. Magnification CC (**L**) and mediolateral (**M**) views show the scar and a few faint fat necrosis calcifications with adjacent skin thickening just beneath the metallic linear scar marker, typical for a scar.

the skin is compressed away from the underlying breast parenchyma during the mammogram. If a spiculated mass is seen far from the metallic scar marker, that mass might be cancer rather than a scar. The radiologist reviews the preoperative mammograms to see where the biopsy occurred and correlates the prebiopsy and current mammograms to make this determination (see Fig. 8-8L and M).

Fat necrosis is common after a breast biopsy and usually appears as a radiolucent lipid-filled mass. Mammography is pathognomonic for fat necrosis if it shows lipid cysts or typical calcified eggshell-type rims around a radiolucent center (Fig. 8-9A). The fat necrosis, lipid cyst, and calcifications usually form in the scar, so these findings should be located near any linear metallic scar markers on the skin (see Fig. 8-9B and C).

On ultrasound, the immediate postoperative site shows a seroma or hematoma, breast edema, and focal skin thickening. The fluid collection occasionally contains air. More commonly, the seroma is completely filled with fluid, sometimes containing septa or debris that has varying appearances on ultrasound (Fig. 8-10). Usually the incision can be traced from the biopsy cavity up to the skin and is shown as a linear scar that disturbs the normal breast architecture (Box 8-6).

Later, the fluid in the biopsy cavity resolves and only the fibrotic scar remains. In these cases, ultrasound shows the scar as a hypoechoic spiculated mass that simulates breast cancer, but it should correlate with the postoperative site (Fig. 8-11). Correlating biopsy histories and the physical finding of a scar on the skin distinguishes normal postoperative scarring from cancer. On ultrasound, the spiculated scar often has a "tail" that extends from the scar to the skin, representing the healing biopsy

---

BOX 8-6. Postbiopsy Ultrasound Findings

EARLY
Seroma/hematoma
Focal skin thickening
Ability to trace incision from the biopsy cavity to the skin
Fibrin in the seroma (strands, balls)

LATE
Spiculated mass (simulates cancer)
± Acoustic shadowing
May see healed incision from the scar to the skin

All ultrasound-detected scars should be correlated to the skin scar and mammographic findings. If there is a mass near the scar *but separated by normal tissue,* be worried about cancer.

---

cavity and its adjacent subcutaneous tissue anastomosis (Fig. 8-12).

Whole-Breast, External Beam Radiotherapy and Accelerated Partial Breast Irradiation

An integral part of breast conservation therapy is radiation therapy. Conventional whole-breast, external beam radiotherapy (WB-XRT) with the postradiotherapy boost dose to the biopsy cavity achieves effective local control of disease within the remaining breast. WB-XRT lowers the frequency of IBTR after breast-conserving therapy. The percentages of local recurrence after lumpectomy in the NSABP, Milan, Swedish, and Canadian studies without WB-XRT were 39%, 23%, 24%, and 35%, respectively.

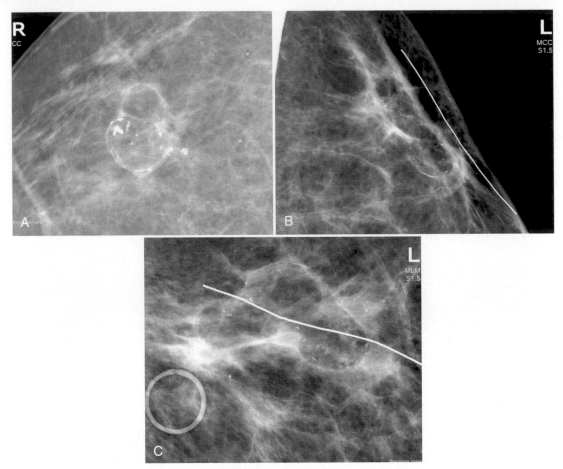

FIGURE 8-9. Benign postbiopsy calcifications. **A,** A spot compression magnification mammogram shows a calcifying oil cyst in fat necrosis calcifications in a biopsy site. Note the radiolucent center and the calcifications rimming the oil cyst borders. Magnification craniocaudal (**B**) and mediolateral (**C**) views of a postbiopsy scar show fat surrounded by curvilinear calcifications representing fat necrosis just under the linear metallic scar marker. There are also a few punctate dense calcifications from accelerated partial breast irradiation (APBI). Note that the round punctuate calcifications are very dense, almost metallic-like, and are very typical for APBI associated calcifications. The round structure in the lower left corner of the image is a skin mole marker.

With WB-XRT, recurrences were lower—14%, 6%, 8%, and 11%, respectively, and the difference was statistically significant. From 60% to 90% of local recurrences develop near the original primary tumor, so-called *true recurrences*, whereas other recurrences, or *elsewhere failures*, are uncommon. These elsewhere failures occur at the same rate with (0.5% to 3.8%) or without (0.5% to 3.6%) WB-XRT.

Thus, it is important that little or no residual tumor remains after breast surgery and that any residual microscopic tumor foci receive therapeutic doses of radiation. Whole-breast irradiation takes 6 to 7 weeks, during which the dose is fractionated. During WB-XRT the breast becomes edematous and reddened. The skin becomes slightly pitted (*peau d'orange*) due to skin edema; the breast can become tender. This is due to small vessel leakage and edema from radiotherapy. Because studies have shown that up to 85% of IBTR after lumpectomy occurs in the vicinity of the lumpectomy site, a postradiotherapy electron beam boost to the biopsy cavity helps eradicate residual tumor foci at the place where IBTR is most likely to occur. After WB-XRT and the electron beam boost, the breast edema slowly subsides, and the skin becomes less edematous and more normal in appearance as the breast heals.

APBI is a treatment option for selected women with limited early stage breast cancer after breast-conserving surgery. APBI occurs over a significantly shorter period (*accelerated*) than WB-XRT and targets the tumor bed and defined margin (*partial breast*) rather than the whole breast (Box 8-7).

The shortened time course of radiotherapy increases accessibility of breast conservation treatment and may increase the proportion of women who receive appropriate adjuvant radiotherapy after breast-conserving surgery. In addition, limiting the treatment field to the local tumor bed should, in theory, reduce treatment-related morbidities such as radiation pneumonitis, lymphedema, and radiation-induced sarcoma. Because only a part of the breast is irradiated, it is also possible that IBTR after APBI could be treated with repeat breast-conserving surgery and radiation therapy rather than mastectomy. Finally, some investigators suggest that a single fraction of high-dose radiotherapy applied to tumor endothelial cells is more lethal to cancers than fractionated dosing. Accordingly, single-fraction intraoperative radiotherapy (IORT) is potentially the most convenient form of APBI for patients, could provide the most accurate targeting of tissue at risk, and might spare normal tissue.

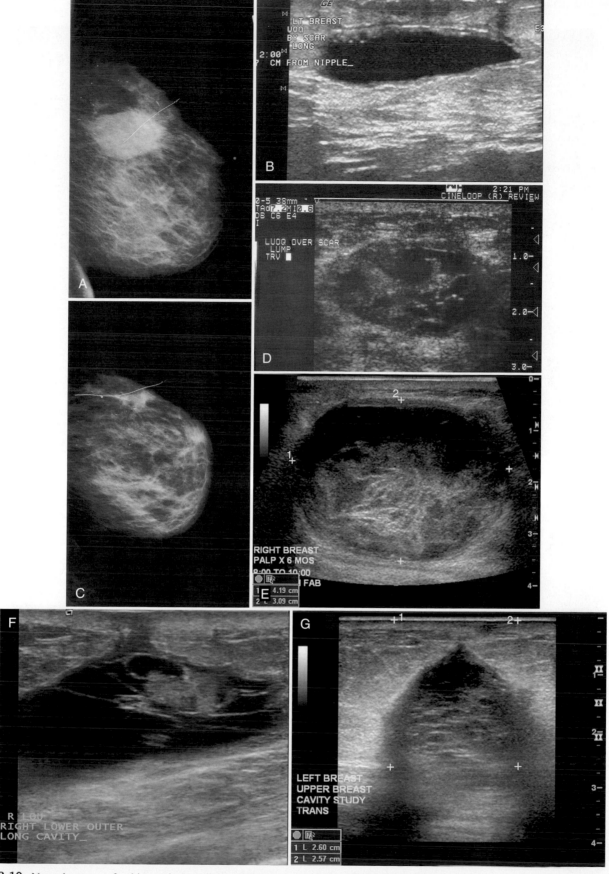

FIGURE 8-10. Normal seromas after biopsy. **A,** A mediolateral oblique mammogram after biopsy shows a mass in the biopsy site under the scar marker. **B,** Ultrasound under the scar shows a typical fluid collection representing the seroma. The collection was aspirated. **C,** Two years later, the fluid collection has resolved, with only scarring remaining. **D,** A septated seroma is seen in a second patient. **E,** Another normal seroma with debris and fluid 6 months after biopsy in a third patient. **F,** Normal 16-week-old seroma with septations and a fibrin ball in a fourth patient. **G,** Normal large seroma cavity with septations in a fifth patient.

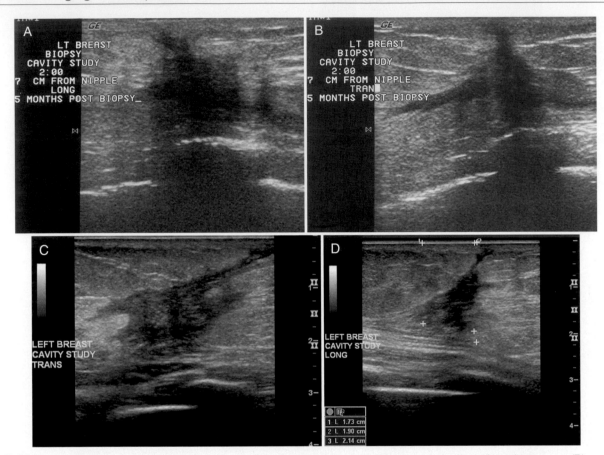

FIGURE 8-11. New biopsy scars on ultrasound. Five months after biopsy and radiation therapy, longitudinal (**A**) and transverse (**B**) scans show a hypoechoic triangular-shaped scar containing fluid, with the incision (filled with fluid) extending to the skin surface. Note the skin thickening and acoustic shadowing of the scar in this case. In another patient, three months after biopsy and radiation therapy, transverse (**C**) and longitudinal (**D**) scans show a typical, spiculated hypoechoic fluid-filled scar and its incision extending from the scar to the skin surface, similar to the biopsy scar in parts **A** and **B**. Note that there is no acoustic shadowing in this case. Note also that the longitudinal study shows distance measurements from the skin surface to the bottom of the cavity and to the chest wall for electron beam boost planning. The radiation oncologist uses these measurements to sterilize the biopsy cavity with an electron beam boost.

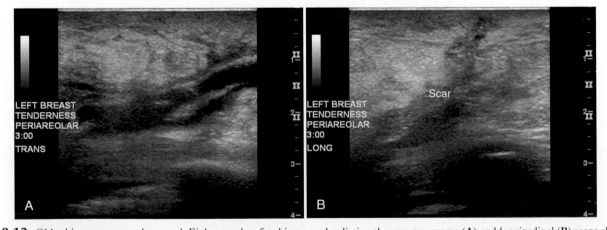

FIGURE 8-12. Older biopsy scars on ultrasound. Eight months after biopsy and radiation therapy, transverse (**A**) and longitudinal (**B**) scans show fluid in the scar, but note that the margins are less sharp than those in Figure 8-11, indicating scar healing and fluid resorption. Note the typical appearance of breast edema on ultrasound in part **A**, shown by the indistinct skin line, gray fat between the skin line and the scar, and dark linear fluid-filled lymphatics in the subcutaneous tissues.

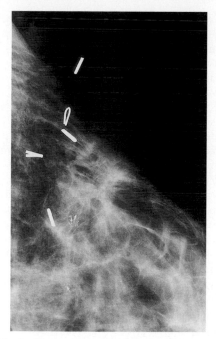

FIGURE 8-13. Residual tumor. After biopsy of pleomorphic calcifications showing invasive ductal cancer, the postbiopsy mammogram shows residual calcifications in the biopsy site surrounded by metallic clips in the cavity.

Several different techniques of APBI are used, including interstitial brachytherapy, intracavitary brachytherapy (balloon or multicatheter brachytherapy), IORT, and 3-D conformal external beam radiation (3D-CRT). An attractive feature common to IORT and 3D-CRT is that neither requires an invasive procedure separate from lumpectomy. IORT, which delivers radiation directly to the lumpectomy cavity at the time of surgery, is the only ABPI technique that allows completion of the surgical and radiation treatment in one hospital visit, resulting in saving time for both the patient and the hospital. 3D-CRT is noninvasive and can be performed over 5 to 7 days with twice-daily treatments. All types of APBI use a higher dose per fraction to achieve an effective total dose. Given the higher fractionated dose, post-treatment changes in the breast after APBI may be different from that seen after WB-XRT.

However, the main concern with WB-XRT and APBI is local recurrence, because IBTR may impact overall survival. This is particularly true with the use of APBI, in which the entire breast does not receive therapeutic doses of radiation. This means that it is especially important to identify appropriate patients for APBI to prevent elsewhere failures. Several ongoing Phase III trials are investigating the role of APBI in selected patients.

BREAST IMAGING BEFORE RE-EXCISION LUMPECTOMY OR RADIOTHERAPY

For patients who have undergone an initial cancer excision but have close or involved tumor margins, additional imaging is warranted before re-excision. If, for some reason, ultrasound was not performed for a palpable lesion, ultrasound may visualize previously unanticipated residual disease around the cavity margins or unsuspected satellite lesions. If a specimen radiograph from the original excision had shown microcalcifications at or near the specimen edge and involved margins were seen histologically, repeat mammography (with wire localization) may be helpful in guiding re-excision. Given the difficulty in identifying microscopic residual disease at the time of reoperation, the treatment team should attempt to utilize any advantage possible to identify residual areas of disease with the intent of targeting them for the surgeon at the time of re-excision.

Patients who have undergone therapeutic excision demonstrating tumor-free margins may still benefit from additional imaging. This is particularly true for women whose lesions presented initially as microcalcifications. Such imaging helps determine the completeness of tumor excision. There is some controversy in the literature as to whether preradiotherapy mammography of the affected breast should become standard to identify possible multifocal disease before committing to radiotherapy. Because the main concern with breast conservation is local recurrence, and because IBTR may affect overall survival, physicians may order postbiopsy mammograms to determine the completeness of tumor excision if there is any question about residual gross disease or residual microcalcifications (Fig. 8-13). These mammograms are particularly appropriate before the initiation of breast irradiation to make sure there is no residual tumor.

When the biopsy shows unexpected cancer, magnification views of the lumpectomy site and remaining breast before re-excision are especially helpful to show unsuspected, suspicious calcifications or masses. Calcifications are important because they could be cancer, but they do not always represent tumors. Dershaw and colleagues found the positive predictive value of residual microcalcifications representing residual tumor to be 69%, with the likelihood that they represent residual tumor being greatest in cases with DCIS and in those with more than five microcalcifications.

When considering radiation therapy, the number and extent of any calcifications is important even when they do not indicate tumor. The radiation oncologist must gauge whether they will be able to detect early recurrences on the post–WB-XRT or APBI mammogram. The presence of extensive innumerable calcifications that limit the radiologist's ability to find early cancer is a consideration in patient exclusion from breast conservation.

Pre-ABPI MRI aids patient selection by excluding patients with multifocal or multicentric disease. In one study, Horst and colleagues showed that, by using MRI, 9.8% of 51 patients ($n = 5$) had unsuspected disease, including multifocal (3) or multicentric (1) disease, or pectoral fascia involvement (1), precluding enrollment into APBI studies. It is also important to recognize typical magnetic resonance findings in post-ABPI patients and to distinguish these findings from recurrent or new disease.

■ NORMAL IMAGING CHANGES AFTER RADIATION THERAPY

Mammography

Recommendations for follow-up mammography after radiation therapy vary by institution. Most facilities obtain a unilateral mammogram immediately after the conclusion of radiation therapy, with further follow-up bilateral mammograms at 6- to 12-month intervals. Obtaining a mammogram relatively soon after completion of radiation therapy establishes a baseline for future reference (Fig. 8-14A to F).

Normal lumpectomy and WB-XRT changes alter the normal mammogram. These include the usual postbiopsy changes in the surgical site plus diffuse skin thickening and breast edema from WB-XRT (Box 8-8; see also Fig. 8-14G to J). Unlike normal focal postoperative edema, breast edema from WB-XRT encompasses the entire breast and not just the region around the postoperative site. On physical examination, the breast commonly shows *peau d'orange*, a large swollen areola or nipple, occasional brownish or red skin, and occasional breast tenderness and swelling. Skin thickening in the immediate postradiation therapy period is due to breast edema from small-vessel damage; later, it is due to fibrotic change. Findings of breast edema are most obvious when compared with the contralateral side or older mammograms.

On the mammogram, the indications of breast edema are skin and stromal thickening, diffuse increased

breast density, and trabecular thickening in subcutaneous fat. The usual changes of the postbiopsy scar are superimposed on the findings of whole-breast edema. The biopsy cavity, seen initially as a fluid-filled mass, may be partially obscured by surrounding breast edema from radiation therapy. These changes usually decrease somewhat over a period of 2.5 to 3 years or may remain stable. With resolution of the surrounding breast edema, the biopsy cavity may become more apparent but should not grow in size.

Progression of breast edema is abnormal and should be investigated. Other etiologies of unilateral breast edema outside the radiation therapy setting are inflammatory breast cancer, mastitis, lymphoma, and obstructed breast lymphatic or venous drainage.

After completion of whole-breast irradiation, many facilities use an electron beam boost to sterilize the operative site. Some facilities line the cavity with radiopaque markers to guide the electron beam boost and use x-ray imaging for guidance (Fig. 8-15). Other facilities use breast ultrasound to delineate and mark the skin over the breast biopsy cavity for the electron beam boost.

In about 25% of women, calcifications develop in the treated breast at the biopsy site; these calcifications can be extreme if the radiation therapy was done many years ago with higher orthovoltage radiation compared to current therapy (Fig. 8-16A and B). Although most of these calcifications will be due to benign dystrophic calcification, fat necrosis, or calcifying suture material, magnification views of calcifications in the biopsy site are required to distinguish them from the pleomorphic calcifications of cancer recurrence. Fat necrosis may be evident if it has dystrophic appearance or forms around a radiolucent center. The dystrophic calcifications in fat necrosis can simulate malignancy, but magnification orthogonal projections may show the beginnings of the typical curvilinear shape of fat necrosis not evident on only one view. Careful inspection of the previous mammogram may also help by showing that the calcifications are forming around a radiolucent center of fat. Sometimes, when there are no distinguishing features to diagnose dystrophic or fat necrosis calcifications, these calcifications cannot be distinguished from cancer and prompt biopsy (see Fig. 8-16C to I).

Biopsy should be performed on suspicious pleomorphic calcifications. Some suspicious calcifications represent incompletely resected tumor, especially in the absence of postbiopsy, preradiotherapy mammograms or if the specimen radiograph suggested that the calcifications were incompletely excised. Comparison to the original prebiopsy mammograms is important to determine whether the original microcalcifications were not totally excised and should undergo re-excision.

Nonspecific microcalcifications forming in or near the biopsy site are a problem. Such calcifications may be benign or malignant. Calcifications that diminish or disappear may represent resolving benign calcifications as a result of changes in the calcium phosphate product in the breast or they may represent residual tumor that has responded to therapy. Disappearing calcifications are worrisome if they are replaced by a suspicious mass.

Unchanging nonspecific calcifications should be monitored or biopsied because they may represent incompletely

---

Box 8-8. Mammographic Findings after Breast Conservation and Radiation Therapy

Whole-breast edema
Postbiopsy scar
Skin retraction/deformity (variable)
Axillary node dissection distortion (if performed)
Metallic clips outlining the biopsy cavity (variable)

The findings are worst at 6 months, diminish, and then stabilize at 2 to 3 years.

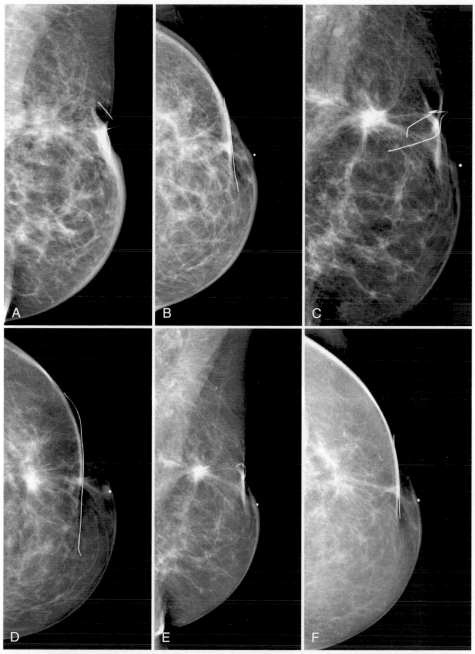

FIGURE 8-14. Normal postbiopsy/radiation therapy changes over time. Mediolateral oblique (MLO) (**A**) and craniocaudal (CC) (**B**) mammograms immediately after biopsy and radiation therapy for cancer show architectural distortion in the biopsy site and overlying skin retraction; metallic markers are seen on the scar. Edema is present, as shown by skin thickening, especially in the lower breast on the MLO view (**A**). MLO (**C**) and CC (**D**) mammograms 1 year later show diminishing breast edema and retraction of the biopsy scar, which is more apparent than the year before and looks like a spiculated mass or cancer. Note that its proximity to the metallic linear skin scar markers shows that it clearly corresponds to the biopsy site. MLO (**E**) and CC (**F**) mammograms 3 years later show resolution of breast edema, with some residual skin thickening. Further retraction of the skin over the biopsy scar has occurred, and the scar still looks like a spiculated mass, simulating cancer, but is unchanged, indicating its benign etiology.

Continued

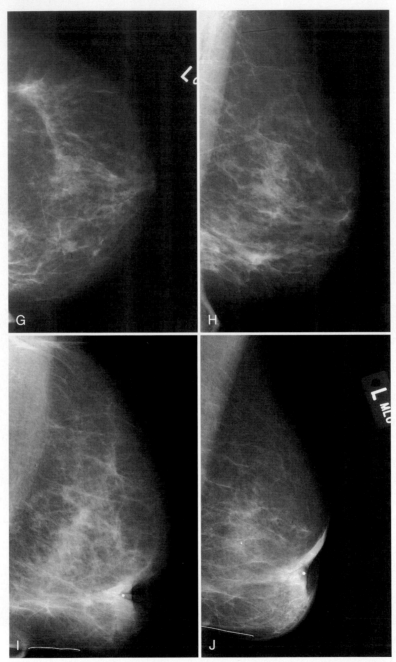

FIGURE 8-14, cont'd. CC (**G**) and MLO (**H**) views show a round invasive ductal cancer (*arrow*) in the lower inner aspect of the left breast. **I**, One year after biopsy and radiation therapy, note the skin deformity, edema, and skin thickening in the lower portion of the breast on an MLO view. **J**, At 3 years the edema has diminished, but the skin thickening and deformity persist. This mammogram is the new baseline appearance for the rest of this woman's life.

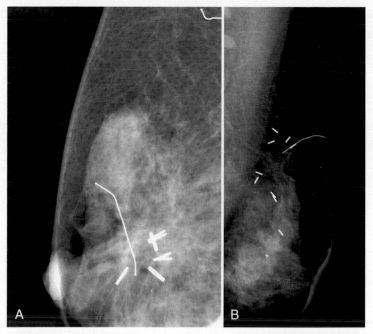

FIGURE 8-15. Markers in the biopsy site for electron beam boost. **A,** Mediolateral oblique (MLO) cropped mammogram shows postbiopsy change in the upper outer portion of the right breast, with metallic markers lining the biopsy site. The markers are used as a guide for radiation therapy ports. **B,** In another patient, MLO mammogram shows postbiopsy change in the upper left breast, with metallic markers lining a large biopsy site and a linear metallic marker showing the skin scar.

resected tumor. Increasing microcalcifications are suggestive of breast cancer recurrence and should prompt biopsy unless they are specific for dystrophic calcifications or fat necrosis.

Because investigators have been exploring the use of APBI in lieu of standard WB-XRT, the higher doses per fraction used with APBI have led to a variety of findings in several phase I/phase II studies. Some groups have reported a higher incidence of post-treatment calcifications, leading to fairly high rates of early postlumpectomy biopsy. It has not been clear from these studies whether a lower threshold for biopsy was set because of the experimental nature of APBI. Other studies have suggested that the incidence of calcifications, attributed to asymptomatic fat necrosis, increases with time after APBI. There has been no systematic evaluation of mammographic findings after APBI either with prior phase I or phase II studies, or from the limited reports from phase III studies published to date. It is fairly clear, however, that APBI will likely become a standard treatment option for at least some women with early-stage breast cancer pursuing breast conservation. Because radiologists may see the findings of a large seroma cavity extending from the skin surface to the chest wall (Fig. 8-17) or increased calcifications in and around the lumpectomy cavity resulting from fat necrosis, it will be important to contrast this to "normal" postbiopsy changes in which the scar is small (Fig. 8-18). Recognition of post-ABPI findings will minimize both false-positive, as well as false-negative, interpretations of post-APBI mammograms as this new paradigm emerges.

MRI

On MRI, the breast biopsy scar enhances for up to 18 months and is a common cause for false-positive readings.

Normal postbiopsy fat necrosis produces a spiculated mass that enhances rapidly and washes out on the kinetic curve; this common false-positive MRI finding can result in biopsy unless the radiologist investigates the patient's history and correlates the MRI to the mammogram (Fig. 8-19).

Recurrent invasive cancers usually appear as a mass in or near the biopsy site in the first few years. Cancers recurring as DCIS are more difficult to identify because DCIS may not produce the characteristic rapid enhancement and late-phase plateau or washout kinetic curve types and may show a nonspecific segmental or regional pattern of enhancement. Moreover, chemotherapy changes the enhancement pattern of the breast in that it diminishes enhancement of normal breast parenchyma and tumor alike.

Chemotherapy can change a suspicious kinetic late-phase plateau or washout curve pattern to a late-phase benign persistent pattern even when an invasive breast cancer is still present. The change in the kinetic curve pattern should not be mistaken for total tumor destruction by chemotherapy in the face of abnormal enhancement morphology. Investigators have shown that viable invasive breast cancers that previously showed late-phase plateaus or washout can change to a benign persistent late-phase kinetic pattern after chemotherapy. If one has any doubt regarding a controversial finding on MRI in the post-chemotherapy setting, biopsy should be considered.

APBI using either IORT or 3D-CRT results in characteristic post-treatment MRI changes, which extend from the skin to the chest wall. Typically, there is only localized skin thickening in the APBI area and an absence of generalized skin thickening. In addition, signal voids are common in the postoperative breast after APBI. These signal voids may persist up to 25 months after treatment. Some signal voids may resolve between 6 and 33 months

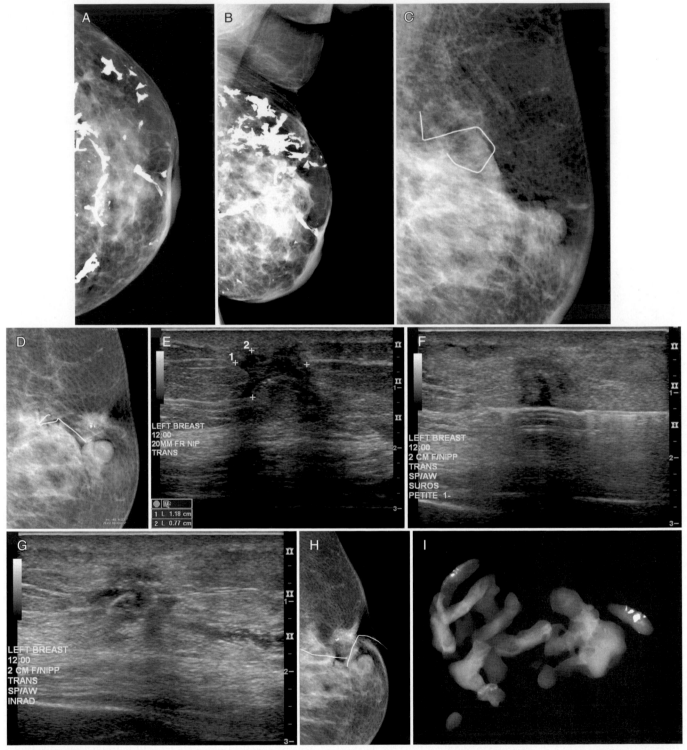

FIGURE 8-16. Dystrophic calcifications after radiation therapy. Craniocaudal (**A**) and mediolateral oblique (**B**) views after an older type of whole-breast radiation therapy that used a higher orthovoltage radiation compared to current methods shows a small left breast, skin thickening, and large, coarse, bizarre dystrophic calcifications. Breast shrinkage and these types of calcifications are not usually seen with whole-breast radiation therapy today. **C,** In another patient, cropped mammogram shows scarring in the upper left breast and skin thickening from radiation therapy after cancer biopsy. **D,** Two years later, a new spiculated mass containing dystrophic calcifications is noted near the scar, worrisome for cancer. **E,** Ultrasound shows the spiculated mass and calcifications corresponding to the mammographic finding. **F,** Ultrasound shows a core biopsy needle through the mass and calcifications. **G,** Postbiopsy ultrasound shows the residual mass, a marker and surrounding hematoma. **H,** Postbiopsy mammogram shows removal of the calcifications, a hematoma and the marker. Note the linear scar markers and skin deformity from the prior biopsy. **I,** Specimen radiograph shows the calcifications within the core biopsy samples. Histology showed fat necrosis and scar. This demonstrates how fat necrosis can simulate recurrent cancer when it forms a spiculated mass and calcifications.

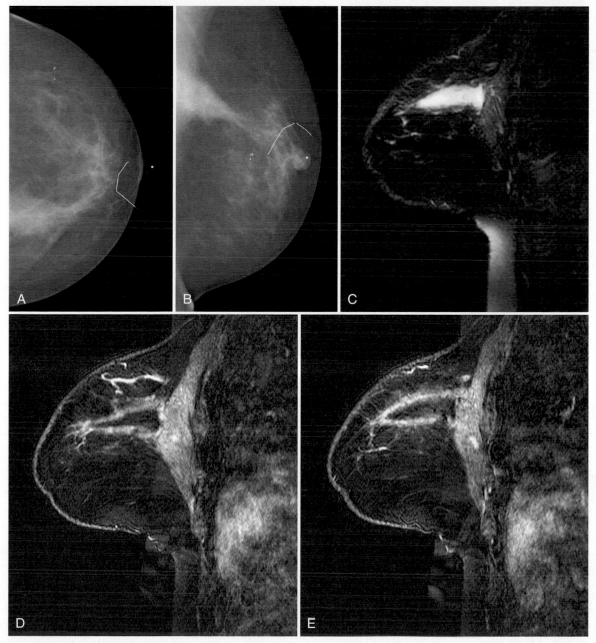

FIGURE 8-17. Mammography and magnetic resonance imaging (MRI) after accelerated partial breast irradiation (APBI). Craniocaudal (**A**) and medio-lateral oblique (**B**) views show postbiopsy change in a cylindrical scar extending from the skin surface (marked by a metallic linear scar marker) to the chest wall of the left breast after intraoperative radiation therapy. Note that skin deformity, edema, and skin thickening is limited to the operative site and is mixed down to the medial breast, unlike whole breast irradiation changes. **C,** Sagittal fat-suppressed T2-weighted MRI shows the fluid-filled biopsy site extending from the skin to the chest wall, corresponding to the scar seen on the mammogram. **D** and **E,** Sagittal postcontrast three-dimensional magnetization transfer MRIs show the fluid-filled biopsy site extending from the skin to the chest wall, with enhancement on the periphery of the biopsy cavity. Note that, unlike with whole-breast irradiation, after ABPI there is very little breast edema or skin thickening.

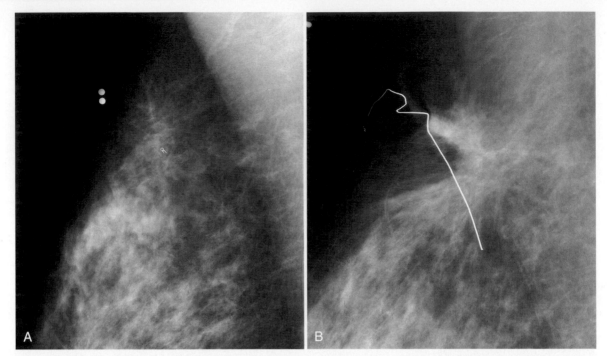

FIGURE 8-18. Scarring at a biopsy site. **A,** A prebiopsy cropped mediolateral oblique (MLO) view shows a clip where cancer was biopsied by stereotaxis; two BBs show the previous needle entry site. **B,** A postbiopsy cropped MLO view shows limited architectural distortion and skin deformity at the biopsy scar after definitive cancer surgery. Contrast part **B** to the scarring after accelerated partial breast irradiation in Figure 8-17. Cancer recurrences display pleomorphic calcifications, increasing density, or masslike change in the scar, which are not present here. Contrast part **B** to the cancer recurrence in Fig. 8-20A.

after treatment, whereas others persist. The reason for persistent signal voids in the breast lumpectomy cavities not containing metal at 25 months is uncertain but may be related to altered paramagnetic properties of the treated biopsy site. Radiologists should be aware of the characteristic MRI appearance of the APBI field to accurately detect IBTR and find new primary carcinomas elsewhere in the breast, as well as avoid false-positive diagnoses.

■ TREATMENT FAILURE OR IPSILATERAL BREAST TUMOR RECURRENCE

The incidence of treatment failure is approximately 1% per year. Women who are at greatest risk for failure include those younger than age 35 (and especially those younger than age 30); women treated for invasive cancer with an extensive intraductal component or infiltrating ductal carcinoma with a large intraductal component; women with intraductal carcinoma of the comedo type; women with intraductal cancer measuring 2.5 cm or greater in diameter; women with multicentric lesions, as suggested in the studies discussed in this chapter, and those treated for more than one synchronous cancer in the same breast; and women with angiolymphatic invasion. Gross residual tumor also has a poor prognosis, but microscopic residual disease may not infer a greater risk of IBTR. Despite the slightly higher tendency for recurrence in these groups, no risk factor is an absolute contraindication to breast conservation; data on lesions with these features in randomized studies more often than not suggest a trend for increased recurrence rather than a statistically significant association.

For women who choose lumpectomy, IBTR rates are approximately 5% at 5 years and between 10% and 15% at 10 years after therapy. Invasive IBTR is most common between 18 months and 7 years after treatment; during this period IBTR more commonly occurs in or around the lumpectomy cavity. IBTR after 7 years more frequently is a random event in any quadrant of the affected breast, not necessarily at the original site, and is usually unrelated to the original lesion in the breast.

Late ipsilateral breast treatment failures consisting of DCIS or invasive tumors smaller than 2 cm may have a better prognosis; thus, some feel it is important to diagnose recurrences near the original tumor or new cancers elsewhere in the breast as early as possible. However, there is no clinical trial evidence supporting this belief. Treatment failures after lumpectomy and WB-XTR are usually treated by salvage mastectomy.

Treatment failures detected on mammography manifest as new pleomorphic calcifications or masses developing in the biopsy site. At times, a breast cancer recurrence is hard to distinguish from the normal postbiopsy scar, which mimics cancer. However, unlike cancer recurrences, the normal postbiopsy scar becomes smaller and less apparent over time on the mammogram, with stabilization at 2 to 3 years. Central fat necrosis may produce a radiolucent center in the biopsy cavity. Thus, it is not normal if the scar grows in size or becomes denser or more masslike. The radiologist suspects recurrent carcinoma and prompts biopsy if the "scar" develops new pleomorphic calcifications or becomes more dense, if the "scar" edge becomes rounder, or if the "scar" grows (Fig. 8-20).

Recurrent tumor in the irradiated breast may arise at the site of the original tumor or elsewhere in the breast

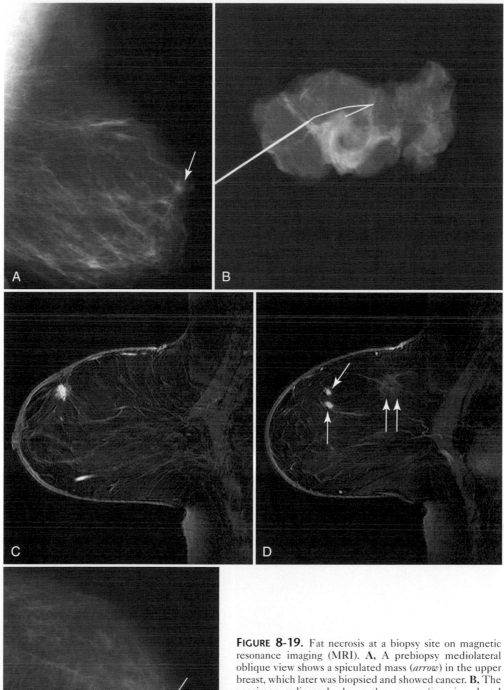

FIGURE 8-19. Fat necrosis at a biopsy site on magnetic resonance imaging (MRI). **A,** A prebiopsy mediolateral oblique view shows a spiculated mass (*arrow*) in the upper breast, which later was biopsied and showed cancer. **B,** The specimen radiograph shows the cancer (invasive ductal cancer) and localizing wire. **C,** Six months later, a postcontrast sagittal 3-D spectral-spatial excitation magnetization transfer (3DSSMT) MRI shows an enhancing spiculated mass in the upper breast and skin thickening. **D,** On another slice, the postcontrast sagittal 3DSSMT MRI shows two enhancing masses (*arrows*) and a posterior nonenhancing architectural distortion representing an old biopsy scar (*double arrows*). Scarring older than 18 months does not enhance, so the old biopsy scar in the posterior breast is of low signal intensity. **E,** Craniocaudal mammogram after the MRI shows the old architectural distortion in the central breast (*double arrows*) and postbiopsy scarring closer to the nipple (*arrow*), corresponding to the spiculated enhancing mass on MRI, which represented normal fat necrosis. Note how fat necrosis can simulate cancer on MRI.

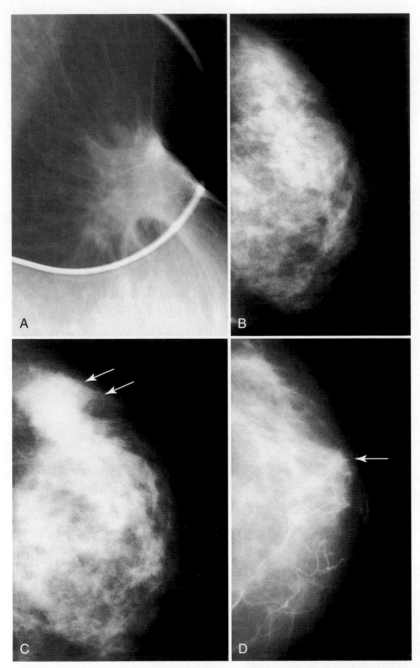

FIGURE 8-20. Breast cancer occurring at a biopsy site. **A,** A postbiopsy spot mediolateral oblique view shows architectural distortion, skin retraction, and deformity at a biopsy scar. Unlike normal biopsy scars, which have a little density in their central part, this spot view shows a moderately masslike area in the scar, which was invasive ductal cancer. Contrast this tumor with the normal postbiopsy scar in Figure 8-18B. **B,** In another patient, a postbiopsy craniocaudal (CC) view shows architectural distortion in the outer portion of the breast after biopsy and radiation therapy for cancer. **C,** Five years later, a developing density (*arrows*) is present in the outer part of the breast. Biopsy showed recurrent cancer. **D,** In a third patient, a postbiopsy CC view shows minimal architectural distortion near the nipple after biopsy and radiation therapy for cancer (*arrow*).

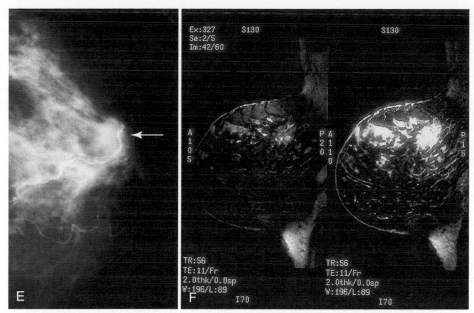

FIGURE 8-20, cont'd. E, The next year a developing mass (*arrow*) was noted in the biopsy site. Biopsy showed recurrent cancer. **F,** Sagittal 3-D spectral-spatial excitation magnetization transfer noncontrast-enhanced (*left*) and contrast-enhanced (*right*) magnetic resonance images show segmental enhancement in a cancer recurrence in the upper part of the breast long after biopsy and radiation therapy.

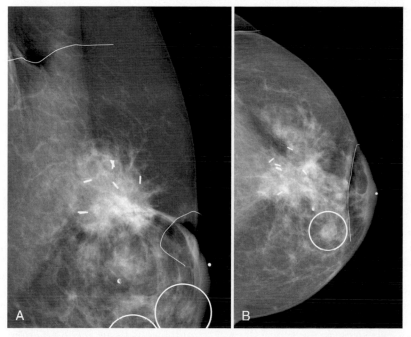

FIGURE 8-21. Ipsilateral breast tumor recurrence. Mediolateral oblique (**A**) and craniocaudal (CC) (**B**) mammograms 2 years after radiation therapy show postbiopsy scarring and surgical clips in the retroareolar region, with skin thickening. There is a new round mass in the medial left breast best seen and circled on the CC view (**B**), and seen and circled in the MLO view (**A**), separated from the old biopsy site by normal tissue. Additional views confirmed that a mass was present, and biopsy showed a new invasive ductal cancer.

(Fig. 8-21). Recurrences at the original tumor site are usually due to failure to eradicate the original cancer and represent true treatment failures; they occur sooner than a tumor developing elsewhere in the breast. Tumors developing outside the treated area occur at the same rate as tumors forming in the contralateral breast and represent new cancers. Breast irradiation does not lead to an increased incidence of breast cancer in the opposite breast or in the boosted area of the treated breast.

Recurrent disease is diagnosed by mammography or physical examination. About half of the recurrences are detected by mammography and half by physical examination. Those that are mammographically detected usually contain pleomorphic microcalcifications or masses (Box 8-9). Palpable recurrences are usually manifested as masses, are more frequently invasive cancer, and may be displayed on the mammogram as developing densities or masses. On ultrasound, an IBTR shows as a mass separate

---

Box 8-9. Benign and Suspicious Mammographic Findings Developing in the Biopsy Site after Breast Conservation and Radiation Therapy

Pleomorphic calcifications (cancer recurrence or residua)
Nonspecific calcifications (benign or malignant)
Dystrophic calcifications (benign)
Suture calcifications (benign)
Oil cyst (benign)
Developing density or mass (suspicious)

---

from or in continuity with the biopsy scar (Fig. 8-22A to D) if it occurs near the original biopsy site.

On mammography, breast cancer recurrences contain pleomorphic calcifications (see Fig. 8-22E and F) or are shown as masses with or without calcifications. This is why radiologists investigate any new mass, because even benign new solid masses may represent a new cancer (Figs. 8-23 to 8-25).

There are no absolute guidelines for management of an IBTR after lumpectomy and radiotherapy. Traditionally, because the breast can only tolerate the doses used for WB-XTR once, most IBTRs are treated with completion mastectomy with or without reconstruction. Some patients and physicians will attempt repeat lumpectomy without additional radiotherapy but little long-term data on the safety and effectiveness of this approach are available. Recently, investigators have treated patients with IBTR using repeat lumpectomy and APBI. Here as well, isolated case reports alone exist and little long-term data on safety or effectiveness are available. Thus, generally, recurrent tumor is usually treated with salvage mastectomy.

Mastectomy

Mastectomy is used when it is not possible to excise the entire breast tumor with a good cosmetic result, if there is a contraindication to radiotherapy, or if it is the patient's desire to have a mastectomy. Although there is no strict size cut-off when choosing lumpectomy or mastectomy, lesions larger than 5 cm or patients with multifocal disease are usually approached with mastectomy.

There are exceptions to this. For a patient with newly diagnosed breast cancer, if the workup were to reveal an invasive tumor larger than 5 cm, neoadjuvant chemotherapy may be offered before surgery because it might decrease tumor size and facilitate breast conservation.

Also, the demonstration of multifocal disease is now considered a relative contraindication to breast conservation rather than an absolute contraindication.

Various types of mastectomies are performed today. With a traditional mastectomy, the nipple–areolar complex is removed with an ellipse of skin and underlying breast tissue. A skin-sparing mastectomy suggests that some of the breast skin that would normally have been removed is allowed to remain. The postoperative appearance of a skin-sparing mastectomy is variable in terms of the amount of skin remaining. In some patients the skin left behind may simply be in one quadrant; at its extreme, a total skin-sparing mastectomy removes the nipple–areolar complex but leaves all the remaining breast skin intact.

In the case of a subcutaneous mastectomy, the breast tissue is removed as with a simple (total) mastectomy, except that the nipple–areolar complex is preserved. This is occasionally requested by patients who are having mastectomy for prophylactic reasons and do not want to lose the nipple–areolar complex.

More recently areolar-sparing and nipple-sparing mastectomies have been offered to patients with invasive breast cancer; hence the slightly differing nomenclature in contrast to subcutaneous mastectomy. There is more oncologic soundness in areolar-sparing mastectomy, because breast ductal tissue does not involve the skin of the areola and therefore can be removed with the underlying breast as part of the mastectomy. In nipple-sparing mastectomy, by definition, some ductal tissue may remain within the nipple itself, as well as in the underlying bud of tissue, which ensures adequate vascularity to the nipple. Although the risk of direct nipple involvement varies among patient subgroups, it is important to point out that that no randomized trials have demonstrated the safety of nipple-sparing mastectomy compared with a traditional simple mastectomy. Typically, no radiotherapy is performed after a nipple-sparing mastectomy to help reduce local recurrence.

After mastectomy, breast reconstruction options include an implant, a latissimus dorsi flap with a tissue expander when significant breast skin has been lost, or a transverse rectus abdominis myocutaneous (TRAM) flap or one of its derivative procedures, such as a deep inferior epigastric perforator (DIEP) flap. Images of reconstructed breasts are shown in Chapter 9. In the case of skin-sparing subcutaneous mastectomy, the surgeon removes the breast tissue as for simple (total) mastectomy but preserves the nipple–areolar complex and inserts a tissue expander. Unless there is a medical contraindication to breast reconstruction, patients who choose mastectomy are always offered breast reconstruction with a tissue expander or autologous tissue flap. Imaging of the reconstructed breast is typically not performed after expander or implant placement or after autologous tissue reconstruction.

Sometimes, reduction mammoplasty may be required on the contralateral, unaffected breast to achieve symmetry with the treated breast. The appearances of breasts reconstructed with autologous tissue and contralateral normal breasts that have undergone reduction mammoplasty are characteristic and should not be mistaken for cancer. These are shown in Chapter 9.

Breast cancer recurrences in the unreconstructed mastectomy site are usually detected by physical examination. Because of the low yield of breast cancer detection due to the small amount of breast tissue remaining, surveillance mammography of the mastectomy site is usually not performed.

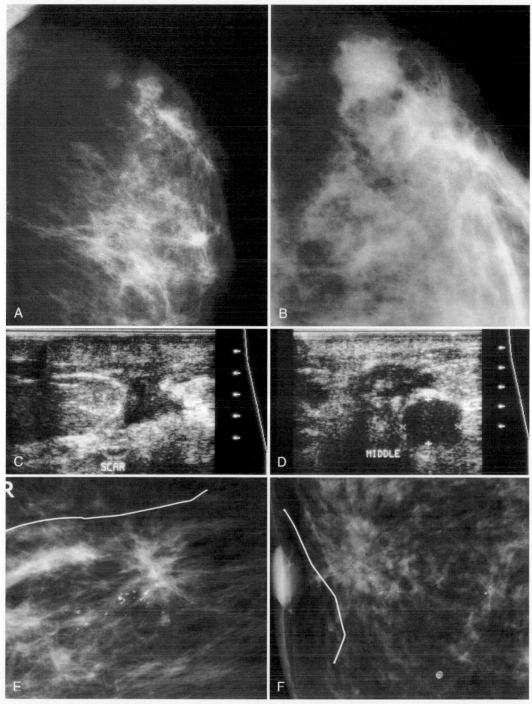

FIGURE 8-22. Treatment failure. Mediolateral oblique views 1 year (**A**) and 1.5 years (**B**) after radiation therapy show a palpable mass in the biopsy site in the upper part of the breast. **C,** Ultrasound at 1.5 years shows a fluid-filled scar at the biopsy site. Separate from the biopsy site is a round hypoechoic solid mass marked by calipers (**D**). Note that because the round mass is separated from the fluid collection, it cannot represent a part of the biopsy scar and must be considered suspicious. Biopsy showed an invasive ductal cancer. **E,** Magnified cropped mammogram shows a linear metallic scar marker overlying a spiculated but stable postlumpectomy scar. However, there are new pleomorphic calcifications in and near the scar, representing ductal carcinoma in situ in the biopsy site. **F,** In another patient, a stable spiculated scar is seen under the linear metallic marker in the periareolar region. Note the pleomorphic calcifications in and extending posteriorly to the scar, representing recurrent cancer.

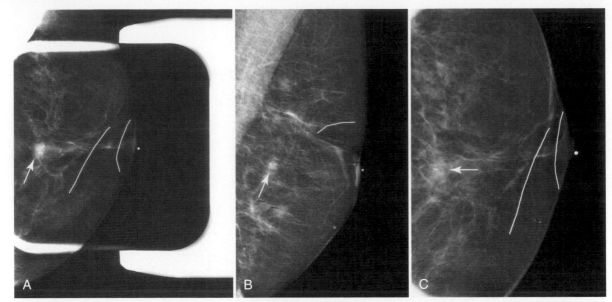

FIGURE 8-23. Treatment failure. Craniocaudal (**A**) and mediolateral oblique (**B**) views show architectural distortion near a linear scar marker in the 12-o'clock position of the left breast after biopsy and radiation therapy for cancer. Inferior to the scar in the retroareolar region there is a suspicious irregular mass with calcifications representing ipsilateral breast tumor recurrence (*arrow*). **C,** Spot compression magnification mammogram shows the mass and calcifications (*arrow*). Biopsy showed invasive ductal cancer and the patient underwent mastectomy.

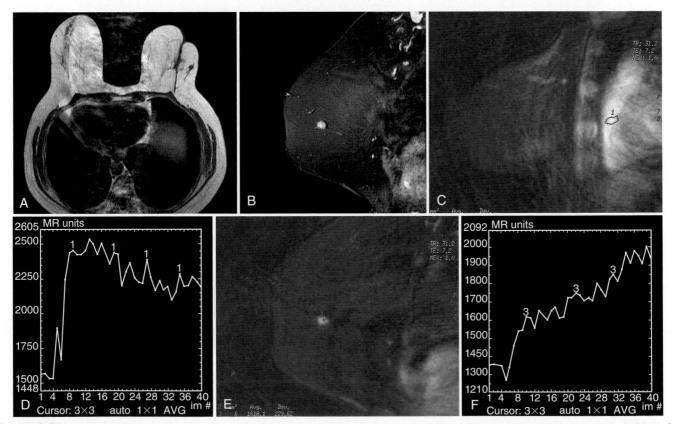

FIGURE 8-24. Atypical ipsilateral breast tumor recurrence on magnetic resonance imaging (MRI), mammography, and ultrasound. **A,** Axial nonfat-suppressed T1-weighted localizer shows architectural distortion in skin from the prior biopsy for cancer and a small round, low signal intensity mass in the outer right breast. **B,** Sagittal postcontrast 3-D spectral-spatial excitation magnetization transfer (3DSSMT) shows an enhancing round mass against a fatty background. Spiral dynamic sagittal MRI with an ROI over the heart (**C**) and dynamic kinetic curve (**D**) show that there was a good contrast bolus, as shown by the rapid initial rise and washout. Spiral dynamic sagittal MRI with an ROI over the outer breast mass (**E**) and kinetic curve (**F**) show a benign mass characterized by a slow initial rise and persistent late phase. However, because the mass was not present previously, it was considered suspicious.

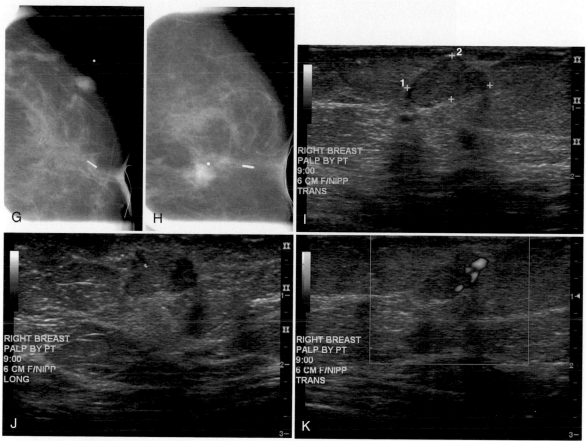

FIGURE 8-24, cont'd. In the same patient, craniocaudal (**G**) and mediolateral (**H**) views show architectural distortion and a marker in the retroareolar region after biopsy and radiation therapy for cancer. In the outer left breast, lateral to the scar, there is a palpable oval mass, marked by a BB and corresponding to the mass seen on MRI in Figure 8-24B. **I,** Transverse ultrasound over the mass shows an oval lobulated solid mass that shows microlobulated margins on longitudinal scan (**J**) and marked vascularity on color Doppler ultrasound (**K**). Biopsy showed invasive ductal cancer and the patient underwent mastectomy.

▬ KEY ELEMENTS

Immediate postsurgical breast changes on mammography include increased density (local edema), oval or round masses (seroma/hematoma) with or without air, and skin thickening.

The fluid in the surgical site resolves over the next few weeks and months in most cases.

Postsurgical changes diminish in severity over time and are stable at 3 to 5 years.

From 50% to 55% of patients undergoing surgical breast biopsy for benign disease have no mammographic findings at 3 years.

The remaining 45% to 50% of patients show architectural distortion, parenchymal changes (scarring) that may be spiculated, or increased density that can simulate breast cancer.

To determine whether a spiculated density on the mammogram is a postbiopsy scar or cancer, it is important to correlate the postsurgical site with the location of the spiculated finding.

Fat necrosis occurring in a biopsy site is visualized as radiolucent lipid-filled masses, with occasional curvilinear calcifications forming around the lucent center.

On ultrasound, the immediate postsurgical site appears as a fluid-filled mass representing the seroma; it occasionally displays septa, debris, or fluid tracking up to the skin incision.

If only the fibrotic scar remains, ultrasound reveals a hypoechoic spiculated mass that simulates breast cancer, but it should correlate with the postoperative site.

On MRI, the immediate postbiopsy cavity is a fluid-filled structure with surrounding tissue enhancement.

Postbiopsy scarring enhancement persists for up to 18 months and should then subside.

Breast tumors are staged by the TNM (tumor, lymph node, metastasis) classification of breast cancer from the American Joint Committee on Cancer.

Local control of breast cancer requires surgical eradication of tumor by mastectomy or lumpectomy, followed by radiotherapy.

The breast imager aids the surgeon in selecting candidates for breast-conserving surgery by determining the extent of tumor.

Relative contraindications to radiation therapy include previous radiation therapy, pregnancy, collagen vascular disease, and multicentric or diffuse disease.

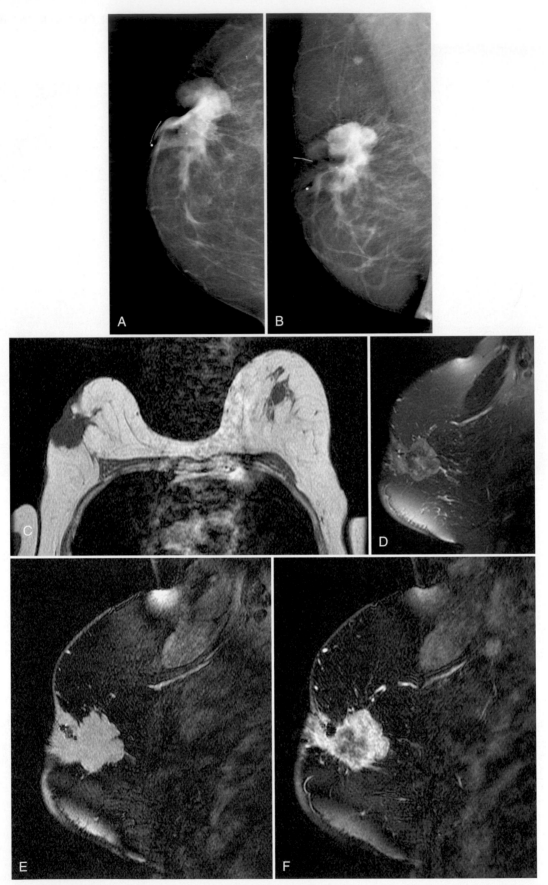

FIGURE 8-25. Ipsilateral breast tumor recurrence on mammography, ultrasound, and magnetic resonance imaging (MRI). Craniocaudal (**A**) and mediolateral (**B**) views show a dense, lobulated, suspicious mass growing in the biopsy site of a cancer that had been resected years ago, worrisome for cancer recurrence. **C,** Axial nonfat-suppressed T1-weighted MRI localizer shows the large mass in the outer right breast. **D,** Sagittal fat-suppressed T2-weighted noncontrast MRI shows the outer right breast cancer as a gray lobulated heterogeneous mass that extends to and infiltrates the skin. **E,** Sagittal T1-weighted precontrast 3-D spectral-spatial excitation magnetization transfer (3DSSMT) MRI shows the outer right breast mass that enhances on the postcontrast sagittal 3DSSMT MRI (**F**). Note the central necrosis. A round signal void is seen in the anterior aspect of the mass from a recent fine-needle biopsy resulting in air or methemoglobin.

Ipsilateral breast tumor recurrences are reported in 5% of women at 5 years and in 10% to 15% at 10 years after completion of therapy.

Treatment failures after breast conservation are managed by salvage mastectomy.

The sentinel lymph node biopsy technique identifies the lymph node most likely to harbor metastasis. Radionuclide tracers or blue dye is injected into the breast and later carried into the breast lymphatics draining the tumor or biopsy cavity.

A "hot" node, a blue node, or an abnormal palpable node identified at surgery is a sentinel lymph node.

The sentinel lymph node may be examined by hematoxylin and eosin staining, as well as by immunohistochemistry staining for low-molecular-weight cytokeratins.

The sentinel lymph node may be identified at surgery even with nonvisualization of a sentinel lymph node at lymphoscintigraphy.

MRI has been used for predicting the extent of tumor before the initial breast cancer surgical procedure, with some false-negative results in women with invasive lobular carcinoma and ductal carcinoma in situ.

If preoperative needle localization has been performed, specimen radiography or specimen sonography is used to determine whether the suspicious finding has been adequately removed.

As needed, postbiopsy mammograms determine the completeness of tumor excision, are particularly appropriate before the initiation of breast irradiation, and should be performed if residual tumor is suspected.

Most facilities obtain a unilateral mammogram immediately after the conclusion of radiation therapy, with further follow-up bilateral mammograms at 6- to 12-month intervals.

Breast edema from whole breast radiation therapy encompasses the entire breast and is manifested as diffuse increased parenchymal density, skin thickening, and trabecular thickening in subcutaneous fat.

Postsurgical and postradiation therapy changes usually decrease somewhat over a period of 2.5 to 3 years or may remain stable.

Calcifications in the biopsy site in an irradiated breast represent fat necrosis, dystrophic calcifications, calcifying suture material, or breast cancer recurrence.

Chemotherapy changes the MRI enhancement pattern of the breast by diminishing enhancement of normal breast parenchyma and tumor alike.

On MRI, suspicious postchemotherapy kinetic late-phase plateau or washout curve patterns can change to a benign persistent late-phase pattern despite the presence of viable breast cancer.

Recurrent cancer on mammography shown by pleomorphic microcalcifications is frequently ductal carcinoma in situ.

Palpable recurrences are usually manifested as mammographic masses and are more frequently invasive cancers.

Breast reconstruction includes an implant, a latissimus dorsi flap, or a transverse rectus abdominis myocutaneous flap.

Breast cancer recurrence in an unreconstructed mastectomy site is usually detected by physical examination.

■ SUGGESTED READINGS

Abe H, Schmidt RA, Kulkarni K, et al: Axillary lymph nodes suspicious for breast cancer metastasis: sampling with US-guided 14-gauge core-needle biopsy—clinical experience in 100 patients, *Radiology* 250:41–49, 2009.

Alazraki NP, Styblo T, Grant SF, et al: Sentinel node staging of early breast cancer using lymphoscintigraphy and the intraoperative gamma-detecting probe, *Semin Nucl Med* 30:56–64, 2000.

Al-Hallaq HA, Mell LK, Bradley JA, et al: Magnetic resonance imaging identifies multifocal and multicentric disease in breast cancer patients who are eligible for partial breast irradiation, *Cancer* 113:2408–2414, 2008.

American College of Radiology: *ACR Breast Imaging Reporting and Data System*, Breast Imaging Atlas. Reston, VA, 2003, American College of Radiology.

American Joint Committee on Cancer: *AJCC cancer staging manual*, ed 7, New York, 2010, Springer.

Bauer TW, Spitz FR, Callans LS, et al: Subareolar and peritumoral injection identify similar sentinel nodes for breast cancer, *Ann Surg Oncol* 9:169–176, 2002.

Bedrosian I, Mick R, Orel SG, et al: Changes in the surgical management of patients with breast carcinoma based on preoperative magnetic resonance imaging, *Cancer* 98:468–473, 2003.

Bedrosian I, Reynolds C, Mick R, et al: Accuracy of sentinel lymph node biopsy in patients with large primary breast tumors, *Cancer* 88:2540–2545, 2000.

Bevilacqua JL, Gucciardo G, Cody HS, et al: A selection algorithm for internal mammary sentinel lymph node biopsy in breast cancer, *Eur J Surg Oncol* 28:603–614, 2002.

Birdwell RL, Smith KL, Betts BJ, et al: Breast cancer: variables affecting sentinel lymph node visualization at preoperative lymphoscintigraphy, *Radiology* 220:47–53, 2001.

Bleicher RJ, Ciocca RM, Egleston BL, et al: Association of routine pretreatment magnetic resonance imaging with time to surgery, mastectomy rate, and margin status, *J Am Coll Surg* 209:180–187, 2009.

Bleicher RJ, Morrow M: MRI and breast cancer: role in detection, diagnosis, and staging, *Oncology (Williston Park)* 21:1521–1533, 2007.

Boughey JC, Middleton LP, Harker L, et al: Utility of ultrasound and fine-needle aspiration biopsy of the axilla in the assessment of invasive lobular carcinoma of the breast, *Am J Surg* 194:450–455, 2007.

Brennan ME, Houssami N, Lord S, et al: Magnetic resonance imaging screening of the contralateral breast in women with newly diagnosed breast cancer: systematic review and meta-analysis of incremental cancer detection and impact on surgical management, *J Clin Oncol* 27:5640–5649, 2009.

Brenner RJ, Pfaff JM: Mammographic features after conservation therapy for malignant breast disease: serial findings standardized by regression analysis, *AJR Am J Roentgenol* 167:171–178, 1996.

Brenner RJ, Pfaff JM: Mammographic changes after excisional breast biopsy for benign disease, *AJR Am J Roentgenol* 167:1047–1052, 1996.

Budrukkar A: Accelerated partial breast irradiation: an advanced form of hypofractionation, *J Cancer Res Ther* 4:46–47, 2008.

Chen PY, Vicini FA, Benitez P, et al: Long-term cosmetic results and toxicity after accelerated partial-breast irradiation: a method of radiation delivery by interstitial brachytherapy for the treatment of early-stage breast carcinoma, *Cancer* 106:991–999, 2006.

Choi YJ, Ko EY, Han BK, et al: High-resolution ultrasonographic features of axillary lymph node metastasis in patients with breast cancer, *Breast* 18:119–122, 2009.

Clarke M, Collins R, Darby S, et al: Effects of radiotherapy and of differences in the extent of surgery for early breast cancer on local recurrence and 15-year survival: an overview of the randomised trials, *Lancet* 366(9503):2087–2106, 2005.

Cody HS 3rd, Fey J, Akhurst T, et al: Complementarity of blue dye and isotope in sentinel node localization for breast cancer: univariate and multivariate analysis of 966 procedures, *Ann Surg Oncol* 8:13–19, 2001.

Cody HS 3rd, Urban JA: Internal mammary node status: a major prognosticator in axillary node-negative breast cancer, *Ann Surg Oncol* 2:32–37, 1995.

Cote RJ, Peterson HF, Chaiwun B, et al, for the International Breast Cancer Study Group: Role of immunohistochemical detection of lymph-node metastases in management of breast cancer, *Lancet* 354:896–900, 1999.

Cox BW, Horst KC, Thornton S, Dirbas FM: Impact of increasing margin around the lumpectomy cavity to define the planning target volume for 3D conformal external beam accelerated partial breast irradiation, *Med Dosim* 32:254–262, 2007.

Crivellaro M, Senna G, Dama A, et al: Anaphylaxis due to patent blue dye during lymphography, with negative skin prick test, *J Investig Allergol Clin Immunol* 13:71–72, 2003.

Damle S, Teal CB: Can axillary lymph node dissection be safely omitted for early-stage breast cancer patients with sentinel lymph node micrometastasis? *Ann Surg Oncol* 16(12):3215–3216, 2009.

Dang CM, Zaghiyan K, Karlan SR, Phillips EH: Increased use of MRI for breast cancer surveillance and staging is not associated with increased rate of mastectomy, *Am Surg* 75:937–940, 2009.

Denison CM, Ward VL, Lester SC, et al: Epidermal inclusion cysts of the breast: three lesions with calcifications, *Radiology* 204:493–496, 1997.

Dershaw DD, Shank B, Reisinger S: Mammographic findings after breast cancer treatment with local excision and definitive irradiation, *Radiology* 164:455–461, 1987.

Dirbas FM: Accelerated partial breast irradiation: where do we stand? *J Natl Compr Canc Netw* 7:215–225, 2009.

Dirbas FM, Jeffrey SS, Goffinet DR: The evolution of accelerated, partial breast irradiation as a potential treatment option for women with newly diagnosed breast cancer considering breast conservation, *Cancer Biother Radiopharm* 19:673–705, 2004.

Dowlatshahi K, Fan M, Anderson JM, Bloom KJ: Occult metastases in sentinel nodes of 200 patients with operable breast cancer, *Ann Surg Oncol* 8:675–681, 2001.

Dowlatshahi K, Fan M, Snider HC, Habib FA: Lymph node micrometastases from breast carcinoma: reviewing the dilemma, *Cancer* 80:1188–1197, 1997.

Dupont EL, Kuhn MA, McCann C, et al: The role of sentinel lymph node biopsy in women undergoing prophylactic mastectomy, *Am J Surg* 180:274–277, 2000.

Evans SB, Kaufman SA, Price LL, et al: Persistent seroma after intraoperative placement of MammoSite for accelerated partial breast irradiation: incidence, pathologic anatomy, and contributing factors, *Int J Radiat Oncol Biol Phys* 65:333–339, 2006.

Fischer U, Kopka L, Grabbe E: Breast carcinoma: effect of preoperative contrast-enhanced MR imaging on the therapeutic approach, *Radiology* 213:881–888, 1999.

Fisher B, Dignam J, Wolmark N, et al: Lumpectomy and radiation therapy for the treatment of intraductal breast cancer: findings from National Surgical Adjuvant Breast and Bowel Project B-17, *J Clin Oncol* 16:441–452, 1998.

Freedman GM, Fowble BL, Nicolaou N, et al: Should internal mammary lymph nodes in breast cancer be a target for the radiation oncologist? *Int J Radiat Oncol Biol Phys* 46:805–814, 2000.

Garcia-Barros M, Paris F, Cordon-Cardo C, et al: Tumor response to radiotherapy regulated by endothelial cell apoptosis, *Science* 300:1155–1159, 2003.

Godinez J, Gombos EC, Chikarmane SA, et al: Breast MRI in the evaluation of eligibility for accelerated partial breast irradiation, *AJR Am J Roentgenol* 191:272–277, 2008.

Golshan M, Martin WJ, Dowlatshahi K: Sentinel lymph node biopsy lowers the rate of lymphedema when compared with standard axillary lymph node dissection, *Am Surg* 69:209–212 2003.

Gorechlad JW, McCabe EB, Higgins JH, et al: Screening for recurrences in patients treated with breast-conserving surgery: is there a role for MRI? *Ann Surg Oncol* 15:1703–1709, 2008.

Goyal S, Khan AJ, Vicini F, et al: Factors associated with optimal cosmetic results at 36 months in patients treated with accelerated partial breast irradiation (APBI) on the American Society of Breast Surgeons (ASBrS) MammoSite Breast Brachytherapy Registry Trial, *Ann Surg Oncol* 16:2450–2458, 2009.

Heywang SH, Hilbertz T, Beck R, et al: Gd-DTPA enhanced MR imaging of the breast in patients with postoperative scarring and silicone implants, *J Comput Assist Tomogr* 14:348–356, 1990.

Hill AD, Tran KN, Akhurst T, et al: Lessons learned from 500 cases of lymphatic mapping for breast cancer, *Ann Surg* 229:528–535, 1999.

Holwitt DM, Swatske ME, Gillanders WE, et al: Scientific Presentation Award: The combination of axillary ultrasound and ultrasound-guided biopsy is an accurate predictor of axillary stage in clinically node-negative breast cancer patients, *Am J Surg* 196:477–482, 2008.

Horst KC, Ikeda DM, Birdwell RL, et al: Breast magnetic resonance imaging alters patient selection for accelerated, partial breast irradiation. Proceedings of the American Society for Therapeutic Radiology and Oncology 47th annual meeting, *Int J Radiat Oncol Biol Phys* 63(Suppl 1):S4–S5, 2005.

Houssami N, Hayes DF: Review of preoperative magnetic resonance imaging (MRI) in breast cancer: should MRI be performed on all women with newly diagnosed, early stage breast cancer? *CA Cancer J Clin* 59:290–302, 2009.

Huvos AG, Hutter RV, Berg JW: Significance of axillary macrometastases and micrometastases in mammary cancer, *Ann Surg* 173:44–46, 1971.

Jannink I, Fan M, Nagy S, et al: Serial sectioning of sentinel nodes in patients with breast cancer: a pilot study, *Ann Surg Oncol* 5:310–314, 1998.

Jothy Basu KS, Bahl A, Subramani V, et al: Normal tissue complication probability of fibrosis in radiotherapy of breast cancer: accelerated partial breast irradiation vs conventional external-beam radiotherapy, *J Cancer Res Ther* 4:126–130, 2008.

Jozsef G, Luxton G, Formenti SC: Application of radiosurgery principles to a target in the breast: a dosimetric study, *Med Phys* 27:1005–1110, 2000.

Karamlou T, Johnson NM, Chan B, et al: Accuracy of intraoperative touch imprint cytologic analysis of sentinel lymph nodes in breast cancer, *Am J Surg* 185:425–428, 2003.

Keshtgar MR, Ell PJ: Clinical role of sentinel lymph node biopsy in breast cancer, *Lancet Oncol* 3:105–110, 2002.

Kiluk JV, Ly QP, Meade T, et al: Axillary recurrence rate following negative sentinel node biopsy for invasive breast cancer: long-term follow-up, *Ann Surg Oncol* Sept. 24, 2009 [epub ahead of print].

Krag D, Weaver D, Ashikaga T, et al: The sentinel node in breast cancer—a multicenter validation study, *N Engl J Med* 339:941–946, 1998.

Kuzmiak CM, Zeng D, Cole E, Pisano ED: Mammographic findings of partial breast irradiation, *Acad Radiol* 16(7):819–825, 2009.

Lacour J, Le M, Caceres E, et al: Radical mastectomy versus radical mastectomy plus internal mammary dissection. Ten year results of an international cooperative trial in breast cancer, *Cancer* 51:1941–1943, 1983.

Lagios MD: Clinical significance of immunohistochemically detectable epithelial cells in sentinel lymph node and bone marrow in breast cancer, *J Surg Oncol* 83:1–4, 2003.

Langer I, Guller U, Viehl CT, et al: Axillary lymph node dissection for sentinel lymph node micrometastases may be safely omitted in early-stage breast cancer patients: long-term outcomes of a prospective study, *Ann Surg Oncol* 16(12): 3366–3374, 2009.

Lehman CD, DeMartini W, Anderson BO, Edge SB: Indications for breast MRI in the patient with newly diagnosed breast cancer, *J Natl Compr Canc Netw* 7:193–201, 2009.

Liberman L: Lymphoscintigraphy for lymphatic mapping in breast carcinoma, *Radiology* 228:313–315, 2003.

Liberman L, Van Zee KJ, Dershaw DD, et al: Mammographic features of local recurrence in women who have undergone breast-conserving therapy for ductal carcinoma in situ, *AJR Am J Roentgenol* 168:489–493, 1997.

Lu WL, Jansen L, Post WJ, et al: Impact on survival of early detection of isolated breast recurrences after the primary treatment for breast cancer: a meta-analysis, *Breast Cancer Res Treat* 114:403–412, 2009.

Mamounas EP: Sentinel lymph node biopsy after neoadjuvant systemic therapy, *Surg Clin North Am* 83:931–942, 2003.

Mariani L, Salvadori B, Marubini E, et al: Ten year results of a randomised trial comparing two conservative treatment strategies for small size breast cancer, *Eur J Cancer* 34:1156–1162, 1998.

Martin RC, Derossis AM, Fey J, et al: Intradermal isotope injection is superior to intramammary in sentinel node biopsy for breast cancer, *Surgery* 130:432–438, 2001.

McCarter MD, Yeung H, Fey J, et al: The breast cancer patient with multiple sentinel nodes: when to stop? *J Am Coll Surg* 192:692–697, 2001.

McCarter MD, Yeung H, Yeh S, et al: Localization of the sentinel node in breast cancer: identical results with same-day and day-before isotope injection, *Ann Surg Oncol* 8:682–686, 2001.

McMasters KM, Chao C, Wong SL, et al: Sentinel lymph node biopsy in patients with ductal carcinoma in situ: a proposal, *Cancer* 95:15–20, 2002.

McMasters KM, Tuttle TM, Carlson DJ, et al: Sentinel lymph node biopsy for breast cancer: a suitable alternative to routine axillary dissection in multi-institutional practice when optimal technique is used, *J Clin Oncol* 18:2560–2566, 2000.

McMasters KM, Wong SL, Martin RC 2nd, et al: Dermal injection of radioactive colloid is superior to peritumoral injection for breast cancer sentinel lymph node biopsy: results of a multi-institutional study, *Ann Surg* 233:676–687, 2001.

Mendelson EB: Evaluation of the postoperative breast, *Radiol Clin North Am* 30:107–138, 1992.

Montague ED: Conservation surgery and radiation therapy in the treatment of operable breast cancer, *Cancer* 53(Suppl):700–704, 1984.

Montague ED, Fletcher GH: Local regional effectiveness of surgery and radiation therapy in the treatment of breast cancer, *Cancer* 55(Suppl):2266–2272, 1985.

Morris EA, Schwartz LH, Drotman MB, et al: Evaluation of pectoralis major muscle in patients with posterior breast tumors on breast MR images: early experience, *Radiology* 214:67–72, 2000.

Morrow M: Should routine breast cancer staging include MRI? *Nat Clin Pract Oncol* 6:72–73, 2009.

Mortellaro VE, Marshall J, Singer L, et al: Magnetic resonance imaging for axillary staging in patients with breast cancer, *J Magn Reson Imaging* 30:309–312, 2009.

Mumtaz H, Hall-Craggs MA, Davidson T, et al: Staging of symptomatic primary breast cancer with MR imaging, *AJR Am J Roentgenol* 169:417–424, 1997.

Nathanson SD, Wachna DL, Gilman D, et al: Pathways of lymphatic drainage from the breast, *Ann Surg Oncol* 8:837-843, 2001.

Nelson JC, Beitsch PD, Vicini FA, et al: Four-year clinical update from the American Society of Breast Surgeons MammoSite brachytherapy trial, *Am J Surg* 198(1):83–91, 2009.

Offersen BV, Overgaard M, Kroman N, Overgaard J: Accelerated partial breast irradiation as part of breast conserving therapy of early breast carcinoma: a systematic review, *Radiother Oncol* 90:1–13, 2009.

Ollila DW, Klauber-DeMore N, Tesche LJ, et al: Feasibility of breast preserving therapy with single fraction in situ radiotherapy delivered intraoperatively, *Ann Surg Oncol* 14:660–669, 2007.

Orel SG, Schnall MD, Powell CM, et al: Staging of suspected breast cancer: effect of MR imaging and MR-guided biopsy, *Radiology* 196:115–122, 1995.

Orel SG, Troupin RH, Patterson EA, Fowble BL: Breast cancer recurrence after lumpectomy and irradiation: role of mammography in detection, *Radiology* 183:201–206, 1992.

Pendas S, Dauway E, Giuliano R, et al: Sentinel node biopsy in ductal carcinoma in situ patients, *Ann Surg Oncol* 7:15–20, 2000.

Pernas S, Gil M, Benitez A, et al: Avoiding axillary treatment in sentinel lymph node micrometastases of breast cancer: a prospective analysis of axillary or distant recurrence, *Ann Surg Oncol* 17:772–777, 2010.

Philpotts LE, Lee CH, Haffty BG, et al: Mammographic findings of recurrent breast cancer after lumpectomy and radiation therapy: comparison with the primary tumor, *Radiology* 201:767–771, 1996.

Polgar C, Strnad V, Major T: Brachytherapy for partial breast irradiation: the European experience, *Semin Radiat Oncol* 15:116–122, 2005.

Rao R, Lilley L, Andrews V, et al: Axillary staging by percutaneous biopsy: sensitivity of fine-needle aspiration versus core needle biopsy, *Ann Surg Oncol* 16:1170–1175, 2009.

Sandrucci S, Mussa A: Sentinel lymph node biopsy and axillary staging of T1–T2 N0 breast cancer: a multicenter study, *Semin Surg Oncol* 15:278–283, 1998.

Schwartz GF, Giuliano AE, Veronesi U: Proceedings of the consensus conference of the role of sentinel lymph node biopsy in carcinoma of the breast, 19–22 April 2001, Philadelphia, *Breast J* 8:124–138, 2002.

Shen P, Glass EC, DiFronzo LA, Giuliano AE: Dermal versus intraparenchymal lymphoscintigraphy of the breast, *Ann Surg Oncol* 8:241–248, 2001.

Sickles EA, Herzog KA: Mammography of the postsurgical breast, *AJR Am J Roentgenol* 136:585–588, 1981.

Singletary SE, Greene FL: Revision of breast cancer staging: the 6th edition of the TNM Classification, *Semin Surg Oncol* 21:53–59, 2003.

Smith BD, Arthur DW, Buchholz TA, et al: Accelerated partial breast irradiation consensus statement from the American Society for Radiation Oncology (ASTRO), *Int J Radiat Oncol Biol Phys* 74:987–1001, 2009.

Steinhoff MM: Axillary node micrometastases: detection and biologic significance, *Breast J* 5:325–329, 1999.

Tendulkar RD, Chellman-Jeffers M, Rybicki LA, et al: Preoperative breast magnetic resonance imaging in early breast cancer: implications for partial breast irradiation, *Cancer* 115:1621–1630, 2009.

Tuli R, Christodouleas J, Roberts L, et al: Prognostic indicators following ipsilateral tumor recurrence in patients treated with breast-conserving therapy, *Am J Surg* 198:557–561, 2009.

Turner RR, Ollila DW, Krasne DL, Giuliano AE: Histopathologic validation of the sentinel lymph node hypothesis for breast carcinoma, *Ann Surg* 226:271–278, 1997.

Veronesi U, Luini A, Del Vecchio M, et al: Radiotherapy after breast-preserving surgery in women with localized cancer of the breast, *N Engl J Med* 328:1587–1591, 1993.

Veronesi U, Orecchia R, Luini A, et al: Full-dose intraoperative radiotherapy with electrons during breast-conserving surgery: experience with 590 cases, *Ann Surg* 242:101–106, 2005.

Veronesi U, Paganelli G, Viale G, et al: Sentinel lymph node biopsy and axillary dissection in breast cancer: results in a large series, *J Natl Cancer Inst* 91:368–373, 1999.

Veronesi U, Paganelli G, Viale G, et al: A randomized comparison of sentinel-node biopsy with routine axillary dissection in breast cancer, *N Engl J Med* 349:546–553, 2003.

Veronesi U, Zurrida S, Mazzarol G, Viale G: Extensive frozen section examination of axillary sentinel nodes to determine selective axillary dissection, *World J Surg* 25:806–808, 2001.

Vicini FA, Kestin L, Huang R, Martinez A: Does local recurrence affect the rate of distant metastases and survival in patients with early-stage breast carcinoma treated with breast-conserving therapy? *Cancer* 97:910–919, 2003.

Vicini FA, Remouchamps V, Wallace M, et al: Ongoing clinical experience utilizing 3D conformal external beam radiotherapy to deliver partial-breast irradiation in patients with early-stage breast cancer treated with breast-conserving therapy, *Int J Radiat Oncol Biol Phys* 57:1247–1253, 2003.

Wazer DE, Kaufman S, Cuttino L, et al: Accelerated partial breast irradiation: an analysis of variables associated with late toxicity and long-term cosmetic outcome after high-dose-rate interstitial brachytherapy, *Int J Radiat Oncol Biol Phys* 64:489–495, 2006.

Yarbro JW, Page DL, Fielding LP, et al: American Joint Committee on Cancer prognostic factors consensus conference, *Cancer* 86:2436–2446, 1999.

Zafrani B, Fourquet A, Vilcoq JR, et al: Conservative management of intraductal breast carcinoma with tumorectomy and radiation therapy, *Cancer* 57:1299–1301, 1986.

Quizzes

8-1. Fill in the contraindications to whole-breast radiation therapy.

_____

_____

_____

_____

_____

For answers, see Box 8-1.

8-2. Fill in the factors affecting the frequency of in-breast tumor recurrence after radiation therapy.

_____

_____

_____

_____

_____

For answers, see Box 8-2.

8-3. Fill in the sentinel lymph node biopsy identification techniques.

_____

_____

_____

For answers, see Box 8-3.

8-4. Fill in the enhancement on MRI after biopsy.

_____

_____

_____

For answers, see Box 8-4.

8-5. Fill in the normal postoperative findings for benign disease.

_____

_____

_____

_____

_____

_____

_____

_____

For answers, see Box 8-5.

8-6. Fill in the postbiopsy ultrasound findings.

EARLY

_____

_____

_____

LATE

_____

_____

For answers, see Box 8-6.

8-7. Fill in the principles for whole-breast, external beam irradiation (WB-XRT) and accelerated partial breast irradiation (APBI).

WB-XRT

_____

_____

_____

APBI

_____

_____

For answers, see Box 8-7.

8-8. Fill in the mammographic findings after breast conservation and radiation therapy.

For answers, see Box 8-8.

8-9. Fill in the benign and suspicious mammographic findings developing in the biopsy site after breast conservation and radiation therapy.

For answers, see Box 8-9.

8-10. Fill in the TNM staging classification for breast cancer.

PRIMARY TUMOR (T)

REGIONAL LYMPH NODES (N)

DISTANT METASTASES (M)

PATHOLOGIC (pN)

_____ _____

_____ _____

_____ _____

_____ _____

_____ _____

_____ _____

_____ _____

_____ _____

_____ _____

_____ _____

_____ _____

_____ _____

_____ _____

_____ _____

_____ _____

_____ _____

POST-TREATMENT ypN

_____

_____

_____

ANATOMIC STAGE/PROGNOSTIC GROUP

_____ _____ _____ _____

_____ _____ _____ _____

_____ _____ _____ _____

_____ _____ _____

_____ _____ _____ _____

_____ _____ _____

_____ _____ _____

_____ _____ _____ _____

_____ _____ _____

_____ _____ _____ _____

_____ _____ _____

_____ _____ _____

_____ _____ _____

_____ _____ _____ _____

_____ _____ _____ _____

_____ _____ _____

_____ _____ _____ _____

_____ _____

For answers, see Table 8-1.

8-11. Fill in the location of lymph nodes draining the breast.

LEVEL   **LOCATION**

_____   _____

_____   _____

_____   _____

For answers, see Table 8-2.

8-12. Fill in the breast imaging relating to breast-conserving therapy.

TIMING   **REASON**   **TECHNIQUE**

_____   _____   _____

                              _____

_____   _____   _____

                              _____

          _____   _____

          _____   _____

          _____   _____

          _____   _____

          _____   _____

          _____   _____

          _____   _____

For answers, see Table 8-3.

CHAPTER 9

Breast Implants and the Reconstructed Breast

Silicone breast implants were introduced in 1962. An estimated 2 million women in the United States have silicone breast implants, with approximately 80% placed for breast augmentation and the remainder for breast reconstruction after mastectomy. On April 16, 1992, the U.S. Food and Drug Administration (FDA) restricted the use of silicone implants to women undergoing breast reconstruction for mastectomy because of concern about implant rupture and a possible association with connective tissue disease.

Addressing these concerns, an article by Tugewell and colleagues in 2001 reported a U.S. District Court order establishing a national science panel to assess whether existing scientific studies showed an association between silicone breast implants and connective tissue disease. They concluded that no scientific evidence of such a relationship exists, nor is there evidence of a relationship between silicone breast implants and breast cancer. At this time, silicone gel breast implants were used for breast reconstruction after mastectomy in the United States. Saline-filled implants were used for cosmetic breast augmentation.

In 2006, a review article by McLaughlin and colleagues restated that there was no "causal association between breast implants and breast or any other type of cancer, definite or atypical connective tissue disease, adverse offspring effects, or neurologic disease." The FDA re-approved silicone breast implants for both augmentation and reconstruction after extensive study and analysis, but still requires careful patient tracking. This chapter reviews breast implants, implant rupture, and the reconstructed breast.

IMPLANT TYPES

The most common breast implants are single-lumen and filled with either silicone or saline. Silicone implants are composed of a silicone elastomer shell filled with silicone made from a synthetic polymer of cross-linked chains of dimethylsiloxane that makes the implant soft and movable (Box 9-1 and Fig. 9-1). The outer envelope can be textured or smooth, polyurethane-coated or uncoated. The inner silicone can be a gel, a liquid, or a solid form. Saline implants are composed of an outer silicone shell and an inner envelope filled with saline (Fig. 9-2A to D). Of note, newer generation silicone implants have had a very small rupture rate in augmentation patients. Double- or triple-lumen implants have two or more envelopes inside one another, and each can contain saline or silicone gel. A common double-lumen implant is the saline outer, silicone inner implant. More recent common double-lumen implants have silicone outer and saline inner components.

All implants are placed behind the breast tissue, and some implants are placed behind the pectoralis muscle.

Less common implants include those filled with a polyvinyl alcohol sponge or a lipid substance (Trilucent implant), the latter of which may show a serous/lipid level on magnetic resonance imaging (MRI) if ruptured. "Stacked" implants are two single-lumen implants placed one on top of the other in the breast for aesthetic purposes. An implant type that is no longer used was covered with a finely textured meshlike surface over the outer envelope that was composed of a polyurethane-coated material to prevent fibrous capsular formation. This implant was banned because of the release of 2,4-toluenediamine (TDA), a byproduct suspected to cause cancer in laboratory animals.

MAMMOGRAPHY OF NORMAL IMPLANTS

Surgeons place silicone gel-filled implants behind the breast tissue on the chest wall in the subglandular or subpectoral position (see Fig. 9-2E and F). In either case, the body generally forms a fibrous capsule around the implant. The fibrous capsule is usually soft, nonpalpable, and undetectable to physical examination, but with time, the capsule hardens or calcifies in some individuals. If a silicone implant ruptures, this fibrous capsule holds the silicone within as long as it, too, does not rupture.

A normal silicone implant is quite dense and completely opaque, and obscures and displaces much of the surrounding breast tissue. On mammography the implant appears as a smooth white oval opacity near the chest wall (Fig. 9-3). The pectoralis muscle curves over the implant in subpectoral implants and lies underneath the implant in subglandular implants. A silicone gel-filled implant is not as compressible as breast tissue and can be ruptured if compressed too hard during mammography or closed capsulotomy. Because limited compression decreases visualization of the surrounding breast tissue for breast cancer screening, the Mammography Quality Standards Act (MQSA) recommends four views of each implanted breast. Two views are implant-displaced views, in which the technologist pinches the breast tissue in front of the implant to compress it, and two views include the implant but do not use much compression (Box 9-2). Breast tissue is evaluated on the implant-displaced views; implant integrity is evaluated on limited-compression mammograms in which the implant is surrounded by noncompressed breast tissue. Even with the implant-displaced views, the radiologist sees only about 80% of the breast tissue because it is hidden by the implant.

The implant-displaced technique does not completely resolve the problem of imaging small breast cancers, but it does optimize the amount of breast tissue displayed on the mammogram. Both physical examination and breast ultrasound as an adjunct to mammography are helpful in evaluating mammographically detected breast masses or palpable findings because mammography is limited with implants in place. Ultrasound can be especially helpful in determining whether a true mass exists, because ultrasound can evaluate the entire breadth of the breast tissue down to the implant. Ultrasound also distinguishes breast masses from the snowstorm appearance of silicone granulomas caused by ruptured implants (Fig. 9-4).

BOX 9-1. Implant Types

Single-lumen silicone
Single-lumen saline
Double-lumen: saline outer, silicone inner
Single-lumen silicone, outer polyurethane mesh
  coating
Single-lumen, lipid-filled
Complex or custom implants
Stacked implants
Direct silicone or paraffin injections

BOX 9-2. Mammography of Implants

Four views of each breast:
  CC and ML or MLO with the implant
  CC and ML or MLO implant-displaced views
Magnification, spot, and other fine-detail views can be
  performed in the implanted breast
5% of screenings show asymptomatic rupture

CC, craniocaudal; ML, mediolateral; MLO, mediolateral oblique.

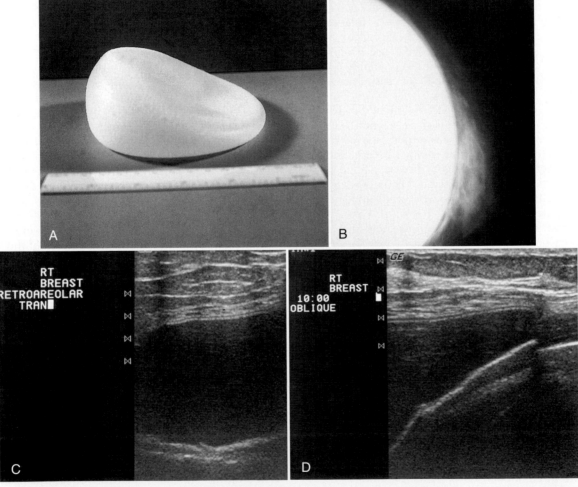

FIGURE 9-1. Normal silicone implant. **A,** A silicone gel implant photographed from the side. The implant will be placed underneath the breast tissue and either on top of or underneath the pectoralis muscle at surgery. **B,** Mammogram shows a dense structure near the chest wall and a little breast tissue around it. **C,** Ultrasound of a typical intact silicone implant shows the breast tissue in the near-field and the oval hypoechoic implant near the chest wall. Note that the appearance of a normal silicone implant is almost anechoic and simulates a very, very large cyst. **D,** Ultrasound of an intact silicone implant shows a typical normal edge artifact causing shadowing where the edge of the implant meets breast tissue. Typical normal reverberation artifact is seen in the near-field of the implant, similar to artifacts seen in a normal urinary bladder.

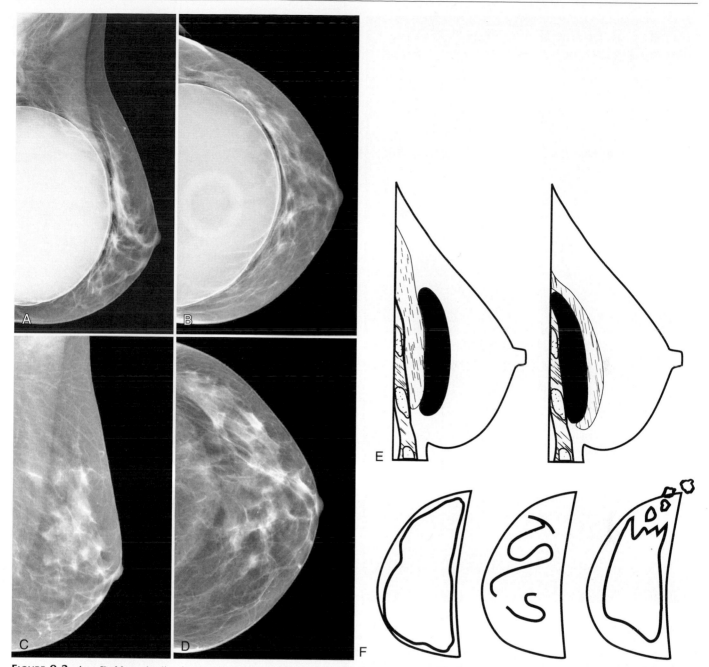

FIGURE 9-2. **A** to **D,** Normal saline implant: standard and implant-displaced mammograms. Mediolateral oblique (MLO) (**A**) and craniocaudal (CC) (**B**) mammograms with a saline implant show the implant behind the pectoralis muscle. The silicone envelope surrounds the lucent saline filling, so that the wrinkles within its envelope and the ringlike injection port are visible. In contrast, a silicone implant is completely white. MLO (**C**) and CC (**D**) implant-displaced mammograms show well-compressed breast tissue anterior to the implant. The technologist obtains the implant-displaced view by pinching the breast tissue in front of the implant, compressing the breast tissue for optimal visualization without rupturing the implant. **E,** Schematic of implant placement: subglandular implant placement (*left*) and subpectoral implant placement (*right*). **F,** Schematic of implant complications. On the *left*, a fibrous capsule forms around an intact implant. In the *middle*, the implant shell may rupture, but the silicone is contained in the fibrous capsule—called *intracapsular rupture*. On the *right*, the implant capsule and the fibrous capsule are ruptured, with silicone outside the fibrous capsule—called *extracapsular rupture*.

Unlike opaque silicone implants, saline implants contain radiolucent saline surrounded by a dense silicone outer envelope, in which small wrinkles may be seen. When a saline implant ruptures, the saline diffuses into the breast tissue and the envelope shrinks back against the chest wall (Fig. 9-5). In contradistinction, when a silicone implant ruptures, most of the silicone may be contained by the fibrous capsule and the implant retains much of its shape and volume. Saline outer, silicone inner double-lumen implants have an outer envelope containing saline surrounding a dense inner silicone implant filling.

The fibrous capsule surrounding implants of any type is not usually visible unless it calcifies. A calcified fibrous capsule contains dystrophic sheetlike calcifications and

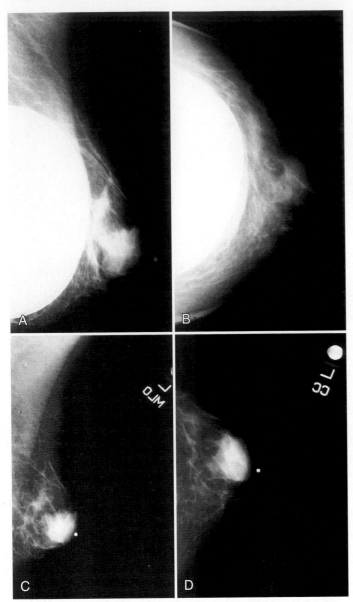

FIGURE 9-3. Normal silicone implant: standard and implant-displaced mammograms. Mediolateral oblique (MLO) (**A**) and craniocaudal (CC) (**B**) mammograms with subglandular silicone implants show the implant as a white structure near the chest wall and the relatively uncompressed breast tissue anterior to it. The technologist uses very little compression on these images to avoid rupturing the implant, but it is hard to find breast cancer in uncompressed breast tissue. Implant-displaced MLO (**C**) and CC (**D**) mammograms show well-compressed breast tissue anterior to the implant. Note that the breast tissue is spread apart on the implant-displaced views, making it easier to find early cancer. However, even with the best implant-displaced views, the radiologist can see at most only 80% of the breast tissue because the implant obscures the rest.

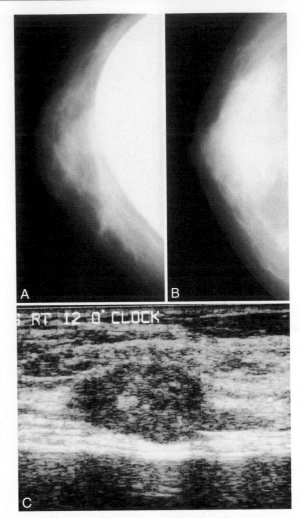

FIGURE 9-4. Mammogram with standard and implant-displaced views, with cancer present. **A,** Notice that the dense silicone implant near the chest wall obscures most of the breast tissue in this patient with a palpable mass at the 12-o'clock position of the right breast. **B,** Even when the implant is displaced, not all the breast tissue can be seen. **C,** At the 12-o'clock position of the right breast, ultrasound shows a suspicious irregular mass containing calcification on the fibrous capsule of the implant, not seen on the mammogram because it was pushed away from the field of view on the compressed images. Biopsy revealed invasive ductal cancer.

appears bumpy on the nondisplaced-implant views (Fig. 9-6A). Implant-displaced views displace the capsular calcifications away from the implant for analysis if one is concerned that the calcifications are in breast parenchyma rather than in the implant capsule. Spot magnification mammograms also help the radiologist analyze intraparenchymal calcifications and distinguish them from capsular calcifications.

If an implant ruptures, the surgeon removes the ruptured implant but does not always remove the fibrous capsule. If the fibrous capsule has calcified, the mammogram shows dystrophic calcifications in a sheetlike curvilinear pattern because they reside in the retained fibrous capsule. These calcifications can be hard to distinguish from cancer and can prompt biopsy (see Fig. 9-6B). Another specific type of capsular calcification that can be mistaken for cancer and will sometimes prompt biopsy is from calcifying polyurethane-covered implants. These implants are covered with a spongelike material, and when they calcify produce a typical fine meshlike calcification that can mimic ductal carcinoma in situ (see Fig. 9-6C and D).

When evaluating breast tissue for cancer in women with implants, it is important to inspect both the implant-displaced views and the breast tissue adjacent to the implant on the nonimplant-displaced views. The standard

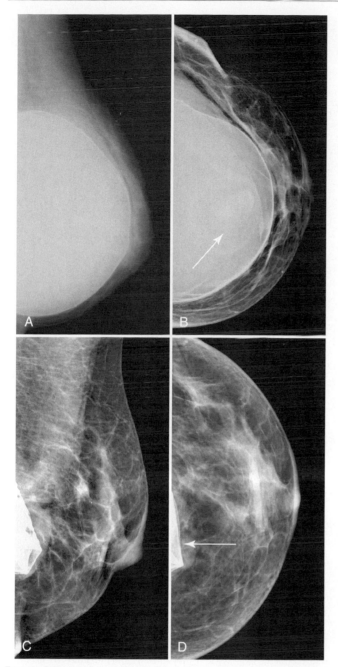

FIGURE 9-5. Ruptured saline implant. Mediolateral oblique (MLO) (**A**) and craniocaudal (CC) (**B**) mammogram with a saline implant in place shows the saline implant near the chest wall and a typical ringlike portion of the implant (*arrow*). A year later, the patient thought her breast suddenly got smaller after a car accident. MLO (**C**) and CC (**D**) mammograms show that the saline implant ruptured. Note the collapsed saline envelope at the chest wall (*arrow*).

TABLE 9-1. Baker Classification

Grade	Breast Firmness	Implant	Implant Visibility
I	Soft	Nonpalpable	Nonvisible
II	Minimal	Palpable	Nonvisible
III	Moderate	Easily palpable	Distortion visible
IV	Severe	Hard, tender, cold	Distortion may be marked

From Baker JL Jr: Augmentation mammaplasty. In Owsley JQ Jr, Peterson RA, editors: *Symposium on aesthetic surgery of the breast, 1978.* St. Louis, 1978, CV Mosby.

from the woman, including implant rupture as a possible complication for percutaneous biopsies.

IMPLANT COMPLICATIONS AND RUPTURE

Untoward complications associated with silicone gel-filled breast implants include contracture of the fibrous capsule, calcification of the fibrous capsule, hematoma, infection, implant rupture, and the controversial silicone gel "bleed," in which silicone gel leaks outside the implant through an intact envelope (Box 9-3). Capsular contracture is the most common complication, with a reported incidence of more than 70% in some older series and only about a 20% incidence in more recent series.

Implants can undergo capsular contraction, becoming hard and resistant, leading to a round, hard appearance and feel. The Baker classification of capsular formation on implants describes increasing levels of capsular contracture (Table 9-1). The incidence of capsular contracture may be diminished by the use of textured submuscular implants, although the use of such implants remains controversial. Open surgical capsulotomy, in which the hardened implant capsule is removed, was used to solve the problem of capsular contracture. Alternatively, surgeons would squeeze the implant to break the hardened fibrous capsule to allow the implant to become soft and pliable again, called *closed capsulotomy*. Unfortunately, closed capsulotomy could result in implant rupture.

Different types of fillers for implants were examined in trials, resulting in varying rates of fibrous capsule contracture. Munker and colleagues reported on Trilucent implants in 27 patients who elected to exchange their implants for a fourth-generation cohesive silicone implant. Of these 27 patients, 14 had a change in the volume of

---

views may display a mass near the implant or the fibrous capsule not evident on implant-displaced views. Masses on the fibrous capsule can be pushed away from the field of view with the implant-displaced views (Fig. 9-7). However, for masses or suspicious calcifications, spot compression or other fine-detail views can be used in women with implants, just as with any other woman. Needle localization, ultrasound-guided core biopsy, and stereotactic core biopsy all can be performed in women with implants as well. The radiologist just has to obtain informed consent

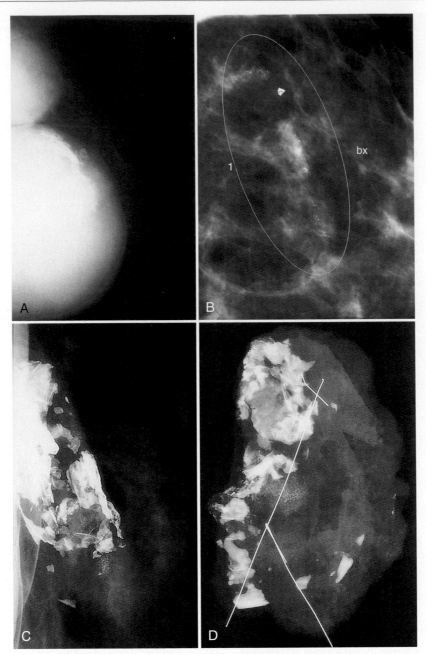

FIGURE 9-6. Calcifications near implants. **A,** Mediolateral oblique (MLO) mammogram shows two "stacked" implants in close proximity to each other with dense calcifications in the fibrous capsule that make the implant surface look bumpy. **B,** In another patient, capsular calcifications in a line mimic ductal carcinoma in situ. Biopsy showed dystrophic calcifications in the retained fibrous capsule after the implant was removed. **C,** An implant-displaced MLO mammogram shows a subpectoral saline implant in another patient and a calcified fibrous capsule from a previously removed subglandular polyurethane-covered implant. Notice the dystrophic sheetlike calcifications around the previous implant cavity. **D,** Tiny meshlike microcalcifications were seen near the dystrophic implant capsule and were removed by preoperative needle localization, as seen on specimen radiography; these microcalcifications represented the calcifying mesh of the outer polyurethane coating.

their implants but not all were aware of the change, and capsular contracture was not present (Baker grade II) (see Table 9-1); 55% of the implants had thickening or color changes caused by peroxidation of the triglyceride contents, and the implant capsule was adherent to breast tissues—in particular, the pectoralis muscle, which led to prolonged operative times. Rizkalla and colleagues reported similar results, with a reoperation rate of 20% (10/50) and an implant deflation rate of 10% (5/50). The Medical Devices Agency in the United Kingdom (which merged with the Medicines Control Agency in April 2003

to form the Medicines and Healthcare Products Regulatory Agency) withdrew the Trilucent implant from the market in March 1999, with a subsequent recommendation in June 2000 that the implants be removed from patients. A new type of alloplastic material for implants that contains carboxymethylcellulose, called Hydrogel, was introduced into the European market. Of 12 patients with 20 implants placed between 1996 and 1997, as reported by Cicchetti and colleagues, none showed immediate complications and had Baker grade I or II capsular contracture at 3.5 years of follow-up.

Implant Rupture

Reports attribute implant failure to a subpectoral location and implant age, especially implants manufactured in the late 1970s and early 1980s (i.e., second-generation implants). Closed capsulotomy, or manual breaking of the fibrous capsule, is also associated with implant rupture.

Implant integrity is classified as intact, intact with gel bleed, intracapsular rupture, or extracapsular rupture (Table 9-2). *Extracapsular rupture* is defined as implant rupture with silicone gel extruded outside a broken fibrous

TABLE 9-2. Implant Rupture Types

Rupture Types	Silicone Location	Envelope Status
Intracapsular rupture	Fibrous capsule contains silicone gel	Envelope ruptured
Extracapsular rupture	Silicone gel outside fibrous capsule	Envelope ruptured
Gel bleed (controversial)	Silicone outside envelope	Envelope intact

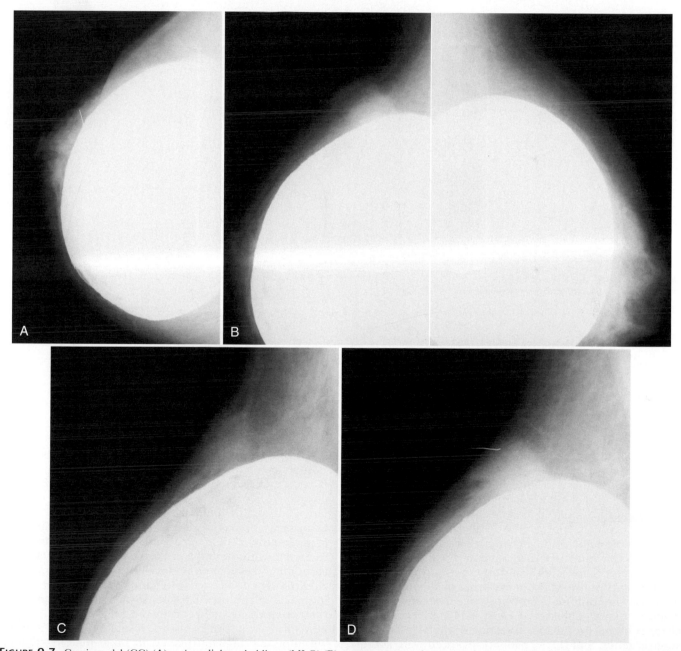

FIGURE 9-7. Craniocaudal (CC) (**A**) and mediolateral oblique (MLO) (**B**) mammograms; a dense mass is seen near the implant in the upper portion of the right breast on the MLO view only. The mass is obscured by the implant on the CC view. **C** and **D**, Photographically magnified views of the upper portion of the right breast taken in 1999 (**C**) and 2002 (**D**) show that the mass is new and developing in a previous biopsy site; the mass was not seen on implant-displaced views because it was pushed away with the implant, thus showing the importance of analyzing mammograms that include the implant as well as the implant-displaced view.

Continued

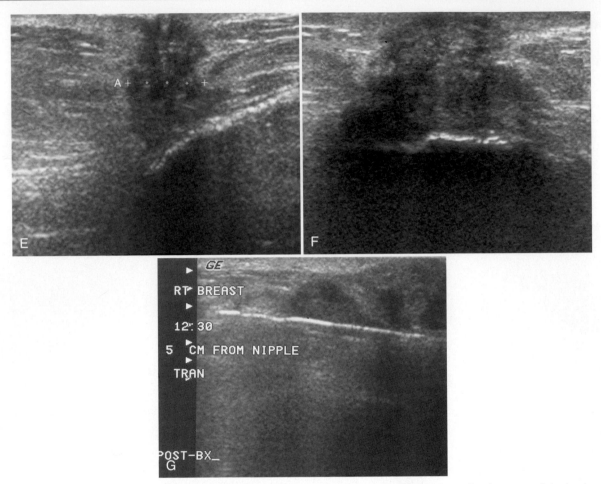

FIGURE 9-7, cont'd. Transverse (**E**) and longitudinal (**F**) ultrasound images show a spiculated mass immediately on top of the implant. **G,** Core biopsy under ultrasound guidance revealed invasive ductal cancer.

capsule. *Intracapsular rupture* is defined as implant rupture with silicone gel still contained within an intact fibrous capsule. *Gel bleed* is defined as silicone gel leakage through an intact implant envelope, although the existence of gel bleed versus small, undetected ruptures remains controversial.

A clinical diagnosis of implant rupture is often difficult to make. Feng and Amini report significant risk factors for implant rupture as an older implant ages: retroglandular location, capsular contracture, local symptoms, implant type (double-lumen and polyurethane-covered implants rupture less frequently than smooth gel implants), and manufacturer. The clinical history, signs, and symptoms are frequently nonspecific. In one series of 19 symptomatic patients with ruptured implants, women complained of palpable axillary, breast, or chest wall masses; pain; or changes in the size, shape, or texture of the breast. In one surgical series, 3 of the 32 patients reviewed were asymptomatic. Because physical examination misses approximately 50% of ruptures, clinicians have turned to imaging to help diagnose ruptured implants when the clinical findings are questionable.

IMPLANT IMAGING

Mammography

A retrospective review of screening mammograms in 350 asymptomatic women with breast implants showed an incidence of asymptomatic implant rupture of 5%. Mammography shows extracapsular rupture as silicone extravasation outside the implant envelope with blobs of silicone in the breast tissue (Fig. 9-8A and B), within implant ducts, or as a contour abnormality caused by extruded silicone in contiguity with the implant (Table 9-3). After extracapsular rupture, the surgeon removes the implant. Removal of all extravasated silicone is often impossible without removing much of the breast tissue, so the surgeon may leave some extravasated silicone in the breast. Later, when a new silicone implant is placed, residual silicone from the old ruptured implant makes it impossible to tell on mammography if the new implant has ruptured (see Fig. 9-8C). Silicone within axillary lymph nodes implies extravasation of silicone outside the fibrous capsule, because the silicone has traveled to the lymph nodes. This means that

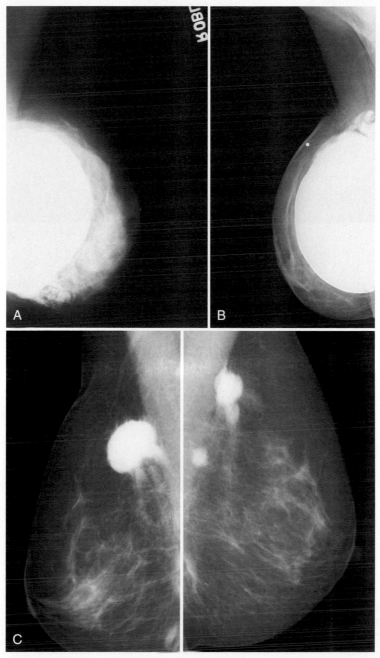

FIGURE 9-8. Implant rupture. **A,** Mediolateral oblique (MLO) mammogram shows blobs of silicone extruded into tissue inferior to the implant on an analog mammogram. **B,** This patient felt a mass in her upper right breast, marked by a BB and showing extruded silicone above the implant on a digital mammogram. **C,** In another patient, digital MLO mammograms show retained silicone in the upper breasts after removal of ruptured bilateral silicone implants. If the patient replaces the silicone implants, new ruptures would be impossible to diagnose.   *Continued*

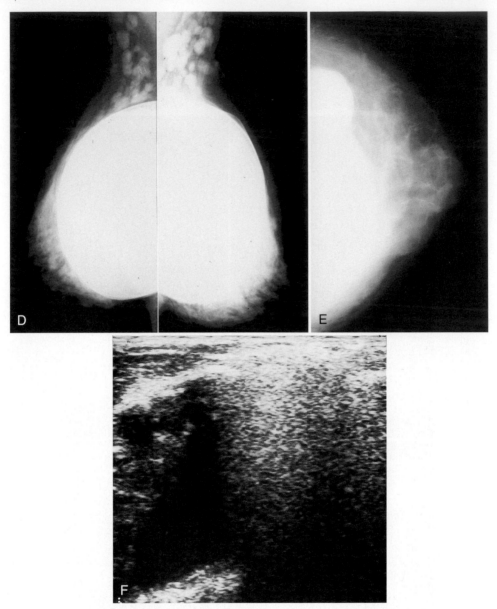

FIGURE 9-8, cont'd. D, After rupture and removal of silicone implants and replacement with saline implants, this patient has retained silicone in her lymph nodes bilaterally. **E,** A craniocaudal mammogram shows an unusual bulge of the implant's outer contour that represents either rupture or a herniation of the implant through a tear in the fibrous capsule; surgery showed rupture. **F,** Ultrasound shows echodense noise or snowstorm sign over the bulge in part **E,** confirming a rupture.

TABLE 9-3. Imaging Findings with Rupture

Imaging Modality	Intracapsular	Extracapsular	Gel Bleed
Mammography	Not present	Silicone globs in breast tissue Silicone in lymph nodes Silicone in ducts Implant contour deformity (occasionally seen)	Occasionally seen
Ultrasound	Stepladder sign	Snowstorm or echodense noise	Snowstorm or echodense noise
MRI	Linguine sign Teardrop/keyhole sign Subcapsular lines Water droplets (occasionally seen)	Silicone outside the envelope Signs of intracapsular rupture	Teardrop/keyhole sign Subcapsular lines

there must be an extracapsular rupture as well (see Fig. 9-8D).

Silicone implant contour lobulation indicates either capsular contracture, herniation of an intact implant envelope through a break in the surrounding fibrous capsule, or a contained implant leak (Table 9-4). Because intracapsular rupture is defined as implant rupture with silicone gel still contained within an intact fibrous capsule, mammography may show an intracapsular rupture as a normal-looking or bulging implant, depending on the shape of the fibrous capsule. Because both implant lobulation and a contained leak have the same mammographic appearance, radiologists use ultrasound and MRI to make the diagnosis of a rupture (see Fig. 9-8E and F). Mammography cannot identify intracapsular ruptures when the implant contour is normal, nor can it show posterior implant ruptures on the chest wall.

Direct silicone or paraffin injections were used overseas for breast augmentation; free silicone, paraffin, or other materials were injected directly into the breast tissue. The injections are foreign bodies and therefore result in multiple tiny round eggshell-type calcifications that obscure the underlying breast tissue. Because these silicone or injection granulomas may become quite hard, both physical examination and mammography of the underlying tissue are nearly impossible (Fig. 9-9). Ultrasound of patients with silicone injections shows multiple areas of snowstorm or echodense noise that cast shadows

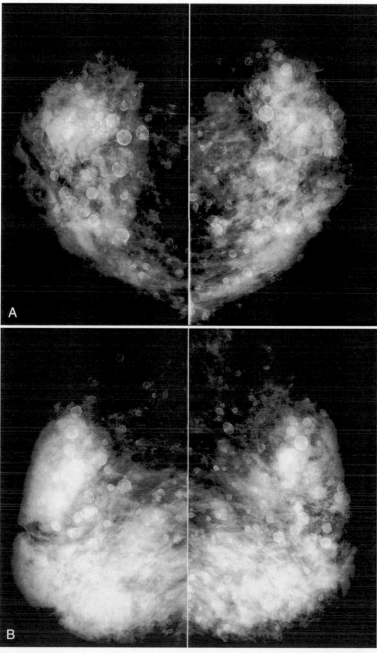

FIGURE 9-9. Direct silicone/paraffin injections. Craniocaudal (**A**) and mediolateral oblique (**B**) mammograms show dense tissue and multiple eggshell-type calcifications compatible with paraffin or silicone injections.

TABLE 9-4. False-Positive Imaging Findings for Rupture

Imaging Modality	Sign	Differential Diagnosis
Mammography	Implant contour deformity	Contained rupture Capsular contracture Herniation through a capsule tear
	Intraparenchymal silicone	Previous leak with the ruptured implant removed
Ultrasound	Stepladder sign	Intracapsular rupture Intact multilumen implant
MRI	Linguine sign Water droplets (occasionally seen)	Intracapsular rupture Intact multilumen implant

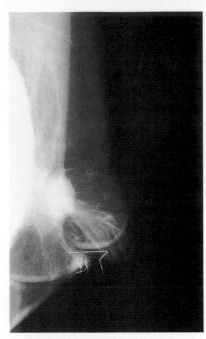

FIGURE 9-10. After removal of a subglandular implant and placement of a subpectoral implant, this patient has a characteristic "removed-implant cavity" on her chest wall, now filled with fluid. The fluid-filled implant cavity has produced a small, smooth oval mass in the prior implant site. Note the metallic linear scar markers showing the scars in the lower part of the breast associated with skin distortion and deformity.

throughout the breast and obscure the breast tissue, thus rendering evaluation for breast cancer difficult.

Some women have their implants removed and not replaced. When surgeons remove the implants, they often leave the fibrous capsules in the breasts. After implant removal the mammogram shows distortion from the implant cavity, usually located on the chest wall. The implant cavity may become unapparent on mammography, may scar, or may fill with fluid and look like a mass (Fig. 9-10).

Ultrasound

Ultrasound is an adjunct to mammography in the diagnosis of ruptured breast implants. The normal single-lumen implant has a smooth echogenic edge, and the inside of the implant is anechoic, similar to a cyst. The implant may have infoldings of the intact envelope, called *radial folds*, which look like white lines extending to the periphery of the envelope. Minor contour abnormalities and short radial folds are incidental findings. Normal reverberation artifacts on ultrasound appear as short gray echoes in the near-field of an intact implant. Reverberation artifacts are the same width as the breast tissue anterior to the implant and are easily distinguished from ruptures (Fig. 9-11).

Ultrasound signs of rupture have varying sensitivities of 25% to 65% and specificities of 57% to 98%. Ultrasound is less expensive than MRI and is more cost-effective than MRI in diagnosing ruptures. On ultrasound, extracapsular rupture has the classic snowstorm sign or echodense noise, a characteristic echogenic finding caused by the slow velocity of sound in silicone with respect to the surrounding breast parenchyma. Snowstorm, or echodense noise, looks like air in the bowel, has an intense echogenic appearance, and obscures all findings beneath it (Fig. 9-12A to E). It can be distinguished from edge artifact by scanning at different angles, because snowstorm produces the echogenic snowstorm appearance when scanned from all angles whereas edge artifact changes or disappears.

Another sign of extracapsular rupture is a hypoechoic mass corresponding to large globules of silicone extruded away from the implant (see Fig. 9-12F). In this situation, so much silicone is extruded that the silicone glob appears

as a hypoechoic mass, similar to the intact implant. To ensure the correct diagnosis, the sonographer places a skin marker on the hypoechoic mass and repeats the mammogram to correlate the silicone on the radiograph with the ultrasound finding. Silicone or paraffin injections have an appearance similar to extracapsular rupture and are characterized by echodense noise. Usually there is so much artifact from the snowstorm with silicone/paraffin injections that the ultrasound is nondiagnostic.

Gel bleed is defined as silicone gel outside an intact implant envelope. Ultrasound shows gel bleed as snowstorm or echodense noise. By definition, gel bleed indicates extracapsular silicone surrounding an intact implant, but this definition is controversial because some investigators believe that there will always be a tiny rupture accompanying gel bleed. Given that ultrasound examinations demonstrating echodense noise can be caused by severe gel bleed, it is controversial whether the scan should be classified as a true- or false-positive examination. Patients with gel bleed usually have their implants removed because silicone is outside the implant and is in direct contact with breast tissue.

Intracapsular rupture means that the envelope is ruptured but the silicone is still inside an intact fibrous capsule. This means that there will be no snowstorm, unless silicone has leaked into the surrounding tissue (making it an *extracapsular* rupture). Intracapsular rupture produces stepladder sign, which represents the collapsing ruptured implant shell within the intact fibrous capsule. The stepladder sign is characterized by multiple thin echogenic lines within the implant that do not extend to the periphery of the implant. The thin lines represent echoes of the collapsing implant wall folding in on itself. The stepladder

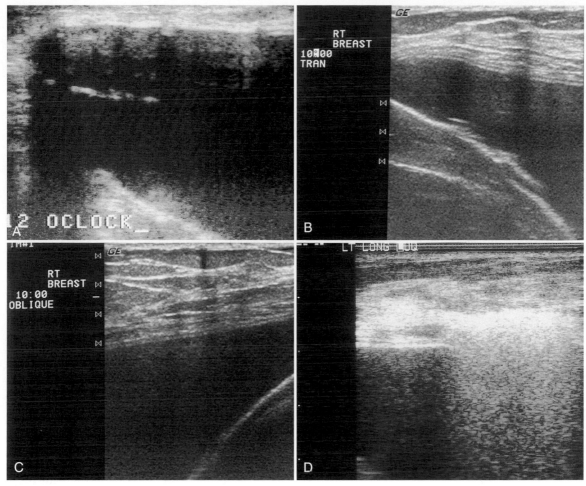

FIGURE 9-11. Reverberation artifact versus rupture on ultrasound. **A,** Ultrasound shows a normal anechoic implant with normal reverberation artifacts in the near-field of the implant that are as thick as the breast tissue above it; the bright line within the implant represents a normal radial fold that extends to the periphery of the implant when scanned from multiple angles. **B,** Reverberation artifact is shown as gray speckles in the near-field of a normal silicone implant with normal radial folds on its inferior aspect. **C,** Normal intact implant on ultrasound. **D,** Ultrasound shows echodense noise or snowstorm artifact, representing extracapsular silicone. Compare with normal implants and normal reverberation artifact in parts **A** to **C**. Note that rupture produces a bright shadow that obscures all features of structures deep to the extruded silicone, whereas reverberation artifact occurs only in the near-field and does not obscure deeper structures.

sign is seen with both intracapsular and extracapsular rupture (Fig. 9-13).

Normal radial folds can simulate the stepladder sign. However, radial folds always extend to the implant periphery whereas stepladder lines do not. False-positive stepladder signs are also caused by intact multilumen implants producing multiple linear echoes in the implant, similar to an intracapsular rupture.

Diffuse linear echoes, debris, or diffuse low-level echoes within the implant may also indicate intracapsular rupture, but they are less definitive. In a small percentage of studies, the ultrasound is false-negative for rupture.

Magnetic Resonance Imaging

In a study of implants imaged by MRI for rupture by Cher and colleagues, the summary MRI sensitivity for rupture was 78% and summary specificity was 91%, with an odds ratio for overall test accuracy of 40.1 (range, 18.8–85.4), using receiver operating characteristics meta-analysis methodology.

BOX 9-4. MRI Techniques for Implants

T1-weighted spin-echo
Gradient echo
T2-weighted fast spin-echo
Short tau inversion recovery
Modified three-point Dixon

In the setting of ruptured implants, MRI distinguishes breast tissue from leaking silicone, contrasting fat and water in glandular tissue from silicone in the implant, and various signs of implant rupture (Fig. 9-14). MRI techniques that evaluate silicone breast implants include T1-weighted spin-echo imaging, gradient echo imaging, T2-weighted fast spin-echo (FSE) imaging, short tau inversion recovery (STIR) imaging, and the modeled three-point Dixon technique, which yield sensitivities and specificities of 95% to 98% and 50% to 93%, respectively (Box 9-4). The modeled three-point Dixon chemical shift

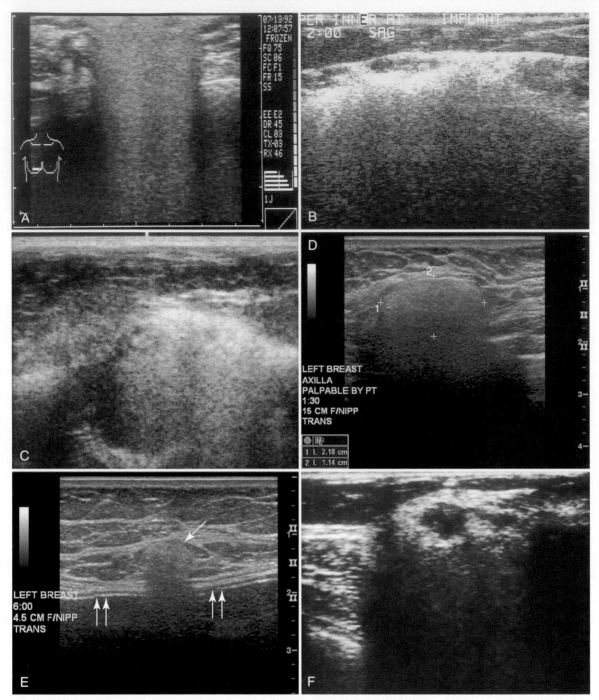

FIGURE 9-12. Implant rupture on ultrasound. **A,** Ultrasound of extracapsular silicone shows the bright gray echodense noise or snowstorm artifact that obscures the implant below. **B,** In another patient with a large extracapsular rupture, the snowstorm fills the image and obscures all adjacent structures, including the breast tissue and implant below. **C,** The snowstorm appearance on the right side almost obscures the implant below. **D,** This silicone granuloma was palpable, forming a round mass that had the snowstorm appearance. **E,** Another silicone granuloma (*arrow*) above the normal intact implant (*double arrows*). **F,** An extracapsular rupture in a patient who had a glob of silicone is producing a hypoechoic mass in the breast tissue above the implant, but surrounded by echodense noise. The extruded glob of silicone was confirmed by placing a marker over the finding and obtaining a mammogram, which showed silicone. Note that the larger silicone glob produces a mass similar to the intact implant in the lower right corner of the image.

technique has the distinct advantage of allowing selective imaging of silicone by separation of the signal of silicone from that of fat and water based on the chemical shift of silicone (1.3–1.6 parts per million lower than that of lipid). Inversion recovery fast spin-echo (IRFSE) sequences combine the speed of a T2-weighted FSE sequence with homogeneous fat suppression.

Patients are scanned prone in a dedicated breast coil to diminish breathing artifacts from chest wall movement. The implant is usually scanned in the axial and sagittal/oblique planes to look at all implant contours and to see radial folds versus ruptured envelopes. MRI of a normal single-lumen silicone implant shows high signal from the silicone with a smooth oval implant border. Minor implant

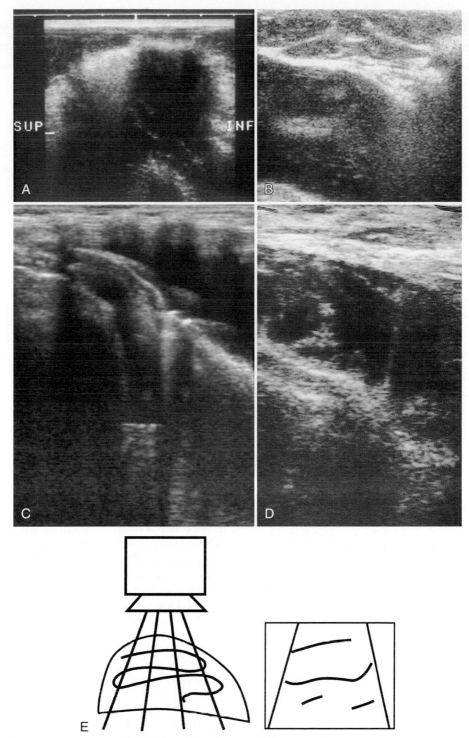

FIGURE 9-13. Stepladder sign on breast ultrasound. **A,** Stepladder sign within the inferior breast is shown as thin white lines within the implant on the right side of the image. There is a snowstorm sign on the left side of the image, representing extracapsular silicone. **B,** Stepladder sign and multiple tiny linear echoes in the implant in a patient with an extracapsular rupture and a snowstorm artifact on the right. **C,** False-positive stepladder sign in a multilumen saline implant in which multiple lines represent the multiple envelopes in this intact multilumen implant. **D,** A true stepladder sign in intracapsular rupture consists of multiple thick and thin linear echoes in the implant that do not always extend to the periphery. **E,** Schematic of an intracapsular rupture showing the stepladder sign. The transducer shows the collapsing implant envelope, which is producing multiple lines, or a stepladder, on ultrasound.

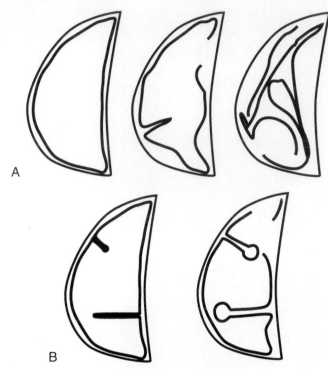

FIGURE 9-14. Schematic of intracapsular rupture. **A,** On the *left* is an intact implant in a fibrous capsule. When the implant shell breaks, the shell pulls away from the fibrous capsule and produces the subcapsular line (*middle*). Later, when the entire shell collapses into the fibrous capsule, the linguine sign is produced, which looks like a loose thread (*right*). **B,** Schematic of radial folds versus keyholes. As seen on the *left*, an intact implant can fold on itself and produce dark lines called radial folds that extend to the periphery of the implant but are totally black inside. With a rupture, silicone intersperses between the collapsing envelope and the fibrous capsule and produces a white center inside the fold called a keyhole or an inverted teardrop, indicative of intracapsular rupture (*right*).

bulges or herniations, short and long radial folds are noted as incidental findings. Radial folds are dark lines that extend to the periphery of the implant and represent folds in the implant envelope (Fig. 9-15). Reactive fluid around the implant and water droplets are classified as nonspecific findings but are noted in the report, particularly if the findings are marked or implant infection is suspected. MRI of a normal saline implant shows the intact implant envelope filled with water.

Intracapsular rupture is diagnosed by the linguine sign, which consists of dark lines inside the implant that do not extend to the periphery. The *linguine* is the curvy noodle-shaped dark lines of the collapsing ruptured implant shell contained within an intact fibrous capsule (Fig. 9-16). Another indication of intracapsular rupture is the teardrop or keyhole sign, which represents silicone outside the implant envelope within a short radial fold outside the implant envelope. Other signs of intracapsular rupture include an intracapsular mottled appearance of the silicone or a dark subcapsular line paralleling the implant shell that cannot be traced to the periphery of the implant. A subcapsular line represents incomplete shell collapse.

Silicone outside the fibrous capsule, within the breast parenchyma or axilla, represents extracapsular rupture (Fig. 9-17). Signs of intracapsular rupture will always be present with the finding of extracapsular rupture. Severe

gel bleed is diagnosed if a thin coating of silicone is identified around the periphery of the implant but the implant is intact.

In an early series of 143 patients with 281 silicone implants, MRI showed a sensitivity of 76% and a specificity of 97% for implant rupture. This series used a T2-weighted FSE technique, a T2-weighted FSE technique with water suppression, and a T1-weighted spin-echo technique with fat suppression.

In another series of 30 patients with 59 implants, MRI had a sensitivity of 100%, a specificity of 63%, a positive predictive value of 71%, a negative predictive value of 100%, and an accuracy of 81% in the detection of rupture/bleed. The linguine sign was the most sensitive (93%) and specific (65%) finding for rupture. The nonspecific sign of water droplets within the implant had a sensitivity of 92% and a low specificity of 44% (Box 9-5). Linear extension of silicone along the chest wall and the presence of reactive fluid were neither sensitive nor specific for rupture. Nonspecific signs such as contour deformity (77%, 10/13), water droplets (54%, 7/13), and reactive fluid (23%, 3/13) were common. In this series, MRI was shown to be more sensitive and accurate than mammography and ultrasound in detecting breast implant rupture or bleed.

The modest MRI specificity noted in most series was predominantly due to pitfalls in imaging interpretation—namely, misinterpreting contour abnormalities and over-interpreting findings within the implant. Knowing the implant type before imaging is crucial for accurate interpretation (Fig. 9-18) because one can overdiagnose ruptures if complex multilumen implants, stacked implants, or a history of previous ruptures is present (see Table 9-4).

Finally, patients should understand that breast MRI for the diagnosis of implant rupture is not the same as for the diagnosis of breast cancer. Specifically, implant MRI examinations do not use intravenous contrast, which is essential for the diagnosis of breast cancers (Box 9-6).

■ BREAST RECONSTRUCTION

After mastectomy, the breast may be reconstructed with a tissue expander followed by an implant, autologous tissue, or a combination of the two. Implant reconstruction usually requires placement of a tissue expander at the time of mastectomy and subsequent expansion of the skin. At a

Text continued on p 360

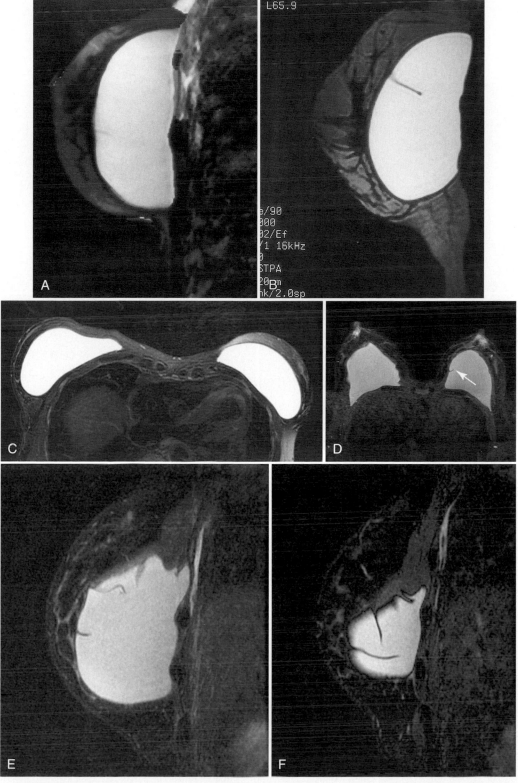

FIGURE 9-15. Intact implants on magnetic resonance imaging (MRI). **A,** Normal silicone implant on MRI. **B,** Normal silicone implant on MRI with a normal radial fold. **C,** Axial T2-weighted MRI of normal bilateral saline implants shows normal smooth implant contours and a small amount of pericapsular fluid on the medial aspect of the right implant. Fluid around the implant does not necessarily mean the implant is infected or ruptured. **D,** Axial MRI in another patient shows bilateral intact silicone implants and a small radial fold (*arrow*). **E,** Sagittal MRI of the intact implant shown in part **D** shows radial folds. Note that the dark radial folds extend all the way to the implant periphery. **F,** Sagittal MRI slice further laterally of the patient shown in parts **D** and **E** shows the intact implant with the radial folds more pronounced in the lateral implant edge. Note that each radial fold is dark throughout its course and tip.

Continued

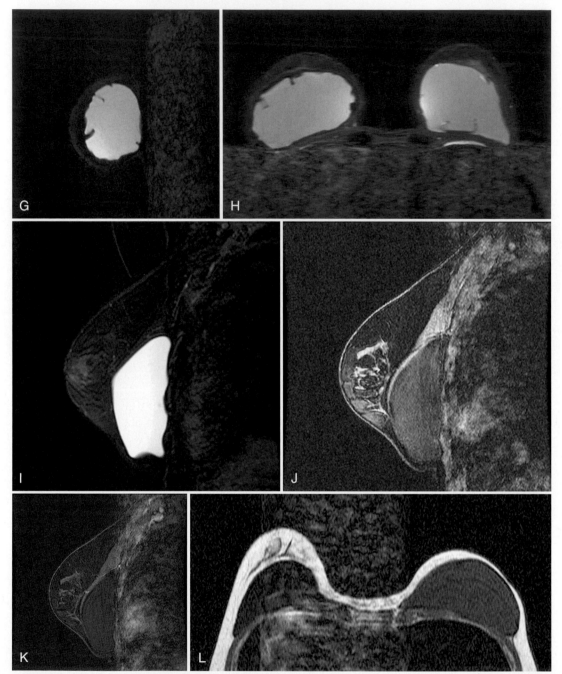

FIGURE 9-15, cont'd. G, Intact silicone implant on sagittal MRI with radial folds. **H,** Bilateral intact silicone implants on axial MRI with radial folds. **I to L,** Intact saline implants on sagittal MRI at different pulse sequences. **I,** Sagittal water-specific sequence shows a smooth intact saline subpectoral implant contour and the bright signal of saline within. **J,** Precontrast sagittal 3-D spectral-spatial excitation magnetization transfer (3DSSMT) MRI shows the saline implant as dark gray underneath the pectoralis muscle. **K,** Postcontrast sagittal 3DSSMT MRI shows the saline implant as black underneath the pectoralis muscle and the enhancing heart behind it. **L,** After reconstruction for cancer, when a silicone implant was placed on the right and a saline implant was placed on the left for cosmesis, an axial nonfat-suppressed T1-weighted localizer MRI shows the intact implants.

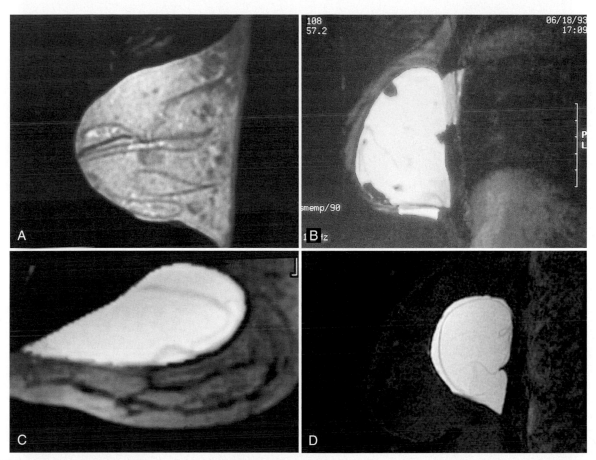

FIGURE 9-16. Intracapsular rupture findings on magnetic resonance imaging (MRI). **A,** Linguine sign on sagittal three-point Dixon MRI, with water droplets. **B,** Linguine sign, water droplets (round low signal findings in the implant), and keyhole sign on sagittal MRI. **C,** Linguine sign on axial MRI. **D,** Subcapsular line and keyhole sign on sagittal three-point Dixon MRI.

Continued

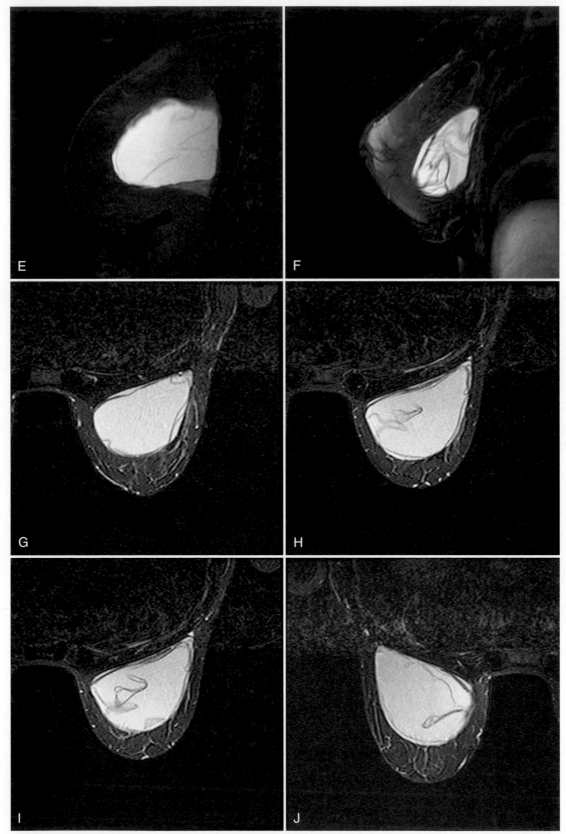

FIGURE 9-16, cont'd. E, Linguine sign, subcapsular line, and keyhole sign on sagittal MRI. **F,** Linguine sign on sagittal MRI. **G,** Axial MRI shows subcapsular lines from an intracapsular rupture. **H** and **I,** Two superior slices on axial MRI show subcapsular lines, linguine sign, and keyhole sign from intracapsular rupture. **J,** Intracapsular rupture on the contralateral side on axial MRI. Contrast the intracapsular rupture to the normal radial folds of the intact implant shown in Figure 9-15H.

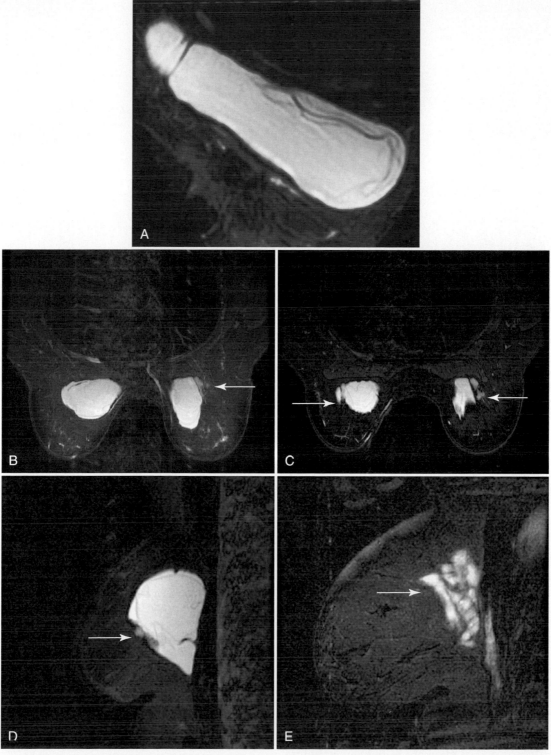

FIGURE 9-17. Extracapsular on magnetic resonance imaging (MRI). **A,** Axial MRI of an extracapsular rupture shows extravasated silicone, seen as a bulge in the axillary portion of the implant. The linguine sign is seen within the implant. **B,** In a different patient, axial three-point Dixon MRI shows bilateral extracapsular rupture with the linguine sign and extravasated silicone in the lateral aspect of the implant (*arrow*). **C,** A more inferior slice on the axial three-point Dixon MRI shows the bilateral extracapsular rupture with extravasated silicone in the lateral aspects of the implants (*arrows*). **D,** Sagittal three-point Dixon MRI shows intracapsular and extracapsular rupture, with extravasated silicone anterior to the implant (*arrow*). **E,** Sagittal three-point Dixon MRI shows extravasated silicone far lateral to the implant within the breast tissue (*arrow*).

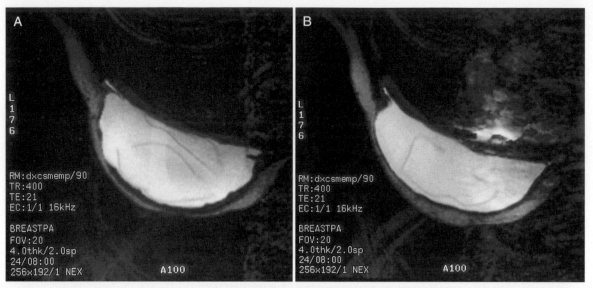

FIGURE 9-18. Intact complex silicone-silicone double-lumen implant simulating intracapsular rupture. Multiple lines simulating the linguine sign are seen in the implant on axial magnetic resonance imaging (MRI) (**A**), but other axial images (**B**) show the multiple lumens in this silicone outer lumen, silicone inner lumen, custom complex implant. This case illustrates the importance of knowing the implant type before MRI interpretation.

subsequent surgery, the surgeon removes the tissue expander and places a permanent implant. The transverse rectus abdominis myocutaneous (TRAM) flap remains the most common form of autologous tissue reconstruction, and it may be performed as a pedicle or free flap. Finally, a latissimus dorsi myocutaneous flap with an implant may be used when additional skin is needed to close the wound or additional soft tissue is required. Although other flaps are used for breast reconstruction, these three methods remain the most popular. The reconstructive method selected depends on the patient's goals, medical history, body habitus, physical examination, and potential need for adjuvant therapy.

In the case of subcutaneous, or skin-sparing, mastectomy, the breast tissue is excised with a small shell of tissue left under the skin. Surgeons then place an implant under the skin. The small amount of breast tissue underneath the skin maintains skin vascularity, and the nipple may or may not be resected. Because of high rates of cancer recurrence, this operation is not routinely performed for cancer treatment or for prophylactic prevention of cancer in high-risk patients.

In patients undergoing tissue expansion after mastectomy, very little, if any, breast tissue has been left in the mastectomy site, and the breast is left with little or no glandular tissue to image on mammography. Usually, a saline expander is left in the mastectomy site and gradually enlarged until the space is adequate to hold an appropriately sized implant. Patients with subcutaneous mastectomies or mastectomies with implant placement may undergo mammography if there is enough breast tissue to compress around the implant, but frequently, too little tissue is left to compress for an adequate view. Breast cancer recurrences appear as suspicious calcifications or masses when breast tissue is adequately seen.

In the case of TRAM, latissimus dorsi, and free flap reconstructions, fat and muscle are transferred to the mastectomy site with attachments to vascular structures and shaped to form a breast. Traditionally, autologous flaps are not imaged by mammography, but mammography can be helpful in evaluating these structures when there are clinical questions. The most common findings in autologous flaps are fat centrally, with or without density from muscle fibers around the edges of the TRAM or latissimus dorsi flaps (Fig. 9-19A to E). Common mammographic findings in TRAM flaps are calcifications from fat necrosis, benign dermal calcifications, calcified hematoma, and clustered microcalcifications. Areas of increased or decreased density without calcifications are also common and appear to be related to postsurgical changes and fat necrosis. A nipple can be reconstructed out of skin and tattooed to provide color similar to the contralateral side. Rarely, the tattoo can be seen on mammography (see Fig. 9-19F to I).

Mammography is a useful diagnostic tool in patients who have undergone TRAM flap breast reconstruction and have suspicious physical findings postoperatively. In a 2001 article by Shaikh and colleagues, breast cancer recurrence in TRAM flaps appeared as masses with a differential diagnosis of granulomas or fat necrosis. In another study, Helvie and colleagues found six breast cancers in women undergoing TRAM flap reconstruction; they appeared as four suspicious masses and two suspicious microcalcification clusters.

REDUCTION MAMMOPLASTY

Reduction mammoplasty and mastopexy are done for aesthetic purposes. Reduction mammoplasty is most commonly performed for macromastia. After cancer surgery, patients often undergo breast reduction or mastopexy (breast lift) of the contralateral breast. This surgery matches the "normal" breast to the operated, conserved breast. To perform reduction mammoplasty, the surgeon removes skin and breast parenchyma from the lower breast and relocates the nipple superiorly. The resulting scar runs

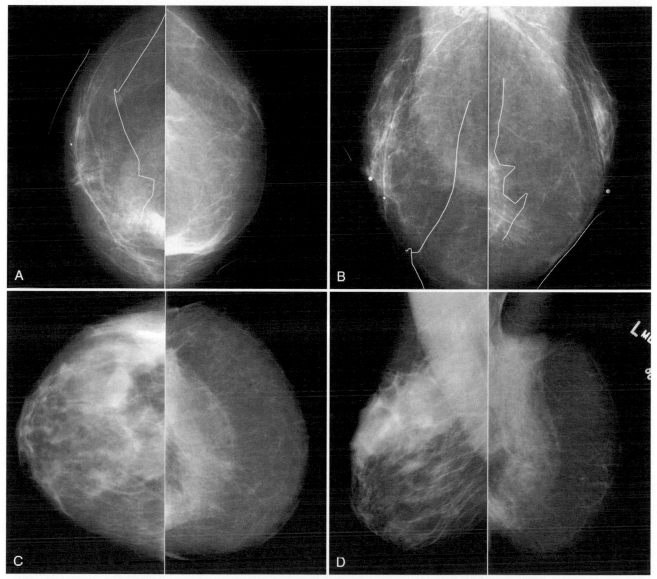

FIGURE 9-19. Transverse rectus abdominis musculocutaneous (TRAM) flap reconstruction on mammography. Craniocaudal (CC) (**A**) and mediolateral oblique (MLO) (**B**) mammograms show fatty tissue and focal density in the breasts reconstructed from abdominal tissue. Note the relative fatty composition of the reconstructed breast and lack of normal glandular elements. Linear metallic scar markers show the location of the scars. **C** and **D**, TRAM flap reconstruction in the left breast and a normal mammogram on the right breast. CC (**C**) and MLO (**D**) mammograms show a normal breast on the right and the TRAM reconstruction on the left. Note the anterior fatty portion and the muscular posterior portion of the TRAM reconstruction.

Continued

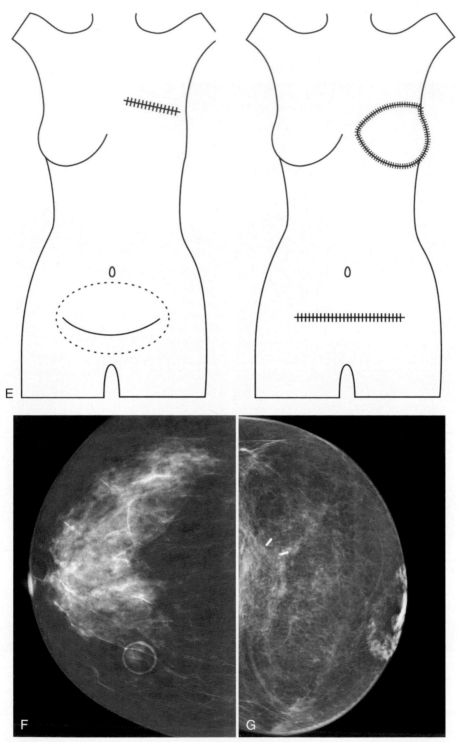

FIGURE 9-19, cont'd. **E,** Schematic of TRAM reconstruction showing the abdominal pedicle removed from the lower portion of the abdomen and tunneled under the skin to the mastectomy site where the breast is reconstructed. Right (**F**) and left (**G**) CC mammogram and right (**H**) and left (**I**) MLO mammograms of a left TRAM flap breast reconstruction and normal right breast. Note the fatty left TRAM reconstructed breast, clips at TRAM flap pedicle, and tattooed nipple–areolar complex on the left.

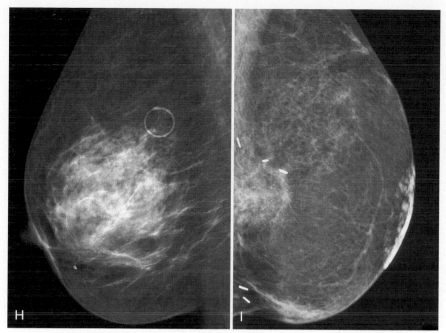

FIGURE 9-19, cont'd.

around the areola, vertically down to the inframammary fold, and often within the inframammary fold.

The reduction mammoplasty mammogram shows characteristic skin thickening over the lower breast in the region of the scars, most evident on the mediolateral oblique or mediolateral view. The breast ducts terminate lower than the replaced nipple because the nipple has been moved to a higher location. The lower portion of the breast shows architectural distortion, and the overall pattern of the lower portion of the breast will be distorted from scarring. Depending on the amount of tissue removed from various areas of the breast, the breast parenchymal pattern can be patchy and much different from the pre-reduction mammogram (Figs. 9-20 and 9-21).

Reduction mammoplasty or any breast surgery can result in focal fat necrosis or oil cysts that have a characteristic appearance, or they may be atypical and form a palpable mass (Fig. 9-22). Epidermal inclusion cysts can also form in biopsy scars and produce a dense smooth round or oval mass near the skin surface but not connected to it. These masses represent epidermal cells that are displaced into breast tissue during biopsy. The epithelial cells can grow and form a round benign-appearing mass. In the case of fat necrosis, breast ultrasound may be helpful, but biopsy may be needed.

■ KEY ELEMENTS

No scientific evidence has shown a definite association between silicone breast implants and connective tissue disorders or breast cancer.

In the United States, silicone breast implants are approved for breast reconstruction after mastectomy, and saline implants are approved for breast augmentation.

Breast implants may have single or multiple lumens, each containing silicone or other materials in the different shells.

Implants are placed in subpectoral or subglandular (above the pectoral muscle) locations.

Fibrous capsules form around all implants, sometimes becoming hard or calcified and impairing the implant's look and feel.

Implant complications include rupture, infection, hematoma, and capsular contraction.

Closed capsulotomy, or manual breaking of a hardened fibrous capsule, can result in implant rupture.

Implant rupture is classified as intracapsular (silicone contained in the fibrous capsule) or extracapsular (silicone outside the fibrous capsule).

Symptoms associated with silicone implant rupture are nonspecific and include axillary, breast, or chest wall masses; pain; and changes in breast size, shape, or texture.

Mammography includes standard and implant-displaced craniocaudal and mediolateral or mediolateral oblique views of each breast, for a total of four views of each breast.

Approximately 5% of asymptomatic women have implant ruptures detected on screening mammography.

Extracapsular ruptures appear on mammography as silicone outside the implant in breast tissue, lymph nodes, or ducts or as a deformity in implant contour.

Direct silicone or paraffin injections are used outside the United States for augmentation and cause eggshell-type calcifications or dense masses on mammography, snow-storm or echodense noise on ultrasound, and hard palpable silicone granuloma masses on physical examination.

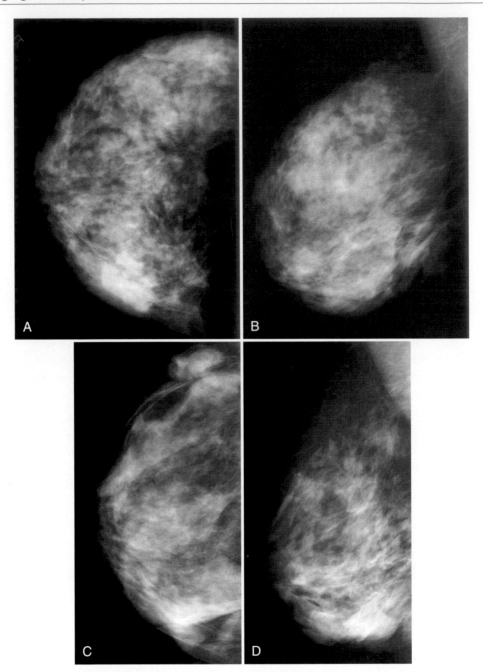

FIGURE 9-20. Reduction mammoplasty on mammography. Craniocaudal (CC) (**A**) and mediolateral oblique (MLO) (**B**) mammograms show heterogeneously dense tissue. After reduction mammoplasty, CC (**C**) and MLO (**D**) mammograms show smaller and less dense breasts, with a parenchymal pattern different from that on the previous mammogram. Distortion is apparent in the outer, inner, and lower portions of the breast, and the breast ducts no longer terminate at the reconstructed nipple.

Ultrasound of extracapsular rupture shows the snowstorm sign, or echodense noise.

Ultrasound of intracapsular rupture shows the stepladder sign.

MRI of extracapsular rupture shows blobs of silicone outside the implant and signs of intracapsular rupture.

MRI of intracapsular rupture shows the linguine sign, subcapsular lines, teardrops, or the keyhole sign.

Nonspecific findings on MRI are water droplets, reactive fluid, and implant contour abnormalities.

False-positive findings of rupture on ultrasound and MRI are due to intact multiple-lumen implants simulating the stepladder and linguine signs.

False-positive findings of rupture on all imaging methods include previous rupture with implant replacement but without removal of all intraparenchymal silicone.

To avoid false-positive diagnoses of rupture, know the implant type and whether previous rupture and removal of the implant have occurred.

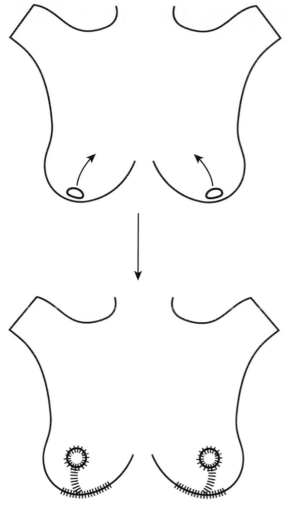

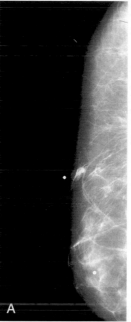

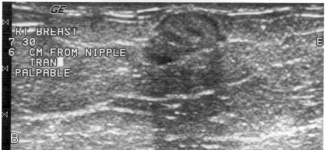

FIGURE 9-21. Reduction mammoplasty. Schematic of reduction mammoplasty. Breast tissue is removed from the lower portion of the breast, and the nipple is elevated and moved cranially to the upper part of the breast. Below are the typical reduction mammoplasty scars.

FIGURE 9-22. Fat necrosis producing a mass after transverse rectus abdominis musculocutaneous (TRAM) reconstruction. **A,** A lateral mammogram shows fatty tissue from a TRAM reconstruction with a skin marker over an upper oval equal-density palpable mass. The second skin marker in the lower portion of the breast shows the location of the reconstructed nipple. **B,** Ultrasound shows a hypoechoic mass near the skin surface. The differential diagnosis includes recurrence of cancer, an epidermal inclusion cyst, and fat necrosis. Biopsy showed fat necrosis.

Autologous tissue reconstructions consist of transverse rectus abdominis or latissimus dorsi myocutaneous flaps performed as a pedicle or a free flap.

Mammographic findings of autologous tissue reconstruction include fat and muscle and, commonly, calcifications from fat necrosis and densities from postsurgical changes.

Cancer in reconstructed breasts is often detected by physical examination, with occasional mammographic findings of suspicious masses or calcifications.

Reduction mammoplasty produces a characteristic distortion of the lower portion of the breast and scarring, with relocation of the nipple higher on the breast.

Beware of cancer.

▬ SUGGESTED READINGS

Ahn CY, DeBruhl ND, Gorczyca DP, et al: Comparative silicone breast implant evaluation using mammography, sonography, and magnetic resonance imaging: experience with 59 implants, *Plast Reconstr Surg* 94:620–627, 1994.

Ahn CY, Shaw WW, Narayanan K, et al: Residual silicone detection using MRI following previous breast implant removal: case reports, *Aesthetic Plast Surg* 19:361–367, 1995.

Baker JL Jr: Augmentation mammaplasty. In Owsley JQ Jr, Peterson RA editors: *Symposium on Aesthetic Surgery of the Breast, 1978*, St Louis, 1978, CV Mosby.

Beahm EK, Walton RL: Discussion. Patient satisfaction with mastectomy breast reconstruction: a comparative evaluation of DIEP, TRAM, latissimus flap, and implant techniques. *Plast Reconstr Surg* 125(6):1596–1598, 2010.

Beekman WH, Hage JJ, Taets van Amerongen AH, Mulder JW: Accuracy of ultrasonography and magnetic resonance imaging in detecting failure of breast implants filled with silicone gel, *Scand J Plast Reconstr Surg Hand Surg* 33:415–418, 1999.

Berg WA, Caskey CI, Hamper UM, et al: Diagnosing breast implant rupture with MR imaging, US, and mammography, *Radiographics* 13:1323–1336, 1993.

Berg WA, Caskey CI, Hamper UM, et al: Single- and double-lumen silicone breast implant integrity: prospective evaluation of MR and US criteria, *Radiology* 197:45–52, 1995.

Breiting VB, Holmich LR, Brandt B, et al: Long-term health status of Danish women with silicone breast implants, *Plast Reconstr Surg* 114:217–228, 2004.

Brown SL, Middleton MS, Berg WA, et al: Prevalence of rupture of silicone gel breast implants revealed on MR imaging in a population of women in Birmingham, Alabama, *AJR Am J Roentgenol* 175:1057–1064, 2000.

Carlson GW, Moore B, Thornton JF, et al: Breast cancer after augmentation mammaplasty: treatment by skin-sparing mastectomy and immediate reconstruction, *Plast Reconstr Surg* 107:687–692, 2001.

Cher DJ, Conwell JA, Mandel JS: MRI for detecting silicone breast implant rupture: meta-analysis and implications, *Ann Plast Surg* 47:367–380, 2001.

Chung KC, Wilkins EG, Beil RJ Jr, et al: Diagnosis of silicone gel breast implant rupture by ultrasonography, *Plast Reconstr Surg* 97:104–109, 1996.

Cicchetti S, Leone MS, Franchelli S, Santi PL: [Evaluation of the tolerability of Hydrogel breast implants: A pilot study,] *Minerva Chir* 57:53–57, 2002.

Collis N, Coleman D, Foo IT, Sharpe DT: Ten-year review of a prospective randomized controlled trial of textured versus smooth subglandular silicone gel breast implants, *Plast Reconstr Surg* 106:786–791, 2000.

Collis N, Sharpe DT: Silicone gel-filled breast implant integrity: a retrospective review of 478 consecutively explanted implants, *Plast Reconstr Surg* 105:1979–1989, 2000.

Collis N, Litherland J, Enion D, Sharpe DT: Magnetic resonance imaging and explantation investigation of long-term silicone gel implant integrity, *Plast Reconstr Surg* 120:1401–1406, 2007.

Cunningham B: The Mentor Core Study on silicone MemoryGel breast implants, *Plast Reconstr Surg* 120(7 Suppl 1):19S–32S, 2007.

Cunningham B: The Mentor Study on contour profile gel silicone MemoryGel breast implants, *Plast Reconstr Surg* 120(7 Suppl 1):33S–39S, 2007.

Destouet JM, Monsees BS, Oser RF, et al: Screening mammography in 350 women with breast implants: prevalence and findings of implant complications, *AJR Am J Roentgenol* 159:973–981, 1992.

Di Benedetto G, Cecchini S, Grassetti L, et al: Comparative study of breast implant rupture using mammography, sonography, and magnetic resonance imaging: correlation with surgical findings, *Breast J* 14:532–537, 2008.

Eidelman Y, Liebling RW, Buchbinder S, et al: Mammography in the evaluation of masses in breasts reconstructed with TRAM flaps, *Ann Plast Surg* 41:229–233, 1998.

Eklund GW, Busby RC, Miller SH, Job JS: Improved imaging of the augmented breast, *AJR Am J Roentgenol* 151:469–473, 1988.

Fajardo LL, Roberts CC, Hunt KR: Mammographic surveillance of breast cancer patients: should the mastectomy site be imaged? *AJR Am J Roentgenol* 161:953–955, 1993.

Fajardo LL, Harvey JA, McAleese KA, et al: Breast cancer diagnosis in women with subglandular silicone gel-filled augmentation implants, *Radiology* 194:859–862, 1995.

Feng LJ, Amini SB: Analysis of risk factors associated with rupture of silicone gel breast implants, *Plast Reconstr Surg* 104:955–963, 1999.

Ganott MA, Harris KM, Ilkhanipour ZS, Costa-Greco MA: Augmentation mammoplasty: normal and abnormal findings with mammography and US, *Radiographics* 12:281–295, 1992.

Gorczyca DP: MR imaging of breast implants, *Magn Reson Imaging Clin North Am* 2:659–672, 1994.

Gorczyca DP, Schneider E, DeBruhl ND, et al: Silicone breast implant rupture: comparison between three-point Dixon and fast spin-echo MR imaging, *AJR Am J Roentgenol* 162:305–310, 1994.

Gui GP, Kadayaprath G, Tan SM, et al: Long-term quality-of-life assessment following one-stage immediate breast reconstruction using biodimensional expander implants: the patient's perspective, *Plast Reconstr Surg* 121:17–24, 2008.

Harris KM, Ganott MA, Shestak KC, et al: Silicone implant rupture: detection with US, *Radiology* 187:761–768, 1993.

Hayes MK, Gold RH, Bassett LW: Mammographic findings after the removal of breast implants, *AJR Am J Roentgenol* 160:487–490, 1993.

Heden P, Nava MB, van Tetering JP, et al: Prevalence of rupture in inamed silicone breast implants, *Plast Reconstr Surg* 118:303–312, 2006.

Heden P, Bone B, Murphy DK, et al: Style 410 cohesive silicone breast implants: safety and effectiveness at 5 to 9 years after implantation, *Plast Reconstr Surg* 118:1281–1287, 2006.

Heden P, Bronz G, Elberg JJ, et al: Long-term safety and effectiveness of style 410 highly cohesive silicone breast implants, *Aesthetic Plast Surg* 33:430–436, 2009.

Helvie MA, Bailey JE, Roubidoux MA, et al: Mammographic screening of TRAM flap breast reconstructions for detection of nonpalpable recurrent cancer, *Radiology* 224:211–216, 2002.

Helvie MA, Wilson TE, Roubidoux MA, et al: Mammographic appearance of recurrent breast carcinoma in six patients with TRAM flap breast reconstructions, *Radiology* 209:711–715, 1998.

Henriksen TF, Holmich LR, Fryzek JP, et al: Incidence and severity of short-term complications after breast augmentation: results from a nationwide breast implant registry, *Ann Plast Surg* 51:531–539, 2003.

Herborn CU, Marincek B, Erfmann D, et al: Breast augmentation and reconstructive surgery: MR imaging of implant rupture and malignancy, *Eur Radiol* 12:2198–2206, 2002.

Hogge JP, Zuurbier RA, de Paredes ES: Mammography of autologous myocutaneous flaps, *Radiographics* 19(Spec No):S63–S72, 1999.

Holmich LR, Friis S, Fryzek JP, Vejborg IM, et al: Incidence of silicone breast implant rupture, *Arch Surg* 138:801–806, 2003.

Holmich LR, Fryzek JP, Kjoller K, et al: The diagnosis of silicone breast-implant rupture: clinical findings compared with findings at magnetic resonance imaging, *Ann Plast Surg* 54:583–589, 2005.

Holmich LR, Vejborg I, Conrad C, et al: The diagnosis of breast implant rupture: MRI findings compared with findings at explantation, *Eur J Radiol* 53:213–225, 2005.

Hsu W, Sheen-Chen SM, Eng HL, Ko SF: Mammographic microcalcification in an autogenously reconstructed breast simulating recurrent carcinoma, *Tumori* 94:574–576, 2008.

Hulka BS, Kerkvliet NL, Tugwell P: Experience of a scientific panel formed to advise the federal judiciary on silicone breast implants, *N Engl J Med* 342:812–815, 2000.

Ikeda DM, Borofsky HB, Herfkens RJ, et al: Silicone breast implant rupture: pitfalls of magnetic resonance imaging and relative efficacies of magnetic resonance, mammography, and ultrasound, *Plast Reconstr Surg* 104:2054–2062, 1999.

Janowsky EC, Kupper LL, Hulka BS: Meta-analyses of the relation between silicone breast implants and the risk of connective-tissue diseases, *N Engl J Med* 342:781–790, 2000.

Kang BJ, Jung JI, Park C, et al: Breast MRI findings after modified radical mastectomy and transverse rectus abdominis myocutaneous flap in patients with breast cancer, *J Magn Reson Imaging* 21:784–791, 2005.

Kessler DA: The basis of the FDA's decision on breast implants, *N Engl J Med* 326:1713–1715, 1992.

Kirkpatrick WN, Jones BM: The history of Trilucent implants, and a chemical analysis of the triglyceride filler in 51 consecutively removed Trilucent breast prostheses, *Br J Plast Surg* 55:479–489, 2002.

Kreymerman P, Patrick RJ, Rim A, et al: Guidelines for using breast magnetic resonance imaging to evaluate implant integrity, *Ann Plast Surg* 62:355–357, 2009.

Kwek JW, Choi H, Ma J, Miller MJ: Gel-gel double-lumen silicone breast implant: mimic of intracapsular implant rupture, *AJR Am J Roentgenol* 187:W436–W437, 2006.

Lee JM, Georgian-Smith D, Gazelle GS, et al: Detecting nonpalpable recurrent breast cancer: the role of routine mammographic screening of transverse rectus abdominis myocutaneous flap reconstructions, *Radiology* 248:398–405, 2008.

Leibman AJ, Kossoff MB, Kruse BD: Intraductal extension of silicone from a ruptured breast implant, *Plast Reconstr Surg* 89:546–547, 1992.

Marotta JS, Widenhouse CW, Habal MB, Goldberg EP: Silicone gel breast implant failure and frequency of additional surgeries: analysis of 35 studies reporting examination of more than 8,000 explants, *J Biomed Mater Res* 48:354–364, 1999.

Mason AC, White CS, McAvoy MA, Goldberg N: MR imaging of slipped stacked breast implants: a potential pitfall in the diagnosis of intracapsular rupture, *Magn Reson Imaging* 13:339–342, 1995.

McKeown DJ, Hogg FJ, Brown IM, et al:. The timing of autologous latissimus dorsi breast reconstruction and effect of radiotherapy on outcome, *J Plast Reconstr Aesthet Surg* 62:488–493, 2009.

McLaughlin JK, Lipworth L, Murphy DK, Walker PS: The safety of silicone gel-filled breast implants: a review of the epidemiologic evidence, *Ann Plast Surg* 59:569–580, 2007.

Middleton MS: Magnetic resonance evaluation of breast implants and soft-tissue silicone, *Top Magn Reson Imaging* 9:92–137, 1998.

Mitnick JS, Vazquez MF, Plesser K, Colen SR: "Ductogram" associated with extravasation of silicone from a breast implant, *AJR Am J Roentgenol* 159:1126–1127, 1992.

Mitnick JS, Vazquez MF, Plesser K, et al: Fine needle aspiration biopsy in patients with augmentation prostheses and a palpable mass, *Ann Plast Surg* 31:241–244, 1993.

Monticciolo DL, Nelson RC, Dixon WT, et al: MR detection of leakage from silicone breast implants: value of a silicone-selective pulse sequence, *AJR Am J Roentgenol* 163:51–56, 1994.

Monticciolo DL, Ross D, Bostwick J 3rd, et al: Autologous breast reconstruction with endoscopic latissimus dorsi musculosubcutaneous flaps in patients choosing breast-conserving therapy: mammographic appearance, *AJR Am J Roentgenol* 167:385–389, 1996.

Mund DF, Wolfson P, Gorczyca DP, et al: Mammographically detected recurrent nonpalpable carcinoma developing in a transverse rectus abdominis myocutaneous flap. A case report, *Cancer* 74:2804–2807, 1994.

Munker R, Zorner C, McKiernan D, Opitz J: Prospective study of clinical findings and changes in 56 Trilucent implant explantations, *Aesthetic Plast Surg* 25:421–426, 2001.

Muzaffar AR, Rohrich RJ: The silicone gel-filled breast implant controversy: an update, *Plast Reconstr Surg* 109:742–748, 2002.

Palmon LU, Foshager MC, Parantainen H, et al: Ruptured or intact: what can linear echoes within silicone breast implants tell us? *AJR Am J Roentgenol* 168:1595–1598, 1997.

Patani N, Devalia H, Anderson A, Mokbel K: Oncological safety and patient satisfaction with skin-sparing mastectomy and immediate breast reconstruction, *Surg Oncol* 17:97–105, 2008.

Piza-Katzer H, Pulzl P, Balogh B, Wechselberger G: Long-term results of MISTI gold breast implants: a retrospective study, *Plast Reconstr Surg* 110:1425–1465, 2002.

Rieber A, Schramm K, Helms G, et al: Breast-conserving surgery and autogenous tissue reconstruction in patients with breast cancer: efficacy of MRI of the breast in the detection of recurrent disease, *Eur Radiol* 13:780–787, 2003.

Rivero MA, Schwartz DS, Mies C: Silicone lymphadenopathy involving intramammary lymph nodes: a new complication of silicone mammaplasty, *AJR Am J Roentgenol* 162:1089–1090, 1994.

Rizkalla M, Duncan C, Matthews RN: Trilucent breast implants: a 3-year series, *Br J Plast Surg* 54:125–127, 2001.

Rizkalla M, Webb J, Chuo CB, Matthews RN: Experience of explanation of Trilucent breast implants, *Br J Plast Surg* 55:117–119, 2002.

Rosculet KA, Ikeda DM, Forrest ME, et al: Ruptured gel-filled silicone breast implants: sonographic findings in 19 cases, *AJR Am J Roentgenol* 159:711–716, 1992.

Saint-Cyr M, Nagarkar P, Schaverien M, et al: The pedicled descending branch muscle-sparing latissimus dorsi flap for breast reconstruction, *Plast Reconstr Surg* 123:13–24, 2009.

Shaikh N, LaTrenta G, Swistel A, Osborne FM: Detection of recurrent breast cancer after TRAM flap reconstruction, *Ann Plast Surg* 47:602–607, 2001.

Silverstein MJ, Handel N, Gamagami P, et al: Mammographic measurements before and after augmentation mammaplasty, *Plast Reconstr Surg* 86:1126–1130, 1990.

Silverstein MJ, Handel N, Gamagami P: The effect of silicone-gel-filled implants on mammography, *Cancer* 68(Suppl):1159–1163, 1991.

Soo MS, Kornguth PJ, Walsh R, et al: Intracapsular implant rupture: MR findings of incomplete shell collapse, *J Magn Reson Imaging* 7:724–730, 1997.

Spear SL, Mardini S: Alternative filler materials and new implant designs: what's available and what's on the horizon? *Clin Plast Surg* 28:435–443, 2001.

Stevens WG, Pacella SJ, Gear AJ, et al: Clinical experience with a fourth-generation textured silicone gel breast implant: a review of 1012 Mentor MemoryGel breast implants, *Aesthet Surg J* 28(6):642–647, 2008.

Stewart NR, Monsees BS, Destouet JM, Rudloff MA: Mammographic appearance following implant removal, *Radiology* 185:83–85, 1992.

Stralman K, Mollerup CL, Kristoffersen US, Elberg JJ: Long-term outcome after mastectomy with immediate breast reconstruction, *Acta Oncol* 47:704–708, 2008.

Tugewell P, Wells G, Peterson J, et al: Do silicone breast implants cause rheumatologic disorders? A systematic review for a court-appointed national science panel, *Arthritis Rheum* 44:2477–2484, 2001.

Wong JS, Ho AY, Kaelin CM, et al: Incidence of major corrective surgery after post-mastectomy breast reconstruction and radiation therapy, *Breast J* 14:49–54, 2008.

Young VL, Bartell T, Destouet JM, et al: Calcification of breast implant capsule, *South Med J* 82:1171–1173, 1989.

Young V, Watson M: Breast implant research: where we have been, where we are, where we need to go, *Clin Plast Surg* 28:451–483, 2001.

Quizzes

9-1. Fill in the implant types.

_____

_____

_____

_____

_____

_____

_____

For answers, see Box 9-1.

9-2. Fill in the mammography of implants.

_____

_____

_____

_____

For answers, see Box 9-2.

9-3. Fill in the untoward effects of breast implants.

_____

_____

_____

_____

_____

For answers, see Box 9-3.

9-4. Fill in the MRI techniques for implants.

_____

_____

_____

_____

_____

For answers, see Box 9-4.

9-5. Fill in the nonspecific findings on MRI.

_____

_____

_____

_____

For answers, see Box 9-5.

9-6. Fill in the reducing false-positive MRI studies.

_____

_____

For answers, see Box 9-6.

9-7. Fill in the Baker classification.

GRADE	BREAST FIRMNESS	IMPLANT	IMPLANT VISIBILITY
___	___	___	___
___	___	___	___
___	___	___	___
___	___	___	___

For answers, see Table 9-1.

9-8. Fill in the implant rupture types.

RUPTURE TYPE	SILICONE LOCATION	ENVELOPE STATUS
_____	_____	_____
_____	_____	_____
_____	_____	_____

For answers, see Table 9-2.

9-9. Fill in the image findings with rupture.

IMAGING MODALITY	INTRACAPSULAR	EXTRACAPSULAR	GEL BLEED
Mammography	_____	_____	_____
		_____	
		_____	
		_____	
Ultrasound	_____	_____	_____
MRI	_____	_____	_____
	_____	_____	_____
	_____		
	_____		

For answers, see Table 9-3.

9-10. Fill in the false-positive imaging findings for rupture.

IMAGING MODALITY	SIGN	DIFFERENTIAL DIAGNOSIS
Mammography	_____	_____
		_____
		_____
		_____
	_____	_____
Ultrasound	_____	_____
		_____
MRI	_____	_____
	_____	_____

For answers, see Table 9-4.

CHAPTER 10

Clinical Breast Problems and Unusual Breast Conditions

Various breast symptoms and clinical problems are encountered in both benign breast conditions and breast cancer. This chapter briefly describes these conditions and elucidates how to distinguish them from malignancy.

THE MALE BREAST: GYNECOMASTIA AND MALE BREAST CANCER

The incidence of breast cancer in males is less than 1% of all breast cancers and less than 1% of all male cancers in the United States. Male breast patients seek clinical attention for unilateral or bilateral breast enlargement, breast pain, or a palpable breast lump. Most of these complaints are related to benign gynecomastia and are not due to breast cancer. Gynecomastia is an abnormal proliferation of benign ducts and supporting tissue that causes breast enlargement or a subareolar mass, with or without associated breast pain. It is reversible in its early stages if the cause of the gynecomastia is corrected. Unchecked, the reversible phase of gynecomastia progresses to late periductal edema with irreversible stromal fibrosis.

Broad categories of conditions causing gynecomastia include high serum estrogen levels from endogenous or exogenous sources, low serum testosterone levels, endocrine disorders (hyperthyroidism or hypothyroidism), systemic disorders (cirrhosis, chronic renal failure with maintenance by dialysis, chronic obstructive pulmonary disease), drug-induced (cimetidine, spironolactone, ergotamine, marijuana, anabolic steroids, estrogen for prostate cancer), tumors (adrenal carcinoma, testicular tumors, pituitary adenoma), or idiopathic (Box 10-1). Gynecomastia can occur at any age, but it may be seen in particular in neonates as a result of maternal estrogens circulating to the fetus through the placenta, in healthy adolescent boys 1 year after the onset of puberty because of high estradiol levels, or in older men as a result of decreasing serum testosterone levels.

The normal male breast contains major breast ducts only and otherwise has mostly fatty tissue. Under a stimulus producing gynecomastia, breast enlargement occurs as a result of ductal proliferation and stromal hyperplasia, occasionally accompanied by ductal multiplication and elongation, which may be reversible in the active phase if the stimulus is removed. If the stimulus persists, irreversible stromal fibrosis and ductal epithelial atrophy develop, and the breast enlargement may decrease but not completely resolve. Pseudogynecomastia is a fatty proliferation of the breasts without proliferation of glandular tissue that simulates gynecomastia clinically, but unlike true gynecomastia, proliferation of glandular breast tissue does not occur.

Mammography is performed in men in the same fashion as in women. On the mammogram, the normal male breast consists of fat without obvious fibroglandular tissue, and the pectoralis muscles are usually larger than in women (Fig. 10-1A to D). In both pseudogynecomastia and in women with Turner syndrome, mammograms consist mostly of fat, similar to the normal male breast (see Fig. 10-1E and F).

On the mammogram, gynecomastia is shown as glandular tissue in the subareolar region that is symmetric or asymmetric, unilateral or bilateral. In a large series by Gunhan-Bilgen and colleagues, gynecomastia was unilateral in 45% and bilateral in 55% of 206 cases on mammograms. In the early phases of gynecomastia, the glandular tissue takes on a flamelike dendritic appearance consisting of thin strands of glandular tissue extending from the nipple, similar to fingers extending posteriorly toward the chest wall (Table 10-1). With continued proliferation of breast ducts, the glandular tissue takes on a triangular nodular shape behind the nipple in the subareolar region that can be symmetric or asymmetric (Fig. 10-2). If the etiology of the gynecomastia is not eliminated, the proliferation may progress to the appearance of diffuse dense tissue in the later stromal fibrotic phase that is irreversible (Fig. 10-3). On ultrasound, gynecomastia shows hypoechoic flamelike, fingerlike, or triangular structures extending posteriorly toward the chest wall from the nipple (Fig. 10-4). Pseudogynecomastia shows only fatty tissue on the mammogram and is distinguished from gynecomastia by the absence of glandular tissue.

Male breast cancer accounts for less than 1% of all cancers found in men and is usually diagnosed at or around age 60, older than the mean age for the diagnosis of breast cancer in women (Box 10-2). Male breast cancer has the same prognosis as breast cancer in women, but it is often detected at a higher stage than in women because of delay in diagnosis; up to 50% of men have axillary adenopathy at initial evaluation. Risk factors include Klinefelter syndrome, high estrogen levels such as from prostate cancer treatment, and the development of mumps orchitis at an older age. Male breast cancer is generally manifested as a hard, painless, subareolar mass eccentric to the nipple. When not subareolar, cancers in men are usually found in the upper outer quadrant. Clinical symptoms of nipple discharge or ulceration are not rare in association with male breast cancer.

Text continued on p 376

Box 10-1. Causes of Gynecomastia

PHYSIOLOGIC
Liver disease
Renal failure
Chronic obstructive pulmonary disease
Diabetes
Hyperthyroidism
Hypothyroidism
Starvation/refeeding

DRUG-RELATED
Sertraline (Zoloft)
Marijuana
Tricyclic antidepressants
Cimetidine
Spironolactone
Reserpine
Digitalis

HORMONAL
Neonates
Adolescence
Older men
Estrogen therapy
Testicular failure
Klinefelter syndrome
Hypogonadism

TUMORS
Lung
Pituitary
Adrenal
Hepatoma
Testicular

Box 10-2. Male Breast Cancer

Average age: 60 years
Hard, painless subareolar mass
Mass eccentric to the nipple or upper outer quadrant
Nipple discharge or ulceration not uncommon
Noncalcified round mass, variable border
Cancer usually ductal in origin
Treatment and prognosis identical to women's cancers

TABLE 10-1. Mammographic Appearance of Gynecomastia

Type	Mammography	Gynecomastia
Normal	Fatty breast	N/A
Pseudogynecomastia	Fatty breast	N/A
Dendritic	Prominent radiating extensions	Epithelial hyperplasia
Nodular	Fan-shaped triangular density	Later phase
Diffuse	Diffuse density	Dense fibrotic phase

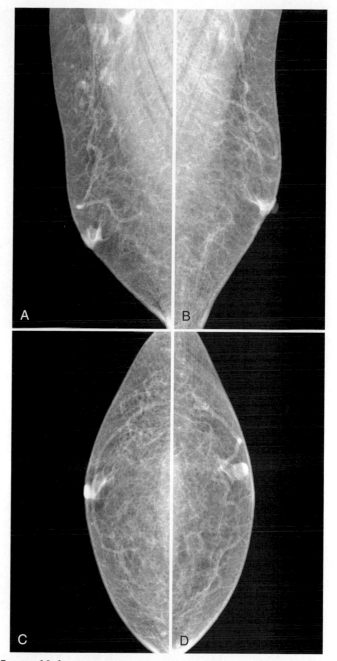

FIGURE 10-1. A to D, Mammograms in a man showing normal findings. Right (A) and left (B) mediolateral oblique (MLO) views and right (C) and left (D) craniocaudal (CC) mammograms show mostly fatty tissue and normal, scant, flamelike strands of glandular tissue in the subareolar regions. In some men, only normal fatty tissue is seen; in others, there are more faint strands of retroareolar tissue. In either case there is never as much tissue as in a woman in the normal male. *Continued*

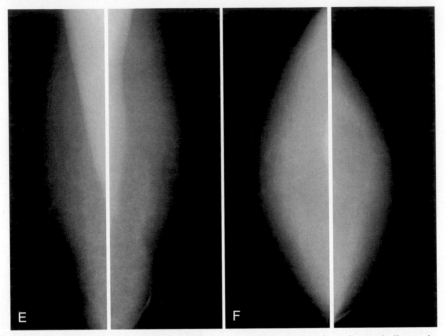

FIGURE 10-1, cont'd. **E** and **F,** Turner syndrome. MLO **(E)** and CC **(F)** views show mostly fatty tissue, similar to the normal male breast, in this female patient with Turner syndrome.

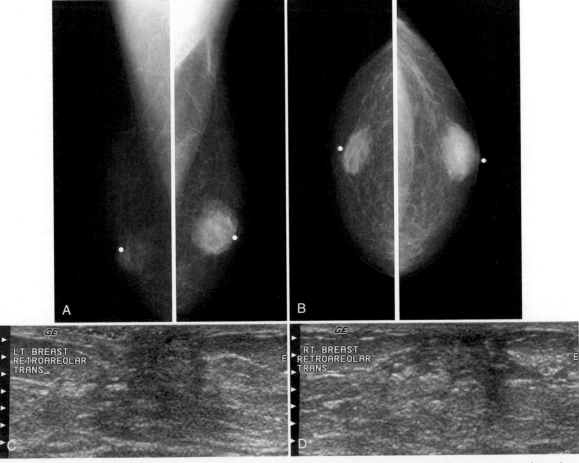

FIGURE 10-2. **A** to **D,** Triangular nodular gynecomastia. Mediolateral oblique (MLO) **(A)** and craniocaudal **(B)** mammograms show triangular, focally dense breast tissue behind the nipple. Ultrasound of the left **(C)** and right **(D)** breast shows hypoechoic dark strands of tissue extending from the nipple in a fingerlike triangular distribution in this male with gynecomastia.

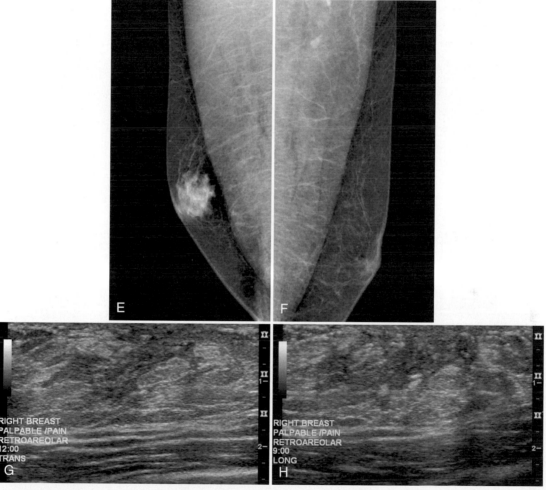

FIGURE 10-2, cont'd. E to H, Asymmetric nodular gynecomastia. Right (E) and left (F) MLO mammograms show triangular focal asymmetric subareolar glandular breast tissue behind the right nipple, representing right gynecomastia, and a left normal mammogram. Ultrasound of the right retroareolar region on transverse (G) and longitudinal (H) scans show the typical, normal "fingerlike" hypoechoic dark strands of tissue from gynecomastia extending from the right nipple.

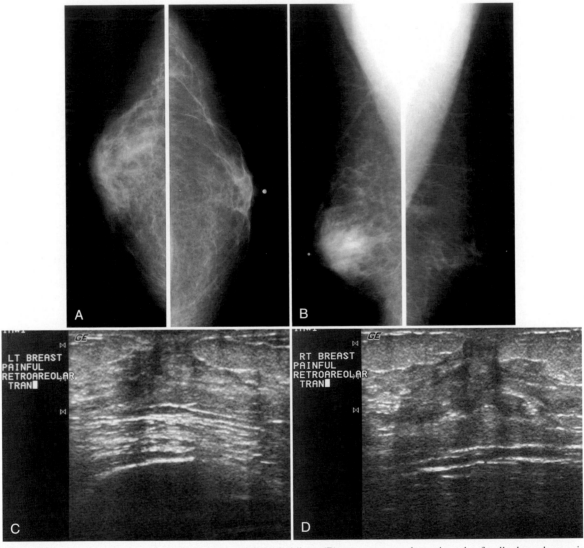

FIGURE 10-3. Diffuse gynecomastia. Craniocaudal (**A**) and mediolateral oblique (**B**) mammograms show triangular, focally dense breast tissue behind the nipple. Ultrasound of the left (**C**) and right (**D**) breast reveals hypoechoic dark triangular strands of tissue extending down from the nipple.

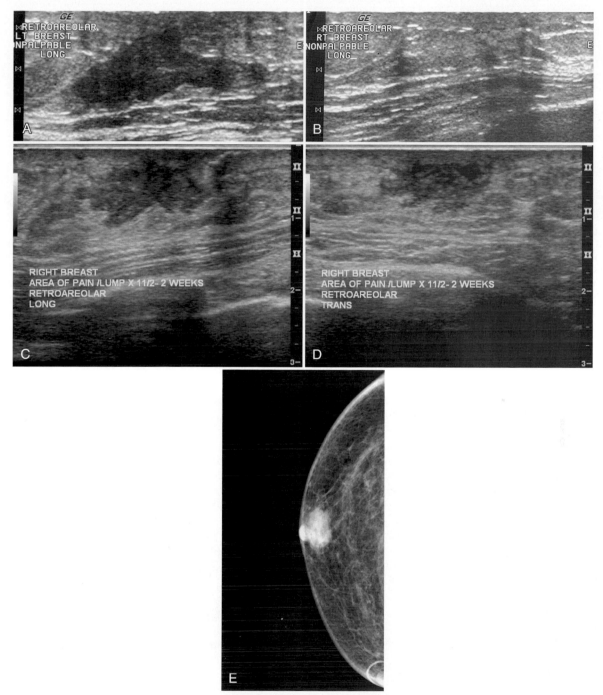

FIGURE 10-4. **A** and **B,** Varying appearance of gynecomastia on ultrasound. **A,** Ultrasound of painful, but nonpalpable left gynecomastia shows a triangle of hypoechoic tissue extending to the chest wall from the nipple. **B,** The right breast ultrasound is normal appearance and shows no glandular tissue. Longitudinal (**C**) and transverse (**D**) ultrasounds show triangular ductlike gynecomastia in a right retroareolar region that contains a painful lump. **E,** Corresponding right craniocaudal mammogram shows a focal glandular tissue in the right subareolar region, compatible with gynecomastia.

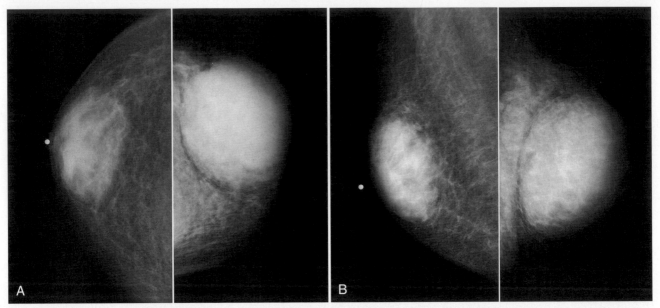

FIGURE 10-5. Male breast cancer. In a patient with a palpable mass in the retroareolar region of the left breast, craniocaudal (**A**) and mediolateral oblique (**B**) mammograms show diffuse bilateral gynecomastia with a large oval retroareolar mass on the left. Contrast the gynecomastia on the right, which shows indistinct breast tissue interfacing with fat, with the sharp smooth-bordered mass of the left breast cancer. Ultrasound-guided fine-needle aspiration of a portion of the mass showed invasive ductal cancer.

On mammography, male breast cancers are generally dense noncalcified masses with variable margin patterns located in the subareolar region (Figs. 10-5 and 10-6). Calcifications are less common in male than female breast cancer, although calcifications may be present. On ultrasound, male breast cancers are described as masses with well-circumscribed or irregular margins. Concomitant findings of skin thickening, adenopathy, and skin ulceration are associated with a poor prognosis. Breast cancers in men have the histologic appearance of invasive ductal cancer in 85% of cases, with most of the remaining tumors being medullary, papillary, and intracystic papillary tumors. An associated component of ductal carcinoma in situ (DCIS) may be present. Invasive lobular carcinoma is rare. Treatment of breast cancer is the same for men as for women and consists of surgery, axillary node dissection, chemotherapy, radiation therapy for invasive tumors, or any combination of these treatments; the prognosis is identical as that for women.

■ PREGNANT PATIENTS AND PREGNANCY-ASSOCIATED BREAST CANCER

Pregnancy produces a proliferation of glandular breast tissue that results in breast enlargement and nodularity; rarely, the condition progresses to gigantomastia or enlargement of multiple fibroadenomas. Breast masses are difficult to manage in a pregnant patient because of the surrounding breast nodularity and size increase over time. Most masses occurring in pregnancy are benign and include benign lactational adenomas, fibroadenomas, galactoceles, and abscesses (Box 10-3), but the diagnosis of exclusion is pregnancy-associated breast cancer.

Pregnancy-associated breast cancer is defined as breast cancer discovered during pregnancy or within 1 year of delivery (Box 10-4). The incidence of breast cancer in pregnant women is 0.2% to 3.8% of all breast cancers, or 1 in every 3000 to 10,000 pregnancies. Most pregnancy-associated breast cancers are invasive ductal cancer. These cancers are generally manifested as a hard mass, but they may be associated with bloody nipple discharge or findings of breast edema. The usual initial imaging test in a pregnant patient is breast ultrasound. Many patients are reluctant to undergo mammography because of concern about the effect of radiation on the fetus. However, if cancer is a clinical concern, it is important to perform mammography as part of the evaluation and in particular to detect the presence of suspicious calcifications that are often

---

BOX 10-3. Pregnancy and Lactational Breast Problems

Growing fibroadenoma (rare)
Lactational adenoma (rare)
Cancer (rare)
Mastitis/abscess (common)
Galactocele (uncommon)
Benign bloody nipple discharge (uncommon)

BOX 10-4. Pregnancy-Associated Breast Cancer

Cancer diagnosed during pregnancy or within 1 year postpartum
Stage for stage, same prognosis as in nonpregnant patients
Mammography and ultrasound are indicated
Chemotherapy possible after the second trimester
Radiation therapy absolutely contraindicated

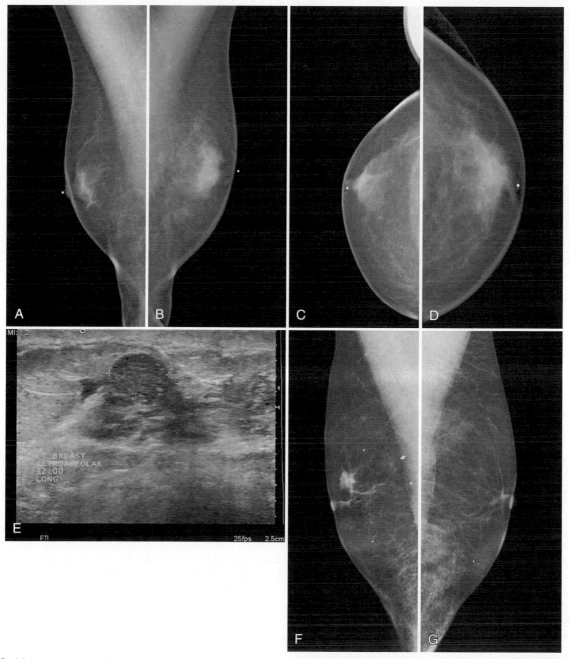

FIGURE 10-6. Male breast cancer. In a patient with bilateral gynecomastia and a palpable mass in the left breast, right (**A**) and left (**B**) mediolateral oblique (MLO) and right (**C**) and left (**D**) craniocaudal mammograms show bilateral benign-appearing gynecomastia, with markers on the right nipple and on an invisible palpable left breast mass that is obscured by the glandular tissue. **E,** Longitudinal ultrasound shows a round, homogeneous, hypoechoic mass corresponding to the palpable finding within the gynecomastia. Biopsy showed invasive ductal cancer. In another patient, right (**F**) and left (**G**) MLO mammograms show a palpable asymmetric spiculated mass superior to the right nipple that looks like cancer. Gynecomastia is usually directly behind the nipple; because the mass is in the upper breast, away from the nipple, it most likely represents cancer. Biopsy showed invasive ductal cancer.

Continued

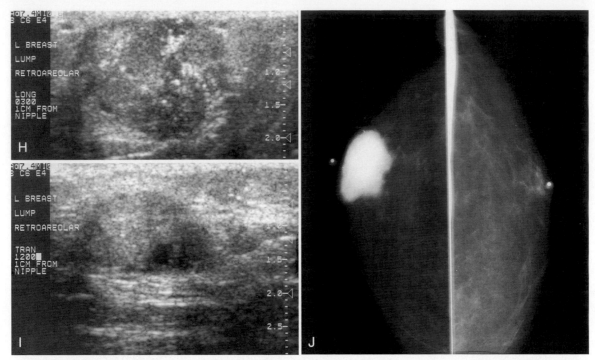

FIGURE 10-6, cont'd. Longitudinal (**H**) and transverse (**I**) ultrasounds of a palpable mass in a man shows a suspicious hypoechoic oval mass with calcifications. **J,** The mammogram shows a round, irregular mass with faint calcifications in the left breast. Biopsy showed invasive ductal cancer.

nonpalpable. The amount of scattered radiation delivered to the fetus is minimal and can be further reduced with lead shielding. Swinford and colleagues showed that breast density on mammography ranges from scattered fibroglandular density in pregnant patients to heterogeneously dense or dense breasts in a lactating patient. In their series, mammography was as useful as it is in nonpregnant women with clinical signs and symptoms of breast disease. In lactating patients, breast density can be reduced on the mammogram by pumping milk from the breasts before the study.

Mammography revealed signs of pregnancy-associated breast cancer in 78% of 23 pregnant women reported by Liberman and colleagues and in 86% of 15 cases reported by Ahn and colleagues. Mammograms showed masses, pleomorphic calcifications (or both masses and calcifications), asymmetries, and breast edema, but occasionally they were negative because of dense breast tissue. Axillary lymphadenopathy, asymmetries, and skin or trabecular thickening have been reported as primary or associated findings. In both series, ultrasound was positive in all cases in which it was performed and showed irregular solid masses with irregular margins. In the series by Ahn and colleagues, four masses also contained "complex echo patterns" or cystic components, and most showed acoustic enhancement.

Magnetic resonance imaging (MRI) of a normal lactating breast shows dense, enhancing, diffuse glandular tissue and widespread high signal throughout the tissue on T2-weighted images. Breast cancer in a lactating breast on MRI shows higher signal intensity in the initial enhancement phase than in the surrounding lactational breast tissue, with a washout or plateau pattern in the late phases in the rare reported cases in the radiology literature.

Pregnancy-associated breast cancers have a prognosis similar to that in nonpregnant women when matched for age and stage. In pregnancy, diagnostic delays may cause breast cancer to be detected at a later stage, thereby leading to a worse prognosis. Modified radical mastectomy was the usual treatment for pregnant women, but more recently, breast-conserving surgery is becoming more common. Chemotherapy has been used safely in women after the first trimester. Pregnancy is an absolute contraindication for radiation therapy.

Benign conditions are the most frequent cause of breast masses in pregnant or lactating patients, and cancer is much less common. Lactational mastitis is a common complication of breast-feeding in which the breast becomes painful, indurated, and tender, usually as a result of *Staphylococcus aureus* infection. A cracked nipple may be the port of entry for the infecting bacteria, but it can be prevented by good nipple hygiene and care, along with frequent nursing to avoid breast engorgement. Treatment is administration of antibiotics and continuation of breast-feeding. On occasion, antibiotic therapy is not sufficient to treat mastitis. If a hot, swollen, painful breast does not respond to antibiotics, ultrasound may identify an abscess and guide percutaneous drainage. On mammography, an abscess is a developing asymmetry or mass in a background of breast edema; it does not usually contain gas and is frequently located in the subareolar region (Fig. 10-7A and B). On ultrasound, abscesses are fluid-filled structures with irregular margins in the early phase, but circumscribed margins develop in the later phase as the walls of the abscess form. The abscess may contain debris or multiple septations, which may be drained under ultrasound guidance, but some residua may remain because of thick debris. Ultrasound-guided percutaneous drainage may be curative

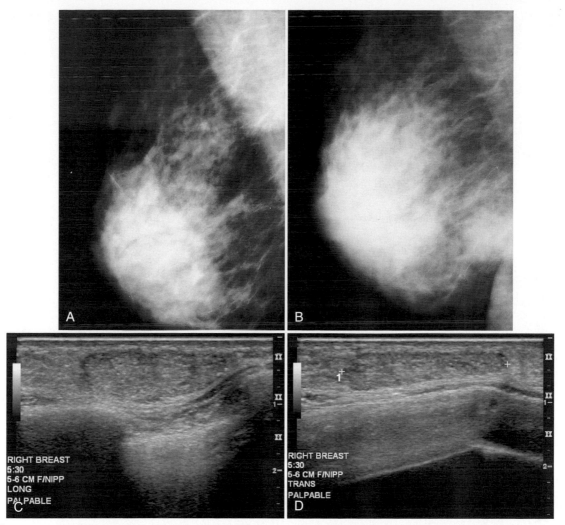

FIGURE 10-7. Pregnancy-associated findings: abscess and lactating adenoma. **A,** Mediolateral oblique mammogram in a lactating patient shows dense tissue. **B,** After the development of mastitis and a lump near the chest wall, the mammogram shows a developing density representing an abscess near the chest wall. Longitudinal (**C**) and transverse (**D**) ultrasounds in a patient with a palpable mass during pregnancy show an oval, homogeneous, well-circumscribed, palpable mass in the right breast that was larger during pregnancy and smaller after pregnancy. The differential diagnosis included fibroadenoma, adenoma of pregnancy, and well-circumscribed cancer. Biopsy showed lactating adenoma.

in small abscesses or palliative until surgical drainage can be performed in large abscesses. Some investigators report using ultrasound-guided aspiration, with abscess irrigation and instillation of antibiotics directly into the abscess cavity, to aid in resolution of the abscess.

Both fibroadenomas and lactating adenomas are solid benign tumors diagnosed during pregnancy. Growth of preexisting fibroadenomas may be stimulated by the elevated hormone levels of pregnancy, and the fibroadenoma may become clinically apparent. Infarction of fibroadenomas has been reported in the literature during pregnancy as well. Presenting as a firm, painless palpable lump that occurs late in prgenancy or during lactation, the lactating adenoma is a circumscribed, lobulated mass containing distended tubules with an epithelial lining. The mass can enlarge rapidly and regress after cessation of lactation. Ultrasound typically shows an oval, well-defined hypoechoic mass that may contain echogenic bands representing the fibrotic bands seen on pathology (see Fig. 10-7C and D). Whether lactating adenoma

represents change stimulated by hormonal alterations in a fibroadenoma or tubular adenoma or whether the tumors arise de novo has not been resolved.

Sampling of solid masses for histologic examination in a pregnant or lactating patient can be accomplished by either percutaneous core biopsy or surgery. Milk fistula produced by damage to the breast ducts is an established, but uncommon complication of these biopsy procedures in women in the third trimester of pregnancy or those who are lactating.

A galactocele produces a fluid-filled breast mass that can mimic a benign or malignant solid breast mass. On mammography, a galactocele is a round or oval, circumscribed mass of equal- or low-density (Fig. 10-8A and B). Because a galactocele is filled with milk, the creamy portions of the milk may rise to the nondependent part of the galactocele and produce a rare, but pathognomonic fluid-fluid or fat-fluid appearance on the horizontal beam image (lateral-medial view) at mammography. Ultrasound shows a fluid-filled mass that can have a wide range of sonographic

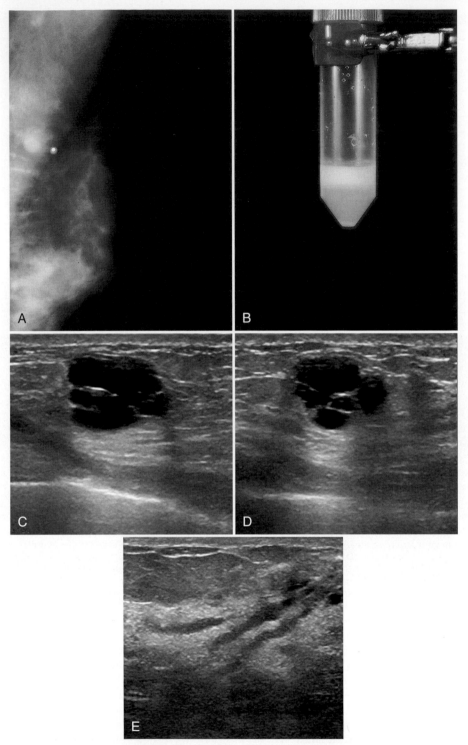

FIGURE 10-8. Galactocele. **A,** Mediolateral oblique mammogram in a lactating patient with a marker over a palpable mass shows a low-density mass in the upper portion of the left breast. **B,** Aspiration produced milky fluid with a fat-fluid level. **C** to **E,** Ultrasound of galactocele shows septated fluid-filled structure with enhanced through-sound transmission in transverse (**C**) and longitudinal (**D**) scans. This galactocele had very little solid material in it. Prominent fluid-filled ducts during lactation are seen on ultrasound (**E**), showing the milk in the ducts before galactocele formation.

appearances, depending on the relative amount of fluid and solid milk components within it. Galactoceles that are mostly fluid-filled have well-defined margins with thin echogenic walls (see Fig. 10-8C to E). Galactoceles containing more solid components of milk show variable findings, ranging from homogeneous medium-level echoes to heterogeneous contents with fluid clefts. Both distal acoustic enhancement and acoustic shadowing may be seen. The diagnosis is made by an appropriate history of childbirth and lactation, with aspiration yielding milky fluid and leading to resolution of the mass. Aspiration is usually therapeutic.

■ PROBABLY BENIGN FINDINGS (BI-RADS® CATEGORY 3)

Mammography detects small cancers, but it can also uncover nonpalpable benign-appearing lesions indeterminate for malignancy. Fine-detail diagnostic mammographic views and ultrasound in appropriate cases show that some indeterminate findings are typically benign and the patient can therefore resume screening. Other findings have a low probability (<2%) of malignancy after an appropriate workup that serves as a baseline for follow-up studies (Box 10-5). Sickles, Varas and colleagues, and Yasmeen and colleagues have independently provided data that Breast Imaging Reporting and Database System (BI-RADS®) category 3, or *probably benign*, findings carry a less than 2% chance of malignancy. Probably benign BI-RADS® category 3 lesions were found in 5%, 3%, and 5% of all screening studies after recall in their series, respectively. Probably benign findings included single or multiple clusters of small, round or oval calcifications; nonpalpable and noncalcified, round or lobulated, circumscribed solid masses; and nonpalpable focal asymmetry containing interspersed fat and concave scalloped margins that resemble fibroglandular tissue at diagnostic evaluation (Fig. 10-9).

For a mass to be considered circumscribed, at least 75% of the mass margin must be visualized as circumscribed; the remaining 25% may be obscured but must not show any signs of malignancy, such as ill-defined or spiculated margins. Rather than assessing as probably benign, multiple bilateral similar-appearing circumscribed or partially circumscribed masses may be considered BI-RADS® category 2 (benign), because it has been shown that the rate of malignancy among multiple masses is 0.14%, which was lower than the age-matched U.S. incident breast cancer rate of 0.24%. Importantly, if a focal asymmetry is to be considered probably benign, it should not be associated with any mass, suspicious calcifications, or architectural distortion. Probably benign findings are often detected on a baseline screening mammogram without comparison films and are managed by short-term mammographic follow-up (usually at 6-month intervals), but only after full diagnostic evaluation, including diagnostic mammographic views and (in some cases) ultrasound.

The 6-month mammographic follow-up serves as an alternative to percutaneous core or surgical biopsy for probably benign findings, with subsequent yearly follow-up for 2 to 3 years. Because the average breast cancer has a tumor volume doubling time of 100 days, growth should be detectable in 2 to 3 years. However, probably benign breast lesions are selected on the basis that they will most likely not change in the time interval. Lesions in which growth is anticipated should undergo biopsy.

Other inclusion criteria for the probably benign category include a lesion that is nonpalpable and identifiable at imaging, as well as a patient who is likely to complete the follow-up imaging surveillance regimen. Criteria that may exclude patients from short-term follow-up include extreme anxiety affecting the patient's quality of life, pregnancy or planned pregnancy, or a likelihood of noncompliance with follow-up.

Rosen and colleagues reviewed the findings of cancers initially subjected to short-term follow-up to identify imaging criteria that should exclude initial assessment as BI-RADS® category 3 (probably benign). Their series of cancers that were mistakenly classified in the probably benign category included palpable findings, developing densities, architectural distortion, irregular spiculated masses, growing masses, pleomorphic calcifications, workups showing motion blur on magnification, and lesion progression of any type since the previous mammogram. Their results emphasize that lesions should only be assessed as probably benign and assigned to short-term follow-up (instead of immediate biopsy) after optimal diagnostic workup. Data from the Breast Cancer Surveillance Consortium show that the few cancers that were initially assessed as probably benign are of early-stage and favorable prognosis, but only if full diagnostic imaging evaluation was initially performed. In contrast, cancers that were initially assessed as probably benign based on screening mammographic views only were of later-stage (and less favorable prognosis). Recall imaging is indicated before assessing a screen-detected lesion as probably benign for two reasons: to identify subtle features of malignancy that can only be seen through fine-detail diagnostic mammographic views or ultrasound (i.e., such lesions should be interpreted as suspicious and biopsied immediately), or to identify definitively benign findings through fine-detail diagnostic mammographic views or ultrasound (i.e., such lesions should be interpreted as benign and followed with routine rather than short-term interval imaging).

Data on probably benign lesions are derived from women in the screening mammography population, who are nominally asymptomatic. In other words, probably benign lesions identified in this cohort are (at least nominally) nonpalpable. Hence, a paucity of data are available regarding palpable lesions that otherwise fulfill the imaging criteria for probably benign assessment. In other words, rather than data existing indicating that palpable lesions cannot be safely considered probably benign, there is no sufficient data examining whether or not palpable findings that otherwise satisfy the imaging criteria for probably benign lesions may be assessed as BI-RADS® category 3. Indeed, more recent studies found that palpability did not affect the probability of malignancy in lesions that otherwise satisfied the probably benign imaging criteria.

BOX 10-5. Probably Benign Findings (BI-RADS® Category 3)

Nonpalpable findings

<2% chance of malignancy

Found in 5% of all screening cases after recall and diagnostic workup

Clustered small round or oval calcifications at magnification mammography

Noncalcified oval or lobulated, primarily well-circumscribed solid masses

Asymmetric densities resembling fibroglandular tissue at diagnostic evaluation

From Rosen EL, Baker JA, Soo MS: Malignant lesions initially subjected to short-term mammographic follow-up, *Radiology* 223:221–228, 2002.

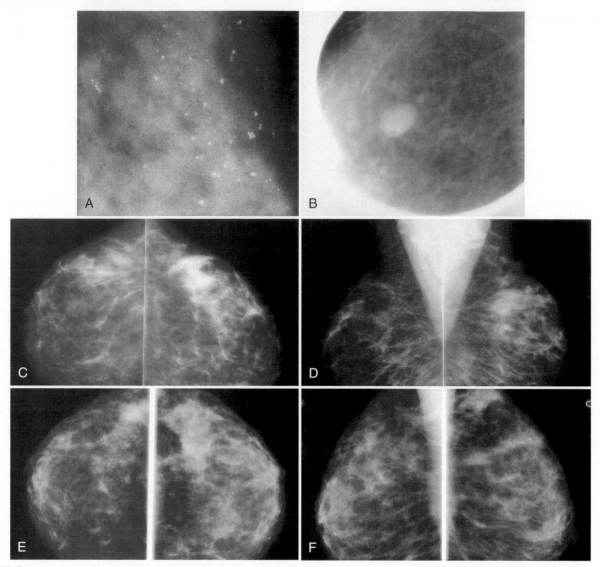

FIGURE 10-9. Probably benign findings on mammography. Findings included scattered and clustered, round punctate, sharply demarcated calcifications (**A**) and a nonpalpable, round, well-circumscribed solid mass (**B**). **C** to **F,** Asymmetries. Craniocaudal (CC) (**C**) and mediolateral oblique (MLO) (**D**) views show global asymmetry consisting of a nonpalpable greater volume of tissue in the upper outer portion of the left breast than in the right. In another patient, a focal asymmetry resembling fibroglandular tissue is seen in the upper part of the left breast on the CC (**E**) and MLO (**F**) views.

Despite the use of these strict criteria, a small number of cancers invariably emerge from BI-RADS® category 3 lesions. It is accepted that such lesions carry a probability of malignancy of less than 2%. In the series by Varas and colleagues, 0.4% of cases that were initially classified as probably benign were determined to be cancer at follow-up. Despite that probably benign lesions were associated with a possibility (albeit small) of malignancy, it is important to note that the few cancers identified were stage 1 or less, of favorable prognosis, and similar to the cancers detected in their mammographic screening series.

The probably benign category was based on imaging features and longitudinal data derived from mammography, which is a well-established imaging modality that has published well-defined standards for the acquisition of images, qualifications of personnel, and criteria for interpretation. In clinical practice, the probably benign category has been used with ultrasound and MRI. However, no specific image criteria, definition of lesions, or longitudinal data that are comparable to mammographic studies have been established for ultrasound or MRI. Emerging data suggest that a round, oval, or gently lobulated mass that appears circumscribed at mammography and ultrasound may be safely followed with short-term interval surveillance imaging, regardless of palpability. Few published reports on the use of the probably benign assessment category in MRI exist, and the probability of malignancy among such lesions ranges widely, from 0.6% to 10%. Caution should be paid regarding inappropriate overuse of the probably benign category in MRI, particularly because MRI is a costly test. Among three single-institutional studies, 17% to 24% of the MRI cases were assessed as probably benign with recommendation for short-term follow-up MRI. These numbers are substantially higher than those reported for mammographic lesions.

▬ NIPPLE DISCHARGE AND GALACTOGRAPHY

Nipple discharge is a common reason for women to seek medical advice. Benign nipple discharge usually arises from multiple ducts, whereas nipple discharge from a papilloma or DCIS usually occurs from a single duct. Nipple discharge is of particular concern if it is spontaneous and from a single duct or if the discharge is bloody. Women may describe intermittent discharge producing tiny stains on their brassiere or nightgown, or they may be able to elicit the discharge themselves. Some women present for imaging evaluation after positive findings from ductal lavage in conjunction with an abnormal cytologic evaluation.

The most frequent causes of both nonbloody and bloody nipple discharge are benign conditions. The most common mass producing a bloody nipple discharge is a benign intraductal papilloma, with only approximately 5% of women found to have malignancy at biopsy. The bloody nipple discharge associated with papillomas is due to twisting of the papilloma on its fibrovascular stalk and subsequent infarction and bleeding. Other causes of bloody discharge are cancer, benign findings such as duct hyperplasia/ectasia, and pregnancy as a result of rapidly proliferating breast tissue. Causes of nonbloody nipple discharge are fibrocystic change, medications acting as dopamine receptor blockers or dopamine-depleting drugs, rapid breast growth during adolescence, chronic nipple squeezing, or tumors producing prolactin or prolactin-like substances (Table 10-2).

Papillomas are benign masses that consist of a fibrovascular stalk with an attachment to the wall and breast duct epithelium; they have a variable cellular pattern and can produce nipple discharge. Papillomas may be single or multiple and may extend along the ducts for quite a distance. When large, papillomas can appear to be encysted and multilobulated. Some pathologists support the theory that peripheral papillomas have an increased risk for the subsequent development of carcinoma, whereas solitary or central papillomas do not. Peripheral papillomas are associated with epithelial proliferation, which may have atypical features, thus raising the possibility that atypia within a peripheral papilloma increases the risk of malignancy rather than the location of the papilloma itself.

The mammogram is frequently negative in the setting of nipple discharge (Table 10-3). Mammographic findings described in association with nipple discharge include a negative mammogram, a single dilated duct in isolation, or a small mass containing calcifications in either papilloma or malignancy (Fig. 10-10A to D). Ultrasound is frequently negative in women with nipple discharge, or fluid-filled dilated ducts without an intraductal mass in the retroareolar region may be seen. Solid masses in a fluid-filled duct may represent debris, a papilloma, or cancer.

Papillomas on MRI deserve special mention because they mimic cancer by producing a round enhancing mass that frequently has rapid initial early enhancement and a late plateau or washout on kinetic curve analysis, indistinguishable from invasive cancer (Fig. 10-11). For this reason, papillomas are a common cause of false-positive MRI-guided breast biopsies. On MRI, intraductal papillomas can have three patterns. The first pattern is a small circumscribed enhancing mass at the terminus of a dilated breast duct, corresponding to the filling defect seen on galactography. The second pattern is an irregular, rapidly enhancing mass with occasional spiculation or rim enhancement in women without nipple discharge; this is the pattern that cannot be distinguished from invasive breast cancer. Finally, despite the presence of a papilloma, MRI may be negative, with the papilloma undetected on both contrast-enhanced and fat-suppressed T1-weighted studies.

Galactography is used to investigate single-duct nipple discharge; when positive, it is helpful in subsequent surgical planning by identifying filling defects and their location and distance from the nipple. Galactography may also show normal duct anatomy, duct ectasia, or fibrocystic change. To perform galactography, the radiologist identifies the discharging duct visually by expressing a small amount of the discharge and pinpointing the location of the discharging duct. The radiologist cleans the nipple, may use a topical anesthetic, and with sterile technique, cannulates the discharging duct with a 30-gauge blunt-tipped sialogram needle connected to tubing and a syringe filled with contrast. Usually, the needle will fall painlessly

TABLE 10-2. Nipple Discharge

Color	Cause
Clear or creamy	Duct ectasia
Green, white, blue, black	Cysts, duct ectasia
Milky	Physiologic (neonatal) Endocrine (lactation/postlactation, pregnancy) Tumor (prolactinoma or other prolactin-producing tumor) Mechanical Drugs (dopamine receptor blockers/dopamine-depleting drugs)
Bloody or blood-related	Hyperplasia Papilloma Ductal carcinoma in situ Pregnancy

TABLE 10-3. Imaging of Nipple Discharge

Modality	Finding
Mammography	Negative (common) Dilated duct Mass with or without calcifications (papilloma or cancer)
Ultrasound	Negative (common) Fluid-filled ducts (normal or pathologic) Intraductal mass (papilloma, cancer, debris)
Galactogram	Filling defect (papilloma, cancer, air bubble, debris) Duct ectasia or cysts
Magnetic resonance imaging	Negative Fluid in dilated ducts Enhancing mass (cancer, papilloma)

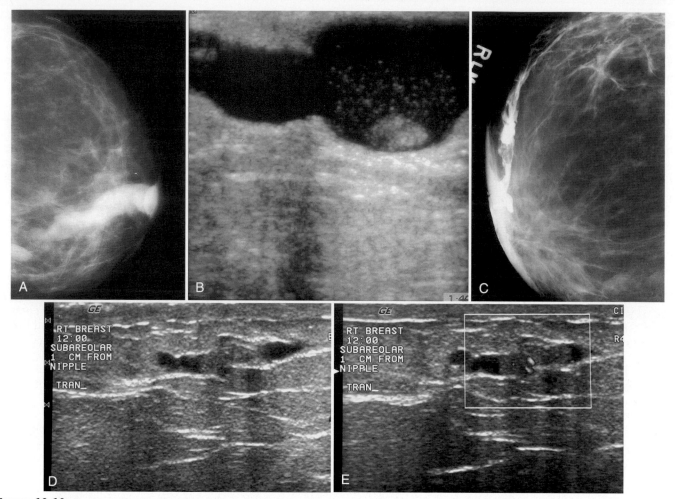

FIGURE 10-10. Papilloma in a dilated duct on mammography and ultrasound. **A,** The mammogram shows a markedly dilated duct (without contrast) extending into the breast from the nipple. **B,** Ultrasound revealed a fluid-filled dilated duct containing a mass, which was found to be a papilloma on biopsy. A papilloma in a contrast-filled duct in another patient has a filling defect (**C**); ultrasound shows the papilloma as a solid mass surrounded by the distended, contrast-filled duct (**D**). A blood vessel is seen in its fibrovascular component on color Doppler ultrasound (**E**).

into the duct, but on occasion, warm compresses are needed to relax the duct opening. A small amount of contrast (0.2–1 mL) is injected into the duct until resistance is felt or the patient feels a sense of fullness in the breast. Because the ducts are quite fragile, pain or burning may indicate perforation or extravasation of contrast, but neither the cannulation nor the injection should be painful. Either symptom is an indication to stop the procedure and re-evaluate the situation.

After the injection, the needle is withdrawn, and the contrast-filled duct is sealed with collodion or the blunt-tipped catheter is taped in place to the nipple. Standard craniocaudal and mediolateral mammograms are obtained; some facilities use magnification views to confirm and evaluate the filling defects. After the mammogram, the contrast is expressed from the breast by gentle massage. If duct filling is incomplete, the contrast is diluted by retained secretions, or if an air bubble is simulating an intraductal filling defect, then the duct can be reinjected immediately for a second study.

A normal duct arborizes from a single entry point on the nipple into smaller ducts extending over almost an entire quadrant of the breast. Normal ducts are thin and smooth-walled and have no filling defects or wall irregularities (Fig. 10-12A). Ductal ectasia is not uncommon; occasionally, normal cysts or lobules fill from the dilated ducts (see Fig. 10-12B). Ectatic ducts without a filling defect are usually normal. However, despite a normal galactogram, surgical excision of the discharging duct may reveal papillomas or cancer (i.e., false-negative study; see Fig. 10-12C).

Ducts containing malignancy or papillomas are typically dilated between the tumor and the nipple. Positive galactograms show a filling defect, an abrupt duct cutoff, or luminal irregularity and distortion. Tumors causing the abnormal findings may be located inside a fluid-filled dilated duct or may compress the duct from outside the duct walls (Fig. 10-13A to D). On occasion, masses, either papilloma or intracystic cancer, may become encysted (see Fig. 10-13D and E). Air bubbles produce filling defects that mimic papilloma or cancer, but they are usually sharply defined and round and change position inside the duct on repeat injection, unlike fixed intraductal tumors. On the galactogram, extravasation is seen as contrast extending outside the duct lumen into the breast tissue and

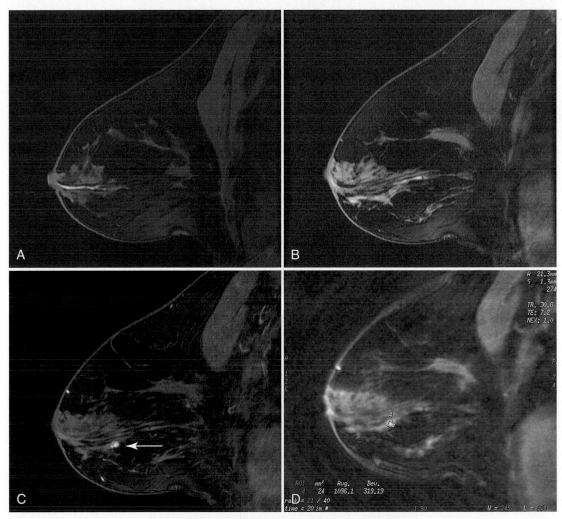

FIGURE 10-11. Papilloma on magnetic resonance imaging (MRI) and ultrasound. **A,** In a patient with nipple discharge, noncontrast T2-weighted sagittal MRI shows a bright fluid-filled duct extending from the nipple into the midbreast. **B,** Noncontrast sagittal 3-D spectral-spatial excitation magnetization transfer (3DSSMT) MRI shows high signal fluid within the lower breast ducts before contrast enhancement. **C,** Postcontrast sagittal 3DSSMT MRI shows a round enhancing mass in a duct (*arrow*), which previously had slight high signal fluid within it on part **B**. ROI over the mass on spiral dynamic scan (**D**) and the corresponding kinetic curve (**E**) show rapid initial enhancement and late washout, identical to kinetic curves in invasive cancer.   *Continued*

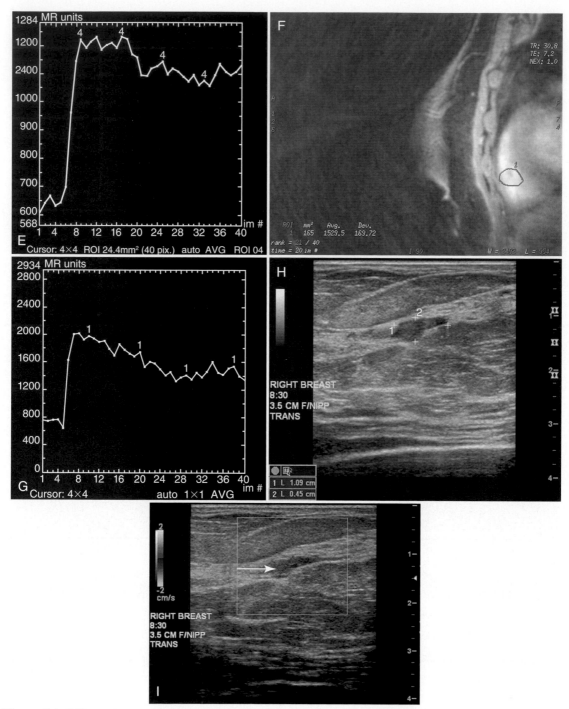

FIGURE 10-11, cont'd. ROI over the heart on spiral dynamic scan (**F**) and the corresponding kinetic curve (**G**) show rapid initial enhancement and late washout occurring in the same timeframe as the enhancing mass, indicating increased vascularity of the mass. **H**, Breast ultrasound shows a mass within a fluid-filled duct. **I**, Doppler ultrasound shows a pulsating blood vessel (*arrow*) within the mass, accounting for the rapid enhancement and washout. Biopsy showed intraductal papilloma.

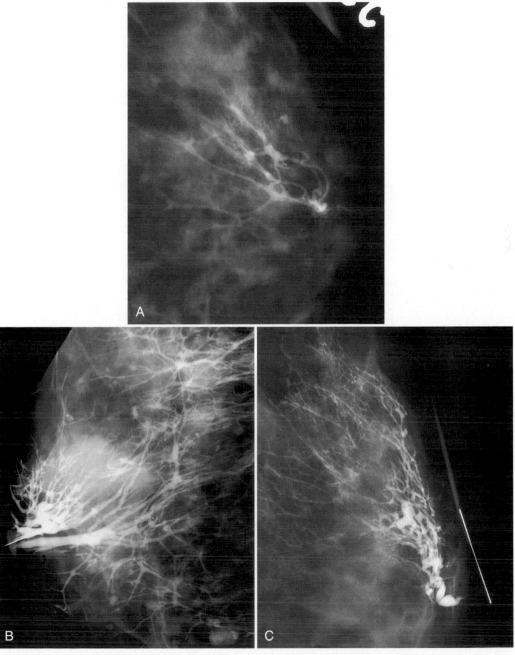

FIGURE 10-12. Normal galactograms. **A,** Normal galactogram showing contrast filling nondilated ducts without an abrupt cutoff or intraductal filling defects to suggest cancer or a papilloma. **B,** Normal galactogram demonstrating acinar filling. The galactogram shows two normally filling ducts, thin in diameter and without filling defects, and rounded acini filling in the periphery. **C,** Normal galactogram showing nondilated contrast-filled ducts in a patient with nipple discharge. Ductoscopy revealed two microscopic papillomas (false-negative galactogram).

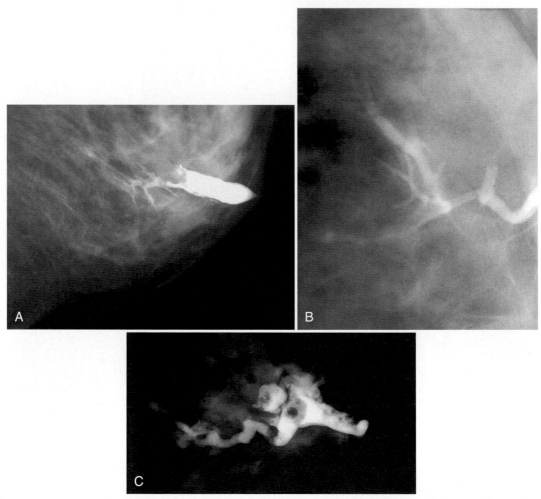

FIGURE 10-13. A to C, Abnormal galactograms. **A,** Papilloma on galactography. A filling defect on the galactogram corresponded to a retroareolar papilloma at surgery. **B,** Galactogram with an abrupt cutoff in a proximal duct. Biopsy showed papilloma. **C,** Galactogram showing cancer. A magnification view of a galactogram reveals an irregular filling defect in the retroareolar region. Biopsy showed ductal carcinoma in situ.

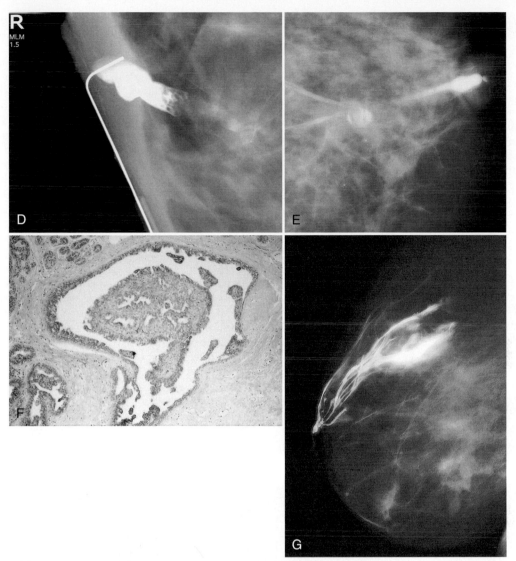

FIGURE 10-13, cont'd. D, Magnified right lateral mammogram after contrast injection into the duct shows the papillary filling defect, representing a papilloma. **E,** Encysted papilloma seen as a filling defect in a cyst. **F,** Photomicrograph of the encysted papilloma. **G,** Extravasation on galactography. The mammogram shows extravasation of contrast outside the normal thin ducts.

obscuring the underlying breast tissue and ducts (see Fig. 10-13F). In the rare instance of lymphatic or venous uptake of extravasated contrast, a draining tubular structure leading away from the extravasation site can be seen.

A positive galactogram usually leads to biopsy, either by preoperative needle localization or by ductoscopy. Preoperative needle localization of filling defects after galactography under x-ray guidance may be helpful for surgical planning, especially if the intraductal mass is deep in the breast. Negative galactograms despite the presence of a papilloma on biopsy have been reported, and galactography has a sensitivity ranging from 69% to 78% for tumors.

In the early 1990s, surgeons reported using a tiny ductoscope to cannulate a discharging duct for identification of papillomas or other intraductal masses intraoperatively to guide surgery. Dooley reported that 16% of women undergoing ductoscopy at surgery had lesions detected by

ductoscopy that were not seen on either ductograms or mammograms before surgery.

▬ BREAST EDEMA

On clinical examination, breast edema may be evident as *peau d'orange* (a term signifying thickening and elevation of the skin around tethered hair follicles, similar in appearance to an orange peel), and the edematous breast may be larger than the contralateral side. The differential diagnosis for breast edema depends on whether the edema is unilateral or bilateral (Box 10-6). Unilateral breast edema is due to mastitis, inflammatory cancer, local obstruction of lymph nodes, trauma, radiation therapy, or coumarin necrosis (Fig. 10-14). Bilateral breast edema is due to systemic etiologies, such as congestive heart failure, liver disease, anasarca, renal failure, or other conditions that can cause edema elsewhere in the body. Alternatively,

Box 10-6. Causes of Breast Edema

UNILATERAL

Mastitis
  Staphylococcus aureus (common)
  Tuberculosis (rare)
  Syphilis (rare)
  Hydatid disease (rare)
  Molluscum contagiosum
Abscess complicating mastitis
Recurrent subareolar abscess
Inflammatory cancer
Trauma
Coumarin necrosis
Unilateral lymph node obstruction
Radiation therapy

BILATERAL

Congestive heart failure
Anasarca
Renal failure
Lymphadenopathy
Superior vena cava syndrome
Liver disease

bilateral lymphadenopathy or superior vena cava obstruction for any reason may cause bilateral breast edema (Fig. 10-15).

The key to diagnosis is to obtain an accurate clinical history and evaluate the breast for any signs of cancer. The mammogram shows breast edema as skin thickening greater than 2 to 3 mm and coarsening of trabeculae in subcutaneous fat because of fluid within subdermal lymphatics. On the mammogram, the subcutaneous fluid produces thick white lines in subdermal fat just below the skin line that have an appearance similar to Kerley B lines at the periphery of the lung on chest radiographs in congestive heart failure. An edematous breast will be much denser and more difficult to penetrate and will appear whiter than the contralateral side because of fluid in the breast tissue.

The differential diagnosis for increased bilateral breast density on mammography includes breast edema, exogenous hormone therapy, and weight loss. Increased breast density from edema is due to fluid overload. Increased breast density from exogenous hormone therapy is due to hormonally driven proliferation of stromal and epithelial breast tissue (Fig. 10-16). Increased breast density due to weight loss is not due to any increase in breast tissue, but

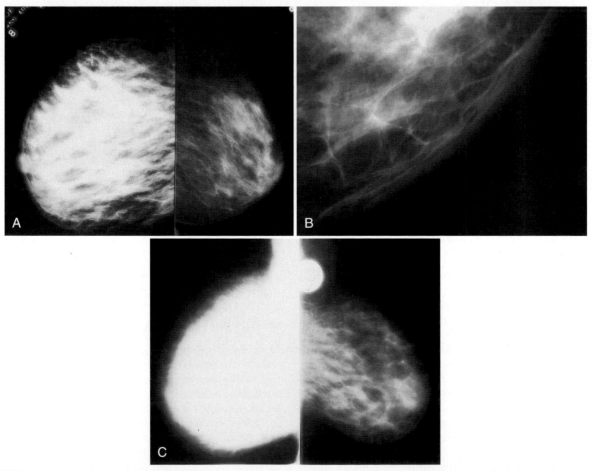

FIGURE 10-14. A, Unilateral breast edema on the right breast secondary to inflammatory cancer. Note the larger and whiter appearance of the right breast than the left, as well as marked coarsening of the trabeculae. **B,** Breast edema. A cropped, magnified mammogram shows skin thickening and atypical engorgement of the subdermal lymphatics in subcutaneous fat causing a trabecular pattern similar to Kerley B lines on a chest radiograph. Inflammatory cancer was the diagnosis. **C,** Unilateral breast edema from Hodgkin lymphoma and obstruction of the right axillary lymphatics. Note the chemotherapy port on the left.

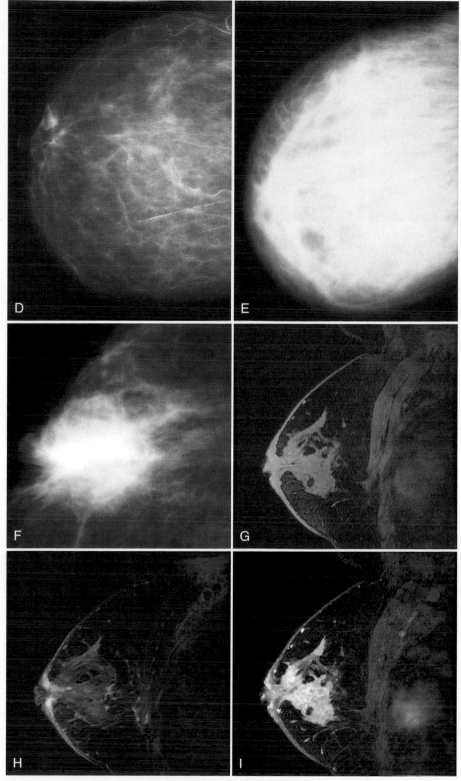

FIGURE 10-14, cont'd. Normal mammogram before the development of inflammatory cancer (**D**) and mammogram with breast edema 8 months later (**E**). **F,** Focal edema and hematoma from trauma. **G** to **I,** Breast cancer, nipple retraction, and breast edema on MRI. **G,** In a patient with a large retroareolar breast cancer, precontrast sagittal 3-D spectral-spatial excitation magnetization transfer (3DSSMT) MRI shows skin thickening, nipple retraction, and dense tissue behind the nipple. **H,** Sagittal precontrast T2-weighted fat-suppressed MRI shows breast edema with fluid in the periareolar region and within thickened skin. **I,** Postcontrast sagittal 3DSSMT MRI shows marked enhancement of a large cancer in the retroareolar region, skin thickening, and enhancement of the areola and skin, which is abnormal. Biopsy showed inflammatory cancer.

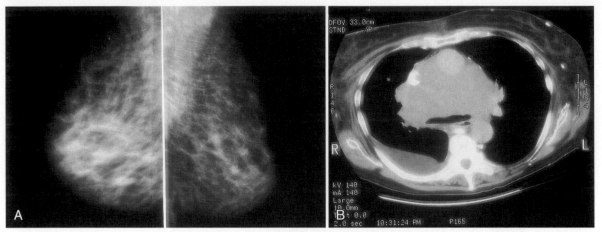

FIGURE 10-15. Bilateral breast edema from superior vena cava (SVC) compression secondary to granulomatous disease. **A,** A bilateral mammogram shows bilateral breast edema, worse on the right because the patient preferentially lies on her right side. **B,** Contrast-enhanced computed tomography shows SVC syndrome from mediastinal adenopathy, collateral vessels in the left chest, and right pleural effusion.

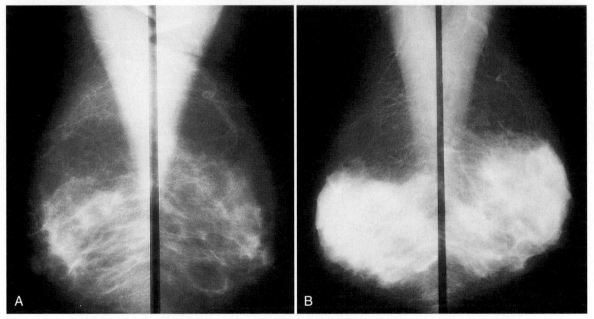

FIGURE 10-16. Exogenous hormone replacement therapy. Bilateral mediolateral oblique mammograms before (**A**) and after (**B**) hormone replacement therapy show increased glandular tissue bilaterally in locations where glandular tissue previously existed. Unlike breast edema, there is no skin thickening or coarsening of trabeculae in subcutaneous fat.

is due to loss of fat (Fig. 10-17). A history of recent weight loss should lead to the correct diagnosis.

To disinguish between breast edema and exogenous hormone therapy or weight loss, the radiologist looks for skin thickening, which is found only with breast edema (Box 10-7). The increased breast density from breast edema can occur anywhere; skin thickening in dependent portions of the breast is often seen. The increased breast density from exogenous hormone therapy is usually bilateral, occurs in regions where breast tissue was previously present, and shows no skin thickening.

On ultrasound, breast edema is characterized by skin thickening, loss of the normal sharp margins of Cooper ligaments, increased echogenicity of surrounding tissues and, in severe cases, fluid in dilated subdermal lymphatics, which are seen as tubular fluid-filled structures just under the skin line. In inflammatory cancer, breast ultrasound

---

BOX 10-7. Hormone Changes versus Breast Edema on Mammography

HORMONE CHANGES
Increased breast density
Breast density increased at sites with glandular tissue
Normal skin
Normal subcutaneous fat
Normal skin on physical examination

BREAST EDEMA
Increased breast density
Diffuse or focal; may develop where no glandular tissue occurred previously
Skin thickening
Subcutaneous trabecular thickening
Peau d'orange on physical examination

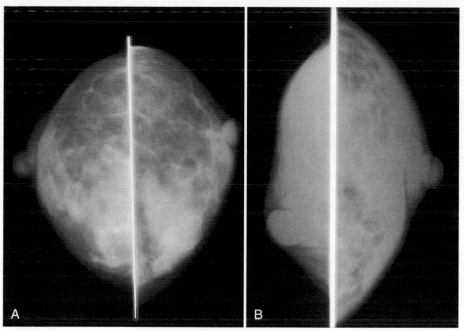

FIGURE 10-17. Weight loss. Bilateral craniocaudal mammograms before (**A**) and after (**B**) weight loss show increased breast density on the mammogram because of loss of fat.

may detect a hypoechoic shadowing mass that may represent an invasive ductal cancer hidden on the mammogram by overlying breast edema.

On MRI, breast edema is manifested as skin thickening and coarsening of breast trabeculae and Cooper ligaments. Locally advanced cancer is usually seen as an irregular mass with rapid initial enhancement, a late plateau or washout phase, and enhancement within the skin if skin invasion has occurred.

Inflammatory cancer, a rare (1% of all cancers) aggressive breast cancer with a poor prognosis, is the most important differential diagnosis for unilateral breast edema. The definition of inflammatory cancer varies, but it usually has the clinical signs of an enlarging erythematous breast with *peau d'orange*, and it should be distinguished from locally advanced breast cancer, producing a focal, red, raised skin metastasis. Inflammatory cancer is often mistaken for mastitis because of its clinical features, but it does not respond to antibiotics. Mammography of inflammatory cancer reveals findings of breast edema (skin thickening, diffuse increased breast density, trabecular thickening), but it may also demonstrate findings of cancer, including a breast mass, asymmetric focal density, microcalcifications, nipple retraction, or axillary adenopathy. Ultrasound may show findings of breast edema in 96% of cases, masses in 80%, and dilated lymphatic channels in 68%. On MRI, one report of inflammatory cancer described a "patch enhancement" pattern with some "areas of focal enhancement" and washout on the late phase of the dynamic curve. The enhancement rate on MRI for inflammatory cancer is reported to be quite rapid in the initial postcontrast phase and slightly less rapid in mastitis. The MRI shows breast edema, skin thickening, and skin enhancement (see Fig. 10-14G to I). On biopsy, breast cancer is present in the dermal lymphatics in 80% of cases.

The usual management is biopsy to make the diagnosis of inflammatory cancer, neoadjuvant chemotherapy with or without subsequent surgery, and radiation therapy, depending on tumor response, or any combination of these modalities.

Mastitis is a common cause of unilateral breast edema, and clinical findings of pain, erythema, and *peau d'orange* are typically noted. The most common cause of mastitis is *S. aureus*. Rare causes of breast infection include tuberculosis, syphilis, hydatid disease, and molluscum contagiosum. Clinically, mastitis produces breast cellulitis, which if untreated, may progress to small focal microabscesses or a larger abscess collection that may become walled off. On mammography, mastitis appears as unlateral breast edema. When mastitis progresses to abscess, abscesses are tender palpable masses, usually in the retroareolar region, on physical examination. On mammography the abscess is an ill-defined or irregular mass without calcifications. Usually, no gas is present in the abscess on the mammogram. Rarely, an abscess contains gas, but most commonly after aspiration has been attempted. On ultrasound, the abscess is an irregular, ill-defined hypoechoic mass, sometimes containing septations or debris, with enhanced through-transmission of sound. Because antibiotics cannot cross abscess walls, larger abscesses require either percutaneous or operative drainage. For this reason, ultrasound is particularly helpful in the setting of mastitis to detect and define abscesses requiring drainage.

A recurrent subareolar abscess is a special entity caused by plugging of the major breast ducts and subsequent infection; it is commonly associated with a fistulous tract that forms from the abscess inside the breast and drains to the skin. The resulting abscess is chronic and may be drained percutaneously or operatively many times without resolution or with frequent recurrence. A recurrent subareolar abscess is treated by surgically removing both the abscess and the fistulous tract.

An extremely rare cause of unilateral breast edema is necrosis of the breast from coumarin (warfarin [Coumadin]) therapy. Necrosis occurs more commonly in the abdomen, buttocks, and thighs, rather than in breast, and it occurs in 0.01% to 1% of coumarin-treated patients (Box 10-8). Although it has been associated with protein C or protein S deficiency, the exact mechanism of coumarin-induced necrosis is unknown. Painful lesions, swelling, and petechiae from thrombosis of small vessels and inflammation occur after the initiation of coumarin treatment; large hemorrhagic bullae result and develop to full-thickness fat and skin necrosis. Discontinuing the use of coumarin is recommended. Heparin or other anticoagulants may be necessary in patients who require sustained anticoagulation in the short term. Heparin-induced skin necrosis has also been reported in association with type II heparin-induced thrombocytopenia, but heparin is often used in the setting of coumarin necrosis. In some cases, the skin lesions heal spontaneously after shallow tissue sloughing. In other cases, skin grafts are required; in extreme cases, mastectomy is required.

Box 10-8. Coumarin Necrosis

Rare cause of breast edema
Exact mechanism unknown
Associated protein C or S deficiency
Painful swelling and petechiae
Hemorrhagic bullae
Full-thickness skin necrosis
Discontinue or change anticoagulants

HORMONE CHANGES

Normal women have extremely dense breast tissue when young that is replaced by fat during the aging process. On mammography, the breasts usually appear very white in younger patients and become darker and darker as glandular tissue is replaced by fatty tissue with age. The overall breast density at any time in the patient's life depends on the patient's age, her genetic predisposition for glandular tissue, and her hormonal status.

Exogenous hormone replacement therapy, pregnancy, and lactation reverse the trend toward fatty breast tissue by causing a proliferation of the glandular elements and periductal stroma of the breast, thereby resulting in a denser mammogram. Unlike breast edema, only the breast tissue becomes denser, and the skin does not become thickened more than 2 to 3 mm as it does with breast edema (Fig. 10-18).

Some women report breast tenderness, pain, fullness, and lumpiness with exogenous hormone replacement therapy. The frequency of increased breast density on mammography in women undergoing exogenous hormone therapy varies from 23% to 34%. The highest percentage of women with increased density were receiving continuous-combined hormone therapy consisting of conjugated equine estrogen, 0.625 mg/day, plus medroxy-progesterone acetate, 2.5 mg/day, or other combinations, with the progestin component most affecting the increase in breast density. In another report, continuous-combined hormone therapy produced increased breast density on mammography, but estrogen-only therapy did not.

Other medications also have effects on breast density. Raloxifene hydrochloride, a drug used for bone mineral density, has been reported to produce increased breast density on mammography in a very small number of women. Case studies of two women undergoing injections

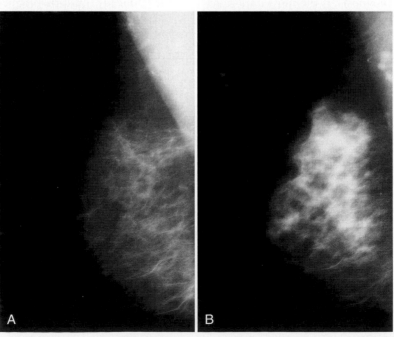

FIGURE 10-18. Exogenous hormone replacement therapy. Mediolateral oblique mammograms before (**A**) and after (**B**) hormone replacement therapy show a denser breast where breast tissue previously existed.

of medroxyprogesterone (Depo-Provera) for contraception reported a decrease in breast density on mammograms during the injections and an increase in breast density when the injections were discontinued. Tamoxifen used for adjuvant or prophylactic treatment of breast cancer has been reported to decrease mammographic tissue density in some women, with one case report describing a return to baseline breast density after termination of drug therapy. Isoflavones are phytoestrogens contained in soy foods and have been reported to have both estrogenic and antiestrogenic effects. A double-blind, randomized trial of women undergoing mammography after isoflavone supplements showed no significant decrease in breast density or change in dense tissue over a 12-month period.

Because breast density changes with hormone therapy, new or focal densities on mammograms are correlated with older films and the clinical history, in addition to being evaluated for a new mass or a developing density as a result of cancer. In questionable cases, spot compression, fine-detail views, and ultrasound may be helpful to exclude the presence of a mass. If questions still remain after additional workup, discontinuing exogenous hormone therapy for 3 months and re-imaging may exclude a mass. Similarly, the increased breast enhancement noted on contrast-enhanced breast MRI in women receiving exogenous hormone replacement therapy is reversible when the therapy is discontinued.

BREAST PAIN

Breast pain is an extremely common complaint. However, in the absence of an associated palpable lump, it is a very infrequent sign of breast cancer. Nevertheless, because both breast pain and breast cancer are common, the purpose of the workup is to reassure the patient and exclude a coexistent cancer. Breast pain may be focal or diffuse. It may vary with the menstrual cycle (i.e., cyclic) or not (i.e., noncyclic). In general, diffuse and cyclic breast pain is a benign symptom that does not warrant imaging evaluation.

Patients with focal breast pain should be evaluated with mammography and breast physical examination. Although focal breast pain is worrisome to the patient, studies have shown that it is most often not caused by cancer. However, because both breast pain and cancer are common, mammography is reasonable to exclude cancer and reassure the patient. Consideration should be given to ultrasound in women with focal pain to exclude a breast cyst that may be causing the pain.

Cyclic mastalgia has many causes, including cyclic enlargement as a result of menses or multiple cysts. Relief from breast pain may be achieved in some cases by aspiration of the cyst, decrease in caffeine intake, or analgesics. Home remedies for breast pain have included 400 U of vitamin E per day, vitamin B$_6$, analgesics, decrease in fat and salt intake, use of sports brassieres, and evening primrose oil. In extreme cases, progestins, danazol, tamoxifen, or bromocriptine is used to relieve mastodynia.

AXILLARY LYMPHADENOPATHY

Axillary lymphadenopathy is visualized on mammography as replacement of the fatty hilum of lymph nodes by dense tissue, a rounded shape of the lymph nodes, and an overall generalized increased density with or without lymph node enlargement (Fig. 10-19). Abnormal lymph nodes may also contain calcifications, gold deposits mimicking calcifications from treatment of rheumatoid arthritis, or silicone

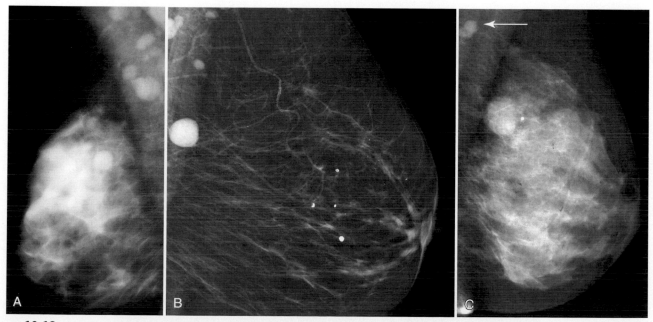

FIGURE 10-19. Axillary lymphadenopathy. **A,** Abnormal dense round lymph nodes in the axilla have lost their fatty hila and are rounder and bigger than normal lymph nodes as a result of lupus and rheumatoid arthritis. **B,** Abnormal round lymph nodes in another patient with lymphoma on digital mammography. **C,** Left mediolateral oblique view shows a mass in the upper breast representing an invasive ductal cancer with an abnormal lymph node (*arrow*) in the left axilla. Even though the lymph node still has its fatty hilum, it is worrisome for cancer metastases because it is rounder, denser, and has a thicker cortex than a normal lymph node. Metastatic disease was found in the lymph node at sentinel lymph node biopsy.

from a previously ruptured breast implant. The differential diagnosis for axillary adenopathy without a definite breast mass varies for unilateral versus bilateral findings (Box 10-9). Causes of unilateral axillary adenopathy include metastatic breast cancer and mastitis. Bilateral axillary adenopathy is usually due to systemic etiologies, such as infection, collagen vascular diseases such as rheumatoid arthritis, lymphoma, leukemia, or metastatic tumor.

"Calcific" particles in abnormal axillary lymph nodes may represent calcified metastasis from breast cancer or calcifying infections such as tuberculosis (Box 10-10). In the case of tuberculous mastitis, patients have axillary swelling and breast enlargement without a breast mass, as well as enlarged dense or matted axillary lymph nodes or breast edema with or without findings of pulmonary tuberculosis. The finding of macrocalcifications rather than pleomorphic microcalcifications in the lymph nodes may suggest tuberculous mastitis, but biopsy is necessary to exclude metastatic breast cancer. Migration of silicone into axillary lymph nodes from ruptured silicone breast implants or migration of gold particles from therapy for rheumatoid arthritis may mimic calcifications in lymph nodes, but the clinical history should provide clues to the correct diagnosis.

Detection of lymphadenopathy on mammography in women with no underlying palpable breast mass or clinical reason for the abnormal lymph nodes should prompt a critical review of the breast for pleomorphic calcifications or other signs of breast cancer. In one clinical series of 21 women with lymphadenopathy detected at screening mammography, 50% was due to malignancy (lymphoma, metastatic carcinoma, leukemia), and the other 50% was due to benign causes (reactive changes, healed granulomatous disease, rheumatoid arthritis, amyloid, infection).

Primary breast cancer presenting as isolated lymph node metastasis in the setting of normal mammographic and physical examination findings is an uncommon clinical problem that accounts for less than 1% of all breast cancers (Fig. 10-20). Both breast ultrasound and contrast-enhanced breast MRI have been used to detect the primary breast cancer in this scenario, with improved results in comparison to mammography, and breast conservation rather than mastectomy is a potential option once the primary tumor is found (Fig. 10-21). Diagnosis of a primary cancer within the breast is clinically contributory, because an occult primary

---

Box 10-9. Axillary Lymphadenopathy

UNILATERAL
Mastitis
Cancer

BILATERAL
Widespread infection
Rheumatoid arthritis
Collagen vascular disease
Lymphoma
Leukemia
Metastatic cancer

Box 10-10. Lymphadenopathy with "Calcifications"

Metastatic calcifying cancer
Granulomatous disease
Gold particles from rheumatoid arthritis therapy
Migrated silicone from implant rupture

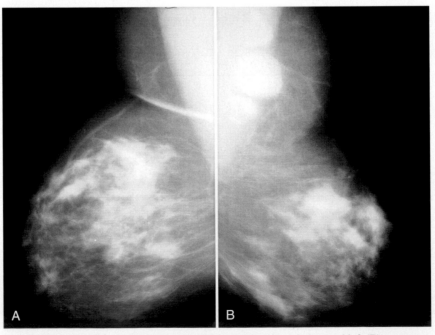

FIGURE 10-20. Breast cancer presenting as axillary lymphadenopathy. Normal right (**A**) and abnormal left (**B**) mammograms show adenopathy in the left axilla, which was consistent with the diagnosis of breast cancer. Additional views of the left breast by mammography and ultrasound did not demonstrate any masses. Examination after mastectomy showed no primary breast cancer. The patient was treated for breast cancer empirically. No breast cancer in the opposite breast and no additional tumors were found elsewhere in 5 years of follow-up.

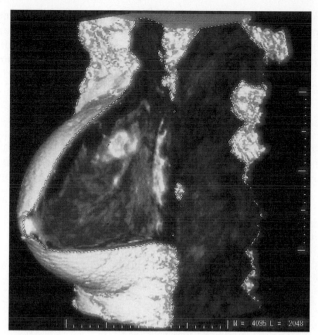

FIGURE 10-21. A shaded, cut-surface display of contrast-enhanced magnetic resonance imaging of the breast shows an irregular-enhancing suspicious mass in the upper part of the breast representing an occult malignancy not seen on mammography. (Image courtesy of Bruce L. Daniel, MD, Stanford University, Stanford, CA.)

malignancy in the breast would be considered locoregional rather than metastatic disease in patients who present with axillary lymphadenopathy of unknown primary. In some cases the primary breast cancer is never identified. In a pathology series by Haupt and colleagues, in which 43 women with this clinical dilemma were reviewed, the primary tumor was found in 31 (72%) specimens but never

identified in the remaining 12. Survival rates between the two groups were similar, and the 12 women in whom a tumor was never discovered did have another primary malignancy detected in the follow-up period.

▬ PAGET DISEASE OF THE NIPPLE

Paget disease of the nipple is a distinct clinical entity that heralds an underlying breast cancer. Ductal carcinoma almost always coexists with Paget disease, either in the ducts beneath the nipple or elsewhere in the breast, and it has a high rate of overexpression of the c-*erb*-B2 oncogene. The underlying pathology is almost always high-grade DCIS, but an invasive component may also be present. Affected women have a bright, reddened nipple and eczematous nipple changes that may extend to the areola, with subsequent ulceration and nipple destruction if the process is unchecked. A delay of several months often occurs before women seek advice, unless associated nipple discharge is present. Paget disease of the nipple may mimic dermatitis of the nipple, resulting in delayed diagnosis. If the patient's symptoms do not respond to a trial of topical steroids, the diagnosis of Paget disease should be considered.

The nipple and mammogram are normal in almost 50% of cases despite clinical signs of Paget disease and the presence of an underlying breast cancer (Box 10-11). On abnormal mammograms, the underlying malignancy has the appearance of suspicious microcalcifications, a spiculated mass, or both. The cancer is often located in the subareolar region or deep in the breast and does not necessarily lie directly adjacent to the nipple or areola (Fig. 10-22A). In women with Paget disease, skin or areolar thickening, nipple retraction, subareolar masses, or calcifications leading to the nipple should be viewed with suspicion on mammography (see Fig. 10-22B). Spot

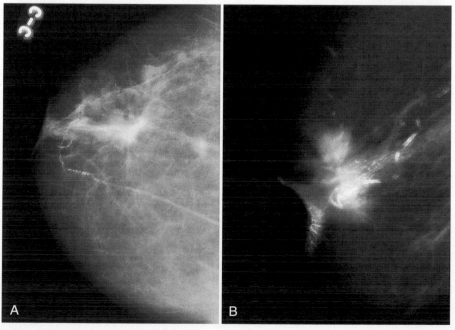

FIGURE 10-22. Paget disease. **A,** Craniocaudal mammogram shows nipple retraction and a second invasive ductal cancer deep in the breast in a patient with Paget disease. **B,** Mediolateral oblique mammogram in a patient with Paget disease shows destruction of the nipple covered with a radiopaque salve and a retroareolar dense mass producing retraction.

Box 10-11. **Paget Disease of the Nipple**

Heralds underlying ductal cancer
Bright red nipple
Eczematous nipple–areolar changes
Ulceration
Cancer location often subareolar, but may be anywhere in the breast
Normal mammogram in 50%
Nipple change, skin/areolar thickening in 30%
Subareolar mass/calcifications suspicious

compression magnification mammography of the nipple and retroareolar region is often helpful in identifying subtle abnormalities. Conversely, nipple–areolar abnormalities or thickening detected at mammography should be correlated with the physical examination to exclude clinical findings of Paget disease.

SARCOMAS

Sarcomas are rare tumors of the breast or the underlying chest wall, and their classification depends on the cell type involved (Fig. 10-23). Ultrasound shows a hypoechoic

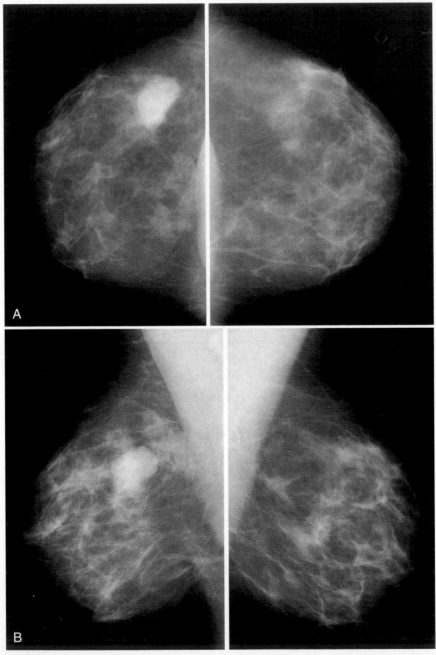

FIGURE 10-23. Carcinosarcoma. Craniocaudal (**A**) and mediolateral oblique (**B**) mammograms in a 37-year-old woman with a palpable mass show a dense lobulated mass in the right breast with an obscured lower border. Pathologic examination demonstrated the epithelial and mesenchymal differentiation required to make the diagnosis. (From Smathers RL: *Mammography: diagnosis and intervention*, Medical Interactive [compact disc]. Copyright Mammography Specialists Medical Group, Inc. Contribution from Suzanne Dintiz, MD, Stanford, CA.)

mass and may be helpful in determining whether the origin of the sarcoma is from the breast or chest wall (Fig. 10-24A and B). Mammography shows high-density masses without calcifications or spiculation, unless the tumor has osseous elements (Fig. 10-25). MRI is useful for demonstrating pectoralis muscle or chest wall involvement, because sarcomas tend to be large and locally invasive.

MRI of angiosarcoma shows low signal intensity on T1-weighted images, higher signal intensity on T2-weighted images, and enhancement of the mass with a low-intensity central region. At pathology, sinusoids containing red blood cells are present. Angiosarcoma of the breast may be primary or secondary to radiation, usually received as adjunctive therapy after breast conservation surgery (i.e., lumpectomy). Secondary angiosarcoma usually occurs approximately one decade after the initial radiation therapy.

▬ MONDOR DISEASE

Mondor disease is acute thrombophlebitis of the superficial veins of the breast (Box 10-12). It is rare, is often associated with trauma or recent surgery, and has been reported to occur after sonography-guided or stereotactic core biopsy, but may also be idiopathic in origin. Patients report acute pain, discomfort, and tenderness along the lateral aspect of the breast, the chest wall, or the region of the thrombosed vein; they may also report a cordlike, painful elongated mass just below the skin. Extension of the arm may produce a long narrow furrow in the skin as a result of retraction from the thrombosed vein, similar to skin dimpling from breast cancer.

Physical examination shows a tender palpable cord extending toward the outer portion of the breast that is produced by fibrosis and obliteration of the superficial

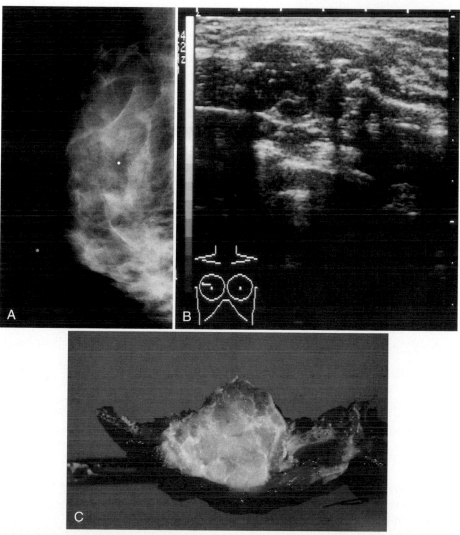

FIGURE 10-24. Chondrosarcoma of the rib. **A,** Mediolateral oblique mammogram shows a marker over a slowly growing mass, which proved to be only dense tissue. **B,** Ultrasound reveals a complex heterogeneous mass invading the chest wall, predominantly posterior to the pectoralis muscle and measuring 6 cm. **C,** Pathologic examination showed a grade 1 chondrosarcoma containing mature hyaline cartilage and reactive bone in continuity with the rib. (From Smathers RL: *Mammography: diagnosis and intervention,* Medical Interactive [compact disc]. Copyright Mammography Specialists Medical Group, Inc. Contribution from Suzanne Dintiz, MD, Stanford, CA.)

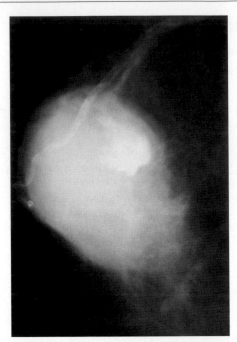

FIGURE 10-25. Fibrosarcoma of the breast with osseous trabeculae. Craniocaudal mammogram shows a dense mass containing dense calcification resembling bone. (From Elson BC, Ikeda DM, Andersson I, Wattsgard C: Fibrosarcoma of the breast: mammographic findings in 5 cases, *AJR* 158:994, 1992.)

Box 10-12. Mondor Disease

Thrombophlebitis of the superficial veins of the breast
Painful, ropelike, palpable cord
Thrombosed vein causes a furrow/dimpling
Self-limited
Related to trauma or surgery
Mammography is negative, or long tubular density is noted
Ultrasound: hypoechoic tube or cord with or without flow

---

vein; in the acute phase, it is occasionally accompanied by discoloration of the overlying skin. Thereafter, the vein diminishes in painfulness over a period of 3 to 4 weeks as a result of either recanalization or complete obliteration of the vein by phlebosclerosis and hyalinization. Because Mondor disease is self-limited and the palpable finding resolves over a 2- to 12-week period, supportive care is the appropriate treatment.

Case reports describe negative mammographic findings in women with Mondor disease or, rarely, a long linear or tubular density on the mammogram corresponding to the thrombosed vein (Fig. 10-26). Case reports of ultrasound in Mondor disease show a noncompressible hypoechoic tubular cord in the subcutaneous tissue, with or without flow on color Doppler imaging, depending on the degree of recanalization.

GRANULOMATOUS MASTITIS

Granulomatous mastitis is a rare disease that occurs in young premenopausal women after their last childbirth. It has been correlated with breast-feeding and oral contraceptive use, and a possible autoimmune component has been implicated in its etiology. Affected patients may have galactorrhea, inflammation, a breast mass, induration, and skin ulcerations.

Women undergoing mammography are found to have asymmetric density, focal asymmetric or ill-defined breast masses, or negative results. Calcifications are not a feature. On ultrasound, findings include irregular masses, focal regions of inhomogeneous patterns associated with hypoechoic tubular/nodular structures, or decreased parenchymal echogenicity with acoustic shadowing, all suggestive of malignancy (Fig. 10-27A to D).

Because the mammographic and sonographic features suggest breast cancer, biopsy is frequently performed on women with this condition. Biopsy shows a chronic granulomatous inflammation composed of giant cells, leukocytes, epithelioid cells, macrophages, and abscesses. Treatment consists of surgical excision, oral steroid therapy, anti-inflammatory drugs or colchicines, or methotrexate, as well as antibiotic treatment of any associated abscesses. Recurrence rates of up to 50% have been reported, but they can be reduced by immunosuppressive treatment until complete remission.

DIABETIC MASTOPATHY

Diabetic mastopathy produces hard, irregular, sometimes painful mobile breast masses that may be recurrent or bilateral in patients with a history of long-term insulin-dependent diabetes, in younger premenopausal diabetic women, or in rare patients with thyroid disease (Box 10-13). Diabetic mastopathy is due to an autoimmune reaction to the accumulation of abnormal matrix proteins caused by hyperglycemia. It leads to atrophy and obliteration of glandular breast tissue and the production of fibrosis, which forms a hard mass simulating breast cancer. Because of the hardness of the mass, needle biopsy is often performed, but it may be insufficient for diagnosis and therefore may necessitate histologic sampling. Pathologic examination reveals fibrosis with a dense lymphocytic infiltration around breast lobules and ducts.

Mammography shows a regional asymmetric density with ill-defined margins but no microcalcifications or dense glandular tissue. Ultrasound demonstrates a hypoechoic mass or region displaying marked acoustic shadowing in most cases, findings suggestive of scirrhous breast cancer (see Fig. 10-27E).

Box 10-13. Diabetic Mastopathy

Long-term insulin-dependent diabetics
Thyroid disease (rare)
Autoimmune reaction causing fibrosis
Periductal and perilobular lymphocytic infiltration
May result in a hard mass
Surgery can result in recurrent masses

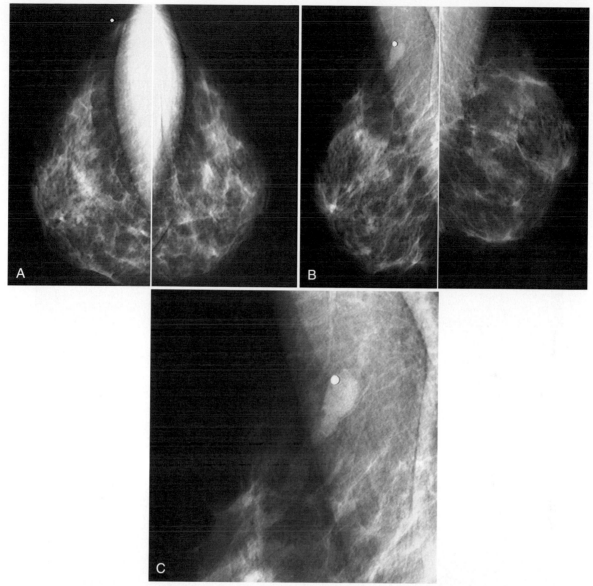

FIGURE 10-26. Mondor disease. Craniocaudal (**A**) and mediolateral oblique (MLO) (**B**) mammograms of a marker over a tender, elongated, dilated ductlike structure in the right axilla of a young woman. **C,** Spot compression on the MLO view shows a tubular mass representing the superficial thrombophlebitis that results in the nodular, superficial tender vein typical of Mondor disease.

Case reports of diabetic mastopathy on MRI describe a decreased area of signal intensity with "poor" or "heterogeneous" enhancement or "nonspecific" enhancement in the initial postcontrast phase. Heterogeneous "spotting enhancement" or a "benign gradual-type dynamic curve" is reported in the late enhancement phase.

On biopsy, fibrosis with perivascular, periductal, or perilobular lymphocytic infiltrates is seen. Frequently, patients will undergo surgical excisional biopsy. Unfortunately, surgery may exacerbate the disease, with recurrences developing in the same location.

DESMOID TUMOR

Desmoid tumor, or extra-abdominal desmoid, is also known as *fibromatosis*. Desmoid tumor is an infiltrative, locally aggressive fibroblastic/myofibroblastic process that may recur locally, may be multicentric, has been associated with previous trauma or surgery, and has been reported in women with breast implants. In the breast, desmoid tumor is manifested as a solitary, hard painless mass, occasionally fixed to the skin or pectoral fascia. Because treatment involves wide surgical excision, the primary tumor is evaluated for its origin within either the breast or the underlying musculo-aponeurotic structures. The extent of invasion into surrounding structures is also evaluated to facilitate surgical planning.

On mammography, desmoid tumors are spiculated masses. Ultrasound shows a hypoechoic shadowing mass. Because these masses simulate spiculated breast cancer, biopsy is required (Fig. 10-28).

Treatment of desmoid tumors is complete local surgical excision. Recurrence of desmoid tumor is less likely with wide excision and clear histologic margins. Tumor

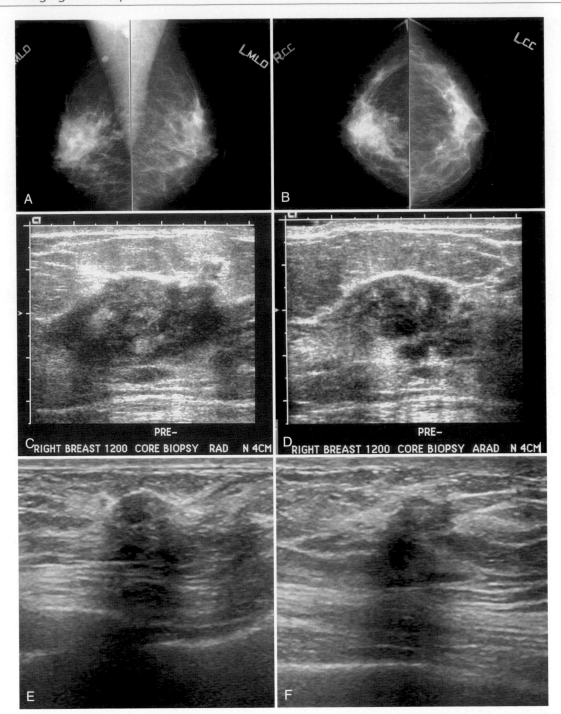

FIGURE 10-27. A to **D,** Granulomatous mastitis. Mediolateral oblique (**A**) and craniocaudal (**B**) mammograms show a marker over a palpable right breast mass shown as a focal asymmetry. Radial (**C**) and antiradial (**D**) ultrasounds show a complex irregular heterogeneous mass corresponding to the palpable finding and the mammographic mass. Biopsy showed granulomatous mastitis. **E** and **F,** Diabetic mastopathy. Ultrasound scans of diabetic mastopathy in longitudinal (**E**) and transverse (**F**) images show an ill-defined shadowing mass mimicking breast cancer. Biopsy showed diabetic mastopathy.

recurrence usually occurs within 3 years of excision, and for this reason breast reconstruction is generally delayed for 3 years. Because surgical trauma has been associated with recurrence, informed consent is necessary before breast reconstruction. Recurrences are treated by radical excision, just as the primary tumor is. Radiation therapy is used as an alternative to surgery for tumors in which complete excision would result in a poor functional outcome or for some tumors with positive margins (Box 10-14).

BOX 10-14. Desmoid Tumor

Synonyms: extra-abdominal desmoid/fibromatosis
Recurrent unless widely resected
Associated with previous trauma or surgery, implants
Solitary spiculated hard painless mass, occasionally fixed
If recurrent, does so within 3 years

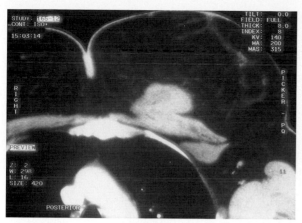

FIGURE 10-28. Computed tomography scan shows a soft-tissue mass adjacent to the pectoralis muscle in the left breast. Biopsy revealed a desmoid tumor.

TRICHINOSIS

Trichinosis is caused by the ingestion of raw or undercooked meat containing encysted larvae of the *Trichinella* genus. Diarrhea is produced during the intestinal phase of adult development, and then myositis, fever, and periorbital edema develop during larval migration (Box 10-15). After gastric digestion releases the encysted larvae, the larvae migrate into the intestinal mucosa, mature, and mate. The adult female releases new larvae into mucosal blood vessels, and the larvae are distributed throughout the body over a period of 4 to 6 weeks. The larvae enter skeletal muscles, most commonly the diaphragm, tongue, periorbital muscles, deltoid, pectoralis, gastrocnemius, and intercostal muscles, where the larvae encyst and calcify in 6 to 18 months, with a further life span of 5 to 10 years in the encysted form. During migration, larvae may also produce myocarditis, pneumonitis, or central nervous system symptoms from vasculitis of small arteries or capillaries, but encystment does not usually occur in these locations. Ingestion of the encysted larvae by a new host perpetuates the life cycle of the organism. In the United States, most *Trichinella* infections are asymptomatic and are acquired by ingesting undercooked pork, feral meat, wild boar, bear, or walrus.

On mammography, the calcified encysted larvae are seen as tiny linear calcifications smaller than 1 mm that are aligned along the long axis of the pectoralis muscle, parallel to the muscular fibers (Fig. 10-29). Because the calcifications are within the muscle, they should not be mistaken for breast cancer. At this point patients are asymptomatic.

Parasitic diseases that have been reported to calcify in breast tissue include hydatid disease, paragonimiasis,

BOX 10-15. Trichinosis

Ingestion of encysted worm larvae in undercooked meat

Tiny linear calcified encysted larvae in the pectoralis muscle

No calcifications in breast tissue

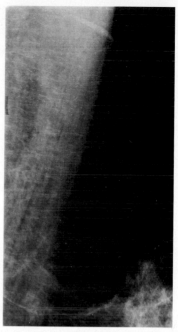

FIGURE 10-29. Trichinosis. A magnified mediolateral oblique view of the upper part of the breast shows innumerable tiny calcifications aligned along the pectoralis muscle that represent the calcified encysted larvae of *Trichinella*.

Dirofilaria repens infection, schistosomiasis, myiasis, and loiasis.

DERMATOMYOSITIS

Dermatomyositis and some collagen vascular diseases can rarely produce calcifications within the soft tissues of the arms and legs. In the breast, bizarre sheetlike calcifications form in a configuration similar to that of fat necrosis; the calcifications align along the breast tissues and generally point at the nipple (Fig. 10-30). Dermatomyositis is not a specific indicator of breast cancer. However, mammography is often performed because of an association of dermatomyositis with malignancies.

FOREIGN BODIES

Foreign bodies can be seen within the breast on mammography. Some acupuncture practitioners break acupuncture needle tips off in the breast tissue after placement, and the tiny sheared-off metallic needle tip fragments can be seen inside the breast tissue (Fig. 10-31A and B).

The most common foreign bodies seen in the breast on mammography are metallic markers placed percutaneously after core needle biopsy guided by stereotaxis, ultrasound, or MRI (see Fig. 10-31C to E). The markers have different shapes, depending on the manufacturer, and may contain a pellet or pellets that are visible by ultrasound. For patients who desire removal of the markers, case reports describe the use of an 11-gauge stereotactic vacuum-assisted probe technique that can remove the markers percutaneously. Percutaneous breast biopsy devices may produce tiny residual metallic shavings or fragments from the biopsy probe or needle itself and are usually not seen on the

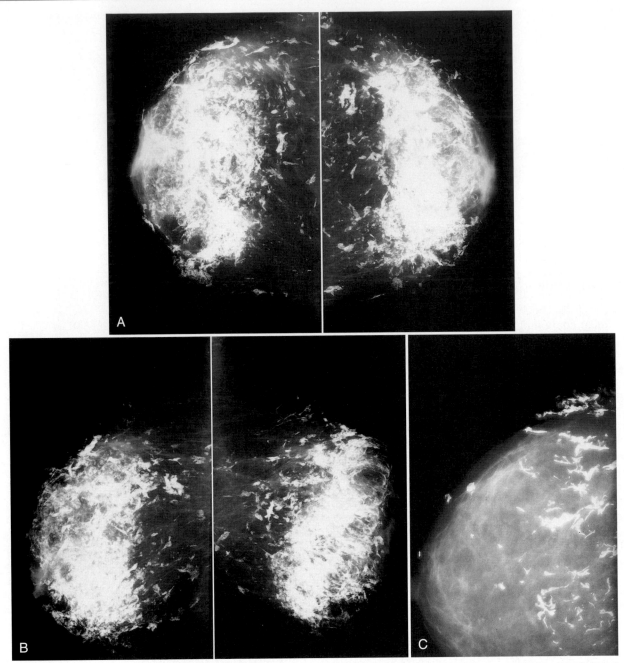

FIGURE 10-30. Mammograms showing dystrophic calcifications in patients with collagen vascular disease. Craniocaudal (**A**) and mediolateral oblique (**B**) mammograms show extensive dystrophic calcifications in both breasts. **C,** Dystrophic calcifications seen in another patient on craniocaudal mammogram. Dermatomyositis with calcifications was the diagnosis.

mammogram. These fragments are ferromagnetic and can occasionally cause signal voids on MRI.

Fragments of preoperatively placed hookwires have been reported in the breast after preoperative needle localization; these fragments may have been transected at surgery or may be due to breakage of the wire at the hooked end. Specimen radiography is used to determine whether the lesion prompting biopsy has been removed, as well as whether the hookwire and hookwire tip are included in the specimen. Information regarding the lesion, hookwire, and hookwire tip should be conveyed to the surgeon in the operating room to ensure complete removal of both the lesion and the hookwire tip. Although

some hookwire fragments have been reported to be stable within the breast 1.5 to 11 years after surgery, other fragments become symptomatic as a result of migration within and through the breast into the soft tissues of other parts of the body.

Round Dacron Hickman catheter cuffs may be left inside the breast after removal of a Hickman catheter. The rounded, short tubelike structure made of Dacron has a characteristic appearance in the upper part of the breast on mammography (see Fig. 10-31F and G).

Sutures used to close breast cancer biopsy sites may calcify after lumpectomy and radiation therapy, thereby delaying absorption of the suture material and promoting

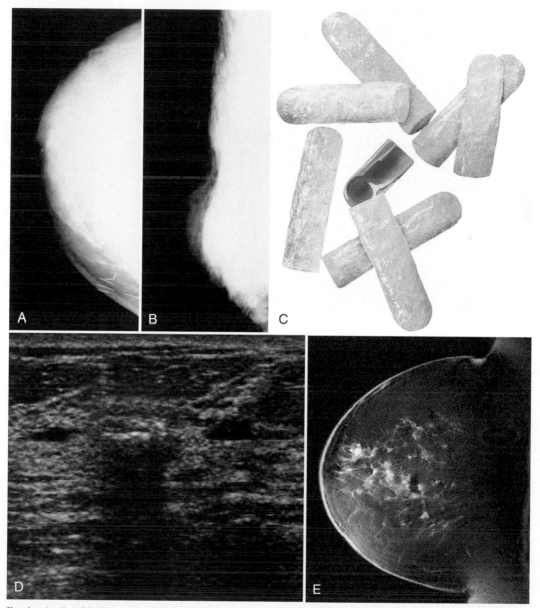

FIGURE 10-31. Foreign bodies. Mediolateral oblique (MLO) (**A**) and craniocaudal (CC) (**B**) mammograms show dense small masses throughout the breast tissue representing silicone injections, as well as thin metallic slivers in the peripheral breast parenchyma representing retained acupuncture needles. **C** to **J**, Metallic clip and ultrasound-visible pellets for marking the biopsy site after percutaneous needle biopsy. **C**, Pellets and a metallic marker. **D**, Echogenic ultrasound appearance after a gel marker is placed. **E**, Magnetic resonance imaging signal void from a metallic marker.

Continued

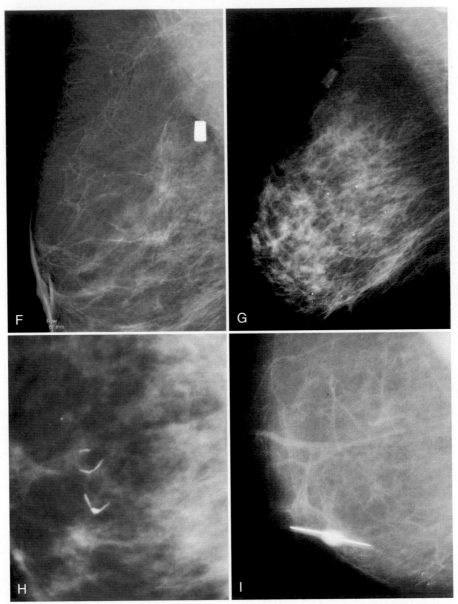

FIGURE 10-31, cont'd. F, Cropped digital mammogram shows an opaque tubelike structure in the upper right breast representing a retained cuff from a prior catheter. **G,** Another retained Dacron Hickman catheter cuff in the upper part of the right breast is seen as a radiopaque tube. **H,** Mammography shows sutures containing knots and a small calcified suture fragment. **I,** A needle was iatrogenically placed by this patient into her own breast, and it subsequently broke and calcified.

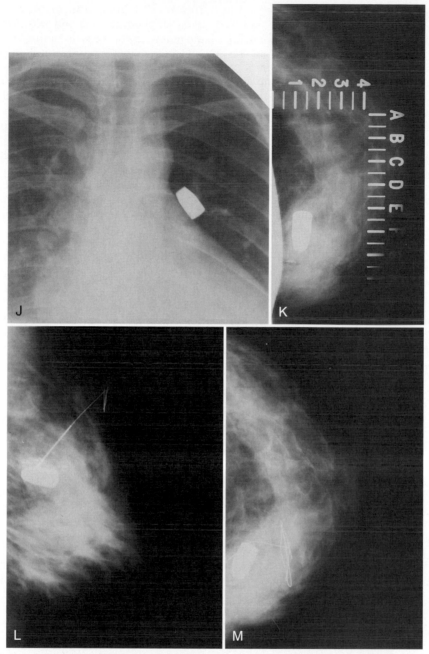

FIGURE 10-31, cont'd. J, Cropped chest radiograph shows a bullet projected over the left breast. **K,** To remove the bullet, the patient underwent needle localization, shown here in the alphanumeric grid. MLO (**L**) and CC (**M**) mammograms show the bullet at the end of the hookwire.

calcification. The result is linear or curvilinear calcification of the suture; the diagnosis can be made if the suture still contains a knot (see Fig. 10-31H).

Surgeons occasionally place metallic surgical clips in breast cancer biopsy cavities to delineate the extent of the tumor site for radiation oncologists to plan electron beam boosts. This practice is becoming less common because of the increasing use of MRI for follow-up and the use of ultrasound to delineate the breast biopsy cavity to guide planning for electron beam boost therapy.

Other materials may lodge in the breast, and the clinical history may help in the diagnosis (see Fig. 10-30I to M).

HIDRADENITIS SUPPURATIVA

This condition involves hidradenitis of the apocrine sweat glands, which are usually located in the axilla and the inguinal region. In the breast, these glands are also found in the inframammary folds, between the breasts, and around the areola. Hidradenitis suppurativa has been reported in obese patients in regions where the skin surfaces of the breasts or chest wall rub together. Severe hidradenitis causes masses with local inflammation. Severe cases are treated by excision of local disease, but local recurrence is common after treatment.

NEUROFIBROMATOSIS

This autosomal dominant disease is composed of two main types, the most common of which is also known as von Recklinghausen disease (type I) and is found in 90% of patients. Affected patients may have café au lait skin lesions, neurofibromas of the neural plexus or peripheral nerve sheaths, and neurilemmomas.

The skin lesions of neurofibroma can mimic a deep breast tissue mass and limit evaluation of the breast. However, like any skin lesion, neurofibromas may be outlined with air, and correlation with the breast history form is advisable. Furthermore, the description of cutaneous findings on the technologist's sheet should enable the radiologist to distinguish neurofibromas on the skin from masses of ductal origin inside the breast (Fig. 10-32).

POLAND SYNDROME

Poland syndrome is an absence of the pectoralis muscle on x-ray. It is usually unilateral. The mammogram shows absence of the pectoralis muscle on one side (Fig. 10-33).

BREAST CANCER MISSED BY MAMMOGRAPHY

Nondetection of breast cancer on mammography is of concern to the patient, the referring physician, and the radiologist. Detection of cancer on mammography is the result of a variety of factors, including the mammographic technique, experience of the radiologist, morphology of the breast tumor, and the background on which it is displayed. Cancers can best be displayed by good mammographic technique, optimal positioning, and a tumor location that can be displayed on the film. Approximately 10% to 15% of breast cancers are mammographically occult, even on good images, and will not be detected on mammography in the best of hands.

Cancer may not be detected on previous mammograms for several reasons (Box 10-16). First, the tumor may have a morphology that is undetectable on the mammographic background on which it is displayed and is therefore mammographically occult.

Second, the tumor may display findings that are visible, but below the threshold of any radiologist for consideration as cancer. Such findings have been termed *nonspecific*, examples of which include mammographic findings suggesting normal islands of fibroglandular tissue, a few benign-appearing calcifications, or a benign-appearing mass among many other benign-appearing masses that do not represent cancer.

Third, the tumor may show subtle findings that represent cancer but are atypical, such as a single dilated duct, a developing density, or other less common features of breast cancer that are perceptible but may have been unrecognized.

Fourth, signs that are classic for breast cancer may have been present on the mammogram but either were not perceived or were misinterpreted at the time of diagnosis.

BOX 10-16. Types of Findings on Previous Mammograms in Patients with Missed Breast Cancer

Occult on mammography (negative)
Nonspecific findings (normal or benign findings)
Atypical findings (subtle)
Classic cancer findings overlooked or misinterpreted

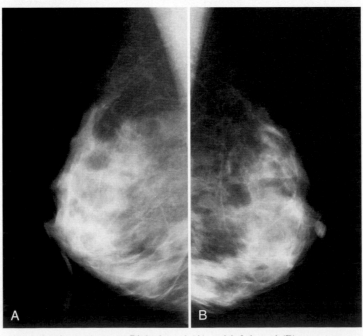

FIGURE 10-32. Neurofibromatosis simulating breast masses. Right lateral (**A**) and left lateral (**B**) mammograms show a neurofibroma simulating a retroareolar mass on the left and a long neurofibroma extending from inferior to the nipple on the right.

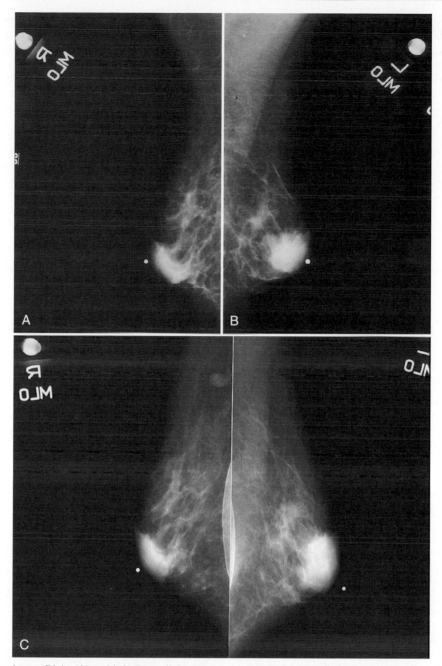

FIGURE 10-33. Poland syndrome. Right (**A**) and left (**B**) mediolateral oblique (MLO) implant-displaced mammograms show a pectoralis muscle on the left and absence of the pectoralis muscle on the right. **C**, Side-by-side MLO implant-displaced mammograms shows symmetry of the glandular tissue to greater advantage.

Box 10-17 shows factors that may contribute to cancer being missed on previous mammograms. Birdwell and colleagues reviewed possible reasons why tumors were not identified on previous mammograms. They postulated that findings were hidden among many other findings ("busy breasts") or that distracting findings other than the cancer were present on the film. Other contributing factors included dense breast tissue, small calcifications or masses that may have been overlooked, cancers hiding in the axilla and simulating lymph nodes, linear microcalcifications simulating vascular calcifications, findings seen on only one mammographic view, and findings at the edge of the film or at the edge of the glandular tissue, producing either a tent sign or concavity that was missed at the time of screening. Of note, most of these cancers were located in the upper outer quadrant, where 50% of all cancers occur. Also of note, not all the cancers that were missed were small, inasmuch as at least half the tumors were 1 cm or larger at the time that they were missed.

To decrease the number of missed breast cancers, the radiologist should use a systematic approach to reviewing the mammogram that minimizes distractions, paper shuffling, or other busy work in the reading room at the time of interpretation. Next, comparison to older films may reveal subtle changes not apparent on only the current examination. Finally, the radiologist should be aware of subtle or nonspecific findings of breast cancer.

ASYMMETRIES

Asymmetries differ from true masses in that they may be seen primarily in one of two standard mammographic views, display concave-outward (rather than convex-outward) margins, and have lucent fat interspersed rather than being densest in the center (Box 10-18). Asymmetries are often normal findings in the breast, but they may occasionally represent a subtle malignancy, particularly lobular carcinoma. Hence, appropriate imaging evaluation is crucial in diagnosing these often subtle cancers while avoiding an unacceptably high false-positive rate.

In the fourth edition of the BI-RADS® lexicon, published in 2003, the terms used to describe asymmetries were changed. Currently, there are four categories of breast asymmetry: *asymmetry*, *global asymmetry*, *focal asymmetry*, and *developing asymmetry*. Formerly known as *density*, an asymmetry is a focus of fibroglandular tissue seen on only one of two standard mammographic views at screening. It is likely the result of superimposition of normal fibroglandular tissues, or a *summation artifact*. This determination may be made by either examination of the other mammographic view or at recall imaging with diagnostic mammographic views, such as spot compression mammography.

Ultrasound is usually not warranted in such cases. Formerly known as *asymmetric breast tissue*, a global asymmetry is asymmetric breast tissue in one breast when compared with a corresponding region in the other breast. It is a sizable finding, usually occupying at least one quadrant of the breast. It is almost always a normal variant, reported in approximately 3% of mammographic examinations. Asymmetric breast tissue has additional clinical significance in possibly denoting malignancy when it is palpable.

Formerly known as *focal asymmetric density*, a focal asymmetry mimics a mass in that it is seen in at least two mammographic projections, but lacks the convex-outward margins of a mass and three-dimensionality of a mass. In the absence of associated calcifications, architectural distortion, sonographic correlate, or palpability, the chance of malignancy in a focal asymmetry is less than 1%. In a retrospective study, Sickles reported that 3% of 300 consecutive nonpalpable breast cancers were initially identified as focal asymmetries. Formerly known as *developing density* or *neodensity*, a developing asymmetry is a focal asymmetry that is new or increasing in size or conspicuity when compared with prior mammographic examinations. This finding differs from hormone-induced increase in density because developing asymmetry is a focal, unilateral finding. In the Sickles study of 300 consecutive nonpalpable breast cancers, 6% were reported as developing asymmetries. Developing asymmetry is a much more alarming finding than focal asymmetry; reported probability of malignancy in a developing asymmetry ranges from 13% when identified at screening versus 27% when identified at diagnostic mammography. Benign causes of developing asymmetry include fibrocystic change, focal fibrosis, pseudoangiomatous stromal hyperplasia, and fibroadenoma.

Once a focal asymmetry or a developing asymmetry has been confidently identified in at least two (ideally orthogonal) projections, ultrasound is helpful in further evaluation. The presence of a sonographic finding will guide management. For example, if a simple cyst is found to correlate to the mammographic finding, only routine mammographic follow-up is indicated. If a suspicious solid sonographic mass is identified, biopsy should be performed, almost always guided by ultrasound. In the absence of any sonographic finding (i.e., lack of a sonographic correlate), a nonpalpable focal asymmetry (without prior mammographic examinations for comparison) may be considered probably benign and assigned to short-term interval imaging surveillance, but a developing asymmetry would still require biopsy. In the latter case, the likelihood of malignancy is less than the case of a developing asymmetry with a sonographic correlate that is not clearly benign. The role of MRI in evaluating asymmetries is unclear at this time, but may be helpful in equivocal cases if the MRI examination is positive in demonstrating a correlate to the mammographic finding. It has not been established with certainty that biopsy may be obviated if MRI is negative.

KEY ELEMENTS

The normal male breast shows only fat on mammography. Gynecomastia is unilateral or bilateral, symmetric or asymmetric, and is shown as glandular tissue in a retroareolar flamelike dendritic, triangular nodular, or diffuse appearance on mammography.

Gynecomastia causes breast lumps and pain and has physiologic, drug-related, and medical-related etiologies.

Breast cancer in men is rare, is manifested as a mass eccentric to the nipple or in the upper outer quadrant, and has the same prognosis as breast cancer in women.

Breast cancer in men develops at 1% of the rate in women, occurs in older men, and on mammography is usually a noncalcified spiculated or circumscribed retroareolar or periareolar mass.

Pregnancy-related conditions include mastitis, lactational adenoma, enlarging fibroadenoma, galactocele, and pregnancy-associated breast cancer.

Pregnancy-associated breast cancer is defined as cancer diagnosed during pregnancy or within 1 year of delivery.

Stage for stage, the prognosis for pregnancy-associated breast cancer is the same as for nonpregnant women.

On mammography, pregnancy-associated breast cancer is detected as masses or pleomorphic calcifications.

Probably benign findings (BI-RADS® category 3) include single or multiple clusters of small, round or oval calcifications, circumscribed masses, and nonpalpable focal asymmetries that resemble fibroglandular tissue at diagnostic evaluation.

To identify subtle signs of malignancy and definitively benign entities, screen-detected findings should be recalled for full diagnostic imaging evaluation (including fine-detail diagnostic mammographic views and often ultrasound) before rendering a BI-RADS® category 3 assessment and assigning to short-term imaging follow-up.

Nipple discharge characteristics that should be investigated are new, bloody, or spontaneously occurring copious serous discharge.

Mammograms and ultrasound are frequently negative in the setting of nipple discharge.

A positive galactogram shows a filling defect, an abrupt duct cutoff, or luminal irregularity.

The differential diagnosis of intraductal masses on galactography includes papilloma, cancer, debris, and an air bubble.

Unilateral breast edema may be caused by mastitis, inflammatory cancer, local obstruction of lymph nodes, trauma, radiation therapy, or coumarin necrosis.

Bilateral breast edema is due to systemic etiologies, such as congestive heart failure, liver disease, anasarca, renal failure, bilateral lymphadenopathy, or superior vena cava syndrome.

Although breast edema, exogenous hormone therapy, and weight loss all result in increased breast density, distinction between these causes is made by the presence of skin thickening, which is seen only with breast edema.

Inflammatory cancer is the most important differential diagnosis for unilateral breast edema and is a rare (1% of all cancers) aggressive breast cancer with a poor prognosis.

The most common cause of mastitis is *S. aureus*; rare causes include tuberculosis, syphilis, hydatid disease, and molluscum contagiosum.

An extremely rare cause of unilateral breast edema is coumarin (warfarin [Coumadin]) therapy, producing necrosis of the breast.

Axillary lymphadenopathy on mammography is shown as replacement of the fatty hilum of lymph nodes by dense tissue, a rounded lymph node shape, and overall generalized increased density with or without lymph node enlargement.

The differential for abnormal lymph nodes containing "calcifications" includes calcifying metastatic disease, granulomatous disease, gold deposits from therapy for rheumatoid arthritis mimicking calcifications, or silicone from a previously ruptured breast implant.

The differential for unilateral axillary adenopathy includes metastatic breast cancer or mastitis.

The differential for bilateral axillary adenopathy is systemic conditions such as infection, collagen vascular diseases such as rheumatoid arthritis, lymphoma, leukemia, and metastatic tumor.

Primary breast cancer manifested as isolated lymph node metastasis in women with normal mammographic findings and normal physical examinations is uncommon and accounts for less than 1% of all breast cancers.

Paget disease of the nipple heralds an underlying breast cancer with a high rate of overexpression of the c-*erb*-B2 oncogene.

Women with Paget disease of the nipple have a bright red nipple, eczematous nipple changes that may extend to the areola, and subsequent ulceration or nipple destruction.

Sarcomas are rare malignant tumors of the breast or underlying chest wall. Their classification depends on the cell type; mammography shows high-density masses without calcifications or spiculation.

Mondor disease is a rare benign and self-limited acute thrombophlebitis of the superficial veins of the breast. It is often associated with trauma or recent surgery and produces a tender palpable cord extending toward the outer portion of the breast.

Mammography is usually negative in women with Mondor disease or rarely shows a long linear or tubular density corresponding to the thrombosed vein.

Granulomatous mastitis is a rare benign cause of a breast mass in young premenopausal women after their last childbirth; it has been correlated with breast-feeding and oral contraceptive use, and a possible autoimmune component has been implicated in its etiology.

Patients with granulomatous mastitis may have galactorrhea, inflammation, a breast mass, induration, and skin ulcerations. Treatment is surgery, but the recurrence rate is high.

Diabetic mastopathy is a benign cause of hard, irregular, sometimes painful mobile breast masses in long-term insulin-dependent diabetes, younger premenopausal diabetic women, or rare patients with thyroid disease.

Diabetic mastopathy is due to an autoimmune reaction to the accumulation of abnormal matrix proteins caused by hyperglycemia. It produces a hard fibrotic mass with a lymphocytic reaction; treatment is surgery, but the recurrence rate is high.

Desmoid tumor is also known as an extra-abdominal desmoid or fibromatosis.

Desmoid tumor is an infiltrative, locally aggressive fibroblastic/myofibroblastic process that is treated by surgery, may recur locally, may be multicentric, is associated with previous trauma or surgery, and has been reported in women with breast implants.

Trichinosis is caused by ingesting raw or undercooked meat containing encysted larvae of the *Trichinella* genus. The larvae give rise to tiny linear calcifications in the pectoralis muscles and not in the breast.

Dermatomyositis and some collagen vascular diseases can rarely produce bizarre sheetlike calcifications that are found to align along the breast tissues on mammography.

Foreign bodies in the breast seen on mammography include percutaneous metallic markers, acupuncture needle tips, hookwire fragments, calcifying sutures, vascular clips to mark breast cancer cavities for planning radiation therapy, Dacron Hickman catheter cuffs, and other foreign objects.

Hidradenitis suppurativa is a benign condition that produces breast lumps representing hidradenitis of the apocrine sweat glands in the axilla, between the breasts, and in the inframammary folds.

Neurofibromatosis is an autosomal dominant disease also known as von Recklinghausen disease (type I); affected patients may have café au lait skin lesions and neurofibromas of the neural plexus or peripheral nerve sheaths. The skin lesions can cause apparent breast masses on mammography.

Missed breast cancers may be due to cancers that are occult on the mammogram, nonspecific findings, atypical findings, or misinterpretation of the classic features of cancer.

Factors influencing why cancers were missed on previous mammograms include findings hidden among many other findings, distracting findings, dense breast tissue, overlooked small calcifications or masses, location simulating lymph nodes, simulation of vascular calcifications, visualization on only one mammographic view, and findings at the edge of the film or at the edge of glandular tissue.

There are four categories of asymmetries in the BI-RADS® lexicon: asymmetry, global asymmetry, focal asymmetry, developing asymmetry. Developing asymmetry is the most suspicious and is associated with a likelihood of malignancy of 13% when identified at screening and 27% when identified at diagnostic mammography.

The absence of a sonographic correlate does not obviate biopsy in cases of developing asymmetry. The role of MRI in the evaluation of asymmetries remains to be defined.

■ SUGGESTED READINGS

Ad-El DD, Meirovitz A, Weinberg A, et al: Warfarin skin necrosis: local and systemic factors, *Br J Plast Surg* 53:624–626, 2000.

Ahn BY, Kim HH, Moon WK, et al: Pregnancy- and lactation-associated breast cancer: mammographic and sonographic findings, *J Ultrasound Med* 22:491–499, 2003.

American College of Radiology: ACR Breast Imaging Reporting and Data System. *Breast Imaging Atlas*, Reston, VA, 2003, American College of Radiology.

Bayer U, Horn LC, Schulz HG: Bilateral, tumorlike diabetic mastopathy—progression and regression of the disease during 5-year follow up, *Eur J Radiol* 26:248–253, 1998.

Bejanga BI: Mondor's disease: analysis of 30 cases, *J R Coll Surg Edinb* 37:322–324, 1992.

Bergkvist L, Frodis E, Hedborg-Mellander C, Hansen J: Management of accidentally found pathological lymph nodes on routine screening mammography, *Eur J Surg Oncol* 22:250–253, 1996.

Berkowitz JE, Gatewood OM, Goldblum LE, Gayler BW: Hormonal replacement therapy: mammographic manifestations, *Radiology* 174:199–201, 1990.

Birdwell RL, Ikeda DM, O'Shaughnessy KF, Sickles EA: Mammographic characteristics of 115 missed cancers later detected with screening mammography and the potential utility of computer-aided detection, *Radiology* 219:192–202, 2001.

Brenner RJ: Follow-up as an alternative to biopsy for probably benign mammographically detected abnormalities, *Curr Opin Radiol* 3:588–592, 1991.

Brenner RJ: Percutaneous removal of postbiopsy marking clip in the breast using stereotactic technique, *AJR Am J Roentgenol* 176:417–419, 2001.

Bruwer A, Nelson GW, Spark RP: Punctate intranodal gold deposits simulating microcalcifications on mammograms, *Radiology* 163:87–88, 1987.

Camuto PM, Zetrenne E, Ponn T: Diabetic mastopathy: a report of 5 cases and a review of the literature, *Arch Surg* 135:1190–1193, 2000.

Chow JS, Smith DN, Kaelin CM, Meyer JE: Case report: galactography-guided wire localization of an intraductal papilloma, *Clin Radiol* 56:72–73, 2001.

Crowe DJ, Helvie MA, Wilson TE: Breast infection. Mammographic and sonographic findings with clinical correlation, *Invest Radiol* 30:582–587, 1995.

Cyrlak D, Wong CH: Mammographic changes in postmenopausal women undergoing hormonal replacement therapy, *AJR Am J Roetgenol* 161:1177–1183, 1993.

Dale PS, Wardlaw JC, Wootton DG, et al: Desmoid tumor occurring after reconstruction mammaplasty for breast carcinoma, *Ann Plast Surg* 35:515–518, 1995.

Daniel BL, Gardner RW, Birdwell RL, et al: Magnetic resonance imaging of intraductal papilloma of the breast, *Magn Reson Imaging* 21:887–892, 2003.

Dershaw DD, Moore MP, Liberman L, Deutch BM: Inflammatory breast carcinoma: mammographic findings, *Radiology* 190:831–834, 1994.

Diesing D, Axt-Fliedner R, Hornung D, et al: Granulomatous mastitis, *Arch Gynecol Obstet* 269(4):233–236, 2004.

Doberl A, Tobiassen T, Rasmussen T: Treatment of recurrent cyclical mastodynia in patients with fibrocystic breast disease. A double-blind placebo-controlled study—the Hjorring project, *Acta Obstet Gynecol Scand* (Suppl 123):177–184, 1984.

Dooley WC: Ductal lavage, nipple aspiration, and ductoscopy for breast cancer diagnosis, *Curr Oncol Rep* 5:63–65, 2003.

Duijm LE, Guit GL, Hendriks JH, et al: Value of breast imaging in women with painful breasts: observational follow up study, *BMJ* 317:1492–1495, 1998.

Eby PR, DeMartini WB, Peacock S, et al: Cancer yield of probably benign breast MR examinations, *J Magn Reson Imaging* 26:950–955, 2007.

Elson BC, Ikeda DM, Andersson I, Wattsgard C: Fibrosarcoma of the breast: mammographic findings in five cases, *AJR Am J Roentgenol* 158:993–995, 1992.

Evans GF, Anthony T, Turnage RH, et al: The diagnostic accuracy of mammography in the evaluation of male breast disease, *Am J Surg* 181:96–100, 2001.

Finder CA, Kisielewski RW, Kedas AM: Residual metal shavings and fragments associated with large-core biopsy needles: a follow-up, *Radiology* 208:833–834, 1998.

Garstin WI, Kaufman Z, Michell MJ, Baum M: Fibrous mastopathy in insulin dependent diabetics, *Clin Radiol* 44:89–91, 1991.

Godwin Y, McCulloch TA, Sully L: Extra-abdominal desmoid tumour of the breast: review of the primary management and the implications for breast reconstruction, *Br J Plast Surg* 54:268–271, 2001.

Graf O, Helbich TH, Hopf G, et al: Probably benign breast masses at US: is follow-up an acceptable alternative to biopsy? *Radiology* 244:87–93, 2007.

Gunhan-Bilgen I, Bozkaya H, Ustun EE, Memis A: Male breast disease: clinical, mammographic, and ultrasonographic features, *Eur J Radiol* 43:246–255, 2002.

Gunhan-Bilgen I, Ustun EE, Memis A: Inflammatory breast carcinoma: mammographic, ultrasonographic, clinical, and pathologic findings in 142 cases, *Radiology* 223:829–838, 2002.

Harenberg J, Hoffmann U, Huhle G, et al: Cutaneous reactions to anticoagulants. Recognition and management, *Am J Clin Dermatol* 2(2):69–75, 2001.

Harvey JA, Nicholson BT, Cohen MA: Finding early invasive breast cancers: a practical approach, *Radiology* 248:61–76, 2008.

Haupt HM, Rosen PP, Kinne DW: Breast carcinoma presenting with axillary lymph node metastases. An analysis of specific histopathologic features, *Am J Surg Pathol* 9:165–175, 1985.

Homer MJ, Smith TJ: Asymmetric breast tissue, *Radiology* 173:577–578, 1989.

Hook GW, Ikeda DM: Treatment of breast abscesses with US-guided percutaneous needle drainage without indwelling catheter placement, *Radiology* 213:579–582, 1999.

Ikeda DM, Birdwell RL, O'Shaughnessy KF, et al: Analysis of 172 subtle findings on prior normal mammograms in women with breast cancer detected at follow-up screening, *Radiology* 226:494–503, 2003.

Ikeda DM, Helvie MA, Frank TS, et al: Paget disease of the nipple: radiologic–pathologic correlation, *Radiology* 189:89–94, 1993.

Ikeda DM, Sickles EA: Mammographic demonstration of pectoral muscle microcalcifications, *AJR Am J Roentgenol* 151:475–476, 1988.

Kedas AM, Byrd LJ, Kisielewski RW: Residual metal shavings and fragments associated with large-core breast biopsy, *Radiology* 200:585, 1996.

Kerlikowske K, Smith-Bindman R, Abraham LA, et al: Breast cancer yield for screening mammographic examinations with recommendation for short-interval follow-up, *Radiology* 234:684–692, 2005.

Kopans DB, Swann CA, White G, et al: Asymmetric breast tissue, *Radiology* 171:639–643, 1989.

Kushwaha AC, Whitman GJ, Stelling CB, et al: Primary inflammatory carcinoma of the breast: retrospective review of mammographic findings, *AJR Am J Roentgenol* 174:535–538, 2000.

Leibman AJ, Kossoff MB: Mammography in women with axillary lymphadenopathy and normal breasts on physical examination: value in detecting occult breast carcinoma, *AJR Am J Roentgenol* 159:493–495, 1992.

Leung JWT, Kornguth PJ, Gotway MB: Utility of targeted sonography in the evaluation of focal breast pain, *J Ultrasound Med* 21:521–526, 2002.

Leung JWT, Sickles EA: Multiple bilateral masses detected on screening mammography: assessment of need for recall imaging, *AJR Am J Roentgenol* 175:23–29, 2000.

Leung JWT, Sickles EA: The probably benign assessment, *Radiol Clin North Am* 23:773–789, 2007.

Leung JWT, Sickles EA: Developing asymmetry identified on mammography: correlation with imaging outcome and pathologic findings, *AJR Am J Roentgenol* 188:667–675, 2007.

Liberman L, Giess CS, Dershaw DD, et al: Imaging of pregnancy-associated breast cancer, *Radiology* 191:245–248, 1994.

Liberman L, Morris EA, Benton CL, et al: Probably benign lesions at breast magnetic resonance imaging: preliminary experience in high-risk women, *Cancer* 98:377–388, 2003.

Liu GJ, Chen WG, Duan G, et al: Mammographic findings of gynecomastia, *Di Yi Jun Yi Da Xue Xue Bao* 22:839–840, 2002.

Matsuoka K, Ohsumi S, Takashima S, et al: Occult breast carcinoma presenting with axillary lymph node metastases: follow-up of 11 patients, *Breast Cancer* 10:330–334, 2003.

Memis A, Bilgen I, Ustun EE, et al: Granulomatous mastitis: imaging findings with histopathologic correlation, *Clin Radiol* 57:1001–1006, 2002.

Montrey JS, Levy JA, Brenner RJ: Wire fragments after needle localization, *AJR Am J Roentgenol* 167:1267–1269, 1996.

Murakami R, Kumita S, Yamaguchi K, Ueda T: Diabetic mastopathy mimicking breast cancer, *Clin Imaging* 33:234–236, 2009.

Murray ME, Given-Wilson RM: The clinical importance of axillary lymphadenopathy detected on screening mammography, *Clin Radiol* 52:458–461, 1997.

Orel SG, Dougherty CS, Reynolds C, et al: MR imaging in patients with nipple discharge: initial experience, *Radiology* 216:248–254, 2000.

Park YM, Kim EK, Lee JH, et al: Palpable breast masses with probably benign morphology at sonography: can biopsy be deferred? *Acta Radiol* 49:1104–1111, 2008.

Parsi K, Younger I, Gallo J: Warfarin-induced skin necrosis associated with acquired protein C deficiency, *Australas J Dermatol* 44:57–61, 2003.

Raza S, Chikarmane SA, Neilsen SS, et al: BI-RADS 3, 4, and 5 lesions: value of US in management—follow-up and outcome, *Radiology* 248:773–781, 2008.

Rieber A, Tomczak RJ, Mergo PJ, et al: MRI of the breast in the differential diagnosis of mastitis versus inflammatory carcinoma and follow-up, *J Comput Assist Tomogr* 21:128–132, 1997.

Rosen EL, Baker JA, Soo MS: Malignant lesions initially subjected to short-term mammographic follow-up, *Radiology* 223:221–228, 2002.

Sachs DD, Gordon AT: Hidradenitis suppurativa of glands of Moll, *Arch Ophthalmol* 77:635–636, 1967.

Sadowski EA, Kelcz F: Frequency of malignancy in lesions classified as probably benign after dynamic contrast-enhanced breast MRI examination, *J Magn Reson Imaging* 21:556–564, 2005.

Sawhney S, Petkovska L, Ramadan S, et al: Sonographic appearances of galactoceles, *J Clin Ultrasound* 30:18–22, 2002.

Schnarkowski P, Kessler M, Arnholdt H, Helmberger T: Angiosarcoma of the breast: mammographic, sonographic, and pathological findings, *Eur J Radiol* 24:54–56, 1997.

Serels S, Melman A: Tamoxifen as treatment for gynecomastia and mastodynia resulting from hormonal deprivation, *J Urol* 159:1309, 1998.

Shin JH, Han BK, Ko EY, et al: Probably benign breast masses diagnosed by sonography: is there a difference in the cancer rate according to palpability? *AJR Am J Roentgenol* 192:187–191, 2009.

Sickles EA: Mammographic features of 300 consecutive nonpalpable breast cancers, *AJR Am J Roentgenol* 146:661–663, 1986.

Sickles EA: Periodic mammographic follow-up of probably benign lesions: results in 3,184 consecutive cases, *Radiology* 179:463–468, 1991.

Sickles EA: Nonpalpable, circumscribed, noncalcified solid breast masses: likelihood of malignancy based on lesion size and age of patient, *Radiology* 192:439–442, 1994.

Sickles EA: Probably benign breast lesions: when should follow-up be recommended and what is the optimal follow-up protocol? *Radiology* 213:11–14, 1999.

Sickles EA: The spectrum of breast asymmetries: imaging features, work-up, management, *Radiol Clin North Am* 45:765–771, 2007.

Stomper PC, Waddell BE, Edge SB, Klippenstein DL: Breast MRI in the evaluation of patients with occult primary breast carcinoma, *Breast J* 5:230–234, 1999.

Swinford AE, Adler DD, Garver KA: Mammographic appearance of the breasts during pregnancy and lactation: false assumptions, *Acad Radiol* 5:467–472, 1998.

Talele AC, Slanetz PJ, Edmister WB, et al: The lactating breast: MRI findings and literature review, *Breast J* 9:237–240, 2003.

Tilanus-Linthorst MM, Obdeijn AI, Bontenbal M, Oudkerk M: MRI in patients with axillary metastases of occult breast carcinoma, *Breast Cancer Res Treat* 44:179–182, 1997.

Varas X, Leborgne JH, Leborgne F, et al: Revisiting the mammographic follow-up of BI-RADS category 3 lesions, *AJR Am J Roentgenol* 179:691–695, 2002.

Woo JC, Yu T, Hurd TC: Breast cancer in pregnancy: a literature review, *Arch Surg* 138:91–99, 2003.

Yasmeen S, Romano PS, Pettinger M, et al: Frequency and predictive value of a mammographic recommendation for short-interval follow-up, *J Natl Cancer Inst* 95:429–436, 2003.

Youk JH, Kim EK, Ko KH, Kim MJ: Asymmetric mammographic findings based on the fourth edition of BI-RADS: types, evaluation, and management, *Radiographics* 29:e33, 2009.

CHAPTER 11

FDG-PET/CT and the Evaluation of Breast Cancer

Andrew Quon

Positron emission tomography (PET) scanning has gained widespread acceptance for the diagnosis, staging, and management of a variety of malignancies, including breast cancer. This has heralded an exciting new era of molecular imaging research, of which the use of 2-deoxy-2-(^{18}F) fluoro-D-glucose (fluorodeoxyglucose, or FDG) as the primary PET tracer is only the beginning. The fundamental strength of PET over conventional imaging is the ability to convey functional information that even the most exquisitely detailed anatomic image cannot provide. The standard PET radiotracer in current clinical use, FDG is a glucose analog that is taken up by cells in proportion to their rate of glucose metabolism. The increased glycolytic rate and glucose avidity of malignant cells in comparison to normal tissue is the basis of the ability of FDG-PET imaging to accurately differentiate cancer from benign tissue regardless of morphology (Gambhir, 2002). The level or intensity of FDG uptake on PET is semi-quantified and reported as the standardized uptake value (SUV).

PET/CT SCANNING PRINCIPLES

The radiotracers employed in PET imaging, such as ^{18}FDG, always emit *pairs* of photons that are 180 degrees apart as they decay. This is the key difference from the conventional radiotracers used in nuclear medicine, which only emit single photons in any direction at each decay event. Accordingly, PET scanners are designed as a ring of multiple pairs of photon detectors arranged 180 degrees apart with the patient lying in the middle of this ring. These pairs of photon detectors, which are made of either bismuth germanium oxide (BGO), gadolinium orthosilicate (GSO), lutetium orthosilicate (LSO) crystals, or lutetium yttrium orthosilicate (LYSO) (Box 11-1) are electronically linked such that they accept only pairs of photons that arrive at both detectors at exactly the same time point and reject scattered photons that arrive at incongruent time points (Fig. 11-1). This design allows for superior photon sensitivity and spatial resolution compared to conventional nuclear medicine scanners, which rely on the use of lead-based collimators that act as filters to reduce scattered photons that hit the camera face at tangential angles.

PET/CT scanners are integrated units with the individual PET and computed tomography (CT) components nearly identical to their stand-alone counterparts. Integrated PET/CT has the added advantage of using the CT data for attenuation correction and anatomic localization;

additionally, more sophisticated PET/CT fusion software can be utilized for interpretation. CT-based attenuation correction, however, may introduce artifacts on PET when imaging high-density materials, such as bowel contrast and metallic prostheses. By comparison, stand-alone PET units do not utilize CT-based attenuation correction, but rely on a transmission scan generated by a built-in germanium-68 rod source within the scanner. The field of view of a modern PET/CT scanner is approximately 16 to 18 cm wide (see Box 11-1). The bed is advanced into the scanner in 6 to 7 increments so the patient can be scanned from the base of the skull to the midthigh. An additional 6 to 7 increments are required for scanning the extremities. Typically, each increment, termed a *bed position*, requires 3 to 7 minutes of acquisition time before moving on to the next section of the body. In contrast to conventional cross-sectional imaging, scanning starts at the pelvis and moves cranially to minimize the amount of urine accumulation in the bladder (Box 11-2).

FDG is the primary radiotracer in clinical use for oncologic PET and PET/CT scanning, including breast cancer screening. Once injected, FDG is transported into cells via the GLUT transport system and is quickly phosphorylated by hexokinase II. After phosphorylation, it is trapped within the cell, where it decays, with a physical half-life of 110 minutes. Typically, imaging commences 45 to 90 minutes after injection of tracer to allow adequate time for tumor accumulation and background washout from renal clearance. The average intensity of FDG uptake in malignant tissue is greater than in normal structures. However, physiologic tracer uptake of moderate intensity is typically seen in the liver, bowel, mediastinal blood pool, myocardium, and lymphoid tissue. Additionally, marked tracer uptake is seen in the kidneys, ureters, and bladder, where FDG is excreted.

Patient preparation before and after FDG PET/CT scanning is critical for high-quality scanning (see Box 11-2). High levels of either endogenous or injected insulin cause significant uptake of FDG in muscle and greatly decrease the sensitivity of the scan. For this reason, diabetic patients who have utilized regular insulin within 4 hours of FDG injection usually require rescheduling, as do patients who have eaten a meal within 8 hours. A less significant and somewhat controversial factor is that high levels of circulating glucose may potentially compete with FDG at tumor sites and, thereby, decrease sensitivity of the scan as well.

Accurate interpretation requires knowledge of the physiology of FDG as well as the limitations of PET scanning

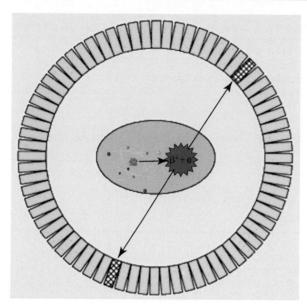

FIGURE 11-1. *Schematic of a positron emission tomography (PET) scanner. Inside a PET scanner, a positron is emitted and annihilated after interaction with an electron. Two gamma rays are emitted 180 degrees apart and detected by paired detectors. (Courtesy of Andrei Iagaru and Andrew Quon, Stanford University School of Medicine, Stanford, CA.)*

Box 11-1. Essentials of PET and PET/CT Instrumentation

Four scintillation crystal types:
  Bismuth germanium oxide (BGO)
  Gadolinium orthosilicate (GSO)
  Lutetium orthosilicate (LSO)
  Lutetium yttrium orthosilicate (LYSO)
Scanner field-of-view: 16–18 cm
Attenuation correction:
  CT-based (integrated PET/CT)
  Germanium-68 rod source (stand-alone PET)

Box 11-2. Imaging Protocol Summary for FDG-PET/CT

PATIENT PREPARATION
Before FDG injection
  Overnight fast (recommend 6- to 8-hour fast)
  Insulin-dependent diabetics:
    Morning scan: Skip morning breakfast and insulin dose
    Afternoon scan: Have morning meal and insulin dose, fast thereafter
  Noninsulin-dependent diabetics:
    Fast overnight and skip morning oral hypoglycemic medication
After FDG injection
  Minimize physical activity and talking
  Minimize visual stimulation
  Drink 3–4 glasses of water
  Urinate immediately before scan

RADIOTRACER
FDG
Intravenous dose
  5–7 mCi (3-D acquisition)
  10–15 mCi (2-D acquisition)

INSTRUMENTATION
Begin scanning at 45–90 min after injection of tracer
Start at pelvis and scan towards head
Field of view per bed position: 16–18 cm
Length of acquisition: 3–7 min/bed position

Box 11-3. Breast Cancer Interpretation Pearls

PRIMARY BREAST LESIONS
Focal lesions more suspicious
Malignancies have SUV beyond background tissue
Lesions < 1 cm difficult to characterized
Invasive ductal carcinoma is FDG-avid
Lobular carcinoma is poorly FDG-avid
Fibrous or dense breasts have greater background FDG activity and hamper lesion detection

DISTANT LESIONS
Axillary metastasis < 1 cm difficult to characterize
Sentinel lymph node dissection superior to PET for staging axilla
Osteolytic bone metastases: high sensitivity
Osteoblastic bone metastases: moderate sensitivity

(Box 11-3). While greater SUV levels suggest a greater likelihood of malignancy, it is not reliable when used alone. Equally important is learning to differentiate focal from non-focal lesions through experience (there is no clinically used quantitative parameter for focality), with focal lesions more likely to be malignant than benign.

A multitude of common physiologic variants can also occur. These include marked fat activity, particularly in the head and neck (termed *brown fat uptake*), skeletal muscle uptake caused by physical activity after the injection of FDG, and increased areolar and ovarian activity, which is dependent on lactation and hormonal cycles. Even with abnormal FDG uptake beyond these physiologic variants, a host of benign processes may cause abnormal findings on PET scanning. These include infection and inflammation, certain benign or adenomatous lesions (including fibroadenomas occasionally), granulomatous disease, as well as other inflammatory conditions (Box 11-4).

Current efforts to improve PET resolution and sensitivity include the development of time-of-flight calculation techniques that account for the slight difference in time at which the pairs of photons arrive at the detectors to further

localize the origin of positron decay within the patient (Surti et al., 2006). On the horizon, the first integrated PET/MRI scanners are being developed at several institutions (Pichler et al., 2006).

■ CLINICAL UTILITY OF FDG-PET AND PET/CT FOR BREAST CANCER

Oncologists have utilized FDG-PET with a great deal of success in imaging lung cancer, lymphoma, and melanoma, and can also be helpful in breast cancer when used judiciously in many common clinical situations. As of June 2009, the Centers for Medicare & Medicaid Services (CMS) approves of coverage for FDG-PET scanning for the following indications in breast cancer:

As an adjunct to standard imaging modalities for staging patients with distant metastasis or restaging patients with locoregional recurrence of metastasis; as an adjunct to standard imaging modalities for monitoring tumor response to treatment for women with locally advanced and metastatic breast cancer when a change in therapy is anticipated.

However, currently CMS has not yet decided to cover FDG-PET for initial diagnosis of primary breast cancer or the staging of axillary lymph nodes, because research studies for these indications have had mixed results. Nevertheless, the role of FDG-PET in clinical diagnosis and management of breast cancer patients is increasing and evolving, and the range of coverage by CMS will likely be expanded in the near future.

Initial Diagnosis

Although noninvasive breast cancer has been previously shown to be poorly imaged by FDG-PET), the majority of FDG-PET studies in the literature have been performed on patients with invasive breast cancer. Significant variations among studies are noted when surveying across several studies; earlier small studies in selected patient groups reported 100% sensitivity and accuracy, which is in contrast to the findings of larger series conducted by Avril and colleagues and Schirrmeister and colleagues, which showed FDG-PET sensitivity ranging from 84% to 93%. The overall specificity of FDG-PET is relatively high, but false positives do occur in patients with some benign inflammatory lesions and fibroadenoma (Jones et al., 1999; Palmedo et al., 1997).

The two major contributing factors that explain the varied statistical results between studies are histopathology and size of the lesion. Invasive breast cancer includes multiple histologic types, including infiltrating ductal, infiltrating lobular, and combined infiltrating ductal carcinoma. Infiltrating ductal carcinoma has a higher level of FDG uptake and therefore is detected at a significantly higher sensitivity than infiltrating lobular breast cancer (Avril et al., 2000; Crippa et al., 1998) (see Box 11-3). This difference in FDG uptake between the two histologic types suggests that tumor aggressiveness is not the sole determinant of FDG uptake but that the mechanism of the variable FDG uptake by breast cancer cells is likely modulated by multiple factors including glucose transport-1 (GLUT-1) expression, hexokinase I activity, tumor microvessel density, amount of necrosis, number of lymphocytes, tumor cell density, and mitotic activity index (Bos et al., 2002).

Not surprisingly, several studies show that breast tumor size significantly affects FDG-PET scan results. Early studies (Adler et al., 1993; Wahl et al., 1993) of lesions larger than 1 cm show that FDG-PET can detect such tumors with both a sensitivity and specificity in the range of 96% to 100%. However, a more recent series by Yutani and colleagues showed that FDG activity was very low or nondetectable in patients with tumor sizes ranging from 0.4 to 1.5 cm. These small lesions are at the limit of the resolution of modern PET systems, which is approximately 6 mm (the newest PET/CT systems possibly have a spatial resolution of 4 mm), and lesions in this size range and smaller will be below the threshold of detectability.

In short, the results of FDG-PET for the initial detection and diagnosis of primary breast cancer vary, largely due to the heterogeneity of the disease and tumor size (Boxes 11-4 to 11-6). Although some nuclear medicine physicians expected that FDG-PET would serve as a "metabolic biopsy" as a means of screening, this is not yet the case for breast cancer. Improvements in spatial resolution and scanner sensitivity, as well as the advent of dual-modality PET/CT scanning, may lead to FDG-PET being more useful for breast cancer diagnosis (Fueger et al., 2005). FDG-PET may also play an important adjunctive role in selected patients with dense breasts, in whom mammography has a much poorer sensitivity (Vranjesevic et al., 2003).

Initial Staging

The performance of FDG-PET imaging in breast cancer staging can be separated into two general categories: staging of axillary lymph nodes, in which use of PET has met with decidedly mixed results, and staging of mediastinal and internal mammary lymph nodes and distant metastatic disease, in which FDG-PET has consistently performed well.

Axillary lymph node involvement in breast cancer patients is an indicator of prognosis and an important factor in determining medical management and therapy. Because conventional anatomic imaging cannot reliably detect axillary nodal metastasis, patients with invasive breast cancer routinely undergo lymphoscintigraphy and axillary lymph node dissection (ALND) for accurate staging. This practice is under debate, because the identification of axillary nodal involvement may not improve overall survival rate, and because ALND is associated with a high incidence of morbidity. Therefore, FDG-PET has been extensively studied for noninvasive staging of the axilla. These results have been promising but mixed. For example, Adler and colleagues tried to achieve high sensitivity using 20 mCi (740 MBq) of FDG (two times the regular dose for an adult patient), and they reported 95% sensitivity in 50 patients, but the specificity in the same series was only 66%. In contrast, a more recent study by Guller and associates evaluated 31 patients using histopathologic correlation of sentinel lymph nodes as the gold standard; the overall sensitivity, specificity, and negative predictive value were 43%, 94%, and 67%, respectively.

The largest and most recent of these studies, by Wahl and colleagues, suggested that FDG-PET may fail to detect tumor in the axilla when few and small nodal metastases are present, but may be highly predictive for nodal tumor involvement when multiple intense foci of tracer uptake are identified. This would suggest that for patients with a highly positive PET, sentinel lymph node (SNL) biopsy might be omitted because ALND will still be required.

Earlier studies suggesting a high sensitivity of FDG-PET for the detection of axillary metastases did not employ the more sensitive methods of serial sectioning and cytokeratin immunohistochemistry currently employed in the assessment of sentinel lymph nodes. With increasing numbers of trials and larger sample sizes, more recent studies are beginning to consistently suggest that FDG-PET may not have a sufficiently high negative predictive value to justify forgoing ALND. In addition, however, studies of FDG-PET together with both SLN biopsy and ALND have been performed in patients with early-stage breast cancer. Such studies have explored the possibility that the combination of SLN biopsy and FDG-PET may have a high enough sensitivity to allow avoidance of ALND, when neither alone is sensitive enough.

It appears that PET is even less sensitive in detecting metastases identified by SLN biopsy than those identified by ALND (Guller et al., 2002). This is presumably because SLN biopsy, with its more detailed pathologic examination of a small number of nodes, is more likely to detect micrometastatic disease that cannot be identified with FDG-PET (Wahl et al., 2004). PET in its current format is not yet sensitive enough to replace SLN biopsy, but its high specificity may be useful in determining the extent of local and systemic disease (see Box 11-3).

In contrast to the mixed results of FDG-PET in axillary lymph node staging, many studies have consistently demonstrated that FDG-PET is superior to CT in the detection of nodal metastases in internal mammary or mediastinal lymph nodes (Jones et al., 1999; Bellon et al., 2004; Eubank et al., 2001). In studies comparing PET to CT staging directly, the overall sensitivity, specificity, and accuracy in detection of mediastinal and internal mammary nodal metastases by PET was 85%, 90%, and 88%, respectively, versus 54%, 85%, and 73%, respectively, by CT. These data are promising for FDG-PET to play a role in staging internal mammary and mediastinal lymph node involvement, which is an important prognostic factor in patient management (Fig. 11-2).

FDG-PET has also proved effective in detecting distant lesions and provides staging information even at the time

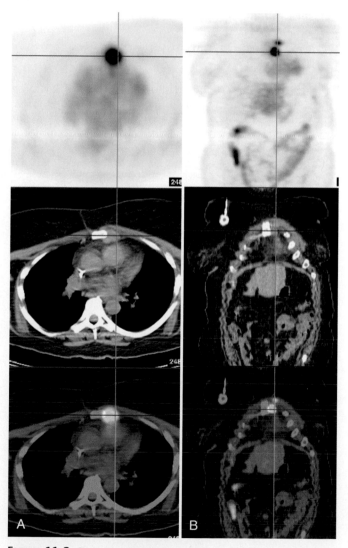

FIGURE 11-2. Fluorodeoxyglucose positron emission/computed tomography (FDG-PET/CT) detection of internal mammary lymph nodes. Dual-modality FDG PET/CT images reveal a metastatic internal mammary lymph node. **A,** Transaxial view. **B,** Coronal view.

of initial diagnosis. Several investigators, including Dose and colleagues, Lonneux and colleagues, and Moon and colleagues, have shown that PET is relatively sensitive (84% to 93%) and has a good negative predictive value (>90%) in the evaluation of distant metastases. Whole-body FDG-PET is able to detect metastases involving liver, lymph nodes, bone, lung, and bone marrow (Fig. 11-3). Specificity and positive predictive values are not quite as high, in the range of 55% to 86% and 82%, respectively, largely due to false-positive findings caused by muscle uptake, inflammation, blood pool activity, and bowel uptake (Moon et al., 1998). In respect to bone metastases, in which technetium-99m methyldisphosphonate (^{99m}Tc-MDP) bone scanning has been the established standard, recent studies by Ohta and colleagues and by Yang and colleagues independently showed that FDG-PET identified bone metastases with similar sensitivity and higher accuracy relative to ^{99m}Tc-MDP bone scanning. Further, a report by Garcia and colleagues and a preliminary study at our center suggests that FDG-PET and particularly dual-modality PET/CT may in fact be superior to bone scanning in the evaluation of lytic bone metastases (Taira et al., 2007).

Treatment Monitoring, Tumor Recurrence, and Restaging

FDG-PET is a metabolic imaging modality that has high sensitivity in the detection of therapy-induced glucose metabolic rate changes, which may not be evident in anatomic images, particularly early after treatment. This concept has naturally led to the evaluation of PET for treatment monitoring. Many groups of investigators (Avril and Weber, 2005; Gennari et al., 2000; Jansson et al., 1995; Schelling et al., 2000; Smith et al., 2000) have reported that FDG-PET can reliably differentiate responding and nonresponding breast cancers as early as after the first cycle of chemotherapy. For example, Schelling and colleagues reported that in a group of 22 patients, all responders were correctly identified, with sensitivity of 100% and specificity of 85%, using a decrease in FDG intensity (i.e., SUV) of greater than 55% compared to baseline. An additional phenomenon has been reported in estrogen receptor-positive tumors, in which metastases may actually show *increased* FDG intensity as a predictive response to successful anti-estrogen treatment, described as *metabolic flare*. This transient increase in FDG activity after hormone therapy initiation may be the result of an initial stimulation of tumor growth by estrogen-like agonist effects induced by increased levels of the hormone (Mortimer et al., 2001). The metabolic flare typically occurs 7 to 10 days after treatment initiation and may be the earliest and most accurate predictor of hormonal therapy response. It should be noted that all of these studies involve relatively small numbers of patients. Clearly more patients need to be evaluated, although there is at least preliminary evidence that FDG-PET may be used for early therapy evaluation of patients with locally advanced or metastatic breast cancer.

FDG-PET can be helpful in evaluating asymptomatic, post-treatment breast cancer patients who may pose a diagnostic challenge for detecting occult recurrences. In a large series of 132 patients being evaluated for disease recurrence,

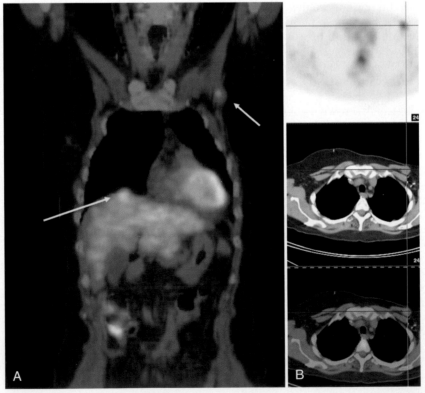

FIGURE 11-3. Positron emission/computed tomography (PET/CT) detection of breast cancer local recurrence and distant disease. The PET/CT fusion image detected local recurrence of breast cancer in the left chest wall (*short arrow*) and a distant metastasis in the liver (*long arrow*), both of which were not detected on CT alone. **A,** Coronal view. **B,** Transaxial view. (Courtesy of Andrew Quon, Osman Ratib, Johannes Czernin, UCLA Department of Pharmacology, 2003.)

Pecking and colleagues reported that FDG-PET detected lesions in 106 patients, with an overall sensitivity of 94% and a positive predictive value of 96%. Published data consistently demonstrate that FDG-PET has a similar or superior diagnostic accuracy, as compared to other conventional imaging modalities, in the detection of occult recurrent breast cancer in patients with rising tumor markers.

An emerging application of PET/CT may be in radiation treatment planning. Fused PET and CT images provide radiation oncologists with two pieces of critical information in a single study: the volume and extent of viable tumor and its exact location. Initial studies in patients with varied tumor types have confirmed that using PET/CT both in pretreatment planning and in follow-up evaluations has a significant impact on radiotherapy management in up to 56% of patients (Ciernik et al., 2003; Giraud et al., 2001). Certainly, evaluation of PET/CT for radiation treatment planning is still in the nascent stages, lacking rigorous randomized trials but nevertheless showing early promise.

▄ KEY ELEMENTS

Patients require adequate fasting to optimize scan quality.
Histologic subtype and lesion size greatly effect sensitivity for malignant breast lesions.
> Infiltrating ductal carcinoma is very FDG avid, whereas lobular variants are only moderately avid.
> Lesions less than 8 to 10 mm may not be reliably characterized by a modern PET/CT.

Many benign breast lesions may have FDG uptake that mimic malignancy.
PET/CT is not appropriate for staging axillary nodal disease. Axilliary lymph node dissection remains the standard.
PET/CT is effective for evaluation of distant sites of disease, response to therapy, and surveillance, particularly in high-risk patients based on family history, histologic features, and/or extent of disease at initial staging.
PET/CT is nearly as sensitive as Tc-99m MDP for identification of osteoblastic metastases and likely superior for identification of osteolytic metastases.

▄ SUGGESTED READINGS

Adler LP, Crowe JP, al-Kaisi NK, Sunshine JL: Evaluation of breast masses and axillary lymph nodes with [F-¹⁸] 2-deoxy-2-fluoro-D-glucose PET, *Radiology* 187:743–750, 1993.

Adler LP, Faulhaber PF, Schnur KC, et al: Axillary lymph node metastases: screening with [F-¹⁸]2-deoxy-2-fluoro-D-glucose (FDG) PET, *Radiology* 203:323–327, 1997.

Avril N, Rose CA, Schelling M, et al: Breast imaging with positron emission tomography and fluorine-18 fluorodeoxyglucose: use and limitations, *J Clin Oncol* 18:3495–3502, 2000.

Avril NE, Weber WA: Monitoring response to treatment in patients utilizing PET, *Radiol Clin North Am* 43:189–204, 2005.

Bellon JR, Livingston RB, Eubank WB, et al: Evaluation of the internal mammary lymph nodes by FDG-PET in locally advanced breast cancer (LABC), *Am J Clin Oncol* 27:407–410, 2004.

Bos R, van Der Hoeven JJ, van Der Wall E, et al: Biologic correlates of ¹⁸fluorodeoxyglucose uptake in human breast cancer measured by positron emission tomography, *J Clin Oncol* 20:379–387, 2002.

Centers for Medicare and Medicaid Services: NCA tracking sheet for positron emission tomography (FDG) for solid tumors (CAG-00181R), April 3, 2009, available at www.cms.gov/mcd/viewtrackingsheet.asp?from2=viewtrackingsheet. asp&id=218&.

Ciernik IF, Dizendorf E, Baumert BG, et al: Radiation treatment planning with an integrated positron emission and computer tomography (PET/CT): a feasibility study, *Intl J Radiat Oncol Biol Physics* 57:853–863, 2003.

Crippa F, Agresti R, Seregni E, et al: Prospective evaluation of fluorine-18-FDG PET in presurgical staging of the axilla in breast cancer, *J Nucl Med* 39:4–8, 1998.

Dose J, Bleckmann C, Bachmann S, et al: Comparison of fluorodeoxyglucose positron emission tomography and "conventional diagnostic procedures" for the detection of distant metastases in breast cancer patients, *Nucl Med Comm* 23:857–864, 2002.

Eubank WB, Mankoff DA, Takasugi J, et al: ¹⁸Fluorodeoxyglucose positron emission tomography to detect mediastinal or internal mammary metastases in breast cancer, *J Clin Oncol* 19:3516–3523, 2001.

Fueger BJ, Weber WA, Quon A, et al: Performance of 2-deoxy-2-[F-¹⁸] fluoro-D-glucose positron emission tomography and integrated PET/CT in restaged breast cancer patients, *Mol Imaging Biol* 7:369–376, 2005.

Gambhir SS: Molecular imaging of cancer with positron emission tomography, *Nature Rev* 2:683–693, 2002.

Garcia JR, Simo M, Perez G, et al: ^{99m}Tc-MDP bone scintigraphy and ¹⁸F-FDG positron emission tomography in lung and prostate cancer patients: different affinity between lytic and sclerotic bone metastases, *Eur J Nucl Med Molecul Imaging* 30:1714, 2003.

Gennari A, Donati S, Salvadori B, et al: Role of 2-[¹⁸F]-fluorodeoxyglucose (FDG) positron emission tomography (PET) in the early assessment of response to chemotherapy in metastatic breast cancer patients, *Clin Breast Cancer* 1:156–163, 2000.

Giraud P, Grahek D, Montravers F, et al: CT and ¹⁸F-deoxyglucose (FDG) image fusion for optimization of conformal radiotherapy of lung cancers, *Intl J Radiat Oncol Biol Physics* 49:1249–1257, 2001.

Guller U, Nitzsche EU, Schirp U, et al: Selective axillary surgery in breast cancer patients based on positron emission tomography with ¹⁸F-fluoro-2-deoxy-D-glucose: not yet! *Breast Cancer Res Treat* 71:171–173, 2002.

Jansson T, Westlin JE, Ahlstrom H, et al: Positron emission tomography studies in patients with locally advanced and/or metastatic breast cancer: a method for early therapy evaluation? *J Clin Oncol* 13:1470–1477, Jun 1995.

Jones A, Bernstein V, Davis N, et al: Pilot feasibility study to assess the utility of PET scanning in the preoperative evaluation of internal mammary nodes in breast cancer patients presenting with medial hemisphere tumors, *Clin Positron Imaging* 2:331, 1999.

Lonneux M, Borbath II, Berliere M, et al: The place of whole-body PET FDG for the diagnosis of distant recurrence of breast cancer, *Clin Positron Imaging* 3:45–49, 2000.

Moon DH, Maddahi J, Silverman DH, et al: Accuracy of whole-body fluorine-18-FDG PET for the detection of recurrent or metastatic breast carcinoma, *J Nucl Med* 39:431–435, 1998.

Mortimer JE, Dehdashti F, Siegel BA, et al: Metabolic flare: indicator of hormone responsiveness in advanced breast cancer, *J Clin Oncol* 19:2797–2803, 2001.

Ohta M, Tokuda Y, Suzuki Y, et al: Whole body PET for the evaluation of bony metastases in patients with breast cancer: comparison with ^{99m}Tc-MDP bone scintigraphy, *Nucl Med Comm* 22:875–879, 2001.

Palmedo H, Bender H, Grunwald F, et al: Comparison of fluorine-18 fluorodeoxyglucose positron emission tomography and technetium-99m methoxyisobutylisonitrile scintimammography in the detection of breast tumours, *Eur J Nucl Med* 24:1138–1145, 1997.

Pecking AP, Mechelany-Corone C, Bertrand-Kermorgant F, et al: Detection of occult disease in breast cancer using fluorodeoxyglucose camera-based positron emission tomography, *Clin Breast Cancer* 2:229–234, 2001.

Pichler BJ, Judenhofer MS, Catana C, et al: Performance test of an LSO-APD detector in a 7-T MRI scanner for simultaneous PET/MRI, *J Nucl Med* 47:639–647, 2006.

Schelling M, Avril N, Nahrig J, et al: Positron emission tomography using [(¹⁸)F] fluorodeoxyglucose for monitoring primary chemotherapy in breast cancer, *J Clin Oncol* 18:1689–1695, 2000.

Schirrmeister H, Kuhn T, Guhlmann A, et al: Fluorine¹⁸ 2-deoxy-2-fluoro-D-glucose PET in the preoperative staging of breast cancer: comparison with the standard staging procedures, *Eur J Nucl Med* 28:351–358, 2001.

Smith IC, Welch AE, Hutcheon AW, et al: Positron emission tomography using [¹⁸F]-fluorodeoxy-D-glucose to predict the pathologic response of breast cancer to primary chemotherapy, *J Clin Oncol* 18:1676–1688, 2000.

Surti S, Karp JS, Popescu LM, et al: Investigation of time-of-flight benefit for fully 3-D PET, *IEEE Trans Medl Imaging* 25:529–538, 2006.

Taira AV, Herfkens RJ, Gambhir SS, Quon A: Detection of bone metastases: assessment of integrated FDG PET/CT imaging, *Radiology* 243:204–211, 2007.

Vranjesevic D, Schiepers C, Silverman DH, et al: Relationship between ¹⁸F-FDG uptake and breast density in women with normal breast tissue, *J Nucl Med* 44:1238–1242, 2003.

Wahl RL, Siegel BA, Coleman RE, Gatsonis CG: Prospective multicenter study of axillary nodal staging by positron emission tomography in breast cancer: a report of the staging breast cancer with PET Study Group, *J Clin Oncol* 22:277–285, 2004.

Wahl RL, Zasadny K, Helvie M, et al: Metabolic monitoring of breast cancer chemohormonotherapy using positron emission tomography: initial evaluation, *J Clin Oncol* 11:2101–2111, 1993.

Yang SN, Liang JA, Lin FJ, et al: Comparing whole body (¹⁸)F-2-deoxyglucose positron emission tomography and technetium-99m methylene diphosphonate bone scan to detect bone metastases in patients with breast cancer, *J Cancer Res Clin Oncol* 128:325–328, 2002.

Yutani K, Shiba E, Kusuoka H, et al: Comparison of FDG-PET with MIBI-SPECT in the detection of breast cancer and axillary lymph node metastasis, *J Computer-assist Tomogr* 24:274–280, 2000.

Index

Note: Page numbers followed by f indicate figures; those followed by t indicate tables; those followed by b indicate boxes.